VOLUME **5**

DISEASE CONTROL PRIORITIES • THIRD EDITION

Cardiovascular, Respiratory, and Related Disorders

DISEASE CONTROL PRIORITIES • THIRD EDITION

Series Editors

Dean T. Jamison

Rachel Nugent

Hellen Gelband

Susan Horton

Prabhat Jha

Ramanan Laxminarayan

Charles N. Mock

Volumes in the Series

Essential Surgery

Reproductive, Maternal, Newborn, and Child Health

Cancer

Mental, Neurological, and Substance Use Disorders

Cardiovascular, Respiratory, and Related Disorders

Major Infectious Diseases

Injury Prevention and Environmental Health

Child and Adolescent Health and Development

Disease Control Priorities: Improving Health and Reducing Poverty

DISEASE CONTROL PRIORITIES

Budgets constrain choices. Policy analysis helps decision makers achieve the greatest value from limited available resources. In 1993, the World Bank published *Disease Control Priorities in Developing Countries* (*DCP1*), an attempt to systematically assess the cost-effectiveness (value for money) of interventions that would address the major sources of disease burden in low- and middle-income countries. The World Bank's 1993 *World Development Report* on health drew heavily on *DCP1*'s findings to conclude that specific interventions against noncommunicable diseases were cost-effective, even in environments in which substantial burdens of infection and undernutrition persisted.

DCP2, published in 2006, updated and extended *DCP1* in several aspects, including explicit consideration of the implications for health systems of expanded intervention coverage. One way that health systems expand intervention coverage is through selected platforms that deliver interventions that require similar logistics but deliver interventions from different packages of conceptually related interventions, for example, against cardiovascular disease. Platforms often provide a more natural unit for investment than do individual interventions. Analysis of the costs of packages and platforms—and of the health improvements they can generate in given epidemiological environments—can help to guide health system investments and development.

DCP3 differs importantly from *DCP1* and *DCP2* by extending and consolidating the concepts of platforms and packages and by offering explicit consideration of the financial risk protection objective of health systems. In populations lacking access to health insurance or prepaid care, medical expenses that are high relative to income can be impoverishing. Where incomes are low, seemingly inexpensive medical procedures can have catastrophic financial effects. *DCP3* offers an approach to explicitly include financial protection as well as the distribution across income groups of financial and health outcomes resulting from policies (for example, public finance) to increase intervention uptake. The task in all of the *DCP* volumes has been to combine the available science about interventions implemented in very specific locales and under very specific conditions with informed judgment to reach reasonable conclusions about the impact of intervention mixes in diverse environments. *DCP3*'s broad aim is to delineate essential intervention packages and their related delivery platforms to assist decision makers in allocating often tightly constrained budgets so that health system objectives are maximally achieved.

DCP3's nine volumes are being published in 2015, 2016, 2017, and 2018 in an environment in which serious discussion continues about quantifying the sustainable development goal (SDG) for health. *DCP3*'s analyses are well-placed to assist in choosing the means to attain the health SDG and assessing the related costs. Only when these volumes, and the analytic efforts on which they are based, are completed will we be able to explore SDG-related and other broad policy conclusions and generalizations. The final *DCP3* volume will report those conclusions. Each individual volume will provide valuable, specific policy analyses on the full range of interventions, packages, and policies relevant to its health topic.

More than 500 individuals and multiple institutions have contributed to *DCP3*. We convey our acknowledgments elsewhere in this volume. Here we express our particular gratitude to the Bill & Melinda Gates Foundation for its sustained financial support, to the InterAcademy Medical Panel (and its U.S. affiliate, the National Academy of Sciences, Engineering, and Medicine), and to World Bank Publications. Each played a critical role in this effort.

Dean T. Jamison
Rachel Nugent
Hellen Gelband
Susan Horton
Prabhat Jha
Ramanan Laxminarayan
Charles N. Mock

VOLUME **5**

DISEASE CONTROL PRIORITIES • THIRD EDITION

Cardiovascular, Respiratory, and Related Disorders

EDITORS

Dorairaj Prabhakaran
Shuchi Anand
Thomas A. Gaziano
Jean-Claude Mbanya
Yangfeng Wu
Rachel Nugent

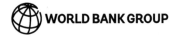 **WORLD BANK GROUP**

Softcover:
ISBN (paper): 978-1-4648-0518-9
ISBN (electronic): 978-1-4648-0520-2
DOI: 10.1596/978-1-4648-0518-9

Hardcover:
ISBN (paper): 978-1-4648-0519-6

DOI: 10.1596/978-1-4648-0519-6

Cover photo: © 2003. Arne Hoel / World Bank. Further permission required for reuse.

Cover design: Debra Naylor, Naylor Design, Washington, DC

Chapter opener photos: **chapter 1:** © WorldFish/M. Yousuf Tushar. Original photo cropped. https://creativecommons.org/licenses/by-nc-nd/2.0/; **chapter 2:** © Frank Spangler/Worldview Images. Used with the permission of Worldview Images. Further permission required for reuse; **chapter 3:** © World Bank. Further permission required for reuse; **chapter 4:** © Frank Spangler/Worldview Images. Used with the permission of Worldview Images. Further permission required for reuse; **chapter 5:** © PAHO/WHO—David Spitz. Used with permission. Further permission required for reuse; **chapter 6:** © Frank Spangler/Worldview Images. Used with the permission of Worldview Images. Further permission required for reuse; **chapter 7:** © Chris Stowers/Panos. Used with permission. Further permission required for reuse; **chapter 8:** © Meghana Kulkarni. Original photo cropped. https://creativecommons.org/licenses/by-nc/2.0/; **chapter 9:** © WHO/Christopher Black. Used with permission. Further permission required for reuse; **chapter 10:** © UNAMID. Used with permission. Further permission required for reuse; **chapter 11:** © World Bank. Further permission required for reuse; **chapter 12:** © WHO/Christopher Black. Used with permission. Further permission required for reuse; **chapter 13:** © WHO/Christopher Black. Used with permission. Further permission required for reuse; **chapter 14:** © Frank Spangler/Worldview Images. Used with the permission of Worldview Images. Further permission required for reuse; **chapter 15:** © WHO/TDR /Julio Takayama. Used with permission. Further permission required for reuse; **chapter 16:** © 2015 Girdhari Bora for IntraHealth International, Courtesy of Photoshare. Used with permission. Further permission required for reuse; **chapter 17:** © 2015 Girdhari Bora for IntraHealth International, Courtesy of Photoshare. Used with permission. Further permission required for reuse; **chapter 18:** © UN Photo/Fardin Waezi. Used with permission. Further permission required for reuse; **chapter 19:** © Department of Foreign Affairs and Trade. Used via a Creative Commons license (https://creativecommons.org/licenses/by-nc-sa/2.0/). Original photo was cropped to fit template; **chapter 20:** © Frank Spangler/Worldview Images. Used with the permission of Worldview Images. Further permission required for reuse; **chapter 21:** © WHO/Quinn Mattingly. Used with permission. Further permission required for reuse; **chapter 22:** © WHO/Christopher Black. Used with permission. Further permission required for reuse.

Library of Congress Cataloging-in-Publication Data has been requested.

Contents

Foreword   *xiii*
Preface   *xv*
Abbreviations   *xvii*

1. **Cardiovascular, Respiratory, and Related Disorders: Key Messages and Essential Interventions to Address Their Burden in Low- and Middle-Income Countries   1**

    Dorairaj Prabhakaran, Shuchi Anand, David A. Watkins, Thomas A. Gaziano, Yangfeng Wu, Jean-Claude Mbanya, and Rachel Nugent, on behalf of the DCP3 CVRD Author Group

2. **Relationships among Major Risk Factors and the Burden of Cardiovascular Diseases, Diabetes, and Chronic Lung Disease   23**

    Vamadevan S. Ajay, David A. Watkins, and Dorairaj Prabhakaran

3. **Early Origins of Cardiometabolic Disease   37**

    Kalyanaraman Kumaran, Clive Osmond, and Caroline H. D. Fall

4. **Tobacco and Cardiovascular Disease: A Summary of Evidence   57**

    Ambuj Roy, Ishita Rawal, Samer Jabbour, and Dorairaj Prabhakaran

5. **Physical Activity for the Prevention of Cardiometabolic Disease   79**

    Fiona Bull, Shifalika Goenka, Vicki Lambert, and Michael Pratt

6. **Effectiveness of Dietary Policies to Reduce Noncommunicable Diseases   101**

    Ashkan Afshin, Renata Micha, Michael Webb, Simon Capewell, Laurie Whitsel, Adolfo Rubinstein, Dorairaj Prabhakaran, Marc Suhrcke, and Dariush Mozaffarian

7. **Obesity Prevention   117**

    Vasanti S. Malik and Frank B. Hu

8. **Ischemic Heart Disease: Cost-Effective Acute Management and Secondary Prevention** 135

   Sagar B. Dugani, Andrew E. Moran, Robert O. Bonow, and Thomas A. Gaziano

9. **Stroke** 157

   Lijing L. Yan, Chaoyun Li, Jie Chen, Rong Luo, Janet Bettger, Yishan Zhu, Valery Feigin, Martin O'Donnell, J. Jaime Miranda, Dong Zhao, and Yangfeng Wu

10. **Heart Failure** 173

    Mark D. Huffman, Greg A. Roth, Karen Sliwa, Clyde W. Yancy, and Dorairaj Prabhakaran

11. **Structural Heart Diseases** 191

    David A. Watkins, Babar Hasan, Bongani Mayosi, Gene Bukhman, J. Antonio Marin-Neto, Anis Rassi Jr., Anis Rassi, and R. Krishna Kumar

12. **Diabetes: An Update on the Pandemic and Potential Solutions** 209

    Mohammed K. Ali, Karen R. Siegel, Eeshwar Chandrasekar, Nikhil Tandon, Pablo Aschner Montoya, Jean-Claude Mbanya, Juliana Chan, Ping Zhang, and K. M. Venkat Narayan

13. **Kidney Disease** 235

    Shuchi Anand, Bernadette Thomas, Giuseppe Remuzzi, Miguel Riella, Meguid El Nahas, Saraladevi Naicker, and John Dirks

14. **Peripheral Artery Disease** 253

    Uchechukwu K. A. Sampson, F. Gerald R. Fowkes, Nadraj G. Naidoo, and Michael H. Criqui

15. **Chronic Lower Respiratory Tract Diseases** 263

    Peter Burney, Rogelio Perez-Padilla, Guy Marks, Gary Wong, Eric Bateman, and Deborah Jarvis

16. **Integrated Public Health and Health Service Delivery for Noncommunicable Diseases and Comorbid Infectious Diseases and Mental Health** 287

    Matthew Magee, Mohammed Ali, Dorairaj Prabhakaran, Vamadevan S. Ajay, and K. M. Venkat Narayan

17. **Innovations in Community-Based Health Care for Cardiometabolic and Respiratory Diseases** 305

    Rohina Joshi, Andre Pascal Kengne, Fred Hersch, Mary Beth Weber, Helen McGuire, and Anushka Patel

18. **Quality Improvement in Cardiovascular Disease Care** 327

    Edward S. Lee, Rajesh Vedanthan, Panniyammakal Jeemon, Jemima H. Kamano, Preeti Kudesia, Vikram Rajan, Michael Engelgau, and Andrew E. Moran

19. **Costs and Cost-Effectiveness of Interventions and Policies to Prevent and Treat Cardiovascular and Respiratory Diseases** 349

   Thomas A. Gaziano, Marc Suhrcke, Elizabeth Brouwer, Carol Levin, Irina Nikolic, and Rachel Nugent

20. **Extended Cost-Effectiveness Analyses of Cardiovascular Risk Factor Reduction Policies** 369

   David A. Watkins, Rachel Nugent, and Stéphane Verguet

21. **Priority-Setting Processes for Expensive Treatments for Chronic Diseases** 375

   Yuna Sakuma, Amanda Glassman, and Claudia Vaca

22. **Management of Hypertension and Dyslipidemia for Primary Prevention of Cardiovascular Disease** 389

   Panniyammakal Jeemon, Rajeev Gupta, Churchill Onen, Alma Adler, Thomas A. Gaziano, Dorairaj Prabhakaran, and Neil Poulter

DCP3 Series Acknowledgments 405
Volume and Series Editors 407
Contributors 411
Advisory Committee to the Editors 415
Reviewers 417
Policy Forum Participants 419
Index 421

Foreword

As the world sets its sights on the avidly aspirational Sustainable Development Goals (SDGs) of 2030, the health goal to secure healthy lives for all and well-being at all ages is especially ambitious. The global health agenda of the Millennium Development Goals (MDGs) has been expanded in the SDGs to include noncommunicable diseases (NCDs)—the greatest public health threat of this century. Concerted action on many areas of health has now been positioned on the platform of universal health coverage (UHC) to ensure equitable and effective provision of essential health services.

In this context, cardiovascular diseases (CVDs) collectively pose the greatest challenge as well as the greatest opportunity to health systems across the world. The challenge arises from the fact that CVDs are the largest overall contributor to global mortality, as well as a major cause of premature mortality below the age of 70 years. The Indian experience, with which I am most familiar, has shown how the escalating epidemics of CVDs and other NCDs not only impose a high cost of healthy life-years lost; they also lead to unaffordable financial burdens on both families and health systems.

With coronary heart disease and stroke as the major manifestations, CVDs present a serious threat to health and development across the world. Low- and middle-income countries (LMICs) now not only join high-income countries (HICs) in suffering high proportional mortality from CVDs; these conditions also account for far higher absolute and premature mortality tolls of CVDs. Rising burdens of renal disease share major risk factors, especially high blood pressure and diabetes, with CVDs. Similarly, respiratory diseases share tobacco as a major risk factor for CVDs. Renal and respiratory diseases join CVDs in posing challenges of preventing, as well as providing appropriate acute and chronic care to health systems everywhere.

However, CVDs also offer a major opportunity to all countries—especially LMICs—to reduce the high burden of disease by averting premature mortality and reducing morbidity through interventions that have proven to be highly effective in preventing disease and death in the prime of productive mid-life. These range from policy instruments, like higher taxes on tobacco products, to health service improvements that expand and intensify the coverage of effective secondary prevention to persons who have survived a cardiovascular event but remain at risk of recurrence. Among the major NCDs, CVDs have the largest array of proven interventions that have demonstrated the benefit of substantial reductions in mortality and morbidity. If the goal of reducing premature mortality from NCDs by one-third between 2015 and 2030 is to be attained, the largest contribution has to come from interventions directed at CVDs, since such a high magnitude of benefit is presently demonstrated only for these interventions in the NCD spectrum.

When positioned in the context of UHC, interventions not only need to demonstrate efficacy but also cost-effectiveness and affordability for accommodation in national budgets—especially in the resource-constrained health systems of LMICs. Hence, economic evaluation has to complement biomedical, epidemiological, clinical, and health systems research to identify high-impact interventions that provide best value for money. This is particularly imperative in an environment of rapid technological advancement, when the seductive appeal of high-profile technologies can misdirect priorities in resource allocation. Unless guided by evidence-informed policy, affairs of the heart can be very costly in more than a poetic sense! Renal and respiratory diseases, too, require prioritization of resource-optimizing health interventions.

The Disease Control Priorities Project (DCP), in its two previous editions, provided the best contemporaneous analysis of major global health challenges and offered policy-enabling cost- effectiveness estimates of interventions that were available to address them. *DCP3* continues that tradition by presenting the best available evidence on cost-effective interventions that will substantially impact and improve global health if earnestly implemented. The reasoned recommendations bridge the often-disconnected realms of rigorous scientific research and real-world policy relevance. Responses to NCDs, long neglected by health systems in LMICs, need to use such evidence to identify prioritized pathways of action and develop efficient delivery systems for the services selected to minimize the health costs of missed or messed opportunities.

This volume on CVDs, renal, and respiratory disorders has particularly high value. It carries the potential to become the most effective game-changer in global health by helping all countries to combat, contain, and control the biggest killer presently prowling the globe and by enabling us to reach the 2030 goals for NCDs and health overall. As one who has witnessed the epidemic of CVDs advance menacingly across the world in the past four decades, I fervently hope that the clear and convincing messages conveyed by the extensively researched and elegantly communicated analyses in this volume will be heard, heeded, and harmonized with policy and practice in all countries. In that hope, this Foreword looks to action moving fast forward.

K. Srinath Reddy
President, Public Health Foundation of India
New Delhi, India

Preface

Cardiovascular, respiratory, and related disorders (CVRDs) and conditions are responsible for a significant portion of the world's health burden. In 2012, 52 percent of global adult deaths were caused by CVRDs, and most occurred in low- and middle-income settings. Most CVRDs and related disorders are preventable or can be treated to reduce morbidity. Doing so, however, requires greater capacity to detect and treat at an early stage, as they are often "silent" diseases. These conditions also threaten economic development due to reduced productivity among those affected with illness and early death, as well as high household treatment costs that are often paid out of pocket in low-resource settings. Combined with the enduring presence of infectious diseases, such as tuberculosis and HIV/AIDS, CVRDs in low-income countries create a double burden of disease.

The *Cardiovascular, Respiratory, and Related Disorders* volume of *DCP3* contributes to existing research efforts in several ways:

- By summarizing the best available evidence for effective and scalable interventions
- By identifying the most effective and cost-effective priority interventions
- By describing the health platforms that can deliver these interventions and thereby curtail the increasing risk for chronic conditions and diseases.

The volume also provides an essential package of policy and health interventions that are cost-effective and feasible in lower-middle-income countries and can significantly reduce the health burden of these diseases.

We focus primarily on cardiovascular diseases and the primary risks—including ischemic heart disease, stroke, and congestive heart failure—as well as secondary risk factors, such as tobacco use, physical activity, and obesity. We also include three other major chronic conditions: respiratory diseases, diabetes, and kidney disease. These conditions share risk factors and are often precursors for one another, and we address treatment and prevention of these conditions together. Cancer and mental health, typically grouped among noncommunicable diseases, are covered in *DCP3* volumes three and four, respectively.

This volume finds that effective prevention strategies are often underused in countries at all income levels. Substantial progress against CVRDs has been achieved in high- and upper-middle-income countries, partly as the result of policies that are applied at the population level—such as tobacco taxation or bans on trans-fats—and partly due to the availability of cost-effective pharmacological treatments. These policies have not been widely implemented in lower-income countries. This volume's essential package recommends 36 policy and health system interventions using primary health service delivery platforms. This set of interventions is focused on population prevention, as well as on targeting high-risk populations in LMICs to prevent and reduce early mortality from CVRDs.

The editors and authors of *Cardiovascular, Respiratory, and Related Disorders* hope that this volume can serve as a basis for universal health care packages. As countries strengthen their health systems and economic resources become more available, this essential package can be expanded to encompass more resource-intensive, life-saving interventions.

We thank the following individuals who provided valuable comments and assistance on this effort: Brianne Adderley, Kristen Danforth, Dean T. Jamison, Shamelle Richards, and Shivali Suri. We particularly acknowledge Jinyuan Qi for her assistance in preparing the Essential Package cost estimates. The editors also thank the reviewers organized by the U.S. National Academy of Medicine (listed separately in this volume), and the Advisory Committee to the Editors of *DCP3* for thoughtful feedback on the essential package.

Dorairaj Prabhakaran
Shuchi Anand
Thomas A. Gaziano
Jean-Claude Mbanya
Yangfeng Wu
Rachel Nugent

Abbreviations

ABI	ankle-brachial index
ABPM	ambulatory blood pressure measurement
ACE	angiotensin-converting enzyme
ACEi	angiotensin-converting enzyme inhibitors
ACS	acute coronary syndrome
AFB	acid fast bacilli
AKI	acute kidney injury
AMPATH	Academic Model Providing Access to Healthcare
ARB	angiotensin receptor blocker
ARF	acute rheumatic fever
BP	blood pressure
BMI	body mass index
CABG	coronary artery bypass graft
CCC	chronic Chagas cardiomyopathy
CCU	coronary care unit
CD	Chagas disease
CDSS	clinical decision support system
CEA	cost-effectiveness analysis
CET-P	cholesteryl ester transfer protein
CHD	coronary heart disease
CHE	catastrophic health expenditure
CHOICE	Choosing Interventions That Are Cost-Effective
CHWs	community health workers
CI	confidence interval
CKD	chronic kidney disease
COBRA	Control of Blood Pressure and Risk Attenuation
COPD	chronic obstructive pulmonary disease
CPACS	Clinical Pathways for Acute Coronary Syndromes
CRT	cardiac resynchronization therapy
CSMBS	Civil Servant Medical Benefit Scheme
CT	computed tomography
CVD	cardiovascular disease
CVRD	cardiovascular, respiratory, and related disorder
DALYs	disability-adjusted life years

DOHaD	developmental origins of health and disease
DPP	Diabetes Prevention Program
ECEA	extended cost-effectiveness analysis
eGFR	estimated glomerular filtration rate
EML	essential medicines list
ESC	European Society of Cardiology
ESH	European Society of Hypertension
ESRD	end-stage renal disease
FCTC	Framework Convention on Tobacco Control
FEV	forced expiratory volume
FRP	financial risk protection
FVC	forced vital capacity
GBD	Global Burden of Disease Study
GDM	gestational diabetes mellitus
GDP	gross domestic product
GINA	Global Initiative for Asthma
GLP-1s	glucagon-like peptide-1 agonists
GNI	gross national income
HCV	hepatitis C virus
HDL	high-density lipoprotein
HHE	home health education
HICs	high-income countries
HITAP	Health Intervention and Technology Assessment Program
HIV	human immunodeficiency virus
HIV/AIDS	human immunodeficiency virus/acquired immune deficiency syndrome
HR	hazard ratio
HTA	health technology assessment
ICD	implantable cardioverter defibrillator
ICER	incremental cost-effectiveness ratio
IDF	International Diabetes Federation
IFG	impaired fasting glucose
IGT	impaired glucose tolerance
IHD	ischemic heart disease
iIFG	isolated IFG
IPF	idiopathic pulmonary fibrosis
kg/m^2	kilogram per square meter
LABA	long-acting beta2-agonist
LDL	low-density lipoprotein
LICs	low-income countries
LMICs	low- and middle-income countries
LSCTC	London Stroke Carers Training Course
LY	life year
MET	metabolic equivalent of task
MET-h	metabolic equivalent hours
MICs	middle-income countries
mHealth	mobile health
MINIMat	Maternal and Infant Nutrition Interventions in Matlab Trial
mmHG	millimeter of mercury
MMS	multimedia message service

NCDs	noncommunicable diseases
NEML	national essential medicines list
NHI	national health insurance
NHSO	National Health Security Office
NICE	National Institute for Health and Care Excellence
NPH	Neutral Protamine Hagedorn
NRT	nicotine replacement therapy
OBPM	office-based blood pressure measurement
OR	odds ratio
PACK	Practical Approach to Care Kit
PAD	peripheral artery disease
PALSA	Practical Approach to Lung Health in South Africa
PCSK9	proprotein convertase subtilisin/kexin type 9
PD	peritoneal dialysis
PFWD	pain-free walking distance
PCI	percutaneous coronary interventions
PD	peritoneal dialysis
QALYs	quality-adjusted life years
RCT	randomized controlled trial
RF	rheumatic fever
RHD	rheumatic heart disease
RR	relative risk
RRT	renal replacement therapy
SAR	special administrative region
SBP	systolic blood pressure
SDG	Sustainable Development Goal
SGLT-2s	sodium-glucose linked transporters-2
SMS	short message service
SSB	sugar-sweetened beverage
SSS	Social Security Scheme
STEMI	ST-elevation myocardial infarction
T2DM	type 2 diabetes mellitus
tPA	tissue plasminogen activator
UCS	Universal Coverage Scheme
UHC	universal health coverage
UMPIRE	Use of a Multi-drug Pill in Reducing Cardiovascular Events
UN	United Nations

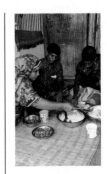

Cardiovascular, Respiratory, and Related Disorders: Key Messages and Essential Interventions to Address Their Burden in Low- and Middle-Income Countries

Dorairaj Prabhakaran, Shuchi Anand, David A. Watkins,
Thomas A. Gaziano, Yangfeng Wu, Jean-Claude Mbanya, and
Rachel Nugent, on behalf of the *DCP3* CVRD Author Group

INTRODUCTION

Adults living today are most likely to die from a cardio-vascular, respiratory, or related disorders (CVRDs). The World Health Organization (WHO) data for 2012 indicate that 44 percent of overall deaths and 52 percent of adult deaths globally were due to CVRDs (WHO 2012). The relative contribution of each disorder differs, but in every region except Sub-Saharan Africa, these closely related disorders are the leading causes of death.

Most of these disorders are preventable or, if they occur, can be medically treated to improve longevity and reduce disability. Optimal prevention and treatment—which require resources, certainly, but also consistent and persistent therapeutic compliance—remain a challenge even in high-income countries (HICs). Additionally, in low- and middle-income countries (LMICs), the limited capacity to detect these silent diseases and provide early treatment contributes to the rapid emergence of advanced complications and premature death.

Cardiovascular, Respiratory, and Related Disorders, volume 5 of the third edition of *Disease Control Priorities (DCP3),* covers three of the four major noncommunicable

diseases (NCDs) prioritized by the United Nations' (UN) high-level meeting on health in 2011:

- Cardiovascular diseases (ischemic heart disease and its risk factors, such as obesity, physical inactivity, tobacco use, high blood pressure and abnormal lipids, stroke, peripheral artery disease, structural heart disease, and congestive heart failure)
- Respiratory diseases
- Diabetes (United Nations 2011).

In addition, we include kidney disease as a related condition; cancers and mental health (also typically grouped among NCDs) are covered in other volumes of *DCP3* (box 1.1). These CVRDs are closely related precursors or sequelae for the others, and they share many risk factors and therefore similar prevention and control measures. Box 1.2 summarizes the key messages from *DCP3*'s volume 5 and provides a framework for systematically addressing CVRDs in LMICs. We present several evidence-based strategies for prevention of CVRDs. We also address the reality that the burden of

Corresponding author: Dorairaj Prabhakaran, Centre for Chronic Disease Control, New Delhi; and Centre for Control of Chronic Conditions, Public Health Foundation of India, Haryana, India; dprabhakaran@ccdcindia.org.

History of the *Disease Control Priorities* Initiative

Budgets constrain choices. Policy analysis helps decision makers achieve the greatest value from limited available resources. In 1993, the World Bank published *Disease Control Priorities in Developing Countries (DCP1)*, an attempt to assess the cost-effectiveness (value for money) of interventions in a systematic way that would address the major sources of disease burden in low- and middle-income countries (Jamison and others 1993). The World Bank's 1993 *World Development Report* on health drew heavily on the findings in *DCP1* to conclude that specific interventions against noncommunicable diseases were cost-effective, even in environments in which substantial burdens of infection and undernutrition persisted (World Bank 1993).

DCP2, published in 2006, updated and extended *DCP1* in several respects, including explicit consideration of the implications for health systems of expanded intervention coverage (Jamison and others 2006). One way that health systems expand intervention coverage is through selected platforms that deliver interventions that require similar logistics but address heterogeneous health problems. Platforms often provide a more natural unit for investment than do individual interventions, but conventional health economics has offered little understanding of how to make choices across platforms. Analysis of the costs of packages and platforms—and the health improvements they can generate in given epidemiological environments—can help guide health system investments and development.

The third edition of *DCP* is being completed. *DCP3* differs substantively from *DCP1* and *DCP2* by extending and consolidating the concepts of platforms and packages, and by offering explicit consideration of health systems' financial risk protection objective. In populations lacking access to health insurance or prepaid care, medical expenses that are high relative to income can be impoverishing. Where incomes are low, seemingly inexpensive medical procedures can have catastrophic financial effects. *DCP3* offers an approach that explicitly includes financial protection as well as the distribution across income groups of financial and health outcomes resulting from policies (for example, public finance) to increase intervention uptake (Verguet, Laxminarayan, and Jamison 2015).

The task in all of the *DCP* volumes has been to combine the available science about interventions implemented in very specific locales and under very specific disorders with informed judgment to reach reasonable conclusions about the impact of intervention mixes in diverse environments. The broad aim of *DCP3* is to delineate essential intervention packages (such as the package for cardiovascular, respiratory, and related disorders in this volume) and their related delivery platforms. This information will assist decision makers in allocating often tightly constrained budgets so that health system objectives are maximally achieved.

DCP3's nine volumes are being published in 2015–18 in an environment in which serious discussion continues about quantifying the Sustainable Development Goal (SDG) for health (United Nations 2015). *DCP3*'s analyses are well-placed to assist in choosing the means to attain the health SDG and assessing the related costs for scaled-up action.

Dean T. Jamison
Rachel Nugent
Hellen Gelband
Susan Horton
Prabhat Jha
Ramanan Laxminarayan
Charles N. Mock

many arguably preventable disorders is likely to remain high in the coming decades, and that health care systems in LMICs will need to identify viable approaches to treat them. Furthermore, implementing treatment strategies for the aforementioned diseases prevents downstream, highly morbid complications such as heart failure, blindness, or end-stage kidney disease as well as premature mortality among those with preexisting disorders.

In this review, we discuss the overarching burden of CVRDs, including reasons why LMICs face disproportionately high premature mortality. We summarize the

Box 1.2

Key Messages Regarding Cardiovascular, Respiratory, and Related Disorders

1. *Adults living in low- and middle-income countries (LMICs) face high risk for death, disability, and impoverishment from cardiovascular, respiratory, and related disorders (CVRDs).* The world is experiencing an increase in the number of deaths from CVRDs at least partly because of population growth and aging (Roth and others 2015). Nearly 80 percent of these deaths occur in LMICs. Furthermore, 39 percent of the CVRD deaths in LMICs occur prematurely—at younger than age 70 years—compared to 22 percent in high-income countries (HICs). In 2015, the United Nations General Assembly agreed to an array of development goals, including a target to reduce premature mortality from NCDs by one-third by 2030 (United Nations 2015). The world is not on track to achieve that goal because premature deaths from CVRDs are declining only very slowly.

Therefore, stronger actions are needed to combat CVRDs, especially in LMICs. Residents of LMICs have not benefited from the astonishing advances in preventing and treating cardiovascular disease—by far the most common cause of death among CVRDs—seen in HICs. In a woman with cardiovascular disease, the annual risk of death attributable to cardiovascular disease is twofold higher if she lives in a LMIC than if she lives in a HIC (Yusuf and others 2014). Should she require hospitalization for a stroke or myocardial infarction, she bears a one-in-two chance that out-of-pocket payments for her health care will push her family into poverty (Huffman and others 2011).

2. *Effective prevention strategies are underutilized.* High- and upper-middle income countries have reduced age-standardized mortality resulting from cardiovascular disease by more than 25 percent since 2000 (WHO 2012), largely by using policy interventions to reduce risk-factor levels,

strengthening the health system at the primary care level, and improving acute care with attention to early initiation of treatment. Policies aimed at reducing population-wide risk factors, such as high taxation of tobacco, reduction of salt in processed foods, or bans on trans fatty acids (trans fats), are effective but have not been widely adopted in LMICs. Targets related to individual-level risk factors (for example, reducing obesity and improving physical activity) are harder to achieve; however, when achieved sustainably, these targets improve health in multiple domains.

3. *Primary care centers require strengthening to treat the current and growing burden of CVRDs.* Medications crucial for individual-level treatment (such as diuretics for hypertension, and metformin or insulin for diabetes) also have long positive track records for efficacy; however, to improve their uptake, innovation is needed with respect to their affordability and delivery in high-volume, resource-poor health systems. Most of the disease-specific interventions recommended in this volume should be delivered in primary care centers because (a) CVRD management requires long-term follow-up and (b) many interventions use medications that can be prescribed and titrated best in primary care centers. Specific needs to shore up this care platform include training primary or non-physician health care providers in the management and follow-up of CVRDs, ensuring availability of inexpensive, generic, or combination drugs in clinics, and creating culturally viable strategies to improve patient adherence. These approaches are being evaluated worldwide and include shifting and sharing tasks with nonphysician health providers and traditional healers (such as village doctors in China and Ayush practitioners in India) and new health platforms to improve access (such as mobile health [mHealth] and telemedicine).

box continues next page

4. *Cost-effective prevention policies and treatments for CVRDs are possible to implement in LMICs.* Because of lower estimated costs, population-level policies to prevent and control CVRDs are generally more affordable than treatments. However, many cost-effective treatment interventions exist that can be delivered at primary care or referral-level hospitals. Evidence for cost-effective CVRD treatment approaches has increased since *Disease Control Priorities in Developing Countries*, second edition, was published in 2006. Yet evidence gaps remain; the need still exists to generalize many findings from middle- and high-income countries to estimate the potential cost-effectiveness of highly effective individual-level treatments (such as secondary prevention) for which coverage is low and technologies are not available in many low-income countries.

5. *Universal health care that includes care for CVRDs provides benefits beyond individual health to financial protection of families.* The household financial burden is particularly relevant in economic analyses related to the disorders covered in this volume, many of which are costly even if cost-effective and often are not part of publicly financed health services. On a value-for-health basis, CVRD interventions—particularly ones that incur ongoing, long-term costs (inhalers for asthma)—are expensive. However, many of the afflicted adults are wage earners, and investing in primary prevention can avert significant disability and acute care costs; the potential to improve economic productivity and avert poverty is clear and large.

effectiveness and cost-effectiveness evidence and propose 36 essential interventions (see tables 1.1 and 1.2) that are feasible for LMICs to pursue that can either reduce the incidence of new disease or delay complications among persons who have developed CVRDs. We also present estimates of the cost of this package in typical low- and lower-middle-income country settings and discuss various aspects of package implementation.

HIGH RISK FOR DEATH, DISABILITY, AND IMPOVERISHMENT

The world's population is aging. Persons older than age 65 years now constitute 10 percent of the world's population and are expected to constitute more than 15 percent by 2030, whereas for most of the twentieth century, 5 percent or fewer persons reached age 65 years (WHO 2011b). Combined with population growth, population aging has led to an overall increase in the number of persons dying from CVRDs, because, although the propensity for these diseases may start *in utero*, their substantive effects are seen in adulthood. From 2000 to 2012, the absolute number of deaths from CVRDs increased 16 percent globally (figure 1.1), although the age-standardized mortality rate for most disorders is declining (WHO 2012).

However, with implementation of population-level risk-reduction measures and advances in acute and chronic care, age-specific mortality has declined to the extent that it counterbalances the absolute increase in number of deaths from population growth and aging (Roth and others 2015; WHO 2012). Thus, age-standardized mortality rates for cardiovascular diseases (CVDs) and respiratory diseases are declining, whereas rates for diabetes and kidney diseases (including kidney disease that is due to diabetes) are unchanged or increasing (Roth and others 2015). In comparison with HICs, LMICs have experienced smaller declines; therefore, inequalities in outcomes are worsening (see annex 1A). For CVD—by far the most common cause of death among the CVRDs—the decline has ranged from 5 percent in low-income countries to 19 percent in upper-middle-income countries versus 28 percent in HICs (figure 1.2). Absolute rates of morbidity and premature mortality, captured in the summary metric of disability-adjusted life-years (DALYs), are increasing rapidly in the poorest regions. From 2000 through 2015, DALYs from CVD and diabetes increased 33 and 72 percent, respectively, in South Asia and 26 and 56 percent, respectively, in Sub-Saharan Africa (GBD 2015 DALYs and HALE Collaborators 2016).

On an individual level, where a person with CVD lives predicts his or her risk for death (Yusuf and others 2014) as strongly as if he or she were overweight (Manson and others 1995) or had hypertension (van den Hoogen and others 2000) (figure 1.3). Residence in a LMIC also predicts higher likelihood of a serious

Table 1.1 Essential Package of Interventions: Interventions Targeted Toward the Prevention or Management of Shared Risk Factors for Cardiovascular and Respiratory Disease

Condition	Fiscal interventions	Intersectoral interventions	Public health interventions	Personal health services, by delivery platform			
				Community based	Primary health center	First-level hospital	Referral and specialized hospitals
All conditions	1. Large excise taxes on tobacco products[a] 2. Product taxes on sugar-sweetened beverages	3. Improvements to the built environment to encourage physical activity[b] 4. School-based programs to improve nutrition and encourage physical activity **5. Regulations on advertising and labeling tobacco products** **6. Actions to reduce salt content in manufactured food products** **7. Ban on trans fatty acids**	8. Nutritional supplementation for women of reproductive age[c] 9. Use of mass media concerning harms of specific unhealthy foods and tobacco products	10. Use of community health workers to screen for CVRD using non-lab-based tools for overall CVD risk, improving adherence, and referral to primary health centers for continued medical management	11. Opportunistic screening for hypertension for all adults[d] **12. Screening for diabetes in all high-risk adults,[e] including pregnant women** 13. Combination therapy[f] for persons with multiple risk factors to reduce risk of CVD	14. Tobacco cessation counseling and use of nicotine replacement therapy in certain circumstances	—

Note: Red type denotes urgent care; blue type denotes continuing care; black type denotes routine care. — = none; CVRD = cardiovascular and respiratory disease; CVD = cardiovascular disease; ACEi = angiotensin-converting-enzyme inhibitors.

a. For fiscal and intersectoral policies that address CVRD attributable to indoor and outdoor sources of air pollution, see chapter 1 of *DCP3* volume 7.

b. Data are from high-income countries only.

c. Aimed at preventing gestational diabetes and low birthweight.

d. Treatment with generic drugs is recommended, guided by the severity of hypertension or the presence of additional risk factors.

e. High risk is typically defined as individuals who are older, have high blood pressure, or are overweight or obese (as measured for example by waist circumference).

f. Where available, fixed dose combination therapy is preferred.

Table 1.2 Essential Package of Interventions: Disease-Specific Interventions

Disease condition	Fiscal, intersectoral, and public health interventions	Community based	Personal health services, by delivery platform		
			Primary health center	First-level hospital	Referral and specialized hospitals
Ischemic heart disease, stroke, and peripheral artery disease[a]	—	—	15. Long-term management with aspirin, beta-blockers,[a] ACEi, and statins (as indicated) to reduce risk of further events 16. Use of aspirin in all cases of suspected myocardial infarction	17. Use of unfractionated heparin, aspirin, and generic thrombolytics in acute coronary events 18. Management for acute critical limb ischemia with unfractionated heparin and revascularization if available, with amputation as a last resort	19. Use of percutaneous coronary intervention for acute myocardial infarction where resources permit
Heart failure	—	—	20. Medical management with diuretics, beta-blockers,[b] ACEi,[b] and mineralocorticoid antagonists[b,c]	21. Medical management of acute heart failure	—
	22. Mixed vertical-horizontal insecticide spray programs to prevent Chagas disease	—	23. Treatment of acute pharyngitis (children) to prevent rheumatic fever[d] 24. Secondary prophylaxis with penicillin for rheumatic fever or established rheumatic heart disease	—	—
Diabetes	—	25. Diabetes self-management education	26. Prevention of long-term complications of diabetes through blood pressure, lipid, and glucose management as well as consistent foot care 27. Screening and treatment for albuminuria	—	28. Retinopathy screening via telemedicine, followed by treatment using laser photocoagulation

table continues next page

Table 1.2 Essential Package of Interventions: Disease-Specific Interventions *(continued)*

Disease condition	Fiscal, intersectoral, and public health interventions	Personal health services, by delivery platform			
		Community based	Primary health center	First-level hospital	Referral and specialized hospitals
Kidney disease	29. If transplantation available, creation of deceased donor programs[c]	—	30. Treatment of hypertension in kidney disease, with use of ACEi or ARBs in albuminuric kidney disease[c]	—	—
Respiratory disease	—	31. Self-management for obstructive lung disease to promote early recognition and treatment of exacerbations 32. Exercise-based pulmonary rehabilitation for patients with obstructive lung disease	33. Annual flu vaccination and five-yearly pneumococcal vaccine for patients with underlying lung disease **34. Low-dose inhaled corticosteroids and bronchodilators for asthma and for selected patients with COPD[e]**	35. Management of acute exacerbations of asthma and COPD using systemic steroids, inhaled beta-agonists, and, if indicated, oral antibiotics and oxygen therapy	36. Management of acute ventilatory failure due to acute exacerbations of asthma and COPD; in COPD, use of bilevel positive airway pressure preferred

Note: Red type denotes urgent care; blue type denotes continuing care; black type denotes routine care. — = none; ACEi = angiotensin-converting enzyme inhibitors; ARB = angiotensin receptor blocker; COPD = chronic obstructive pulmonary disease.

a. Not applicable to peripheral artery disease.

b. Applicable to heart failure with reduced ejection fraction.

c. Data from high-income countries only.

d. Use available treatment algorithms to determine appropriate antibiotic use.

e. Inhaled corticosteroids are indicated in patients with COPD who have severe disease or frequent exacerbations.

Figure 1.1 Share of All Deaths Caused by Cardiovascular, Respiratory, and Related Disorders, and Other Noncommunicable Diseases, by Country Income, 2015

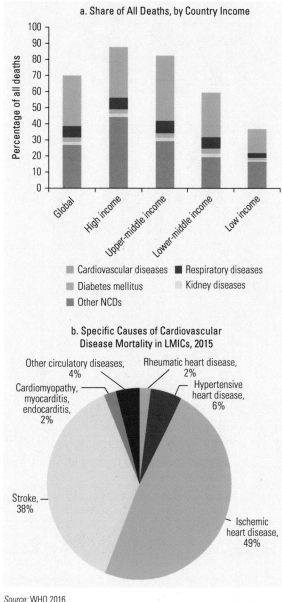

a. Share of All Deaths, by Country Income

Cardiovascular diseases
Diabetes mellitus
Other NCDs
Respiratory diseases
Kidney diseases

b. Specific Causes of Cardiovascular Disease Mortality in LMICs, 2015

Other circulatory diseases, 4%
Rheumatic heart disease, 2%
Cardiomyopathy, myocarditis, endocarditis, 2%
Hypertensive heart disease, 6%
Stroke, 38%
Ischemic heart disease, 49%

Source: WHO 2016.
Note: NCDs = noncommunicable diseases.

Figure 1.2 Trends in Age-Standardized Mortality Rates from Cardiovascular Disease for Both Genders, by Country Income Group, 2000–15

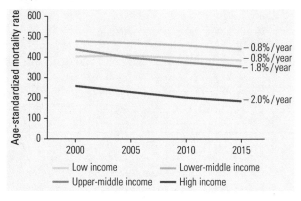

−0.8%/year
−0.8%/year
−1.8%/year
−2.0%/year

Low income
Upper-middle income
Lower-middle income
High income

Figure 1.3 Relative Risk for Mortality from Cardiovascular and Respiratory Disease in LMICs versus HICs, by Age Group, 2015

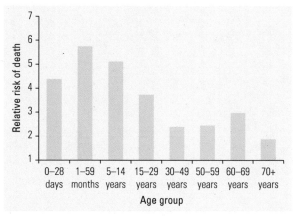

Note: LMIC = low- and middle-income country; HIC = high-income country.

event—for example, myocardial infarction (Yusuf and others 2004) or stroke (Sposato and Saposnik 2012)—at a younger age than in HICs. Acute hospitalizations are expensive and dramatically increase the likelihood of families' falling into poverty (Jaspers and others 2015). More than half of the persons hospitalized for stroke, myocardial infarction, or peripheral artery disease in China, India, or Tanzania experienced catastrophic health spending in the process of receiving care (Huffman and others 2011). Even without acute

complications, paying for routine use of generic medications such as atenolol in the Philippines would impoverish more than 5 percent of the population—and more than 20 percent of the population if brand-name atenolol were used (Niens and others 2010).

Why have LMICs not benefited from advances in CVRD prevention and care? The reasons are many and vary by region, but here we highlight the following: (a) the lack of population-wide strategies to tackle behavioral risk factors, (b) missed opportunities to identify and treat disease in early stages, and (c) inability to provide quality care for advanced complications.

Lack of Population-Wide Strategies to Tackle Behavioral Risk Factors

The attention focused on poor diet, obesity, physical inactivity, and tobacco use through population-wide and individual-level strategies has contributed at least partly to the substantial decline in CVRD mortality in HICs. In contrast, LMICs are experiencing a growing burden of these major behavioral risk factors for the development and progression of CVRDs. For example, most HICs have enacted strict restrictions on public smoking and on advertisements of tobacco products, and they have levied heavy taxes on tobacco consumption. When more than 170 countries signed onto the WHO Framework Convention on Tobacco Control in 2005, optimism grew for a tobacco-free world (Britton 2015). Since that time, the WHO has set a target of reducing the prevalence of smoking by 30 percent by 2025. However, most LMICs are unlikely to meet that goal; the overall number of smokers is growing, and many of the strong evidence-based recommendations of the framework (including taxation, advertising bans, pictorial warnings, and smoking cessation assistance), which are described in the WHO MPOWER package, have not been universally implemented (Bilano and others 2015). Of all tobacco interventions, taxation is the single most effective method of averting tobacco-attributable CVRDs (Jha and Peto 2014). As shown in an extended cost-effectiveness analysis based in China (Verguet, Gauvreau, and others 2015), taxation also provides financial risk protection for low-income families living in LMICs, answering concerns about the potential for a regressive tax on the poor. Yet, tobacco taxes represent less than 40 percent of the average price of cigarettes in LICs, compared with more than 60 percent in HICs, such that cigarettes are relatively more affordable in LMICs and will become even more affordable over time in the absence of drastic price increases (WHO 2010b).

Poor diet, obesity, and physical inactivity are three interlinked risk factors that, when addressed early in life, can lead to lifelong protection from CVRDs in many cases. Based on current trends, the contribution of these risk factors to death and disability is likely to grow in LMICs and diminish in HICs. All countries have experienced a decline in occupation-related physical activity, but leisure-time physical activity is increasing in HICs (Hallal and others 2012). Over the past three decades, deaths attributable to physical inactivity declined 15 percent in HICs but rose 25 percent in LMICs (Institute for Health Metrics and Evaluation [IHME] 2013). In HICs, many stakeholders are working to encourage physical activity: city governments are creating pedestrian plazas, health care organizations are incorporating physical activity assessments in clinic visits, and employers are offering at-work exercise classes (Heath and others 2012). The rapid and haphazard growth of urban metropolises in LMICs, in contrast, impedes the implementation of cost-effective opportunities for physical activity,

such as the preservation of safe, traffic-free space for walking or recreation (Laine and others 2014).

Missed Opportunities to Treat CVRDs in Early Stages

One of the first missed opportunities occurs when a lack of effective care exists for sufferers of an acute event such as myocardial infarction or stroke. Timely emergency response with common, relatively inexpensive medications can save a life until diagnosis and treatment are available. Although optimal treatment for a myocardial infarction requires immediate transport to a health care center, an electrocardiogram, and blood work for proper diagnosis, such response is not always possible in remote locations. Nonetheless, if basic medications such as aspirin and beta-blockers are available and practitioners are empowered to use them appropriately, they can be delivered in a timely and cost-effective fashion at the level of primary care health centers prior to transfer to hospitals (Gaziano 2005).

A second missed opportunity is the failure to provide effective management of hypertension and diabetes; such management can prevent complications such as ischemic heart disease, stroke, peripheral artery disease, retinopathy, and chronic kidney disease. The early use of inhaled corticosteroids decreases frequency of serious attacks, even for those with mild persistent asthma (Pauwels and others 2003). Medications required to treat these disorders overlap across many CVRDs. For example, statins can reduce the risk of first-time and recurrent strokes or myocardial infarctions on average by 21 percent (Collins and others 2016). Aggressive lowering of blood pressure affords a similar degree of protection for heart failure, acute coronary events, and strokes (Wright and others 2015).

The use of these therapies, however, remains dismally low. In a multi-country cross-sectional study of hypertension awareness and control, 49 percent of patients in HICs were aware of their hypertension, compared to 31 percent in LICs; 47 percent of those with hypertension in HICs were treated, compared to 32 percent in LICs (Chow and others 2013). The use of effective therapy in lower-income countries was even lower for those at greatest risk. Since the 2003 Doha Declaration on the Trade-Related Aspects of Intellectual Property Rights Agreement and Public Health, generic cardiovascular medications constitute more than 70 percent of the market in many LMICs (Kaplan, Wirtz, and Stephens 2013). Yet affordability remains a key issue, with large swings in cost even within the same class of drugs (Ait-Khaled and others 2000). Although the WHO Model List of Essential Medicines attempts to focus resources on selected effective and cost-effective medications, conflicting incentives for physicians lead to highly variable prescribing patterns that can increase costs without clear health benefits. One prominent example is the heavier provider reliance on insulin analogs over the cheaper nonanalog form in Brazil, Mexico, and República Bolivariana de Venezuela (Cohen and Carter 2010).

Even if sequelae develop, optimizing their treatment can further delay progression along the disease spectrum to heart failure, limb amputation, blindness, or end-stage kidney disease. Here we note an even larger gap in care provision between HICs and LMICs: fewer than 10 percent of patients in LICs and fewer than 25 percent in lower-middle-income countries take beta-blockers, angiotensin-converting enzyme (ACE) inhibitors, or statins after a myocardial infarction or stroke (Yusuf and others 2011).

Inability to Care for Advanced Complications

Finally, once end-organ damage develops, facilities for caring for advanced conditions are scarce and, when available, have few incentives to ensure high-quality care. The need for specialists or specialized equipment means that some of the advanced conditions covered in this volume (such as heart failure, structural heart disease, and end-stage kidney disease) are expensive to treat. Many middle-income countries and some LICs do have facilities but are not able to take on the large number of persons requiring treatment as a result of either resource scarcity, patient-level financial constraints, or both. In the case of end-stage kidney disease, hemodialysis facilities exist in a majority of countries in the world, but fewer than one-fourth of persons expected to reach end-stage kidney disease annually are able to access therapy (Anand, Bitton, and Gaziano 2013; Liyanage and others 2015). Even for persons who are able to pay for the costly therapy, little to no oversight of the quality of care delivered exists. For example, in a survey of six hemodialysis centers in Lagos, Nigeria, none met accepted standards for microbial decontamination (Braimoh and others 2014). An analysis of patients with rheumatic or congenital heart disease reported that two-thirds of surgical candidates in Uganda did not have access to treatment, and 18 percent died while on the waiting list for surgery (Grimaldi and others 2014). Among those who underwent open-heart surgery, postoperative mortality and loss to follow-up rates were high (19 percent and 22 percent, respectively).

Thus, even as the burden of risk factors for CVRDs increases in LMICs, strategies and facilities to care for persons with these diseases are too rarely available. Evidence also indicates that without oversight, scarce resources are sometimes unnecessarily expended on expensive treatments while cost-effective alternatives go underused (Sakuma, Glassman, and Vaca 2017).

COSTS AND COST-EFFECTIVENESS OF PREVENTION AND TREATMENT INTERVENTIONS FOR CVRDS

We reviewed the costs and cost-effectiveness of various CVRD clinical interventions and policies with the goal of creating a suggested package of interventions that LMICs could adopt to address CVRDs (Gaziano and others 2017). We performed a review of the published literature on the costs of providing preventive care and treatment for cardiovascular and metabolic diseases in LMICs (Brouwer and others 2015), as well as the cost-effectiveness of CVRD interventions in LMICs. We extracted cost and cost-effectiveness data from English-language literature published after 2000 through a bibliometric search, adjusted all reported results to the same currency and year, and ranked the cost and cost-effectiveness outcomes (Gaziano and others 2017). Where necessary to assess priority interventions when evidence from LMICs was lacking, we refer to evidence from HICs. Box 1.3 summarizes use of economic evaluation in *DCP3*.

Overall affordability of individual interventions is an important consideration for country decision making. We found that interventions to prevent and treat conditions at early stages were much less expensive than interventions to treat diseases at advanced stages. Prevention interventions at the population and community levels were the cheapest (less than US$1 per capita in 2012 U.S. dollars), while treatment of end-stage kidney disease was among the most expensive (Gaziano and others 2017). However, affordability is only one measure for policy makers to consider. Preventive treatments or health promotion activities may not have the same efficacy on an individual basis as, for example, appropriate treatment of acute myocardial infarction. Between both population and individual measures, and preventive and treatment measures, policy makers should scrutinize which have the best evidence for being both effective and cost-effective.

Some fairly recent systematic reviews have taken stock of the evidence of cost-effectiveness of interventions to tackle CVD in LMICs specifically (Shroufi and others 2013; Suhrcke, Boluarte, and Niessen 2012). These reviews showed that, while the cost-effectiveness evidence on CVD interventions in LMICs remains modest in comparison to the evidence in HICs, it has been growing. The reviews also noted that a

Box 1.3

Economic Evaluation of Investments in Cardiovascular, Respiratory, and Related Disorder Control

Economic evaluations aim to inform decision making by quantifying the trade-offs between resource inputs required for alternative investments and the resulting outcomes. Four approaches to economic evaluation in health are the following:

- Assessing how much of a *specific health outcome*, such as myocardial infarctions averted, can be attained for a given level of resource input;
- Assessing how much of an *aggregate measure of health*, such as deaths or disability adjusted life years [DALYs], can be attained from a given level of resource inputs applied to alternative interventions. This approach—cost-effectiveness analysis (CEA)—enables comparisons of interventions addressing many different health outcomes (for example, heart disease treatment versus tobacco tax);
- Assessing how much health and financial risk protection can be attained for a given level of public sector finance of a given intervention. This approach, extended CEAs or extended cost-effectiveness analyses (ECEAs), enables assessment not only of efficiency in improving the health of a population but also of efficiency in achieving the other major goal of a health system—protecting the population from financial risk;
- Assessing the *economic benefits*, measured in monetary terms, from investment in a health intervention and weighing that benefit against its cost (benefit-cost analysis [BCA]). BCA enables

comparison of the attractiveness of health investments relative to those in other sectors.

CEAs predominate among economic evaluations in surgery (and for health interventions more generally). Recent overviews of CEA findings for cardiovascular, respiratory, and related disorders (CVRDs) underpin this chapter's conclusion that many CVRD policies and interventions are highly cost-effective even in resource-constrained environments (also see PAHO/*DCP3* companion volume (Alkire, Vincent, and Meara 2015; Chao and others 2014; Legetic and others 2016; Prinja and others 2015; Shroufi and others 2013; Suhrcke, Boluarte, and Niessen 2012). Chapter 19 of *DCP3* Volume 5 also looks at the cost-effectiveness of CVRD interventions (Gaziano and others 2017).

The *Lancet* Commission on Investing in Health applied BCA to broad investments in health and found benefit-cost ratios often in excess of 10 (Jamison and others 2013). Copenhagen Consensus for 2012 used BCAs to rank selected CVRD interventions among the top 15 in a list of 30 attractive priorities for investment in development across all sectors (Kydland and others 2013).

ECEAs remain a relatively new evaluation approach. In chapter 20 of this volume, Watkins and coauthors apply ECEA to several CVRD interventions in different settings and find substantial financial protection benefits (Watkins, Nugent, and Verguet 2017).

substantially larger number of publications assess pharmaceutical interventions, compared with population-level interventions.

Among the most cost-effective ways to reduce CVRD mortality are prevention-oriented *population* policies. The leading types of population policies involve tobacco control, including public smoking bans that are cost-saving/highly cost-effective; for example, taxation that is cost-saving (Vietnam) and

highly cost-effective (US$140 per DALY) (Mexico); public smoking bans that cost US$2.4 to US$136 per life-year saved (India); advertising bans that cost US$2,800 per DALY averted (Mexico); and mass media campaigns that range from cost saving to US$3,200 per DALY averted (Gaziano and others 2017). Evidence is growing for the cost-effectiveness of sugar-sweetened beverage (SSB) taxes but is still inconclusive as to the health effects (Colchero and others 2016; Nakhimovsky and others 2016). The strongest evidence to date comes from Mexico, where an SSB tax reduced consumption of sugary beverages and increased water consumption, especially among the poor (Colchero and others 2016). Longer-term data on changes in obesity, diabetes, and other CVRDs have not yet been reported. Population-level salt reduction strategies range from cost saving (Argentina) to up to US$15,000 per life-year gained (Gaziano and others 2017). Salt reformulation by the food industry appears to be the most cost-effective approach, and salt reduction campaigns to promote health are the least cost-effective (Gaziano and others 2017).

Many important disease prevention or health promotion programs have not been assessed for cost-effectiveness, especially as they might apply to LMICs. Increasing physical activity can, in principle, reduce mortality and improve population health. Governments in many countries have recognized this opportunity, but the evidence on what works best to promote physical activity, let alone what is the best value for the money, remains scarce and largely concentrated on HICs (Ding and others 2016). A study from China shows that combining physical activity with a nutrition program is more effective than either intervention alone (Meng and others 2013), while a review by Laine and others (2014) found that the most efficient interventions to increase physical activity were community rail-trails (US$0.006 per metabolic equivalent hours [MET-h]), pedometers (US$0.014 per MET-h), and school health education programs (US$0.056 per MET-h). How generalizable these findings are to LMIC contexts is unclear.

Screening and pharmacological treatment of hypertension to prevent stroke and ischemic heart disease have been shown to range from cost saving (China) to cost-effective at US$700–US$5,000 per DALY averted or quality-adjusted life year (QALY) gained in South Africa and Argentina (Gaziano and others 2017). Cost-effectiveness of strategies using lipid-lowering therapies have had slightly higher ratios, ranging from as low as US$1,200 per QALY in most large LMICs when part of a multidrug regimen to as much as US$22,000 per DALY in the Philippines (Gaziano and others 2017). The range in cost-effectiveness is wider because the number of generic statins is more limited than the number of blood pressure medications. With more statins coming off patent, the price of statins has dropped, and lipid-lowering therapy is becoming more cost-effective.

Opportunistic screening for prediabetes and diabetes in a high-risk population is more cost-effective than screening for diabetes alone, since prevention of diabetes among those with prediabetes is highly cost-effective or cost saving (Ali and others 2017). Once diagnosed, structured diabetes self-management education programs are cost-effective (Diaz de Leon-Castaneda and others 2012), but self-monitoring of blood glucose among persons not on insulin or an oral hypoglycemic is not (Ali and others 2017). One randomized controlled trial from a HIC supports comprehensive management (for example, attention to blood glucose, blood pressure, and lipids) as being cost-effective (Gaede and others 2008). Similarly, another large randomized trial conducted in India and Pakistan supports comprehensive management delivered through care coordinators enabled with an electronic decision support system (Ali and others 2016). Evidence from both HIC and LMIC settings supports screening for complications of diabetes once diagnosed; screening for foot ulcers is among the most cost-effective (Habib and others 2010). A study in India (Rachapelle and others 2013) suggests that screening for retinopathy via telemedicine ranges from US$1,200 to US$2,400 per QALY gained.

Management of acute ischemic heart disease and stroke can be divided into the prehospital phase and the hospital phase. Prehospital phase management requires an established emergency transport system with trained staff and equipment. When available, prehospital thrombolysis was shown to be cost saving. The use of electrocardiogram machines in primary health centers to triage patients appropriately was shown to be cost-effective in India at US$12 per QALY gained (Gaziano and others 2017). The use of aspirin and beta-blockers is about US$10–US$20 per DALY averted. Streptokinase costs about US$700 per QALY gained, and the use of more fibrin-specific thrombolytics (such as tissue plasminogen activators) costs about US$15,000 per QALY. More advanced treatment includes the use of percutaneous coronary interventions (PCIs), including stents. In China, the availability of PCIs or streptokinase for acute myocardial infarction costs between US$9,000 and US$25,000 per QALY gained. Management of persons undergoing PCI with antiplatelet agents such as prasugrel and clopidogrel is also cost-effective in advanced centers where PCI is conducted. Data on cost-effectiveness of acute ischemic stroke management with a thrombolytic agent are sparse in LMICs, but one study recommends home-based rehabilitation (Sritipsukho and others 2010).

Management of heart failure with oral agents such as ACE inhibitors, beta-blockers, and aldosterone antagonists is cost saving or highly cost-effective (Gaziano and others 2017). Advanced therapy with implantable defibrillators and resynchronization therapy could be cost-effective in advanced centers in middle-income countries, with cost-effectiveness ratios of US$17,000–US$35,000 per QALY gained. The use of low-dose inhaled corticosteroids for mild asthma is an attractive intervention, as it addresses a large disease burden and is cost-effective in lower-middle-income countries (Gaziano and others 2017).

Acknowledging that cost- and cost-effectiveness data rarely translate directly across settings and that each country would need to individually assess its disease burdens and priorities (box 1.3), our review of cost-effectiveness has identified multiple cost-effective and even cost-saving interventions for CVRDs in LMICs, particularly for population-level interventions. Many highly effective clinical interventions—for example, treatment of hypertension or hyperlipidemia—are also cost-effective in some LMICs, whereas others requiring greater technology and specialized care are only cost-effective in MICs.

PATHWAYS TO ADDRESSING CVRDS IN LMICS

After the 2011 UN General Assembly high-level meeting on NCDs highlighted the growing and detrimental impact of NCDs on the health and wealth of nations, the WHO produced a Global Action Plan for the Prevention and Control of NCDs (WHO 2013). Of the eight voluntary targets set to help countries reduce NCD mortality, six focus on prevention and highlight interventions that improve diet and reduce smoking, obesity, and physical inactivity, helping individuals to live longer, healthier lives. To assist countries in meeting those targets, we offer here a set of policies and interventions that form an essential package of prevention actions, primarily delivered at the population level (table 1.1). Further, acknowledging the reality that LMICs continue to struggle with a spectrum of early to advanced cases of these diseases, we propose a set of disease-specific individual-level services appropriate for low-resource settings (table 1.2). These policies and interventions were selected from those deemed most effective and cost-effective by *DCP3* Volume 5 chapter author teams, each using a literature review combined with expert judgment to prioritize among those with the strongest evidence. Interventions included in the essential package were shown to be cost-effective in at least one LMIC setting, or had strong evidence to suggest LMIC cost-effectiveness. This essential package goes beyond the WHO NCD "best buys" (WHO 2011a), but it has a high degree of overlap with priority interventions in the recent revision of appendix 3 of the WHO Global Action Plan (WHO 2013).

Individually and collectively, the 36 actions contained in the essential package can address a large portion of the health burden of these diseases, are proven to be effective, and are expected to be feasible to implement in low-resource settings. Cost-effectiveness is suggested, either by studies from low-income settings or reasonable extrapolation of existing estimates from well-resourced settings. The essential package of recommended interventions is organized by delivery level (or platform).

While all of the interventions in the essential package meet these criteria, not every country can or should implement all of them, and some countries will take years to build a health system that can implement even some of them. As countries expand and scale up their health benefits, the highest-priority interventions are controlling tobacco consumption (especially through tobacco taxation); improving dietary intake; and (when a health system has the capacity to support it) preventing or treating hypertension and promoting health. In addition, LICs with high disease burden (such as Sub-Saharan African countries) may want to consider starting with a suite of cost-effective interventions for endemic CVRDs such as rheumatic heart disease, chronic kidney disease, chronic obstructive pulmonary disease, and heart failure resulting from nonischemic etiologies. The menu chosen must be appropriate for a country's disease burden and feasible given its health system capacity.

Effective Prevention Strategies for Most CVRDs

Effective prevention strategies are available but underutilized. Table 1.1 offers a set of high-priority disease prevention policies that, when implemented effectively, reduce the multiple risk factors of CVRDs. Implementing these actions creates an environment that encourages healthy behavior and reduces involuntary exposure to CVRD risk. Multiple agencies, both public and private, are responsible for establishing this environment.

Fiscal policies are among the most effective and affordable actions that governments can take to create a healthy environment. Tobacco taxation is the best example of a fiscal policy to reduce CVRD risk, with strong evidence from multiple countries (Shibuya and others 2003). Other fiscal policies are being tested in models and in initial LMIC experiences and show promise for improving diet. Recently, taxation on SSBs is gaining steam as a potential deterrent of obesity (Colchero and others 2016; Falbe and others 2016). Another fiscal policy to reduce CVRD risk is subsidizing fruits and vegetables to increase their consumption. When Cecchini and colleagues (Cecchini and others 2010) modeled the subsidy's effects on preventing NCDs (in combination with taxing high-fat food) using a framework jointly developed by the Organisation for Economic Co-Operation and Development and the WHO, they found it to be cost saving in all six LMICs under consideration. This approach lacks broad real-world evidence and therefore was not included in the current iteration of the essential package, but it could be strongly considered if a country is focusing intensively on dietary risk factors for CVRDs.

Policies that are not fiscal (such as regulations to reduce salt or tobacco consumption via labeling or bans on advertisements) can also encourage healthy consumer choices. In the United Kingdom, foods labeled as high in salt saw a marked decline in consumption when coupled with an aggressive public education campaign (Webster and others 2011). In the case of partially hydrogenated oils—the processed form of trans fatty acids (trans fats)—the strength of the data demonstrating improvements in "hard health outcomes" (for example, cardiovascular mortality) warrants bans or mandatory elimination of trans fats from the food supply chain (Restrepo and Rieger 2016).

Health promotion activities aimed at improving risk factors on a population level may have similar effect sizes to fiscal policies but generally require more planning or resources to implement. Mass media health campaigns to improve diet are effective when they offer specific actionable health messages such as increasing fruit and vegetable intake (Afshin and others 2017). Once a country commits to one aspect of the approach, other strategies can be layered on with less additional cost. Cities in Brazil and Colombia committed to providing pedestrian plazas and safe areas for physical activity, allowing them also to offer community exercise classes (Bull and others 2017). Similarly, school-based programs to promote physical activity (but not necessarily weight management) are cost-effective (Malik and Hu 2017); if implemented, however, these programs could include components addressing nutrition as well as physical activity.

Across many of the CVRD health endpoints, establishing absolute risk is a critical first step—both for matching the intensity of prevention effort to the level of risk and for efficient targeting of health system resources. Having community health workers (CHWs) use noninvasive methods to screen for many CVRDs is generally feasible (Gaziano, Abrahams-Gessel, Surka, and others 2015). The most recent data demonstrate that well-trained CHWs can deliver lifestyle modification advice (Jafar and others 2010), can identify high-risk individuals with similar effectiveness as primary care physicians (Falbe and others 2016), can be cost-effective in helping patients adhere to hypertension regimens (Cecchini and others 2010), and can be trained to use mHealth tools effectively (Ajay and others 2016; Gaziano, Abrahams-Gessel, Denman, and others 2015; Gaziano, Abrahams-Gessel, Surka, and others 2015). However, exactly what role these CHWs should play remains

unclear: screening, follow-up, medication prescription, or a component of all of these. Integrating CHWs into the existing health care infrastructure also is a challenge, as their effectiveness depends on their ability to triage the diagnosed cases to appropriate levels of care and to ensure the delivery of medication.

Opportunistic screening for diabetes and hypertension using more sensitive techniques can be done in clinics, especially for higher-risk populations such as pregnant women, obese adults, and persons with multiple risk factors. Generic therapy for preventing secondary diseases is on the WHO's Model List of Essential Medicines and could be made reliably available in primary health settings. Therapy in combination (for example, fixed-dose combinations) or with individual drugs targeting multiple risk factors is especially attractive for high-volume health systems with limited resources for personalization and titration (Gaziano and Pagidipati 2013; Lonn and Yusuf 2009). Data support the use of fixed-dose combinations in secondary prevention, but we await an assessment of their effectiveness in primary prevention. With the widespread availability of drug and disease management algorithms, follow-up and titration of medications may again be possible via CHWs, accompanied by broader prescribing rights, but otherwise should be managed by primary providers (including CHWs, who could be given prescription rights for selected CVRD drugs), rather than specialized physicians. Very few of the essential preventive interventions need to be delivered at first-level hospitals or in more specialized settings, except management of drug therapy for persons with multiple complication, or for persons who need special consideration (such as those with drug intolerance).

CENTRAL ROLE FOR PRIMARY CARE CENTERS

Stronger and better-equipped primary care centers are needed to manage the current and growing burden of CVRDs. Health systems in LMICs do *not* need to be replicas of health systems in HICs. Perhaps more than any other set of diseases, CVRDs require screening, long-term follow-up, and reliable medication delivery (table 1.2). The approach in a majority of HICs (that is, individualized interval screening performed by primary care physicians followed by highly specialized, referral-based care) is unlikely to be viable in most LMICs for a multitude of reasons. Financial and human resource constraints certainly come into play; in addition, the cultural approach to health may be different. For example, LMIC populations may be more amenable to peer counseling or community-based health promotion activities. Therefore, a majority of the medical management interventions (table 1.1) recommended in the essential package can be delivered at the community or primary health care level.

Primary health care clinics could be responsible primarily for delivering and titrating medications. The WHO Health Systems Framework provides a comprehensive approach to their strengthening (WHO 2010a). In addition to ensuring availability of key medications, governments can enable these centers to deliver care effectively by developing national guidelines and targets for specific conditions (table 1.3), which could, in turn, encourage reliance on the available generic medications and standardize follow-up intervals. Structured guidelines for referral to specialized systems could improve efficiency at both the primary and specialized care level. Further, if primary health care centers are the first point of contact in an acute situation (for example, chest pain in a patient likely to be experiencing myocardial infarction), available basic therapy (for example, rapid administration of aspirin), though limited, could be lifesaving. Primary care centers could be empowered to deliver such therapy prior to facilitating transfer to a first-level hospital.

Acute myocardial infarction and stroke are two conditions for which timely intervention is essential. Diagnosis and thrombolytic management of myocardial infarction require a simple electrocardiogram machine; ischemic stroke also benefits from thrombolytic therapy but requires use of computed tomography and on-site radiology to differentiate from hemorrhagic stroke. If built from the ground up to serve only stroke, such approach is unaffordable. However, many first-level hospitals in middle-income countries may have access to these facilities and require

the implementation of a stroke algorithm to help prioritize their timely use in patients presenting within the appropriate time frame.

When specialized centers are used for conditions that are rare or costly to treat, two potential strategies merit consideration: (1) choosing and scaling up one effective treatment from the roster of potential therapies, or (2) creating high-volume centers that specialize in specific diseases. For example, end-stage kidney disease can be treated with relatively equivalent efficacy using either hemodialysis or peritoneal dialysis. After a careful analysis taking into account cost, cultural opinion, and ethics, Thailand has chosen to pay for and scale up the peritoneal form of dialysis (Teerawattananon, Mugford, and Tangcharoensathien 2007); we await long-term outcomes from this strategy, but preliminary data indicate an increase in the availability of treatment with patient survival similar to that in HICs relying mostly on hemodialysis, albeit at quite high cost (Praditpornsilpa and others 2011; Tantivess and others 2013). In children with congenital heart disease that is amenable to a highly technical but relatively effective surgical procedure (such as ventricular septal defect), creating centers especially designed to serve these patients may be a viable approach to treatment (Reddy and others 2015). Similarly, we know that high-volume kidney transplant centers can achieve good outcomes (Axelrod and others 2004; Medina-Pestana 2006).

The essential package does include a few examples of effective specialized care that is potentially immediately feasible and affordable in low-income settings but that is not widespread. Other effective tertiary care services are considered neither feasible nor affordable in low- and most middle-income settings. Advanced treatments such as implantable cardioverter defibrillators or

Table 1.3 Recommendations for Health Systems Improvements That Enable Implementation of the Recommended Interventions

Policy	Platform
Improve access to the following essential medications: aspirin, beta-blockers, diuretics, ACEi, or ARBs, statins, mineralocorticoid agents, nonanalog insulin, bronchodilators, and inhaled corticosteroids	Policy, public health
Develop a category of trained (nonphysician) health worker	Policy, intersectoral
Offer public emergency medical transport services	Policy, intersectoral
Create standardized care pathways for first-level hospitals to manage acute episodes for myocardial infarction, stroke, critical limb ischemia, heart failure, acute kidney injury, chronic obstructive pulmonary disease, or asthma exacerbation	Policy, public health
Issue national targets for secondary prevention to enable primary health centers to manage CVRD effectively	Policy, public health

Note: ACEi = angiotensin-converting enzyme inhibitors; ARB = angiotensin receptor blocker; CVRD = cardiovascular and respiratory disease.

cardiac synchronization therapy are potentially cost-effective in some places (Brazil, for example) but expensive (Ribeiro and others 2010). As costs drop and skilled providers are trained, additional capacity should become available in specialized facilities to diagnose and manage more complex chronic respiratory diseases that are not amenable to treatment using the simple algorithm. Equipment such as continuous positive airway pressure, nebulizers, Doppler ultrasound, and other tools may all be desired depending on the respiratory disease burden.

Costs of Implementing the Package

We estimated the potential cost of implementing the essential package of interventions in stylized low-income and lower-middle-income country settings, reflecting typical costs, demographic and epidemiological characteristics, and coverage gaps in CVRD care (table 1.4). Supplementary annex 1A contains more detail on costing methods and results. We estimated the annual incremental cost of the essential package to be US$21 in a typical low-income country (3.8 percent of current gross national income [GNI] per capita) and US$24 in a typical lower-middle-income country (1.3 percent of current GNI per capita).

Most (60 percent) of the additional investments would need to be in primary health centers that offer preventive services and manage chronic disease. Low-income countries that are particularly resource constrained could focus on achieving full implementation of the bolded interventions in tables 1.1 and 1.2, which we have deemed likely to provide the best value for money in these settings. This high-priority subpackage would only cost an additional US$11 per capita, or 20 percent of current income. This costing exercise suggests that all countries—regardless of resource levels—can begin to put in place at least a few highly effective CVRD interventions at a reasonable cost as they move toward universal health coverage (UHC).

MEASURING THE BENEFITS FROM UNIVERSAL HEALTH CARE FOR CVRDS

In considering whether to expend strained resources on CVRDs, countries can take into account not only the benefits to individual health but also the benefits to outcomes relevant to societal well-being, such as poverty aversion, financial risk protection, and equity. Extended cost-effectiveness analyses (ECEA), developed as part of the Disease Control Priorities effort, attempt to capture some of these outcomes and provide evidence that CVRD care, in particular, offers substantial financial risk protection. Three ECEAs relevant to CVRDs—assessing tobacco taxation in China (Verguet, Gauvreau, and others 2015), salt reduction in processed foods in South Africa (Watkins and others 2016), and treatment of hypertension in Ethiopia (Verguet, Olson, and others 2015)—not only support the cost-effectiveness of these policies but also demonstrate that they could avert thousands of cases of poverty annually.

Treatment of hypertension in Ethiopia illustrates two specific features of universal public finance for CVRD care in LMICs: (1) treatment of CVRDs may be more expensive than interventions in other domains (such as maternal and child health), but (2) because these health policies and interventions protect wage-earning adults from disability or death, universal coverage could reduce financial risk to a greater degree. Further, poor families spend a much larger portion of their household income on hospitalizations or medications for CVRDs than wealthier families, so they could benefit more (Kankeu and others 2013).

For cases of advanced disease, when universal coverage for treatment is not yet affordable or sustainable (that is, complex congenital heart defects, advanced heart failure, or end-stage kidney disease), countries could consider expanding palliative care services. In addition to easing the

Table 1.4 Potential Costs of the Essential Package in a Stylized Typical Low- and Lower-Middle-Income Country

Estimate	LI country	LMI country
Total cost per capita	$22	$39
as a % of current GNI per capita	4.0%	2.1%
Incremental cost per capita	$21	$24
as a % of current GNI per capita	3.8%	1.3%

Note: LI = low-income; LMI = lower-middle-income; GNI = gross national income. GNI estimates taken from the World Bank and deflated to 2012 US dollars. See annex 1A for details of methods, data sources, and assumptions.

emotional and physical burden of disease, palliative care may offer a form of financial risk protection, allowing families to care for their loved ones without exhausting their financial resources on ultimately unsustainable treatments.

CONCLUSIONS

We offer a range of effective and cost-effective policies and interventions to reduce the high and mounting global health burden from the constellation of CVRD. We reviewed the evidence for CVRD interventions to assemble an essential package of the most effective policies and services that could be implemented in LMICs. Modeled studies suggest that countries can expect a high return on investment from prevention and control of CVRD, especially from implementing population prevention policies that cost relatively little (Nugent, Kelly, and Narula 2012). Countries have effective and cost-effective choices available to them. By relying heavily on population-level policies and on services that can be delivered at the community and primary health levels—and by using an effective referral system for the few specialized interventions that meet the essential package criteria—countries may obtain significant health gains at reasonable cost.

Many important issues remain uncertain, especially given the scarcity of LMIC economic evidence. Research in areas likely to produce high public benefit—such as further evaluation of the health gains from taxes on SSBs, agricultural and trade policies to improve fruit and vegetable intake, intersectoral policies to increase physical activity, use of cheaper or faster surveillance techniques, and methods of ensuring a reliable supply of generic medications, including of fixed-dose combination therapy—could be a specific priority in LMICs. New technologies, medications, and delivery platforms on the horizon have the potential to disrupt and shift management paradigms. These issues warrant development of strong priority-setting institutions in LMICs to develop a research agenda and to evaluate new technologies as well as changing disease epidemiology and health system constraints.

Nonetheless, the health benefits of individual medical interventions are clear, and HICs have achieved huge reductions in mortality by making medical treatment widely available. These gains must be extended to LMICs in order for global goals to be achieved. A strong global framework is now in place. Since the 2011 UN high-level meeting on NCDs, a Global Plan of Action for NCD Prevention and Control has been put in place, and the 2015 SDGs have recognized NCDs as a serious threat to development. The *DCP3* essential package provides a pathway to achieving substantial reduction in death, disability, and impoverishment from CVRD in LMICs using evidence-based cost-effective interventions.

ACKNOWLEDGMENTS

The *DCP3* volume 5 author group consists of the following: Alma Adler, Ashkan Afshin, Vamadevan S. Ajay, Mohammed K. Ali, Eric Bateman, Janet Bettger, Robert O. Bonow, Elizabeth Brouwer, Gene Bukhman, Fiona Bull, Peter Burney, Simon Capewell, Juliana Chan, Eeshwar K. Chandrasekar, Jie Chen, Michael H. Criqui, John Dirks, Sagar B. Dugani, Michael Engelgau, Meguid El Nahas, Caroline H. D. Fall, Valery Feigin, F. Gerald R. Fowkes, Amanda Glassman, Shifalika Goenka, Rajeev Gupta, Babar Hasan, Fred Hersch, Frank Hu, Mark D. Huffman, Samer Jabbour, Deborah Jarvis, Panniyammakal Jeemon, Rohina Joshi, Jemima H. Kamano, Andre Pascal Kengne, Preeti Kudesia, R. Krishna Kumar, Kalyanaraman Kumaran, Estelle V. Lambert, Edward S. Lee, Chaoyun Li, Rong Luo, Matthew Magee, Vasanti S. Malik, J. Antonio Marin-Neto, Guy Marks, Bongani Mayosi, Helen McGuire, Renata Micha, J. Jaime Miranda, Pablo Aschner Montoya, Andrew E. Moran, Dariush Mozaffarian, Saraladevi Naicker, Nadraj G. Naidoo, K. M. Venkat Narayan, Irina Nikolic, Martin O'Donnell, Churchill Onen, Clive Osmond, Anushka Patel, Rogelio Perez-Padilla, Neil Poulter, Michael Pratt, Miriam Rabkin, Vikram Rajan, Anis Rassi, Anis Rassi Jr., Ishita Rawal, Giuseppe Remuzzi, Miguel Riella, Greg A. Roth, Ambuj Roy, Adolfo Rubinstein, Yuna Sakuma, Uchechukwu K. A. Sampson, Karen R. Siegel, Karen Sliwa, Marc Suhrcke, Nikhil Tandon, Bernadette Thomas, Claudia Vaca, Rajesh Vedanthan, Stéphane Verguet, Michael Webb, Mary Beth Weber, Laurie Whitsel, Gary Wong, Lijing L. Yan, Clyde W. Yancy, Ping Zhang, Dong Zhao, and Yishan Zhu.

The authors would like to acknowledge Jinyuan Qi for her assistance in preparing the essential package cost estimates, Dean T. Jamison for thoughtful review and guidance, Kristen Danforth for assistance with literature reviews and document preparation, and the World Bank Publisher's office for excellent production support.

ANNEX

The annex to this chapter is as follows. It is available at http://www.dcp-3.org/CVRD.

- Annex 1A. Costing the Essential Package for Cardiovascular, Respiratory, and Related Disorders Notes

NOTE

World Bank Income Classifications as of July 2014 are as follows, based on estimates of gross national income (GNI) per capita for 2013:

- Low-income countries (LICs) = US$1,045 or less
- Middle-income countries (MICs) are subdivided:
  (a) lower-middle-income = US$1,046 to US$4,125
  (b) upper-middle-income (UMICs) = US$4,126 to US$12,745
- High-income countries (HICs) = US$12,746 or more.

REFERENCES

Afshin, A., R. Micha, M. Webb, S. Capewell, L. Whitsel, and others. 2017. "Effectiveness of Dietary Policies to Reduce Noncommunicable Diseases." In *Disease Control Priorities* (third edition): Volume 5, *Cardiovascular, Respiratory, and Related Disorders*, edited by D. Prabhakaran, S. Anand, T. A. Gaziano, J.-C. Mbanya, Y. Wu, and R. Nugent. Washington, DC: World Bank.

Ait-Khaled, N., G. Auregan, N. Bencharif, L. M. Camara, E. Dagli, and others. 2000. "Affordability of Inhaled Corticosteroids as a Potential Barrier to Treatment of Asthma in Some Developing Countries." *International Journal of Tuberculosis and Lung Disease* 4: 268–71.

Ajay, V. S., D. Jindal, A. Roy, V. Venugopal, R. Sharma, and others. 2016. "Development of a Smartphone-Enabled Hypertension and Diabetes Mellitus Management Package to Facilitate Evidence-Based Care Delivery in Primary Healthcare Facilities in India: The mPower Heart Project." *Journal of the American Heart Association* 5.

Ali, M. K., K. R. Siegel, E. Chandrasekar, N. Tandon, P. A. Montoya, and others. 2017. "Diabetes: An Update on the Pandemic and Potential Solutions." In *Disease Control Priorities* (third edition): Volume 5, *Cardiovascular, Respiratory, and Related Disorders*, edited by D. Prabhakaran, S. Anand, T. A. Gaziano, J.-C. Mbanya, Y. Wu, and R. Nugent. Washington, DC: World Bank.

Ali, M. K., K. Singh, D. Kondal, R. Devarajan, S. A. Patel, and others. 2016. "Effectiveness of a Multicomponent Quality Improvement Strategy to Improve Achievement of Diabetes Care Goals: A Randomized, Controlled Trial." *Annals of Internal Medicine* 165 (6): 399–408. doi:10.7326/M15-2807.

Alkire, B., J. Vincent, and J. Meara. 2015. "Benefit-Cost Analysis for Selected Surgical Interventions in Low- and Middle-Income Countries." In *Disease Control Priorities* (third edition): Volume 1, *Essential Surgery*, edited by H. T. Debas, P. Donkor, A. Gawande, D. T. Jamison, M. E. Kruk, and C. Mock. Washington, DC: World Bank.

Anand, S., A. Bitton, and T. A. Gaziano. 2013. "The Gap between Estimated Incidence of End-Stage Renal Disease and Use of Therapy." *PLoS One* 8: e72860.

Axelrod, D. A., M. K. Guidinger, K. P. McCullough, A. B. Leichtman, J. D. Punch, and others. 2004. "Association of Center Volume with Outcome after Liver and Kidney Transplantation." *American Journal of Transplantation* 4: 920–27.

Bilano, V., S. Gilmour, T. Moffiet, E. T. d'Espaignet, G. Stevens, and others. 2015. "Global Trends and Projections for Tobacco Use, 1990–2025: An Analysis of Smoking Indicators from the WHO Comprehensive Information Systems for Tobacco Control." *The Lancet* 385: 966–76.

Braimoh, R. W., M. O. Mabayoje, C. O. Amira, and B. T. Bello. 2014. "Microbial Quality of Hemodialysis Water, A Survey of Six Centers in Lagos, Nigeria." *Hemodialysis International* 18: 148–52.

Britton, J. 2015. "Progress with the Global Tobacco Epidemic." *The Lancet* 385: 924–26.

Brouwer, E. D., D. Watkins, Z. Olson, J. Goett, R. Nugent, and others. 2015. "Provider Costs for Prevention and Treatment of Cardiovascular and Related Conditions in Low- and Middle-Income Countries: A Systematic Review." *BMC Public Health* 15: 1183.

Bull, F., S. Goenka, V. Lambert, and M. Pratt. 2017. "Physical Activity for the Prevention of Cardiometabolic Disease." In *Disease Control Priorities* (third edition): Volume 5, *Cardiovascular, Respiratory, and Related Disorders*, edited by D. Prabhakaran, S. Anand, T. A. Gaziano, J.-C. Mbanya, Y. Wu, and R. Nugent. Washington, DC: World Bank.

Cecchini, M., F. Sassi, J. A. Lauer, Y. Y. Lee, V. Guajardo-Barron, and others. 2010. "Tackling of Unhealthy Diets, Physical Inactivity, and Obesity: Health Effects and Cost-Effectiveness." *The Lancet* 376: 1775–84.

Chao, T. E., K. Sharma, M. Mandigo, L. Hagander, S. Resch, and others. 2014. "Cost-Effectiveness of Surgery and Its Policy Implications for Global Health: A Systematic Review and Analysis." *The Lancet Global Health* 2: e334–45.

Chow, C. K., K. K. Teo, S. Rangarajan, S. Islam, R. Gupta, and others. 2013. "Prevalence, Awareness, Treatment, and Control of Hypertension in Rural and Urban Communities in High-, Middle-, and Low-Income Countries." *Journal of the American Medical Association* 310: 959–68.

Cohen, D., and P. Carter. 2010. "How Small Changes Led to Big Profits for Insulin Manufacturers." *BMJ* 341: c7139.

Colchero, M. A., B. M. Popkin, J. A. Rivera, and S. W. Ng. 2016. "Beverage Purchases from Stores in Mexico under the Excise Tax on Sugar Sweetened Beverages: Observational Study." *BMJ* 352: h6704.

Collins, R., C. Reith, J. Emberson, J. Armitage, C. Baigent, and others. 2016. "Interpretation of the Evidence for the Efficacy and Safety of Statin Therapy." *The Lancet* 388: 2532–61.

Diaz de Leon-Castaneda, C., M. Altagracia-Martinez, J. Kravzov-Jinich, R. Cardenas-Elizalde Mdeland, C. Moreno-Bonett, and others. 2012. "Cost-Effectiveness Study of Oral Hypoglycemic Agents in the Treatment of Outpatients with Type 2 Diabetes Attending a Public Primary Care Clinic in Mexico City." *Journal of ClinicoEconomics and Outcomes Research* 4: 57–65.

Ding, D., K. D. Lawson, T. L. Kolbe-Alexander, E. A. Finkelstein, T. Katzmarzyk, and others. 2016. "The Economic Burden of Physical Inactivity: A Global Analysis of Major Non-Communicable Diseases." *The Lancet* 388: 1311–24.

Falbe, J., H. R. Thompson, C. M. Becker, N. Rojas, C. E. McCulloch, and others. 2016. "Impact of the Berkeley Excise Tax on Sugar-Sweetened Beverage Consumption." *American Journal of Public Health* 106: 1865–71.

Gaede, P., W. J. Valentine, A. J. Palmer, D. M. Tucker, M. Lammert, and others. 2008. "Cost-Effectiveness of Intensified versus Conventional Multifactorial Intervention in Type 2 Diabetes: Results and Projections from the Steno-2 Study." *Diabetes Care* 31: 1510–15.

Gaziano, T. A. 2005. "Cardiovascular Disease in the Developing World and Its Cost-Effective Management." *Circulation* 112: 3547–53.

Gaziano, T. A., S. Abrahams-Gessel, C. A. Denman, C. M. Montano, M. Khanam, and others. 2015. "An Assessment of Community Health Workers' Ability to Screen for Cardiovascular Disease Risk with a Simple, Non-Invasive Risk Assessment Instrument in Bangladesh, Guatemala, Mexico, and South Africa: An Observational Study." *The Lancet Global Health* 3: e556–63.

Gaziano, T. A., S. Abrahams-Gessel, S. Surka, S. Sy, A. Pandya, and others. 2015. "Cardiovascular Disease Screening by Community Health Workers Can Be Cost-Effective in Low-Resource Countries." *Health Affairs* 34: 1538–45.

Gaziano, T. A., and N. Pagidipati. 2013. "Scaling Up Chronic Disease Prevention Interventions in Lower- and Middle-Income Countries." *Annual Review of Public Health* 34: 317–35.

Gaziano, T. A., M. Suhrcke, E. Brouwer, C. Levin, I. Nikolic, and R. Nugent. 2017. "Costs and Cost-Effectiveness of Interventions and Policies to Prevent and Treat Cardiovascular and Respiratory Diseases." In *Disease Control Priorities* (third edition): Volume 5, *Cardiovascular, Respiratory, and Related Disorders*, edited by D. Prabhakaran, S. Anand, T. A. Gaziano, J.-C. Mbanya, Y. Wu, and R. Nugent. Washington, DC: World Bank.

GBD 2015 DALYs and HALE Collaborators. 2016. "Global, Regional, and National Disability-Adjusted Life-Years (DALYs) for 315 Diseases and Injuries and Healthy Life Expectancy (HALE), 1990–2015: A Systematic Analysis for the Global Burden of Disease Study 2015." *The Lancet* 388 (10053): 1603–58.

Grimaldi, A., E. Ammirati, N. Karam, A. C. Vermi, A. de Concilio, and others. 2014. "Cardiac Surgery for Patients with Heart Failure due to Structural Heart Disease in Uganda: Access to Surgery and Outcomes." *Cardiovascular Journal of Africa* 25: 204–11.

Habib, S. H., K. B. Biswas, S. Akter, S. Saha, and L. Ali. 2010. "Cost-Effectiveness Analysis of Medical Intervention in Patients with Early Detection of Diabetic Foot in a Tertiary Care Hospital in Bangladesh." *Journal of Diabetes and Its Complications* 24: 259–64.

Hallal, P. C., L. B. Andersen, F. C. Bull, R. Guthold, W. Haskell, and others. 2012. "Global Physical Activity Levels: Surveillance Progress, Pitfalls, and Prospects." *The Lancet* 380: 247–57.

Heath, G. W., D. C. Parra, O. L. Sarmiento, L. B. Andersen, N. Owen, and others. 2012. "Evidence-Based Intervention in Physical Activity: Lessons from Around the World." *The Lancet* 380: 272–81.

Huffman, M. D., K. D. Rao, A. Pichon-Riviere, D. Zhao, S. Harikrishnan, and others. 2011. "A Cross-Sectional Study of the Microeconomic Impact of Cardiovascular Disease Hospitalization in Four Low- and Middle-Income Countries." *PLoS One* 6: e20821.

IHME (The Institute for Health Metrics and Evaluation). 2013. "GBD Data Tool." IHME, Seattle.

Jafar, T. H., M. Islam, J. Hatcher, S. Hashmi, R. Bux, and others. 2010. "Community Based Lifestyle Intervention for Blood Pressure Reduction in Children and Young Adults in Developing Country: Cluster Randomised Controlled Trial." *BMJ: Overseas and Retired Doctors Edition* 341: 1p.

Jamison, D. T., J. G. Breman, A. R. Measham, G. Alleyne, M. Claeson, D. B. Evans, P. Jha, A. Mills, and P. Musgrove, eds. 2006. *Disease Control Priorities in Developing Countries* (second edition). Washington, DC: World Bank and Oxford University Press.

Jamison, D. T., W. Mosley, A. R. Measham, and J. Bobadilla, eds. 1993. *Disease Control Priorities in Developing Countries* (first edition). New York: Oxford University Press.

Jamison, D. T., L. H. Summers, G. Alleyne, K. J. Arrow, S. Berkley, and others. 2013. "Global Health 2035: A World Converging within a Generation." *The Lancet* 382: 1898–955.

Jaspers, L., V. Colpani, L. Chaker, S. J. van der Lee, T. Muka, and others. 2015. "The Global Impact of Non-Communicable Diseases on Households and Impoverishment: A Systematic Review." *The European Journal of Epidemiology* 30: 163–88.

Jha, P., and R. Peto. 2014. "Global Effects of Smoking, of Quitting, and of Taxing Tobacco." *New England Journal of Medicine* 370: 60–68.

Kankeu, H. T., P. Saksena, K. Xu, and D. B. Evans. 2013. "The Financial Burden from Non-Communicable Diseases in Low- and Middle-Income Countries: A Literature Review." *Health Research Policy and Systems* 11: 31.

Kaplan, W. A., V. J. Wirtz, and P. Stephens. 2013. "The Market Dynamics of Generic Medicines in the Private Sector of 19 Low and Middle Income Countries between 2001 and 2011: A Descriptive Time Series Analysis." *PLoS One* 8: e74399.

Kydland, F. E., R. Mundell, T. Schelling, V. Smith, and J. Bhagwati. 2013. "Expert Panel Ranking." In *Global Problems, Smart Solutions: Costs and Benefits*, edited by B. Lomborg. Cambridge, UK: Cambridge University Press.

Laine, J., V. Kuvaja-Kollner, E. Pietila, M. Koivuneva, H. Valtonen, and others. 2014. "Cost-Effectiveness of Population-Level Physical Activity Interventions: A Systematic Review." *American Journal of Health Promotion* 29: 71–80.

Legetic, B., A. Medici, A. Hernández-Avila, G. Alleyne, and A. Hennis, eds. 2016. *Economic Dimensions of Noncommunicable Diseases in Latin America and the Caribbean*. Washington, DC: Pan American Health Organization.

Liyanage, T., T. Ninomiya, V. Jha, B. Neal, M. P. Halle, and others. 2015. "Worldwide Access to Treatment for End-Stage

Kidney Disease: A Systematic Review." *The Lancet* 385: 1975–82.

Lonn, E., and S. Yusuf. 2009. "Polypill: The Evidence and the Promise." *Current Opinion in Lipidology* 20: 453–59.

Malik, V., and F. Hu. 2017. "Weight Management." In *Disease Control Priorities* (third edition): Volume 5, *Cardiovascular, Respiratory, and Related Disorders*, edited by D. Prabhakaran, S. Anand, T. A. Gaziano, J.-C. Mbanya, Y. Wu, and R. Nugent. Washington, DC: World Bank.

Manson, J. E., W. C. Willett, M. J. Stampfer, G. A. Colditz, D. J. Hunter, and others. 1995. "Body Weight and Mortality among Women." *New England Journal of Medicine* 333: 677–85.

Medina-Pestana, J. O. 2006. "Organization of a High-Volume Kidney Transplant Program—The 'Assembly Line' Approach." *Transplantation* 81: 1510–20.

Meng, L., H. Xu, A. Liu, J. van Raaija, W. Bemelmans, and others. 2013. "The Costs and Cost-Effectiveness of a School-Based Comprehensive Intervention Study on Childhood Obesity in China." *PLoS One* 8: e77971.

Nakhimovsky, S. S., A. B. Feigl, C. Avila, G. O'Sullivan, E. Macgregor-Skinner, and others. 2016. "Taxes on Sugar-Sweetened Beverages to Reduce Overweight and Obesity in Middle-Income Countries: A Systematic Review." *PLoS One* 11: e0163358.

Niens, L. M., A. Cameron, E. Van de Poel, M. Ewen, W. B. F. Brouwer, and others. 2010. "Quantifying the Impoverishing Effects of Purchasing Medicines: A Cross-Country Comparison of the Affordability of Medicines in the Developing World." *PLoS Medicine* 7.

Nugent, R., B. B. Kelly, and J. Narula. 2012. "An Evolving Approach to the Global Health Agenda: Countries Will Lead the Way on NCD Prevention and Control." *Global Heart* 7: 3–6.

Pauwels, R. A., S. Pedersen, W. W. Busse, W. C. Tan, Y. Z. Chen, and others. 2003. "Early Intervention with Budesonide in Mild Persistent Asthma: A Randomised, Double-Blind Trial." *The Lancet* 361: 1071–76.

Praditpornsilpa, K., S. Lekhyananda, N. Premasathian, P. Kingwatanakul, A. Lumpaopong, and others. 2011. "Prevalence Trend of Renal Replacement Therapy in Thailand: Impact of Health Economics Policy." *Journal of the Medical Association of Thailand* 94 Suppl 4: S1–6.

Prinja, S., A. Nandi, S. Horton, C. Levin, and R. Laxminarayan. 2015. "Costs, Effectiveness, and Cost-Effectiveness of Selected Surgical Procedures and Platforms: A Summary." In *Disease Control Priorities* (third edition): Volume 1, *Essential Surgery*, edited by H. T. Debas, P. Donkor, A. Gawande, D. T. Jamison, M. E. Kruk, and C. N. Mock. Washington, DC: World Bank.

Rachapelle, S., R. Legood, Y. Alavi, R. Lindfield, T. Sharma, and others. 2013. "The Cost-Utility of Telemedicine to Screen for Diabetic Retinopathy in India." *Ophthalmology* 120: 566–73.

Reddy, N. S., M. Kappanayil, R. Balachandran, K. J. Jenkins, A. Sudhakar, and others. 2015. "Preoperative Determinants of Outcomes of Infant Heart Surgery in a Limited-Resource Setting." *Seminars in Thoracic and Cardiovascular Surgery* 27: 331–38.

Restrepo, B. J., and M. Rieger. 2016. "Denmark's Policy on Artificial Trans Fat and Cardiovascular Disease." *American Journal of Preventive Medicine* 50: 69–76.

Ribeiro, R. A., S. F. Stella, L. I. Zimerman, M. Pimentel, L. E. Rohde, and others. 2010. "Cost-Effectiveness of Implantable Cardioverter Defibrillators in Brazil in the Public and Private Sectors." *Arquivos Brasileiros de Cardiologia* 95: 577–86.

Roth, G. A., M. H. Forouzanfar, A. E. Moran, R. Barber, G. Nguyen, and others. 2015. "Demographic and Epidemiologic Drivers of Global Cardiovascular Mortality." *New England Journal of Medicine* 372: 1333–41.

Sakuma, Y., A. Glassman, and C. Vaca. 2017. "Priority-Setting Processes for Expensive Treatments for Chronic Diseases." In *Disease Control Priorities* (third edition): Volume 5, *Cardiovascular, Respiratory, and Related Disorders*, edited by D. Prabhakaran, S. Anand, T. A. Gaziano, J.-C. Mbanya, Y. Wu, and R. Nugent. Washington, DC: World Bank.

Shibuya, K., C. Ciecierski, E. Guindon, D. W. Bettcher, D. B. Evans, and others. 2003. "WHO Framework Convention on Tobacco Control: Development of an Evidence Based Global Public Health Treaty." *BMJ* 327: 154–57.

Shroufi, A., R. Chowdhury, R. Anchala, S. Stevens, P. Blanco, and others. 2013. "Cost Effective Interventions for the Prevention of Cardiovascular Disease in Low and Middle Income Countries: A Systematic Review." *BMC Public Health* 13:285.

Sposato, L. A., and G. Saposnik. 2012. "Gross Domestic Product and Health Expenditure Associated with Incidence, 30-Day Fatality, and Age at Stroke Onset: A Systematic Review." *Stroke* 43: 170–77.

Sritipsukho, P., A. Riewpaiboon, P. Chaiyawat, and K. Kulkantrakorn. 2010. "Cost-Effectiveness Analysis of Home Rehabilitation Programs for Thai Stroke Patients." *Journal of the Medical Association of Thailand* 93 Suppl 7: S262–70.

Suhrcke, M., T. A. Boluarte, and L. Niessen. 2012. "A Systematic Review of Economic Evaluations of Interventions to Tackle Cardiovascular Disease in Low- and Middle-Income Countries." *BMC Public Health* 12: 2.

Tantivess, S., P. Werayingyong, P. Chuengsaman, and Y. Teerawattananon. 2013. "Universal Coverage of Renal Dialysis in Thailand: Promise, Progress, and Prospects." *BMJ* 346: f462.

Teerawattananon, Y., M. Mugford, and V. Tangcharoensathien. 2007. "Economic Evaluation of Palliative Management versus Peritoneal Dialysis and Hemodialysis for End-Stage Renal Disease: Evidence for Coverage Decisions in Thailand." *Value in Health* 10: 61–72.

United Nations. 2011. *High-Level Meeting on Non-Communicable Diseases*. New York: United Nations.

———. 2015. *Sustainable Development Goals*. New York: United Nations.

van den Hoogen, P. C., E. J. Feskens, N. J. Nagelkerke, A. Menotti, A. Nissinen, and others. 2000. "The Relation between Blood Pressure and Mortality due to Coronary Heart Disease among Men in Different Parts of the World. Seven Countries Study Research Group." *New England Journal of Medicine* 342: 1–8.

Verguet, S., C. L. Gauvreau, S. Mishra, M. MacLennan, S. M. Murphy, and others. 2015. "The Consequences of Tobacco Tax on Household Health and Finances in Rich and Poor Smokers in China: An Extended Cost-Effectiveness Analysis." *The Lancet Global Health* 3: e206–16.

Verguet, S., R. Laxminarayan, and D. T. Jamison. 2015. "Universal Public Finance of Tuberculosis Treatment in India: An Extended Cost-Effectiveness Analysis." *Health Economics* 24 (3): 318–32. doi:10.1002/hec.3019.

Verguet, S., Z. D. Olson, J. B. Babigumira, D. Desalegn, K. A. Johansson, and others. 2015. "Health Gains and Financial Risk Protection Afforded by Public Financing of Selected Interventions in Ethiopia: An Extended Cost-Effectiveness Analysis." *The Lancet Global Health* 3: e288–96.

Watkins, D. A., R. A. Nugent, and S. Verguet. 2017. "Extended Cost-Effectiveness Analyses of Cardiovascular Risk Factor Reduction Policies." In *Disease Control Priorities* (third edition): Volume 5, *Cardiovascular, Respiratory, and Related Disorders*, edited by D. Prabhakaran, S. Anand, T. A. Gaziano, J.-C. Mbanya, Y. Wu, and R. Nugent. Washington, DC: World Bank.

Watkins, D. A., Z. D. Olson, S. Verguet, R. A. Nugent, and D. T. Jamison. 2016. "Cardiovascular Disease and Impoverishment Averted due to a Salt Reduction Policy in South Africa: An Extended Cost-Effectiveness Analysis." *Health Policy and Planning* 31: 75–82.

Webster, J. L., E. K. Dunford, C. Hawkes, and B. C. Neal. 2011. "Salt Reduction Initiatives around the World." *Journal of Hypertension* 29: 1043–50.

WHO (World Health Organization). 2010a. *Monitoring the Building Blocks of Health Systems: A Handbook of Indicators and Their Measurement Strategies*. Geneva: WHO.

———. 2010b. *WHO Technical Manual on Tobacco Tax Administration*. Geneva: WHO.

———. 2011a. *From Burden to "Best Buys": Reducing the Economic Impact of Non-Communicable Diseases in Low- and Middle-Income Countries*. Geneva: WHO.

———. 2011b. *Global Health and Ageing*. Geneva: WHO.

———. 2012. *Global Health Observatory (GHO) Data*. Geneva: WHO.

———. 2013. *Global Action Plan for the Prevention and Control of Noncommunicable Diseases*. Geneva: WHO.

———. 2016. "Estimates for 2000-2015: Cause-Specific Mortality." WHO, Geneva. http://www.who.int/healthinfo/global_burden_disease/estimates/en/index1.html.

World Bank. 1993. *World Development Report 1993: Investing in Health*. New York: Oxford University Press.

Wright, Jr., J. T., J. D. Williamson, P. K. Whelton, J. K. Snyder, K. M. Sink, and others. 2015. "A Randomized Trial of Intensive versus Standard Blood-Pressure Control." *New England Journal of Medicine* 373: 2103–16.

Yusuf, S., S. Hawken, S. Ounpuu, T. Dans, A. Avezum, and others. 2004. "Effect of Potentially Modifiable Risk Factors Associated with Myocardial Infarction in 52 Countries (The INTERHEART Study): Case-Control Study." *The Lancet* 364: 937–52.

Yusuf, S., S. Islam, C. K. Chow, S. Rangarajan, G. Dagenais, and others. 2011. "Use of Secondary Prevention Drugs for Cardiovascular Disease in the Community in High-Income, Middle-Income, and Low-Income Countries (The PURE Study): A Prospective Epidemiological Survey." *The Lancet* 378: 1231–43.

Yusuf, S., S. Rangarajan, K. Teo, S. Islam, W. Li, and others. 2014. "Cardiovascular Risk and Events in 17 Low-, Middle-, and High-Income Countries." *New England Journal of Medicine* 371: 818–27.

Chapter 2

Relationships among Major Risk Factors and the Burden of Cardiovascular Diseases, Diabetes, and Chronic Lung Disease

Vamadevan S. Ajay, David A. Watkins, and Dorairaj Prabhakaran

INTRODUCTION

Cardiovascular, respiratory, and related disorders (CVRDs) are a subset of noncommunicable diseases (NCDs) that are an important and increasing cause of morbidity and mortality in low- and middle-income countries (LMICs). CVRDs share common risk factors such as smoking, poor diet, and physical inactivity. They also share common interventions at the clinical, public health, and policy levels. Public health professionals and decision makers share a widespread notion that CVRDs are diseases of the affluent (WHO 2010b). Yet recent cross-national studies have demonstrated that the burden of CVRDs falls disproportionately on lower-income countries and disadvantaged groups within countries. Prevention and control of CVRDs, then, have important equity implications. Addressing CVRDs also fits in with the Sustainable Development Goals that focus on reducing poverty and improving health, particularly through mechanisms (such as universal health coverage) that can address the rise in CVRD risk factors and the potential impoverishing effects of chronic illness.

The concept that current or past exposure to specific factors increases the risk of future ischemic heart disease (IHD) was first established in the Framingham Heart study in the United States (Kannel and others 1961), but it has been validated extensively in LMICs (O'Donnell and others 2010; Yusuf and others 2004). These risk factors are now well established globally, not only for IHD (Pearson and others 2003; Perk and others 2013; Yusuf and others 2001; Yusuf and others 2004), but also for stroke (Colditz and others 1988; Markus 2011; O'Donnell and others 2010), other cardiovascular diseases (CVDs) (Greenland and others 2010; Khatibzadeh and others 2013; Mosca and others 2004; Smith and others 2011), diabetes (Caballero 2003; Singh and others 2010; Weber and others 2012; Zimmet and others 1999), chronic lung disease (Madison, Zelman, and Mittman 1980; Palta and others 1991; Salvi and Barnes 2009; Strope and Stempel 1984), and other chronic NCDs (Allender and others 2011; Ezzati and Riboli 2013; Hallal and others 2012). Exposure to these risk factors may occur early in life, including in utero, and continue throughout life or may be limited to only certain phases of the life span. These risk factors may be strongly influenced by socioeconomic and environmental determinants, policy and legislative interventions, lifestyle and behavioral choices, and familial and genetic predisposition. Among modifiable risk factors, reducing the level of individual or population

Corresponding author: Dorairaj Prabhakaran, Centre for Chronic Disease Control, New Delhi; and Centre for Control of Chronic Conditions, Public Health Foundation of India, Haryana, India; dprabhakaran@ccdcindia.org.

risk or discontinuing the exposure leads to corresponding reductions in the magnitude of disease burden and preventable deaths. In-depth knowledge of these relationships as well as the distribution of risk factors in the population provides a sound basis for developing prevention strategies at the individual and population levels.

This chapter describes recent trends in mortality and morbidity from CVRDs in LMICs and the specific conditions (including IHD, structural heart disease, heart failure, stroke, peripheral arterial disease, diabetes, kidney disease, and chronic lung disease) and risk factors covered in this volume. It then reviews the evidence regarding the complex interrelationships between specific risk factors, their early- and late-life determinants, and their corresponding influence on CVRD risk later in life. Finally, it presents steps for addressing CVRD risk factors and for reducing preventable deaths within a socioecological framework.

TRENDS IN CVRD MORTALITY AND MORBIDITY

Of the 55.9 million deaths globally in 2012, 37.9 million were from NCDs, including 23.9 million deaths from CVRDs. A plurality of deaths (17.5 million) were from CVDs, with respiratory diseases (4.0 million) being the second-most frequent cause of death; diabetes mellitus and kidney diseases followed, with 1.5 million and 864,000 deaths, respectively. NCDs not covered in this volume—including mental and neurological disorders

and cancers—constituted 37 percent of total NCD deaths. Table 2.1 presents total deaths by cause and country income group.

Because of a convergence of population size and the epidemiological transition, the vast majority of CVRD deaths occur in LMICs, including 74 percent of cardiovascular deaths, 83 percent of diabetes deaths, 84 percent of respiratory disease deaths, and 76 percent of kidney disease deaths. Figure 2.1 illustrates the proportion of total deaths caused by each group: in low-income countries, 21 percent of deaths were from CVRDs, compared with 30 percent and 54 percent of deaths, respectively, in lower-middle-income and upper-middle-income countries.

Most CVRD deaths occur in LMICs because of disparities in age-specific mortality rates and demographic changes. First, age-specific mortality rates from CVRDs are substantially higher in LMICs than in high-income countries (HICs) (figure 2.2). Although the prevalence of various risk factors is generally lower in LMICs (particularly in low-income countries), case fatality rates are much higher, probably because of the low use of evidence-based prevention and treatment interventions (Yusuf and others 2011; Yusuf and others 2014).

Second, rapid demographic changes are driving the overall increase in observed deaths. Between 2000 and 2012, the total population increased 8 percent in HICs and 17 percent in LMICs. The adult population grew even faster (14 percent and 32 percent, respectively). These trends are probably being driven by persistently high fertility rates in many LMICs as well as lower under-five mortality rates, which together contribute to

Table 2.1 CVRD Deaths, by Cause and Country Income Group, for All Ages and Both Genders, 2012
Thousands, unless otherwise noted

Indicator	Low-income	Lower-middle-income	Upper-middle-income	High-income	World (total)
Population	850,000	2,510,000	2,430,000	1,290,000	7,060,000
Total deaths	7,450	19,900	16,900	11,700	55,900
CVRD deaths	1,540	7,780	9,080	5,530	23,900
CVRD deaths as a percentage of total deaths	21	39	54	47	43
CVRD deaths by cause					
Cardiovascular diseases	999	5,220	6,860	4,440	17,500
Diabetes mellitus	135	549	559	254	1,497
Respiratory diseases	309	1,630	1,460	645	4,040
Kidney diseases	99	378	197	190	864

Source: WHO 2014.
Note: CVRD = cardiovascular, respiratory, and related disorder.

overall population growth and aging. In 1960 less than 5 percent of the global population was older than age 65 years, and 15 percent was younger than age 5 years. By 2015, these proportions had converged and were projected to reverse by 2040. The result of this demographic change is that a larger total number of persons in LMICs are living to older ages and are more exposed to CVRD risk determinants and CVRDs themselves (WHO and U.S. National Institute on Aging 2011).

Age-standardized mortality rates are a useful metric for disentangling epidemiological and demographic changes in CVRD mortality. We calculated age-standardized mortality rates for CVRDs using the 2012 global population structure as a reference for region-specific rates in 2000 and 2012. For CVDs, deaths are rising in all regions because of demographic changes; however, age-standardized mortality rates are declining in HICs much faster than in LMICs, probably because of reductions in risk factors and a decline in case fatality rates (table 2.2).

Age-standardized mortality rates in LMICs are rising for diabetes but declining for respiratory and kidney diseases. The substantial decline in respiratory disease rates is probably related to progress in reducing household air pollution, although this reduction has been offset somewhat by the rise in outdoor air pollution, a subject discussed in volume 7 of *DCP3* (Watkins, Dabestani, and others 2017).

CVDs—the predominant cause of CVRD mortality—demonstrate marked and increasingly disparate trends in age-standardized mortality rates. Rates in high- and low-income countries were similar in 2000, but much more rapid progress had been made in HICs by 2012. Lower-middle-income and upper-middle-income countries had higher rates than HICs in 2000, and their rates have continued to decline modestly, as they have in low-income countries (figure 2.3). Again, this growing inequality in cardiovascular health requires further exploration but, in general, reflects rapid epidemiological change in LMICs and the absence of a health system response to address cardiovascular mortality. Unfortunately, if current trends continue, LMICs are unlikely to meet the Sustainable Development Goal target of achieving a one-third reduction in premature mortality from NCDs.[1]

Finally, the summary metric of disability-adjusted life-years (DALYs) provides insight into the relative impact of CVRD morbidity and mortality. Generally, premature mortality (years of life lost) is the major contributor to total DALYs from CVRDs, but morbidity (years lived with disability) is a particularly important aspect of diabetes and respiratory and kidney diseases. CVDs are responsible for 74 percent of deaths, but

Figure 2.1 Proportion of Total Deaths Caused by Cardiovascular, Respiratory, and Related Disorders and Other Noncommunicable Diseases, by Country Income Group, for All Ages and Both Genders, 2012

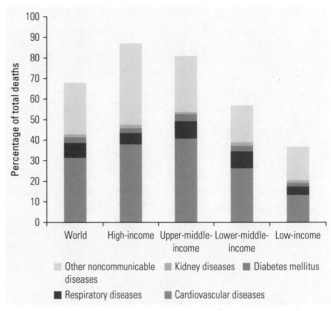

Source: WHO 2014.

Figure 2.2 Age-Specific Mortality Rates from Cardiovascular, Respiratory, and Related Disorders, by Country Income Group, for Both Genders, 2012

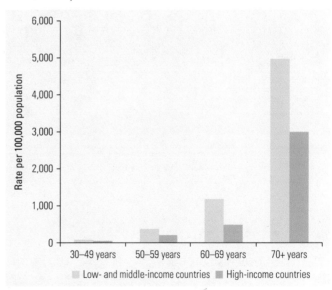

Source: WHO 2014.

only 64 percent of DALYs. Diabetes is responsible for 6 percent of deaths, but 10 percent of DALYs; respiratory diseases are responsible for 17 percent of deaths, but 22 percent of DALYs; and kidney diseases are responsible for 4 percent of deaths, but 5 percent of DALYs.

Table 2.2 Percentage Changes in Total Deaths and Age-Standardized Mortality Rates from Cardiovascular, Respiratory, and Related Disorders, by Country Income Group, for Both Genders, 2000–12

Percentage change

Cause of death	Percentage Change in Total Deaths		Percentage Change in Age-Standardized Mortality Rates	
	Low- and middle-income	High-income	Low- and middle-income	High-income
Cardiovascular diseases	30	–8	–6	–27
Diabetes mellitus	54	7	11	–15
Respiratory diseases	1	15	–28	–10
Kidney diseases	21	41	–9	9

Source: WHO 2014.

Figure 2.3 Age-Standardized Mortality Rates from Cardiovascular Disease, by Country Income Group, for Both Genders, 2000–12

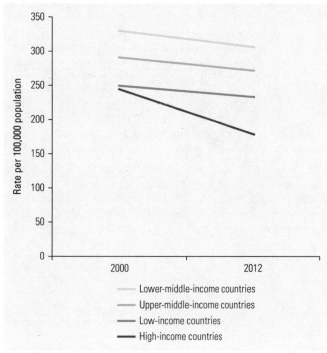

Source: WHO 2014.

SPECIFIC CVRDS

Ischemic Heart Disease

IHD is caused by gradual narrowing of the blood vessels that supply the heart muscles as a result of the buildup of fatty plaques. This narrowing reduces the supply of blood and starves the heart muscles of oxygen, culminating in heart attack. The underlying causes of IHD are predominantly of lifestyle origin, including tobacco use, unhealthy diet, low consumption of fruits and green leafy vegetables, physical inactivity, and harmful use of alcohol.

IHD is a leading cause of death and disability worldwide, accounting for 13 percent of all deaths in 2012. IHD rates vary across populations. The onset of IHD is found to be at least a decade earlier among South Asian populations than among Western populations (McKeigue and others 1993). IHD-related mortality rates are also higher among South Asians. Indeed, in the past few years, IHD rates have been declining in many HICs but rising in LMICs as result of increasing longevity, urbanization, and lifestyle changes.

Stroke

Stroke continues to be a leading cause of death in Africa and major parts of South-East Asia. The causative reasons for stroke in these regions include ethnicity as well as the high prevalence of hypertension among Africans and the high consumption of salt (a precursor of hypertension) among South-East Asians. Stroke can be fatal, but it is more frequently debilitating and has been described as worse than death in some communities. However, stroke is eminently preventable: the single most important modifiable factor for preventing stroke is hypertension. A third of stroke events are attributable to hypertension alone, and hypertension is the entry point for all stroke prevention interventions.

Other Cardiovascular Diseases

Peripheral vascular disease is an important cause of morbidity that shares many risk factors and treatments with IHD and stroke. Hypertensive heart disease, which leads to heart failure without overt ischemia, is particularly relevant in African countries early in the epidemiological transition. Congenital heart disease affects about 1 percent of the world's population, and its frequency is similar in LMICs. It is discussed along with two other structural heart diseases that are endemic in LMICs (rheumatic heart disease and Chagas disease) in chapter 11 of this volume (Watkins, Hasan, and others 2017). Although all of these conditions are relatively neglected compared with IHD and stroke, they accounted for 18 percent of all cardiovascular deaths in LMICs in 2012 (figure 2.4).

Diabetes

Diabetes and metabolic syndrome have emerged as a major problem in many parts of the world, especially LMICs. China and India are home to a large number of people with diabetes. These two countries have an estimated 69 million and 109 million diabetics, respectively, numbers that are projected to increase to 123 million and 150 million, respectively, by 2040 (IDF 2015). Diabetes, in the long term, results in both microvascular and macrovascular complications. Microvascular complications include retinopathy, nephropathy, and neuropathy, and are highly disabling. Macrovascular complications include IHD, ischemic stroke, and amputations as a result of foot infections. Many individuals with diabetes die from IHD or stroke, with the cause of death often being registered as IHD or stroke, not diabetes; therefore, existing estimates likely underestimate the true impact of diabetes on population health.

Chronic Obstructive Pulmonary Disease

Chronic obstructive pulmonary disease (COPD) is a leading cause of morbidity and mortality worldwide. Tobacco smoking is established as a major risk factor, but emerging evidence suggests that other risk factors are also important, especially in LMICs. An estimated 25 percent to 45 percent of patients with COPD have never smoked, so the burden of nonsmoking COPD is much higher than previously believed. Half of the world's population—about 3 billion people—are exposed to smoke from biomass fuel, compared with 1.01 billion people who smoke tobacco, suggesting that exposure to biomass smoke might be the biggest risk factor for COPD globally. At the same time, age-standardized mortality rates from air pollution are declining in areas where indoor biomass fuels are being replaced with cleaner fuels. Other factors associated with COPD are occupational exposure to dusts and gases, history of pulmonary tuberculosis, chronic asthma, respiratory tract infections during childhood, outdoor air pollution, and poor socioeconomic status.

Asthma

Asthma, a disease of the airways, occurs in people of all ages. Globally, 334 million people have asthma, and the

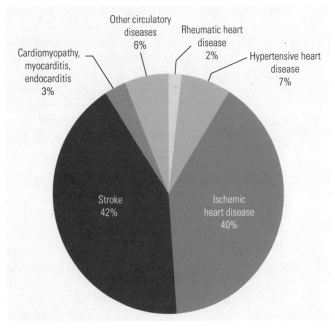

Figure 2.4 Specific Causes of Cardiovascular Death in Low- and Middle-Income Countries, 2012

Source: WHO 2014.

burden of disability is as high as 222 million DALYs; the most affected people are in LMICs (Global Asthma Network 2014; Institute of Health Metrics and Evaluation 2013). Asthma burden is found to have an age-specific gradient. Children ages 10–14 years and elderly persons ages 75–79 years have higher rates of asthma (Global Asthma Network 2014). Asthma symptoms became more common in children in many LMICs between 1993 and 2003; globally, 14 percent of children experience asthma symptoms (Global Asthma Network 2014). Factors responsible for increasing asthma rates are not fully understood, but environmental and lifestyle changes play the key roles.

RELATIONSHIPS BETWEEN RISK EXPOSURE AND DISEASE BURDEN

Nonmodifiable Risk Factors

Risk factors for CVD, diabetes, chronic lung disease, and other chronic NCDs are considered nonmodifiable if their values, once established at birth, cannot be modified. Examples of these nonmodifiable risk factors include age, gender, race, ethnicity, birthweight, prematurity at the time of birth, family medical history, and genetic makeup. Although their actual values cannot be changed, their physiological implications and overall impact on morbidity and mortality can be modified, especially when knowledge of these risk factors appropriately informs strategies for screening for, evaluating, preventing, treating, and controlling NCDs and their modifiable risk factors.

In addition to their individual roles as nonmodifiable risk factors, they have important interactions. Notable examples are the interactions between age, gender, and race or between genes and the environment. These interactions could be taken into account in the prevention and control of disease and risk factors (Ahmad and others 2013; Giolo and others 2010; Hui and others 2013; Lin and others 2009; Schumacher, Hunt, and Williams 1990).

Age is the most important nonmodifiable risk factor for CVRDs. Advancing age is the most powerful independent predictor of death and disability because it effectively integrates the cumulative impact of all modifiable and nonmodifiable risk factor exposures over time. Advancing age is a key factor in the global rise in CVRD mortality (Lozano and others 2012). As a result, interventions designed to address modifiable risk factors early in life and through youth and middle age have the greatest potential to reduce preventable death and disability from CVRDs (WHO 2005). Nonetheless, effective primary and secondary prevention and control of modifiable risk factors in older adults remain important, because these risk factors can still be modified as individuals age, resulting in moderate to large reductions in mortality.

CVDs, diabetes, and chronic lung disease are just as important in women as they are in men. However, at equivalent chronological ages, IHD is two to five times more common in men than in women, depending on the population studied (Jousilahti and others 1999). This gender difference in IHD is particularly prominent before the fifth decade of life; however, the difference reverses and IHD becomes more prominent in women in later decades. More than half of the observed gender-related difference in susceptibility to IHD can be explained by gender-related differences in measured risk factors (Jousilahti and others 1999).

Modifiable Risk Factors

The INTERHEART study showed that high blood pressure, smoking, abnormal lipids, diabetes, abdominal obesity, psychosocial factors, low consumption of fruits and vegetables, physical inactivity, and harmful use of alcohol account for most of the risk of IHD worldwide in both men and women at all ages and in all regions (Yusuf and others 2004). Similarly, the INTERSTROKE study demonstrated that 10 risk factors are associated with 90 percent of the risk of stroke and that targeted interventions that reduce blood pressure and smoking and promote physical activity and a healthy diet could substantially reduce the burden of stroke (O'Donnell and others 2010). Many studies have replicated these findings, and these risk factors are now routinely measured in cardiovascular epidemiology and are tracked in comparative risk assessments conducted for burden of disease studies (GBD 2013 Risk Factors Collaborators 2015).

The prevalence of modifiable risk factors for CVRDs is increasing in many LMICs, particularly middle-income countries, as Western dietary and lifestyle patterns become global dietary and lifestyle patterns (table 2.3).

Tobacco Use

Tobacco use is an important modifiable risk factor for NCD and total mortality. Tobacco use accounted for more than 6.1 million deaths worldwide in 2013 (GBD 2013 Risk Factors Collaborators 2015). This estimate includes exposure to passive smoking (secondhand smoke), which increases the risk of development and progression of atherosclerosis (Law, Morris, and Wald 1997). Cigarettes are the most common smoked form of tobacco, although several other forms are in use. Bidis, small hand-rolled cigarettes widely used in South Asian countries, have levels of nicotine equal to or higher than those in traditional cigarettes and are associated with higher risk for CVRD and cancers (Gupta and Asma 2008). Nearly 80 percent of the world's 1 billion smokers live in LMICs, and that number is projected to rise during the next decade if trends continue (Bilano and others 2015). Most smokers in LMICs are male, which is in contrast to HICs. Tobacco smokers have 2–3 times higher relative risk of IHD, 1.5 times higher risk of stroke, 1.4 times higher risk of COPD, and 12 times higher risk of lung cancer. These risks have an age gradient, with higher relative risk (5–6 times) in younger age groups, although they are similar for men and women (Parish and others 1995; Peto and others 1994). Most of these risks decline within 10 years of quitting smoking (Rosenberg and others 1985). Furthermore, tobacco smoke interacts with other risk factors, and chewable forms of tobacco are as dangerous as cigarettes, causing a range of cancers.

Dyslipidemia (Abnormal Pattern of Blood Fat Level)

Cholesterol in excess, particularly bad cholesterol (low-density lipoprotein), increases the risk of heart disease, stroke, and other vascular diseases. Cholesterol is the key component in the development of atherosclerosis (accumulation of fatty deposits on the inner lining of arteries). The prevalence of high cholesterol among adults in LMICs ranges from 24.3 percent in low-income countries to 45.6 percent in upper-middle-income countries (table 2.3). High cholesterol is estimated to cause 2.6 million deaths and 30 million DALYs annually.

Table 2.3 Prevalence of Selected Cardiovascular, Respiratory, and Related Disorders Risk Factors, by Country Income Group, Various Years

Percent

Indicator	Low-income	Lower-middle-income	Upper-middle-income	High-income
Current tobacco use, males ages 15+ years (2012)	30.5	32.4	42.7	32.8
Current tobacco use, females ages 15+ years (2012)	3.1	2.9	5.2	17.8
Insufficient physical activity, ages 11–17 years (2010)	84.5	77.9	84.4	79.7
Insufficient physical activity, ages 18+ years (2010)	16.6	16.8	25.4	32.7
Overweight (BMI 25 or higher), ages 18+ years (2014)	21.0	27.4	42.7	56.4
Obese (BMI 30 or higher), ages 18+ years (2014)	4.7	7.6	13.0	23.2
High blood pressure (140/90 mmHg or higher), ages 18+ years (2014)	27.6	25.2	20.3	18.5
High blood cholesterol (5.0 mmol/L or higher), ages 25+ years (2008)	24.3	32.4	45.6	58.5
High fasting blood glucose (7.0 mmol/L or higher or on medication), ages 18+ years (2014)	7.4	8.9	9.3	7.0

Source: WHO, various years.

Note: BMI = body mass index; mmHg = millimeters of mercury, a measure of pressure; mmol/L = millimoles per liter. All prevalence ratios are crude estimates except for high fasting blood glucose, which is age-standardized. The most recent estimates are provided, with year of measurement in parentheses.

High Blood Pressure

Globally, high blood pressure (hypertension) is implicated in about 7.5 million deaths (about 13 percent of all deaths) and 57 million DALYs (WHO 2010b). High blood pressure is often without symptoms, silently damaging the arteries that supply blood to the heart, brain, kidneys, and elsewhere and producing a variety of structural changes. High blood pressure increases the risk of stroke, heart attack, kidney failure, and congestive heart failure. When high blood pressure exists with obesity, smoking, high blood cholesterol, or diabetes, the risk of IHD and stroke increases several fold. The relationship of blood pressure to coronary heart disease is linear, positive, and graded, with no discernible lower threshold. Each difference of 20 millimeters of mercury (mmHg, a measure of pressure) in systolic blood pressure is associated with a twofold increase in the relative risk of coronary heart disease, while a 5 mmHg reduction in systolic blood pressure in the population is associated with a 14 percent overall reduction in mortality attributable to stroke, a 9 percent reduction in mortality attributable to coronary heart disease, and a 7 percent decrease in all-cause mortality (Chobanian and others 2003). The prevalence of hypertension among adults in LMICs ranges from 20.3 percent in upper-middle-income countries to 27.6 percent in low-income countries (table 2.3).

Obesity and Overweight

In 2014, more than 1.9 billion adults were estimated to be overweight; of these, more than 600 million were obese (WHO 2016a). The prevalence of overweight and obesity among adults ranges from 21.0 and 4.7 percent, respectively, in low-income countries to 42.7 and 13.0 percent, respectively, in upper-middle-income countries (table 2.3). Obesity is often defined as the accumulation of abnormal or excessive fat in adipose tissue to the extent that health may be impaired (WHO 2000b). People who develop excess body fat, especially at the waist, are more likely to develop heart disease and stroke even if they have no other risk factors. This condition is termed *abdominal obesity* or *central obesity*. The presence of abdominal obesity along with high glucose and high blood pressure and low levels of good cholesterol (high-density lipoprotein) leads to an insulin-resistant state called metabolic syndrome. There is strong evidence that weight loss in overweight and obese individuals reduces the risk of diabetes and CVD. Weight loss lowers blood pressure in overweight individuals with and without hypertension (Appel and others 2006), reduces serum triglycerides, and increases high-density lipoprotein (Miller and others 2011). More important, reductions in blood pressure occur even before attaining a desirable body weight (Appel and others 2006).

Physical Inactivity

According to the World Health Organization, globally, one in four adults is not active enough, and the problem of insufficient physical activity increases as country income rises (WHO 2016b). A concerning counter to this trend is the recent rise in insufficient physical activity among adolescents (table 2.3), a problem that is just as large in low-income countries as in HICs (WHO 2016b). An inactive lifestyle is a risk factor for later overweight and obesity and all of the attendant health consequences. Regular, moderate-to-vigorous physical activity helps prevent CVD over the long term. Specifically, exercise can help control blood pressure, cholesterol, and diabetes as well as lead to weight loss. Even among persons who cannot achieve a normal weight, regular exercise can decrease the number and dosages of drugs to treat these other risk factors, thereby reducing costs and the risk of side effects.

Alcohol

The relationship of alcohol to overall mortality and cardiovascular mortality is thought to be J-shaped. A consistent cardio-protective effect has been observed for moderate consumption of one to two standard drinks per day, but heavy drinkers (including binge drinkers) have higher total mortality than moderate drinkers or abstainers (Srinath Reddy and Katan 2004). Moderate alcohol consumption has also been associated with a lower risk of ischemic stroke in men and women, with exceptions in populations such as South Asians (Sacco and others 1999). In contrast, long-term heavy alcohol consumption increases an individual's risk for all subtypes of stroke (O'Donnell and others 2010). The possible beneficial effects of moderate alcohol consumption must be weighed against the deleterious effects of high intake, including increased risk of hypertension, alcoholic cardiomyopathy, atrial arrhythmias, and hemorrhagic stroke (Klatsky 2015). Alcohol consumption in excess of three drinks per day is associated with a rise in blood pressure and plasma triglyceride levels. Many international guidelines recommend reducing or stopping alcohol consumption for nonpharmacologic therapy of hypertension (Srinath Reddy and Katan 2004).

SOCIAL AND ECOLOGICAL DETERMINANTS OF RISK

During the second half of the twentieth century, health indicators improved in almost all regions of the world. However, striking variations in cause-specific mortality rates, particularly related to NCDs, were observed within and between HICs and LMICs. These differentials suggested that social and ecological determinants of NCD risk were at work across populations.

Studies have found that the rapid rise in CVRD risk in LMICs is shaped largely by globalization and urbanization, which have profound impacts on dietary habits, tobacco consumption, and physical activity. The pathway is further modified by poverty, education, and stress levels. These upstream determinants decisively influence CVRD risk operating through behavioral factors (for example, tobacco use, diet, physical activity), biological factors (for example, blood pressure, cholesterol, blood glucose levels), psychosocial factors (for example, depression, anxiety, acute and chronic life stressors, lack of social support), and health system factors (for example, access to care, screening, diagnosis, quality of care) (Fuster and Kelly 2010).

The biosocial pathway alone cannot explain the cumulative CVRD risk that operates across the life course of individuals and populations. Socioeconomic conditions throughout the life course shape adult health and disease risk. For example, persons living in adverse childhood social circumstances are more likely to be of low birth weight and to be exposed to poor diet, childhood infections, and passive smoking. These exposures may increase their CVRD risk in adult life, perhaps through chains of risk or pathways over time where one adverse (or protective) experience tends to lead to another adverse (or protective) experience in a cumulative way (WHO 2010a). Thus, physical and social exposures during gestation, childhood, adolescence, young adulthood, and later adult life have long-term effects on the risk of NCDs.

Early-Life Determinants

Considerable work in recent years has explored how chronic disease risk begins in fetal life and continues into old age. Multiple studies have shown that adult onset of CVRDs is determined by risks that accumulate throughout life. Such risks are determined largely by what happens in early life and socioeconomic position throughout the life course. There are two major drivers for CVRD risk in adult life: (1) exposures during critical periods in life and (2) accumulation of risks throughout the life course.

Exposures during critical periods such as in the womb, infancy, and childhood have lasting or lifelong adverse effects on body systems that are not modified by any subsequent exposure. The concept of fetal programming explains how and why critical periods are important in the life of an individual, a subject discussed in detail in chapter 3 of this volume (Kumaran, Osmond, and Fall 2017). Furthermore, poverty and chronic undernutrition of women during pregnancy are associated with low birth weight of babies. Given these findings, the importance of the first 1,000 days of life for health and human development has gained greater recognition. The 1,000 days between conception and a child's second birthday offer a unique window of opportunity to shape a healthier and more prosperous future. The right nutrition during this 1,000-day window can have a profound impact on a child's ability to grow, learn, and rise out of poverty.

Risk during Childhood and Adolescence

Growing evidence suggests that environmental exposures do more damage to health and potential long-term health during critical periods of growth and development in childhood and adolescence than they would at other times. Children with low birth weight continue to be underweight up to two years, after which growth catches up and they become prone to childhood obesity (Sachdev and others 2005). Higher rates of obesity in these children increase the risk of adult overweight and obesity and CVRDs. Cohort studies have also found that many children with high blood pressure or obesity become adults with high blood pressure or obesity. The stability of these risk factors over time or the predictability of their future levels through measurements early in life is called *tracking* (Singh and others 2008).

In light of these findings, the impact of socioeconomic status is clearly evident in shaping the environment for CVRD risk of populations. Socioeconomic status bears heavily on household income and nutritional status; it can influence nutrition among pregnant women and their fetuses and affect future cognition, intelligence, schooling, and attainment of optimal height and weight and thus risk of CVRD in the next generation. As a result,

households in lower socioeconomic positions face a vicious intergenerational cycle of poor nutrition, ill health, and poverty. Furthermore, children and adolescents from low socioeconomic backgrounds more frequently experiment with risky behaviors such as smoking and alcohol use and continue to maintain such risky behaviors into adulthood. Poor diet, another risk factor for CVRD, has also been documented among such children. Finally, girls who grow poorly become stunted as adults and are more likely to give birth to low-birth-weight babies who are likely to continue the cycle by being stunted in adulthood.

The relatively larger role played by social, economic, and environmental factors in the epidemic of chronic diseases is explained by several theoretical models that highlight the importance of policy-based approaches for protecting the health of populations. A life course perspective in policies and programs helps identify chains of risk that can be broken and times when intervention may be especially effective. Particularly during key life transitions—for example, late adolescence to early adulthood—not just "safety nets" but "springboards" must be provided that can alter life course trajectories and improve the health of subsequent generations (WHO 2000a). Figure 2.5 outlines the relationships

Figure 2.5 Complex Interplay of Determinants and Risk Factors in the Pathway of Noncommunicable Diseases in the Population

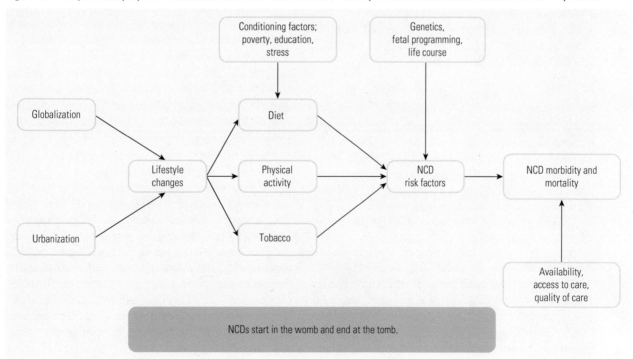

Note: NCD = noncommunicable disease.

between specific risk factors, their early- and late-life determinants, and their contributions to NCD risk.

A FRAMEWORK FOR ADDRESSING THE CHALLENGE OF CVRDS

The growing burden of NCDs in the past few decades clearly indicates that the health systems in LMICs need to focus more on preventing and controlling CVRDs, given that these nations face the major brunt of this epidemic. An integrated life course approach to prevention and control will be needed. The life course approach is an integrated continuum that affects all stages of life, including (but not limited to) the following:

- Addressing nutrition during fetal and early life
- Tackling childhood obesity through policy-level interventions such as banning certain advertisements aimed at schoolchildren, particularly in relation to food products
- Vigorously controlling tobacco, particularly to prevent children from experimenting with and getting habituated to smoking
- Effectively implementing the World Health Organization's Framework Convention on Tobacco Control
- Controlling risk factors in persons with single or multiple risk factors for primary prevention
- Managing diseases for secondary prevention
- Rehabilitating people with impairments and disabilities
- Financially protecting people with acute illness
- Focusing on neglected CVRDs.

It is also important to create an environment that is conducive for individuals to adopt and maintain a healthy life through macro-level policies, including agricultural policies promoting the consumption of fruits and vegetables, an enabling environment for physical activity, public transportation, and access to and affordability of essential drugs and diagnostics. This section describes the socioecological model as a basis for designing interventions for CVRD prevention and control.

Reducing Risk

Intervening in the causal pathway of CVRDs is complex. An ideal but comprehensive approach would follow a socioecological model for intervening that enables identification of interactions between an individual and his or her environment. The socioecological model integrates theories of individual behavior change with an understanding of the role of environmental enhancement in the interactions between an individual and his or her social and physical environments (McLeroy and others 1988). According to this socioecological model, human behaviors are fundamentally determined by five broad categories of factors: intrapersonal factors, interpersonal factors, organizational factors, community factors, and public policy (McLeroy and others 1988).

Multiple pathways and factors are involved in the causal pathway of CVRD risk, and a model that focuses exclusively on individuals is likely to fail. Therefore, efforts to improve individuals' health must be directed simultaneously at multiple levels. The ideal approach would be to take advantage of opportunities for intervention at all stages of the life course by preventing the acquisition and augmentation of risk, detecting and reducing risk, managing NCD events, and preventing the progression of disease and recurrence of NCD events (Fuster and Kelly 2010). Relying on these concepts, the Institute of Medicine has provided a framework for NCD interventions (figure 2.6).

An ideal approach would take advantage of multiple strategies that coordinate across multiple sectors with a mix of interventions that take into account context and locale:

- *An individual-level (high-risk) approach* that focuses on clinical identification of individuals in the population at highest risk of CVRD and intensive treatment through behavior change interventions, pharmacological measures, or both
- *A population-level approach* that focuses on shifting the distribution of risk factors in the population by implementing evidence-based policies, laws, and regulations that favorably affect the consumption of healthier foods, the built environment, and tobacco and alcohol use.

A comprehensive approach takes into account the full range of complex determinants of CVRDs to produce synergies among approaches at the individual and population levels. Concurrent modalities could include health promotion campaigns (for example, in communities, schools, and worksites) and reorientation and strengthening of health systems, with greater use of innovative applications of communications technologies, efficient use of medical therapies and technologies, and integrated clinical programs (Fuster and Kelly 2010).

Figure 2.6 Framework for a Comprehensive Strategy to Address Noncommunicable Diseases

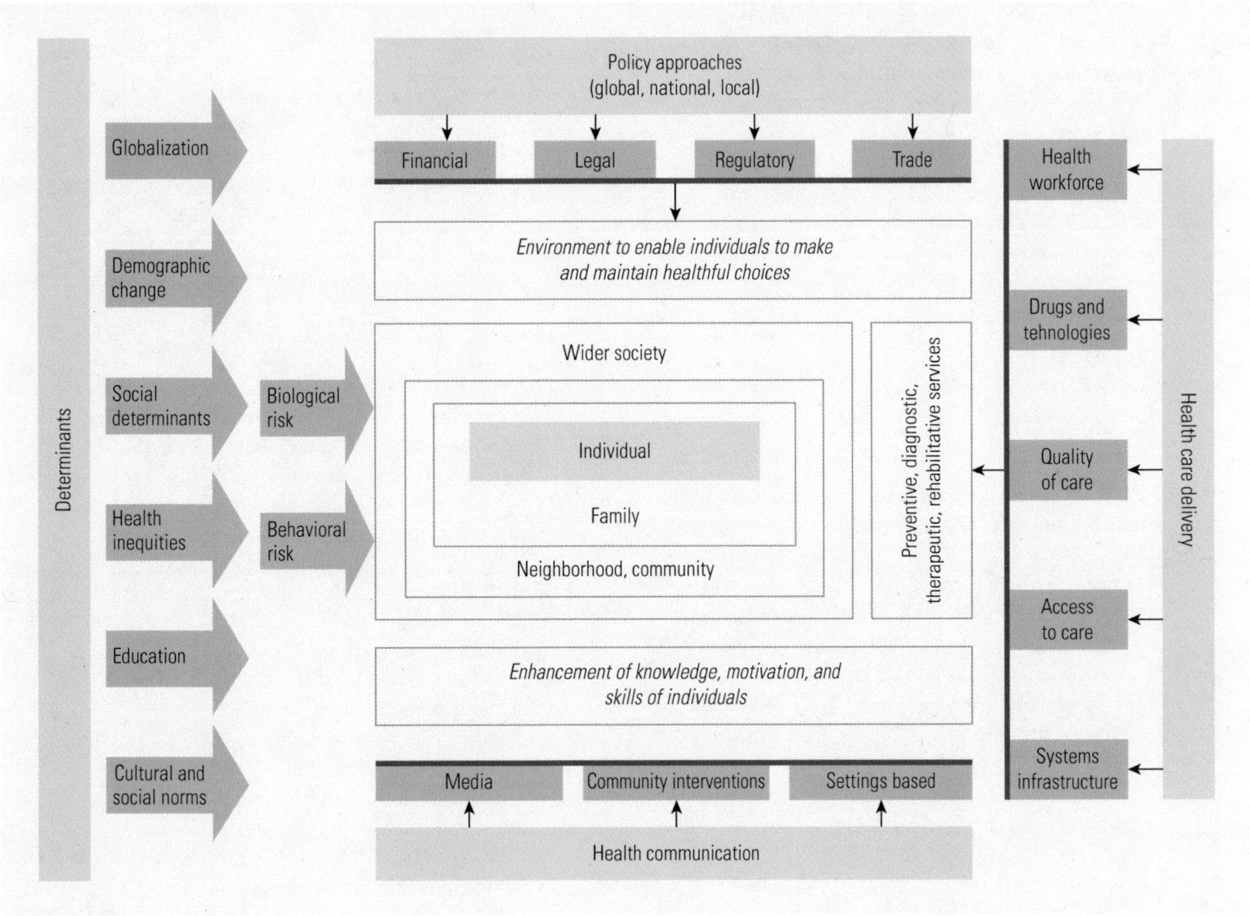

Source: Fuster and Kelly 2010.

Addressing Social Determinants to Prevent the Poor from Acquiring Unhealthy Habits

CVRDs and poverty form a vicious cycle. The poor are more vulnerable to CVRDs and are more likely to use tobacco products, to consume energy-dense food, and to consume fewer fruits and vegetables. These risky behaviors arise from social and economic inequalities such as lack of opportunity, lack of education, psychosocial stress, limited choice of consumption patterns, and inadequate access to health care (WHO 2005). They are exacerbated by aggressive marketing of tobacco products and greater access to cheaper energy-dense fried or processed foods, particularly in middle-income countries. As a result, the poor tend to be more obese than the wealthy and at greater risk of dying prematurely from CVRDs (WHO 2005). Ill health has a direct bearing on the livelihoods of poor

individuals and families because the resulting loss of jobs and wages can exacerbate the poverty trap. Policies for inclusive growth and social protection for poor and marginalized groups are essential to protecting and promoting public health.

CONCLUSIONS

CVRDs are an increasing contributor to poor health in LMICs. The epidemic of CVRDs is being driven by population growth and aging in combination with increasing prevalence of risk factors and inadequate clinical management. Health systems in LMICs, which account for most of the CVRD burden globally, are ill equipped to address this challenge and will require additional investments to strengthen access to evidence-based prevention and treatment. At the same time, public policy could be reoriented with a life course focus so that CVRD prevention and control are not limited to clinical settings but also harness the power of specific policies to improve population health and well-being.

ANNEX

The annex to this chapter is as follows. It is available at http://www.dcp-3.org/CVRD.

- Annex 2A. Updated Estimates of the Burden of CVRD in 2015.

NOTES

World Bank Income Classifications as of July 2014 are as follows, based on estimates of gross national income (GNI) per capita for 2013:

- Low-income countries (LICs) = US$1,045 or less
- Middle-income countries (MICs) are subdivided:
  (a) lower-middle-income = US$1,046 to US$4,125
  (b) upper-middle-income (UMICs) = US$4,126 to US$12,745
- High-income countries (HICs) = US$12,746 or more.

1. Goal 3: Ensure healthy lives and promote well-being for all at all ages, http://www.un.org/sustainabledevelopment /health/.

REFERENCES

Ahmad, S., G. Rukh, T. V. Varga, A. Ali, A. Kurbasic, and others. 2013. "Gene × Physical Activity Interactions in Obesity: Combined Analysis of 111,421 Individuals of European Ancestry." *PLoS Genetics* 9 (7): e1003607.

Allender, S., K. Wickramasinghe, M. Goldacre, D. Matthews, and P. Katulanda. 2011. "Quantifying Urbanization as a Risk Factor for Noncommunicable Disease." *Journal of Urban Health: Bulletin of the New York Academy of Medicine* 88 (5): 906–18.

Appel, L. J., M. W. Brands, S. R. Daniels, N. Karanja, P. J. Elmer, and others. 2006. "Dietary Approaches to Prevent and Treat Hypertension: A Scientific Statement from the American Heart Association." *Hypertension* 47 (2): 296–308.

Bilano, V., S. Gilmour, T. Moffiet, E. T. D'Espaignet, G. A. Stevens, and others. 2015. "Global Trends and Projections for Tobacco Use, 1990–2025: An Analysis of Smoking Indicators from the WHO Comprehensive Information Systems for Tobacco Control." *The Lancet* 385 (9972): 966–76.

Caballero, A. E. 2003. "Endothelial Dysfunction in Obesity and Insulin Resistance: A Road to Diabetes and Heart Disease." *Obesity Research* 11 (11): 1278–89.

Chobanian, A. V., G. L. Bakris, H. R. Black, W. C. Cushman, L. A. Green, and others. 2003. "Seventh Report of the Joint National Committee on Prevention, Detection, Evaluation, and Treatment of High Blood Pressure." *Journal of the American Heart Association* 42 (6): 1206–52.

Colditz, G. A., R. Bonita, M. J. Stampfer, W. C. Willett, B. Rosner, and others. 1988. "Cigarette Smoking and Risk of Stroke in Middle-Aged Women." *New England Journal of Medicine* 318 (15): 937–41.

Ezzati, M., and E. Riboli. 2013. "Behavioral and Dietary Risk Factors for Noncommunicable Diseases." *New England Journal of Medicine* 369 (10): 954–64.

Fuster, V., and B. B. Kelly, eds. 2010. *Promoting Cardiovascular Health in the Developing World: A Critical Challenge to Achieve Global Health.* Washington, DC: National Academies Press.

GBD (Global Burden of Disease) 2013 Risk Factors Collaborators. 2015. "Global, Regional, and National Comparative Risk Assessment of 79 Behavioural, Environmental and Occupational, and Metabolic Risks or Clusters of Risks in 188 Countries, 1990–2013: A Systematic Analysis for the Global Burden of Disease Study 2013." *The Lancet* 386 (10010): 2287–323.

Giolo, S. R., A. C. Pereira, M. de Andrade, J. E. Krieger, and J. P. Soler. 2010. "Evaluating Gene by Sex and Age Interactions on Cardiovascular Risk Factors in Brazilian Families." *BMC Medical Genetics* 11 (January): 132.

Global Asthma Network. 2014. *The Global Asthma Report 2014.* Auckland, New Zealand: Global Asthma Network.

Greenland, P., J. S. Alpert, G. A. Beller, E. J. Benjamin, M. J. Budoff, and others. 2010. "2010 ACCF/AHA Guideline for Assessment of Cardiovascular Risk in Asymptomatic Adults: A Report of the American College of Cardiology Foundation/American Heart Association Task Force on Practice Guidelines." *Circulation* 122 (25): e584–636.

Gupta, P. C., and S. Asma, eds. 2008. *Bidi Smoking and Public Health.* New Delhi: Ministry of Health and Family Welfare, Government of India.

Hallal, P. C., V. L. Clark, M. C. Assunção, C. L. P. Araújo, H. Gonçalves, and others. 2012. "Socioeconomic Trajectories from Birth to Adolescence and Risk Factors for Noncommunicable Disease: Prospective Analyses." *Journal of Adolescent Health* 51 (Suppl 6): S32–37.

Hui, X., K. Matsushita, Y. Sang, S. H. Ballew, T. Fülöp, and others. 2013. "CKD and Cardiovascular Disease in the Atherosclerosis Risk in Communities (ARIC) Study: Interactions with Age, Sex, and Race." *American Journal of Kidney Diseases* 62 (4): 691–702.

IDF (International Diabetes Federation). 2015. *IDF Diabetes Atlas 2015.* 7th ed. Brussels: IDF.

Institute of Health Metrics and Evaluation. 2013. "Global Burden of Disease Study 2013 (GBD 2013) Data Downloads." GHDx, Institute of Health Metrics and Evaluation, University of Washington. http://ghdx .healthdata.org/global-burden-disease-study-2013-gbd -2013-data-downloads.

Jousilahti, P., E. Vartiainen, J. Tuomilehto, and P. Puska. 1999. "Sex, Age, Cardiovascular Risk Factors, and Coronary Heart Disease: A Prospective Follow-Up Study of 14,786 Middle-Aged Men and Women in Finland." *Circulation* 99 (9): 1165–72.

Kannel, W. B., T. R. Dawber, A. Kagan, N. Revotskie, and J. Stokes. 1961. "Factors of Risk in the Development of Coronary Heart Disease—Six-Year Follow-Up Experience. The Framingham Study." *Annals of Internal Medicine* 55: 33–50.

Khatibzadeh, S., F. Farzadfar, J. Oliver, M. Ezzati, and A. Moran. 2013. "Worldwide Risk Factors for Heart Failure: A Systematic Review and Pooled Analysis." *International Journal of Cardiology* 168 (2): 1186–94.

Klatsky, A. L. 2015. "Alcohol and Cardiovascular Diseases: Where Do We Stand Today?" *Journal of Internal Medicine* 278 (3): 238–50.

Kumaran, K., C. Osmond, and C. H. D. Fall. 2017. "Early Origins of Cardiometabolic Disease." In *Disease Control Priorities* (third edition): Volume 5, *Cardiovascular, Respiratory, and Related Diseases,* edited by D. Prabhakaran, S. Anand, T. A. Gaziano, J.-C. Mbanya, Y. Wu, and R. Nugent. Washington, DC: World Bank.

Law, M. R., J. K. Morris, and N. J. Wald. 1997. "Environmental Tobacco Smoke Exposure and Ischaemic Heart Disease: An Evaluation of the Evidence." *British Medical Journal* 315 (7114): 973–80.

Lin, E., D. Pei, Y.-J. Huang, C.-H. Hsieh, and L. S.-H. Wu. 2009. "Gene-Gene Interactions among Genetic Variants from Obesity Candidate Genes for Nonobese and Obese Populations in Type 2 Diabetes." *Genetic Testing and Molecular Biomarkers* 13 (4): 485–93.

Lozano, R., M. Naghavi, K. Foreman, S. Lim, K. Shibuya, and others. 2012. "Global and Regional Mortality from 235 Causes of Death for 20 Age Groups in 1990 and 2010: A Systematic Analysis for the Global Burden of Disease Study 2010." *The Lancet* 380 (9859): 2095–128.

Madison, R., R. Zelman, and C. Mittman. 1980. "Inherited Risk Factors for Chronic Lung Disease." *Chest* 77 (Suppl 2): 255–57.

Markus, H. S. 2011. "Stroke Genetics." *Human Molecular Genetics* 20 (R2): R124–31.

McKeigue, P. M., J. E. Ferrie, T. Pierpoint, and M. G. Marmot. 1993. "Association of Early-Onset Coronary Heart Disease in South Asian Men with Glucose Intolerance and Hyperinsulinemia." *Circulation* 87 (1): 152–61.

McLeroy, K. R., D. Bibeau, A. Steckler, and K. Glanz. 1988. "An Ecological Perspective on Health Promotion Programs." *Health Education Quarterly* 15 (4): 351–77.

Miller, M., N. J. Stone, C. Ballantyne, V. Bittner, M. H. Criqui, and others. 2011. "Triglycerides and Cardiovascular Disease: A Scientific Statement from the American Heart Association." *Circulation* 123 (20): 2292–333.

Mosca, L., L. J. Appel, E. J. Benjamin, K. Berra, N. Chandra-Strobos, and others. 2004. "Evidence-Based Guidelines for Cardiovascular Disease Prevention in Women." *Journal of the American College of Cardiology* 43 (5): 900–21.

O'Donnell, M. J., D. Xavier, L. Liu, H. Zhang, S. L. Chin, and others. 2010. "Risk Factors for Ischaemic and Intracerebral Haemorrhagic Stroke in 22 Countries (the INTERSTROKE Study): A Case-Control Study." *The Lancet* 376 (9735): 112–23.

Palta, M., D. Gabbert, M. R. Weinstein, and M. E. Peters. 1991. "Multivariate Assessment of Traditional Risk Factors for Chronic Lung Disease in Very Low Birth Weight Neonates: The Newborn Lung Project." *Journal of Pediatrics* 119 (2): 285–92.

Parish, S., R. Collins, R. Peto, L. Youngman, J. Barton, and others. 1995. "Cigarette-Smoking, Tar Yields, and Nonfatal Myocardial-Infarction: 14,000 Cases and 32,000 Controls in the United Kingdom." *British Medical Journal* 311 (7003): 471–77.

Pearson, T. A., T. L. Bazzarre, S. R. Daniels, J. M. Fair, S. P. Fortmann, and others. 2003. "American Heart Association Guide for Improving Cardiovascular Health at the Community Level: A Statement for Public Health Practitioners, Healthcare Providers, and Health Policy Makers from the American Heart Association Expert Panel on Population and Prevention Science." *Circulation* 107 (4): 645–51.

Perk, J., G. De Backer, H. Gohlke, I. Graham, Z. Reiner, and others. 2013. "European Guidelines on Cardiovascular Disease Prevention in Clinical Practice (Version 2012). The Fifth Joint Task Force of the European Society of Cardiology and Other Societies on Cardiovascular Disease Prevention in Clinical Practice." *Giornale Italiano di Cardiologia* 14 (5): 328–92.

Peto, R., A. D. Lopez, J. Boreham, M. Thun, and C. Heath Jr. 1994. *Mortality from Smoking in Developed Countries 1950–2000: Indirect Estimates from National Vital Statistics.* Oxford, U.K.: Oxford University Press.

Rosenberg, L., D. W. Kaufman, S. P. Helmrich, and S. Shapiro. 1985. "The Risk of Myocardial Infarction after Quitting Smoking in Men under 55 Years of Age." *New England Journal of Medicine* 313 (24): 1511–14.

Sacco, R. L., M. Elkind, B. Boden-Albala, I. F. Lin, D. E. Kargman, and others. 1999. "The Protective Effect of Moderate Alcohol Consumption on Ischemic Stroke." *JAMA* 281 (1): 53–60.

Sachdev, H. S., C. H. D. Fall, C. Osmond, R. Lakshmy, S. K. Dey Biswas, and others. 2005. "Anthropometric Indicators of Body Composition in Young Adults: Relation to Size at Birth and Serial Measurements of Body Mass Index in Childhood in the New Delhi Birth Cohort." *American Journal of Clinical Nutrition* 82 (2): 456–66.

Salvi, S. S., and P. J. Barnes. 2009. "Chronic Obstructive Pulmonary Disease in Non-Smokers." *The Lancet* 374 (9691): 733–43.

Schumacher, M. C., S. C. Hunt, and R. R. Williams. 1990. "Interactions between Diabetes and Family History of Coronary Heart Disease and Other Risk Factors for Coronary Heart Disease among Adults with Diabetes in Utah." *Epidemiology* 1 (4): 298–304.

Singh, A. S., C. Mulder, J. W. R. Twisk, W. Van Mechelen, and M. J. M. Chinapaw. 2008. "Tracking of Childhood Overweight into Adulthood: A Systematic Review of the Literature." *Obesity Reviews* 9 (5): 474–88.

Singh, S., S. Dhingra, D. D. Ramdath, S. Vasdev, V. Gill, and others. 2010. "Risk Factors Preceding Type 2 Diabetes and Cardiomyopathy." *Journal of Cardiovascular Translational Research* 3 (5): 580–96.

Smith, S. C., E. J. Benjamin, R. O. Bonow, L. T. Braun, M. A. Creager, and others. 2011. "AHA/ACCF Secondary Prevention and Risk Reduction Therapy for Patients with Coronary and Other Atherosclerotic Vascular Disease: 2011 Update: A Guideline from the American Heart Association and American College of Cardiology Foundation." *Journal of the American College of Cardiology* 58 (23): 2432–46.

Srinath Reddy, K., and M. B. Katan. 2004. "Diet, Nutrition, and the Prevention of Hypertension and Cardiovascular Diseases." *Public Health Nutrition* 7 (1A): 167–86.

Strope, G. L., and D. A. Stempel. 1984. "Risk Factors Associated with the Development of Chronic Lung Disease in Children." *Pediatric Clinics of North America* 31 (4): 757–71.

Watkins, D. A., N. Dabestani, C. N. Mock, M. Cullen, K. R. Smith, and others. 2017. "Trends in Morbidity and Mortality Attributable to Injuries and Selected Environmental Hazards." In *Disease Control Priorities* (third edition): Volume 7, *Injury Prevention and Environmental Health,* edited by C. N. Mock, O. Kobusingye, R. Nugent, and K. Smith. Washington, DC: World Bank.

Watkins, D. A., B. Hasan, B. Mayosi, G. Buhkman, J. A. Marin-Neto, and others. 2017. "Structural Heart Diseases." In *Disease Control Priorities* (third edition): Volume 5, *Cardiovascular, Respiratory, and Related Conditions,* edited by D. Prabhakaran, S. Anand, T. A. Gaziano, J.-C. Mbanya, Y. Wu, and R. Nugent. Washington, DC: World Bank.

Weber, M. B., R. Oza-Frank, L. R. Staimez, M. K. Ali, and K. M. Venkat Narayan. 2012. "Type 2 Diabetes in Asians: Prevalence, Risk Factors, and Effectiveness of Behavioral Intervention at Individual and Population Levels." *Annual Review of Nutrition* 32 (August): 417–39.

WHO (World Health Organization). 2000a. *The Implications for Training of Embracing a Life Course Approach to Health.* Geneva: WHO.

———. 2000b. *Obesity: Preventing and Managing the Global Epidemic; Report of a WHO Consultation.* Technical Report Series 894. Geneva: WHO.

———. 2005. *Preventing Chronic Diseases: A Vital Investment.* Geneva: WHO.

———. 2010a. *A Conceptual Framework for Action on the Social Determinants of Health.* Geneva: WHO.

———. 2010b. *Global Status Report on Noncommunicable Diseases.* Geneva: WHO. http://whqlibdoc.who.int /publications/2011/9789240686458_eng.pdf.

———. 2014. "Global Health Estimates." WHO, Geneva.

———. 2016a. "WHO: Obesity and Overweight." Fact Sheet 311, WHO, Geneva. http://www.who.int/mediacentre /factsheets/fs311/en/.

———. 2016b. "WHO: Physical Activity." Fact Sheet 385, WHO, Geneva. http://www.who.int/mediacentre/factsheets/fs385 /en/.

———. Various years. "Global Health Observatory." WHO, Geneva.

WHO and U.S. National Institute on Aging. 2011. *Global Health and Aging.* Geneva: WHO; Bethesda, MD: National Institute on Aging. http://www.who.int/ageing /publications/global_health/en/.

Yusuf, S., S. Hawken, S. Ounpuu, T. Dans, A. Avezum, and others. 2004. "Effect of Potentially Modifiable Risk Factors Associated with Myocardial Infarction in 52 Countries (the INTERHEART Study): Case-Control Study." *The Lancet* 364 (9438): 937–52.

Yusuf, S., S. Islam, C. K. Chow, S. Rangarajan, G. Dagenais, and others. 2011. "Use of Secondary Prevention Drugs for Cardiovascular Disease in the Community in High-Income, Middle-Income, and Low-Income Countries (the PURE Study): A Prospective Epidemiological Survey." *The Lancet* 378 (9798): 1231–43.

Yusuf, S., S. Rangarajan, K. Teo, S. Islam, W. Li, and others. 2014. "Cardiovascular Risk and Events in 17 Low-, Middle-, and High-Income Countries." *New England Journal of Medicine* 371 (9): 818–27.

Yusuf, S., S. Reddy, S. Ounpuu, and S. Anand. 2001. "Global Burden of Cardiovascular Diseases: Part I: General Considerations, the Epidemiologic Transition, Risk Factors, and Impact of Urbanization." *Circulation* 104 (22): 2746–53.

Zimmet, P., E. J. Boyko, G. R. Collier, and M. de Courten. 1999. "Etiology of the Metabolic Syndrome: Potential Role of Insulin Resistance, Leptin Resistance, and Other Players." *Annals of the New York Academy of Sciences* 892 (November): 25–44.

Chapter 3

Early Origins of Cardiometabolic Disease

Kalyanaraman Kumaran, Clive Osmond, and Caroline H. D. Fall

INTRODUCTION: BIRTH WEIGHT AND ADULT CARDIOVASCULAR DISEASE

This chapter discusses the developmental origins of health and disease (DOHaD) and their implications for public health. It summarizes the epidemiological evidence in humans linking low birth weight, infant and childhood growth, adult body mass index (BMI), and maternal weight and nutrition to cardiometabolic risk factors in later life. It describes what is meant by developmental programming and considers alternative explanations for the epidemiological associations. It then evaluates the effects of interventions in pregnancy, infancy, and childhood on later cardiovascular risk and concludes with the public health implications and potential economic benefits of early life interventions.

Forsdahl (1977) discovered that Norwegian counties with the highest infant mortality in 1896–1925 experienced the highest death rates from coronary heart disease in the mid to late twentieth century. He suggested that poverty in childhood caused permanent damage, perhaps due to a nutritional deficit, that resulted in lifelong vulnerability to an affluent lifestyle and high fat intake. A decade later, Barker and Osmond (1986) found a similar phenomenon in the United Kingdom. Using archived birth records from the county of Hertfordshire, they found that lower birth weight and lower weight at age one year were associated with an increased risk of death from coronary heart disease and

stroke in adulthood (Barker and others 1989; Osmond and others 1993). Mortality approximately doubled from the highest to the lowest extremes of birth weight or infant weight (figure 3.1). Barker and others (1989) concluded that processes linked to growth and active in prenatal or early postnatal life strongly influence the risk of adult coronary heart disease.

The association between lower birth weight and increased risk of coronary heart disease has been replicated in many different populations (Andersen and others 2010; Forsen and others 1999; Huxley and others 2007; Leon and others 1998; Stein and others 1996) (figure 3.2). The association is linear and graded across the whole range of birth weight, with an upturn at extremely high birth weight (figure 3.1). The association is independent of adult socioeconomic status, making confounding an unlikely explanation (Leon and others 1998). Studies that include gestational age data indicate that restricted fetal growth, rather than preterm delivery, is associated with coronary heart disease (Leon and others 1998).

RISK FACTORS FOR CARDIOVASCULAR DISEASE

Associations were subsequently found between small size at birth and some of the major risk factors for coronary heart disease, including impaired glucose tolerance

Corresponding author: Kalyanaraman Kumaran, MRC Lifecourse Epidemiology Unit, University of Southampton, United Kingdom; Epidemiology Research Unit, Holdsworth Memorial Hospital, Mysore, India; kk@mrc.soton.ac.uk.

Figure 3.1 Standardized Mortality Ratios for Cardiovascular Disease in Women and Men Younger than Age 65 Years (up to 1992) in Hertfordshire, United Kingdom, by Category of Birth Weight

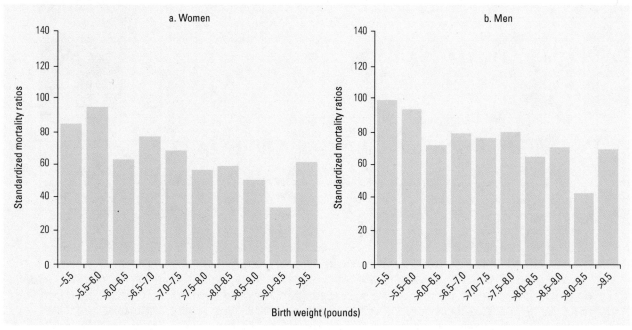

Source: Osmond and others 1993.

Figure 3.2 Forest Plot from a Meta-Analysis of the Relative Risk for a Fatal or Nonfatal Cardiovascular Event per Kilogram Increase in Birth Weight across 18 Studies

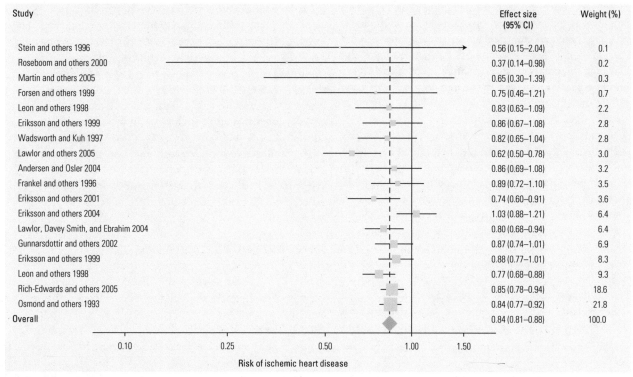

Source: Huxley and others 2007.
Note: CI = confidence interval. Weight (%) refers to the relative weighting of each study in the meta-analysis, based on the study sample size.

and type 2 diabetes mellitus (T2DM) (Hales and others 1991), hypertension (Fall and others 1995), insulin resistance (Phillips 1995), and metabolic syndrome (Barker and others 1993). A systematic review confirmed that the relationship between birth weight and T2DM is inverse, graded, and independent of current body size and socioeconomic class (Whincup and others 2008). The relationship is particularly strong for birth weight under 3 kilograms. For every kilogram increase in birth weight, the odds of diabetes are 0.75 (95 percent confidence interval [CI], 0.70 to 0.81). The inverse relationship between birth weight and blood pressure has also been demonstrated consistently across different populations in both high-income countries (HICs) and low- and middle-income countries (LMICs) and in both childhood and adulthood (Huxley, Neil, and Collins 2002; Huxley, Shiell, and Law 2000; Law and Shiell 1996). The size of the effect is debated, ranging from an estimated fall in systolic blood pressure of 0.6 millimeter of mercury (mmHg) per kilogram increase in birth weight (Huxley, Neil, and Collins 2002) to 2–3 mmHg (Huxley, Shiell, and Law 2000; Law and Shiell 1996). A review (Mu and others 2012) comparing low birth weight (less than 2,500 grams) to high birth weight (more than 2,500 grams) suggested that adult systolic blood pressure is higher by approximately 2 mmHg in the low–birth weight group.

Obesity, as measured by BMI, is not associated with lower birth weight. On the contrary, persons who were small at birth also tend to be thinner as adults (Fall 2011). Evidence indicates that the lower adult BMI associated with lower birth weight reflects lower lean body mass rather than less adiposity (Wells, Chomtho, and Fewtrell 2007). Some evidence suggests that small size at birth is associated with central obesity in later life, as measured by waist circumference, waist-hip ratio, or subscapular-to-triceps skinfold ratio (Fall 2011).

Small size at birth has been shown to predict structural and functional cardiovascular measures such as increased left ventricular size and dysfunction and reduced arterial compliance (Lamont and others 2000; Martyn and others 1995; Vijayakumar and others 1995), although results from LMICs have been inconsistent (Kumaran and others 2000; Norman 2008). Associations between small size at birth and adverse concentrations of plasma lipid or clotting factor have been reported, but they are inconsistent across populations (Lauren and others 2003).

In summary, poor fetal growth resulting in small size at birth is associated with an increased risk of adult coronary heart disease and some of its risk factors. The findings potentially have significance in the context of LMICs, where the prevalence of low birth weight is high.

Approximately one in four newborns in South Asia weighs less than 2,500 grams, and 10 countries account for more than 50 percent of the global burden of low birth weight; India alone accounts for more than 30 percent.[1]

DEVELOPMENTAL ORIGINS OF HEALTH AND DISEASE

Barker proposed that the association between small size at birth and disease in later life reflects the permanent effects of fetal undernutrition (Barker 1998; Barker and others 1993). Fetal undernutrition could occur because the mother is undernourished or because the materno-fetal supply line (uterine blood flow, placenta) is suboptimal. The fetus depends on the transfer of nutrients from the mother and adapts to an inadequate supply of nutrients in various ways: prioritization of brain growth at the expense of other tissues, such as the abdominal viscera; reduction in the secretion of and sensitivity to the fetal growth hormones (for example, insulin); and upregulation of the hypothalamo-pituitary-adrenal (stress) axis. Barker (1998) proposed that, although they occur in response to a transient phenomenon of fetal undernutrition, these changes become permanent or *programmed* because they occur during critical periods of early plasticity. Programmed changes may include different tissues, producing a variety of metabolic effects (figure 3.3), which could lead directly to adult cardiovascular disease or render the individual more susceptible to the adverse cardiometabolic effects of environmental stressors, such as smoking and obesity in later life. Subsequent research in experimental animals has confirmed that it is possible to program high blood pressure and diabetes by manipulating the nutrition of the mother during pregnancy (Duque-Guimaraes and Ozanne 2013).

Research in humans and further studies in experimental animals suggest that environmental influences other than undernutrition can program later disease. These influences include fetal overnutrition (as in maternal diabetes or obesity), maternal smoking, and exposure to environmental pollutants. Many of the body's tissues and organs and its endocrine system may be affected, leading not only to cardiovascular disease and diabetes, but also to renal disease, lung disease, osteoporosis, and impaired mental health (Luyckx and others 2013; Victora and others 2008). While the fetal period may be particularly important because of the rapid growth and development of organs and tissues at this time, evidence suggests that exposures during infancy and childhood also have programming effects. It has become clear that changes in body size, such as low

Figure 3.3 Developmental Origins of Health and Disease Hypothesis

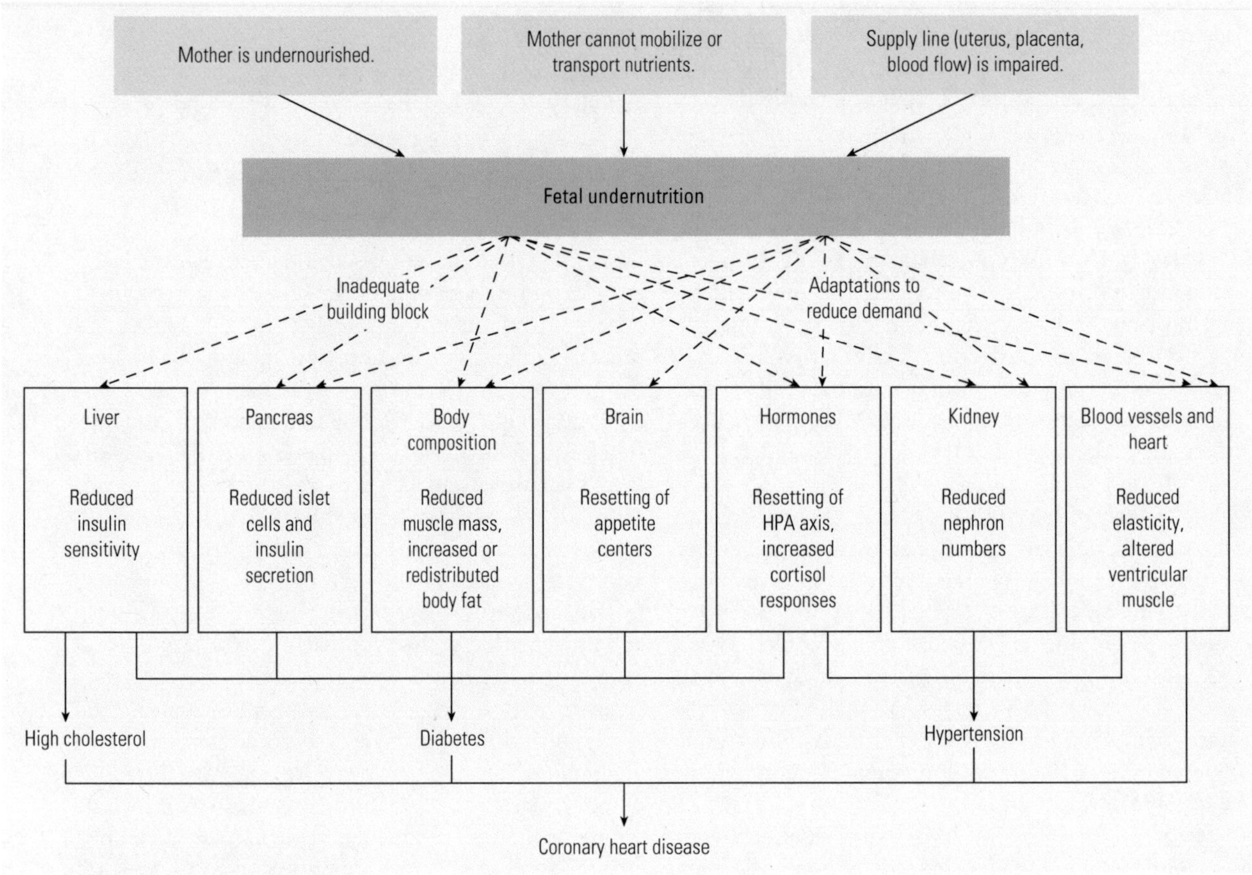

| Mother is undernourished. | Mother cannot mobilize or transport nutrients. | Supply line (uterus, placenta, blood flow) is impaired. |

Fetal undernutrition

Inadequate building block

Adaptations to reduce demand

Liver	Pancreas	Body composition	Brain	Hormones	Kidney	Blood vessels and heart
Reduced insulin sensitivity	Reduced islet cells and insulin secretion	Reduced muscle mass, increased or redistributed body fat	Resetting of appetite centers	Resetting of HPA axis, increased cortisol responses	Reduced nephron numbers	Reduced elasticity, altered ventricular muscle

High cholesterol

Diabetes

Hypertension

Coronary heart disease

Note: HPA = hypothalamo-pituitary-adrenal (stress) axis.

birth weight, do not *cause* later disease. Birth weight is a convenient, frequently measured summary of the *effect* on the fetus of multiple maternal factors, including size, nutritional status, metabolism, pregnancy complications, physical activity, and lifestyle. The effects of these factors on developing fetal organs, resulting in permanently altered structure and function, are thought to be responsible for later disease risk. This new understanding led to what was initially known as the Barker hypothesis or the fetal programming hypothesis, later renamed the DOHaD hypothesis.

A challenge facing DOHaD research is the long lag between early life exposures (such as fetal undernutrition) and the emergence of hard disease outcomes in adult life. This lag means that much of the evidence in humans comes from observational data and from associations between early life factors (usually birth weight) and adult outcomes. However, associations between lower birth weight and higher risk markers for cardiovascular disease, such as blood pressure, glucose, and insulin concentrations,

can be found even in children (Bavdekar and others 1999) and young adults, long before disease becomes apparent, suggesting that the effects of programming and the potential benefit of interventions may be detectable at relatively young ages.

GESTATIONAL DIABETES, MATERNAL OBESITY, AND FUEL-MEDIATED TERATOGENESIS

Fetal overnutrition attributable to maternal hyperglycemia or obesity is thought to program the offspring for obesity and T2DM, strong risk factors for cardiovascular disease. Pedersen (1954) proposed that the transfer to the fetus of excess maternal glucose in gestational diabetes mellitus (GDM) stimulates fetal pancreatic islets to produce fetal hyperinsulinemia, which leads to macrosomia (Pedersen 1954). Freinkel (1980) suggested that a mixture of maternal nutrients (glucose, lipids, and amino acids) affects not only the growth of the fetus, but also its risk of future obesity, diabetes, and neurocognitive development (fuel-mediated teratogenesis). Infants of mothers with GDM are born larger and develop early obesity, central obesity, higher insulin resistance, and impaired glucose tolerance and T2DM (Dabelea and Pettitt 2001). The inheritance of genes responsible for both obesity and GDM could cause such an effect. However, offspring of diabetic mothers have higher rates of obesity and T2DM than do siblings born before the mother developed diabetes (Dabelea and others 2000), suggesting that these higher rates are an effect of the intrauterine diabetic environment.

These findings have been replicated in India, where children born to mothers with GDM were larger at birth and had higher subcutaneous adiposity compared with the newborns of non-GDM mothers (Hill and others 2005). The difference in adiposity in girls continued to increase throughout childhood (figure 3.4). At age nine years, the children of GDM mothers had higher glucose concentrations and insulin resistance (Krishnaveni and others 2010).

Maternal glycemia and insulin resistance are closely linked to maternal adiposity, and there is growing interest in whether maternal obesity, greater pregnancy weight gain, or both also program obesity and increased cardiometabolic risk in children through their effect on fetal nutrition. Studies in HICs have shown that, like diabetic mothers, obese mothers have altered lipid and glucose metabolism, have increased insulin resistance and circulating pro-inflammatory factors (Huda, Brodie, and Sattar 2010), and potentially expose the fetus to fuel-mediated teratogenesis. Newborns of obese women in the United States have increased body fat (Catalano and others 2009), and higher maternal BMI or adiposity during pregnancy is associated with a greater risk of overweight and obesity in children (Oken 2009). Another U.S. study has shown that children of mothers who are obese but do not have GDM are at increased risk of developing metabolic syndrome (Boney and others 2005). Population-based studies in the United Kingdom have shown that children of women who gained excess weight during pregnancy had higher blood pressure, lipids, and body fat percentage (Fraser and others 2010) and that offspring of obese mothers had an increased risk of death from cardiovascular disease in middle age (Reynolds and others 2013).

It is not yet certain that these associations reflect fetal programming by maternal obesity, but the evidence for programming by GDM is strong, with important implications for public health as the world gets fatter. Upward trends in maternal BMI and GDM

Figure 3.4 Median Subscapular Skinfold Thickness for Offspring of Diabetic Mothers, Offspring of Diabetic Fathers, and Controls Ages 0–9.5 Years, in Mysore, India

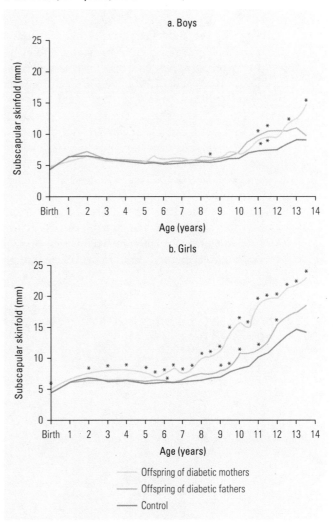

Source: Krishnaveni and others 2010; personal communication.
Note: mm = millimeter.
* = values that were significantly different ($p < 0.05$) from those of control children.

could accelerate the diabetes and obesity epidemics across generations, making young women key targets within strategies to prevent obesity. GDM and obesity are not only a problem in HICs; the prevalence of both conditions is also rising rapidly in LMICs.[2] In Indian cities the prevalence of GDM is now as high as 15 percent to 20 percent (Seshiah and others 2004).

CHILDHOOD WEIGHT GAIN AND GROWTH

Numerous studies have shown that changes in weight or BMI after birth are related to adult cardiovascular disease and its risk factors.

Weight and BMI in Infancy

Greater weight or BMI gain in infancy initially appeared to be protective. In Hertfordshire, men with higher weight at age one year had lower cardiovascular disease mortality (Barker and others 1989) and less T2DM (Hales and others 1991). Higher weight and BMI at age one year were also associated with a lower risk of coronary heart disease and T2DM in both men and women in Finland (Eriksson and others 2001; Eriksson and others 2003). Because there are relatively few adult cohorts with infant data and adult follow-up, the consistency of these findings in other populations is unclear. In India, lower weight or BMI at age one year was associated with a higher risk of diabetes (Bhargava and others 2004) (figure 3.5). However, data from the Consortium of Health-Orientated Research in Transitioning Societies collaboration, combining adult birth cohorts in five LMICs, showed no association between weight or BMI in infancy and later blood pressure or diabetes (Adair and others 2013).

BMI in Childhood and Adolescence

In contrast, greater childhood or adolescent BMI gain is consistently and strongly associated with an increased risk of later cardiovascular disease. In all populations studied—both LMICs and HICs—accelerated childhood or adolescent BMI or weight gain (upward crossing of centiles or rising Z-scores) was associated with an increased risk of coronary heart disease (Eriksson and others 2001; Forsen and others 1999), higher blood pressure (Adair and others 2013), and T2DM (Adair and others 2013; Bhargava and others 2004; Eriksson and others 2003). However, upward crossing of BMI centiles during childhood does not necessarily mean an abnormally high childhood BMI. In Delhi, the children who later developed T2DM had a mean BMI at age 10 years that was similar to the rest of the cohort (figure 3.5) (Bhargava and others 2004).[3] They were on an upward trajectory, becoming "obese relative to themselves," but were not obese in absolute terms. There are no data indicating how many children in LMICs are following this

Figure 3.5 Childhood SD Scores for Height and BMI for Members of the New Delhi Birth Cohort Who Developed Impaired Glucose Tolerance or Diabetes in Young Adulthood

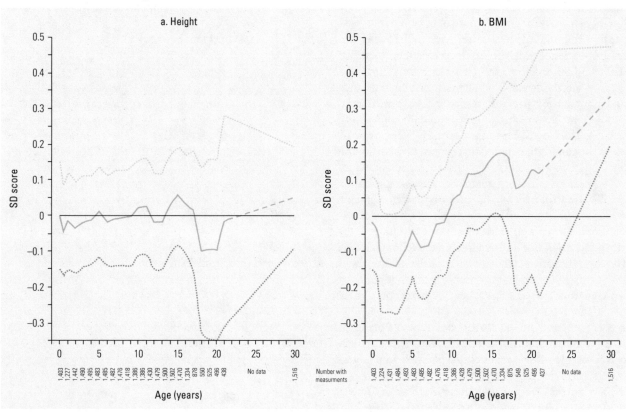

Source: Bhargava and others 2004.
Note: BMI = body mass index; SD = standard deviation. The solid lines indicate mean within-cohort SD scores at each age from birth to age 30 years for height and BMI among the cohort members who developed impaired glucose tolerance or type 2 diabetes mellitus. The dotted lines indicate 95 percent confidence intervals. The dashed line indicates a period between ages 21 years and 30 years in which there was no follow-up. The SD score for the cohort as a whole was set at zero (solid horizontal line).

growth pattern. However, childhood overweight and obesity are certainly rising; of the estimated 42 million children under age five years who were overweight in 2013, 31 million lived in LMICs.[4]

Childhood weight or BMI sometimes interacts with birth weight in the prediction of adult disease. In Finland, an increase in BMI from birth to age seven years was only associated with an increased risk of death from coronary heart disease in persons who were small at birth (figure 3.6).

BMI in Adulthood

Adult obesity adds to, and may interact with, the effects of low birth weight. The most adverse cardiovascular disease risk profile is consistently found across countries and populations in men and women who were small at birth but obese as adults. The effects of adult BMI on coronary heart disease, hypertension, T2DM, and insulin resistance are greater in individuals with low birth weight (Frankel and others 1996; Hales and others 1991). Similar interactive effects have been described between size at birth and other aspects of adult lifestyle—for example, between ponderal index at birth and adult socioeconomic status on coronary heart disease (Barker and others 2001) and between weight in infancy and the effects of smoking on fibrinogen concentrations (Barker and others 1992).

BMI gain in childhood combined with a background of impaired fetal development might be associated with disease for several reasons. Growth-restricted newborns tend to catch up (compensatory weight gain), and the rapidity of postnatal weight gain may indicate greater severity of fetal growth restriction in relation to potential (Leon and others 1996). Alternatively, the catch-up process itself may be disadvantageous. It may place excessive demand on organs that are not capable of compensatory hyperplasia, such as the pancreas or kidneys. It may alter body composition; fat maintains its capacity for growth throughout life, unlike muscle, which develops earlier and loses the capacity for cell division. Several studies have shown that, while lower birth weight and infant weight are associated with reduced adult lean body mass, accelerated BMI gain after infancy is associated with greater gain in fat mass relative to lean mass (Fall 2011). Another possibility is that the hormones driving compensatory weight gain (for example, insulin and insulin-like growth factors) have adverse long-term cardiovascular and metabolic effects.

Height in Childhood

Greater growth in height in childhood has been associated with a higher risk of later coronary heart

Figure 3.6 Hazard Ratios for Death from Coronary Heart Disease of Men Born in Helsinki, 1924–33, According to Ponderal Index at Birth and BMI at Age 11 Years

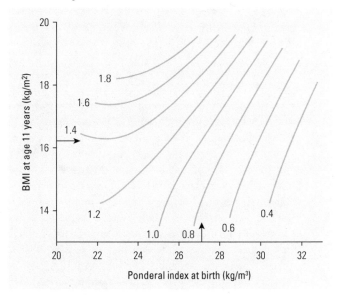

Source: Eriksson and others 1999.
Note: BMI = body mass index; kg/m² = kilograms per square meter; kg/m³ = kilograms per cubic meter. Arrows indicate average values. Ponderal index is a ratio of birth weight to birth length; a lower ponderal index at birth implies a higher degree of thinness.

disease, higher blood pressure, T2DM, and insulin resistance (Bavdekar and others 1999; Eriksson and others 2001; Forsen and others 1999; Leon and others 1996). In contrast, taller height in adulthood has consistently been associated with a lower risk of coronary heart disease. The reasons are unclear. The components of height (leg length and trunk height) show opposite relationships with cardiovascular risk. Longer leg length appears protective, while greater trunk height is associated with an adverse risk profile or with no relationship (Lawlor, Ebrahim, and Davey Smith 2002; Lawlor and others 2004; Schooling and others 2007). Leg length may reflect fetal and infant health and nutrition, while trunk height is thought to be determined during puberty (Gunnell 2001; Wadsworth and others 2002), although the evidence is poor.

Recent statistical modeling techniques using conditional variables have been used to examine separate effects of linear growth and relative weight gain—that is, weight gain independent of linear growth. In five cohorts in LMICs, faster linear growth between birth and mid-childhood was associated with higher adult blood pressure and BMI (mostly lean mass) (Adair and others 2013). It was not associated with T2DM in later life.

OTHER EARLY LIFE EXPOSURES

Other maternal and offspring factors may influence the future risk of cardiometabolic disease. The best studied exposures are diet in infancy, including breastfeeding, and maternal smoking.

Breastfeeding

Compared with formula feeding, breastfeeding has been associated with less obesity and T2DM and lower blood pressure and lipids in later life (Owen and others 2005; Owen and others 2006; Owen, Whincup, and Cook 2011), but the effects appear to be modest. Meta-analyses have shown that mean cholesterol levels in adulthood were 0.04 nanomole per liter lower and systolic blood pressure was 1.4 mmHg lower in persons who were breastfed as infants, compared with those who were bottle fed (Martin, Gunnell, and Davey Smith 2005; Owen and others 2008). The reviews raised the possibility of publication bias. Studies of duration and exclusivity of breastfeeding have shown no evidence that these factors influence later obesity or blood pressure. Most of the evidence on long-term effects of breastfeeding is from observational studies in HICs, and because breastfeeding is strongly associated with higher maternal socioeconomic status and education in these countries, residual confounding is a major issue. Data from five LMICs showed no evidence that breastfeeding is protective against hypertension, diabetes, or obesity (Fall and others 2011). The few randomized controlled trials of breastfeeding interventions have been similarly negative, although none has followed the children into adult life (Fewtrell 2011; Kramer and others 2007; Martin and others 2014).

Maternal Smoking

Maternal smoking has been associated with childhood obesity and behavioral disorders (Swanson and others 2009). In a meta-analysis, the odds ratio for maternal smoking was 1.5 in persons who were obese in later life compared with controls who were not obese (Oken, Levitan, and Gillman 2008). Confounding is an issue because smoking is strongly associated with lower maternal socioeconomic status, which is also strongly related to childhood obesity in HICs. However, it is plausible that maternal smoking could permanently affect fetal development through decreased utero-placental blood flow, hypoxia, direct effects of harmful substances in cigarette smoke, or maternal appetite suppression. Interventions to prevent or stop smoking in pregnancy are effective (Lumley and others 2013), but there are no data on long-term outcomes in the children.

Other Exposures

Prenatal exposure to common environmental pollutants, especially those that have endocrine activity (endocrine disruptors), has been shown to increase adiposity in animals in later life (Heindel, Newbold, and Schug 2015). Chemicals shown to have this effect include estrogenic compounds such as bisphenol A (a weak estrogenic component of polycarbonate plastics used in food containers), polychlorinated biphenyls (used in electrical equipment), dichlorodiphenyl dichloroethene (a breakdown product of the pesticide DDT [dichlorodiphenyltrichloroethane]), and phytoestrogens (derived from soya products). There are few human studies, but prenatal exposure to some of these pollutants has been associated with increased adiposity or weight for height in children in HICs (Vafeiadi and others 2016). More research on this topic is needed in LMICs, where environmental pollution is often poorly regulated and people (especially in low-income groups) are poorly protected.

Stressful experiences in early life may have a role in the programming of adult disease. Although the evidence in humans is limited, children born in Helsinki between 1934 and 1944 who were separated (evacuated) from their parents had higher systolic and diastolic blood pressure and were more likely to be on medication for coronary heart disease than children who were not separated (Alastalo and others 2012, 2013). The age and duration of separation were related to blood pressure levels, suggesting that these early life influences can have lasting effects, perhaps via stress-mediated metabolic or hormonal alterations.

ALTERNATIVE EXPLANATIONS FOR ASSOCIATIONS BETWEEN SIZE IN EARLY LIFE AND LATER HEALTH

Much of the evidence for the early life programming of cardiometabolic disease in humans still rests on observational studies and on associations with crude proxy measures of adverse early life exposures. Such associations could have other explanations, some of which are reviewed briefly here, using birth weight as an example.

Statistical Issues
Selection Effects
Participants recruited into studies in late life may not be representative, either in their early growth and development or in their adult disease, of the original population from which they came. For example, persons with extremely low birth weight may have died earlier. However, bias arises only when the sampling

processes for exposures and outcomes are linked—for example, if the selection of persons with low birth weight was based on whether they had adult coronary heart disease. Moreover, comparisons in these studies were made within the cohort, further reducing the possibility of selection bias.

Measurement Errors

Measurement errors, especially in historical data, may be a source of bias. For example, in the Hertfordshire birth cohort, newborns were measured with agricultural weighing scales to the nearest quarter or even half pound, which could cause misclassification of birth weight. However, such random measurement errors tend to weaken associations rather than create spurious ones.

Confounding

An association between an exposure and an outcome may be induced because of a third variable (known as a confounder) that is related to both exposure and outcome but is not on the causal pathway. For example, confounding by socioeconomic status could induce an association between low birth weight and adult coronary heart disease, because poorer socioeconomic conditions are associated with lower birth weight, poorer childhood and adult diets, and fewer life opportunities, all of which could predispose individuals to adult disease. It is important, therefore, to identify confounders and adjust for them in the analysis. The association between low birth weight and adult coronary heart disease persists even after adjusting for socioeconomic status, although it is possible that some residual confounding remains.

Socioeconomic factors may also operate through behaviors such as differences in maternal diet and stress. Socioeconomic status may be not just a confounder, but also an effect modifier, in that early life effects may have associations with adult disease that differ according to socioeconomic status.

Adjustments

Early size may be associated with adult outcomes in two ways: a direct programming effect and an indirect effect that arises because early size is associated with adult size, which has its own association with adult outcome. A model that only includes early size captures the net effect of these two processes; a model that also includes adult size isolates the direct programming effect. These models address different questions; therefore, they give different answers. This disparity has caused confusion (Tu and others 2005). Theoretically, it is impossible to separate the influences of early size, adult size, and the growth that led from the one to the other (Lucas, Fewtrell, and

Cole 1999) because only two independent observations led to these three variables. Studies that include intermediate time points may be better able to identify the windows of growth that are critical for adult disease (Adair and others 2013). It is important to look for interactions between the effects of early and later size on adult disease (figure 3.6). Data from Finland showed that persons with a lower ponderal index at birth had a higher risk of coronary heart disease and that the risk was greatest in those with higher BMI at age 11 years. Those with a higher ponderal index at birth had a lower risk, and the risk was similar irrespective of their size at age 11 years.

Genetic Effects

The fetal insulin hypothesis suggests a genetic explanation for associations between birth size and adult disease. For example, mutations or polymorphisms in fetal genes influencing insulin secretion, such as the glucokinase gene, could cause lower birth weight, insulin resistance, and later T2DM (Hattersley and Tooke 1999). A large genome-wide association study identified seven loci significantly associated with birth weight, of which two were also related to T2DM and one to blood pressure (Horikoshi and others 2013). However, these loci would not explain the findings from epidemiological studies.

Birth weight is only partly determined by genetic factors, and the relative importance of genes and environment has been an active area of research for the past two decades. It is likely that interactions between genetic and environmental factors influence not only fetal development but also the risk of adult disease. Research suggests that these effects may additionally act through epigenetic mechanisms, which alter the expression of genes without altering the base sequence (Tarry-Adkins and Ozanne 2011).

Randomized controlled trials will provide the best tests of causative links between early life factors and later disease and lead to evidence-based interventions. However, not all interventions are amenable to trials, for ethical and other reasons; even if trials are possible, lengthy follow-up may be needed to see effects. The next section presents what is currently known from intervention studies in early life. Recently developed techniques can strengthen causal inference from observational studies, overcome some of the statistical issues, and lead to new insights into potentially modifiable early life exposures (reviewed in Gage, Munafo, and Davey Smith 2016; Richmond and others 2014). These techniques include the use of cross-cohort comparisons, sibling comparisons, negative control approaches, and instrumental variables (which can be genetic markers, as in the technique known as Mendelian randomization).

EVIDENCE FROM INTERVENTION STUDIES

The DOHaD hypothesis has been tested definitively in humans only recently in studies following up children born during randomized controlled trials of different exposures in utero, in infancy, or in childhood (Hawkesworth 2009). Rather than the immediate effects on birth weight and survival, the focus here is on long-term cardiometabolic effects, which necessarily require prolonged follow-up and for which data are still sparse.

Nutritional Interventions in Pregnancy

Protein and Energy

The trial with the longest follow-up is the cluster randomized trial conducted by the Institute of Nutrition of Central America and Panama in Guatemala, in which pregnant mothers and children up to age seven years received either Atole (a high-energy, high-protein drink) or Fresco (a lower-energy, no-protein drink) as a daily supplement. Both drinks contained micronutrients. Several studies investigating cardiometabolic outcomes in the young adult offspring have shown beneficial effects of prenatal supplementation with Atole on concentrations of high-density lipoprotein cholesterol and triglycerides (Stein and others 2006) and on concentrations of plasma glucose in women (Conlisk and others 2004), but no effect on blood pressure (Webb and others 2005).

In a cluster randomized trial in India, pregnant mothers in intervention villages received food-based energy and protein supplements as part of a package of public health interventions, while those in control villages received standard care. A small increase in birth weight of approximately 61 grams occurred in offspring born to women in the intervention villages, suggesting an effect on fetal development (Kinra and others 2014). Insulin resistance and arterial stiffness were reduced, but not blood pressure, in the adolescent children of women in the intervention villages compared with controls (Kinra and others 2008). These children were also taller by approximately 14 millimeters. A later follow-up found no differences in lean body mass and grip strength between the groups (Kulkarni and others 2014).

Hawkesworth and others have followed up adolescents whose mothers took part in a randomized controlled trial of protein-energy supplementation during pregnancy in The Gambia (Hawkesworth and others 2008, 2009; Hawkesworth and others 2011). They found no differences in blood pressure, body composition, or serum cholesterol concentrations between the intervention and control groups. Plasma glucose was lower in the offspring of mothers who received the protein-energy intervention, but the effect was very small (0.05 millimoles/liter) and unlikely to be clinically significant.

Micronutrients

Micronutrient deficiencies are common among pregnant women in LMICs, and because micronutrient requirements are higher during periods of rapid growth, these deficiencies may impair fetal development. Between 1999 and 2001, 4,926 pregnant women in rural Nepal were cluster randomized to receive daily micronutrient supplements containing vitamin A alone (control) or in combination with folic acid, folic acid plus iron, folic acid plus iron plus zinc, or multiple micronutrients from early pregnancy until three months postpartum. The children were followed up to between ages six and eight years. None of the micronutrient combinations influenced blood pressure, concentrations of cholesterol, triglycerides, glucose, or insulin, or insulin resistance (Stewart, Christian, Schulze, and others 2009). There was a lower risk of microalbuminuria in the folic acid (odds ratio [OR], 0.56; 95 percent CI, 0.33 to 0.93; $p = 0.02$) and folic acid plus iron plus zinc (OR, 0.53; 95 percent CI, 0.32 to 0.89; $p = 0.02$) groups and a reduced risk of metabolic syndrome in the folic acid (OR, 0.63; 95 percent CI, 0.41 to 0.97; $p = 0.03$) group. Maternal supplementation with folic acid plus iron plus zinc resulted in a reduction in triceps thickness (-0.25 millimeter [mm]; 95 percent CI, -0.44 to -0.06), subscapular skinfold thickness (-0.20 mm; 95 percent CI, -0.33 to -0.06), and arm fat area (-0.18 square centimeter [cm^2]; 95 percent CI, -0.34 to -0.01) (Stewart, Christian, Leclerq, and others 2009).

Follow-up data from another multiple micronutrient trial for pregnant women in Nepal showed lower systolic blood pressure in children (N = 917) at age two years (-2.5 mmHg; 95 percent CI, -4.55 to -0.47) compared with children whose mothers received standard iron plus folate tablets (Vaidya and others 2008), and triceps skinfold thickness was increased in the group who received multiple micronutrients (2.0 mm; 95 percent CI, 0.0 to 0.4). However, these differences were not maintained when the children were studied again at age eight years (Devakumar and others 2014).

Several studies have followed up children born to mothers who took part in calcium supplementation trials. Calcium supplementation is a common clinical intervention to prevent pregnancy-induced hypertension (Hawkesworth and others 2009). Overall, there is little evidence of a significant effect on blood pressure.

Combined Protein-Energy and Micronutrients

The Maternal and Infant Nutrition Interventions in Matlab (MINIMat) trial in Bangladesh randomized pregnant women to receive supplementation with either iron and folic acid or multiple micronutrients combined in a factorial design with randomized food-based energy supplementation (608 kilocalories for six days a week), starting either at 9 weeks or at 20 weeks gestation. Follow-up of the children at age 4.5 years showed no effect on body composition of either early energy supplementation or multiple micronutrients (Khan and others 2012). Early pregnancy energy supplementation was associated with a 0.72 mmHg (95 percent CI, 0.16 to 1.28; $p = 0.01$) lower childhood diastolic blood pressure; multiple micronutrient supplementation was associated with higher childhood diastolic blood pressure (0.87 mmHg; 95 percent CI, 0.18 to 1.56; $p = 0.01$) (Hawkesworth and others 2013).

Summary

These results provide little evidence of long-term benefits from supplementing undernourished mothers for their offspring's cardiometabolic risk and little support for the DOHaD hypothesis. More evidence is needed, however, because these trials suffer from limitations related to sample size, losses to follow-up, and age at follow-up (Hawkesworth 2009). Follow-up in childhood or adolescence may be too early. It may be necessary to intervene earlier in pregnancy or even preconceptionally to influence processes such as placentation, organogenesis, and periconceptional epigenetic changes, which may be important for programming later disease.

Interventions to Prevent or Treat Gestational Diabetes

Evidence relating to the efficacy of interventions to prevent gestational diabetes is limited. Recent reviews have concluded that, although dietary counseling and increased exercise may provide some benefits, the quality of evidence is poor and no firm conclusions can be drawn (Han, Middleton, and Crowther 2012; Oostdam and others 2011; Skouteris and others 2014). Evidence suggests that more intensive treatment of gestational diabetes reduces macrosomia and pregnancy complications (Han, Crowther, and Middleton 2012); however, on follow-up, there were no differences in BMI between children at ages four to five years (Gillman and others 2010). Large, well-designed randomized controlled trials are needed to assess the benefits of various interventions on gestational diabetes as well as on downstream outcomes, including newborn size, perinatal complications, and the cardiometabolic health of offspring.

Lifestyle Interventions in Obese Pregnant Women

Several large randomized controlled trials, either recently completed or currently in progress, have studied lifestyle interventions among obese pregnant women (Poston and others 2015). Most of these trials are or have been conducted in HICs. There is little information yet as to whether these interventions alter cardiometabolic outcomes in children. The Lifestyle in Pregnancy and Offspring study in Denmark found no differences in blood pressure, plasma glucose, insulin, lipids, or body composition in children at ages two to three years of obese women who participated in a diet counseling and exercise program compared with controls, but this age may be too young for effects to be observable (Tanvig and others 2014, 2015).

Breastfeeding Interventions

It is clearly unethical to randomize infants to different durations of breastfeeding or to breastfeeding versus formula feeding. However, two large studies have randomized mother-infant pairs to receive additional encouragement to breastfeed, compared with standard care, and have follow-up data on the children. The Promotion of Breastfeeding Intervention Trial in Belarus recruited mother-infant pairs who were cluster randomized to an intervention designed to encourage exclusive breastfeeding for six months or to standard care. Although the intervention increased exclusive breastfeeding compared with controls, it showed no differences between the groups at ages 6 and 11 years in adiposity, blood pressure, plasma glucose, insulin, adiponectin or apolipoprotein A1 concentrations, or prevalence of metabolic syndrome (Kramer and others 2007, 2009; Martin and others 2014). In the MINIMat trial in Bangladesh, 4,436 pregnant women were randomized to six equal-size food and micronutrient groups; 3,214 were randomized during the last trimester of pregnancy to receive either breastfeeding counseling or common health messages. There were no differences in these groups in the growth trajectory or body composition of their children at age five years (Khan and others 2013).

Interventions to Reduce Childhood Obesity and Adiposity

Evidence suggests that BMI and obesity track through childhood and into adulthood. Reversing obesity is difficult, and studies attempting to reduce or prevent childhood obesity have shown varying results; some of these are reviewed in chapter 7 on weight management in this volume (Malik and Hu 2017). Although behavioral changes relating to diet and physical activity are major features of intervention strategies, it is important to consider the wider obesogenic environment and its impact on children. A Cochrane review found evidence that child obesity prevention programs result in reduced

BMI (Waters and others 2011), particularly programs for children ages 6–12 years. These studies used a broad range of components; the authors concluded that it was difficult to disentangle which aspects contributed the most. Overall, school-based interventions that influenced the curriculum, provided support to teachers, and improved the nutritional quality of school food; interventions that provided support to parents; and home activities that encouraged healthy behaviors were effective. No evidence was found to suggest that any of these interventions had adverse effects. Further robust studies with long-term follow-up and cost-effectiveness analysis are needed.

PUBLIC HEALTH IMPLICATIONS

Alternative Preventive Strategy

Current preventive strategies to reduce the burden of cardiovascular disease focus on middle-age individuals with preexisting disease or risk factors but do not address the impact of the disease on future generations. The DOHaD findings have substantial public health implications because they suggest the potential for an alternative primary prevention strategy of optimizing early development to control and prevent the rising burden of cardiovascular disease and break the cycle of intergenerational transmission of susceptibility. Potential interventions include improving the lifestyle, health, and nutrition of future mothers and pregnant women; preventing and reducing exposure to cigarette smoke and other toxins during pregnancy; and optimizing childhood nutrition. The DOHaD findings are likely to have particular significance in LMICs undergoing rapid economic and demographic changes. These transitions include increasing availability of cheap energy-dense but nutrient-poor "fast foods," leading to upward trends in maternal and child BMI, frequently combined with intrauterine and infant undernutrition. Urban environments are often polluted and stressful. Rapid urban development is associated with loss of green spaces and traffic congestion, which militate against healthy physical activity—an important requirement for maintaining a healthy body weight.

Current evidence of long-term benefits to cardiometabolic health of interventions in pregnant women and children is scant. Most of the evidence comes from nutritional interventions, and although these interventions have shown effects on short-term outcomes such as birth weight, they do not suggest significant long-term benefits to the cardiometabolic risk profile in childhood. Longer periods of follow-up are required to assess the effects of these trials. Current knowledge suggests that unless interventions are targeted before conception, it may be difficult to influence programming because key processes such as placentation and organogenesis occur in the first trimester of pregnancy and major epigenetic changes occur around the time of conception.

Potential Size of Effect

Attempts have been made to calculate the potential benefits of improving early life development. Because better markers of adverse intrauterine programming are not available, these attempts focus mainly on birth weight, a major limitation. It has been suggested that the population attributable fraction of diabetes and hypertension due to low birth weight is small compared with adult lifestyle and heredity, respectively (Boyko 2000; Mogren and others 2001). However, these calculations treat birth weight as a dichotomous outcome and do not consider the potential benefit of shifting the birth weight distribution to the right (Ben-Shlomo 2001).

The calculations often ignore combined effects of birth weight and childhood growth. Findings from Finland suggest that if every individual in the cohort had been in the highest third of birth weight and reduced their standard deviation score for BMI between ages 3 and 11 years, the incidence of diabetes would have been reduced by 50 percent and the incidence of hypertension by 25 percent. If each man had been in the highest third of BMI at age 1 year and reduced the standard deviation score for BMI between ages 3 and 11 years, the incidence of coronary heart disease would have been reduced by approximately 40 percent (Barker and others 2002). In an analysis using data from Hertfordshire, United Kingdom, where birth weights were rounded to the nearest 0.5 pound, Joseph and Kramer (1997) showed that if all newborns weighed between 9.0 and 9.5 pounds at birth, 26 percent and 33 percent of deaths from coronary heart disease would be prevented in men and women, respectively. If people within any birth weight category attained birth weights in the next higher category, the decrease in coronary heart disease would be 9 percent, assuming a mean birth weight increase of one pound. It is, however, difficult to identify interventions that can change birth weight by such a large amount.

Although interventions to reduce low birth weight (less than 2,500 grams) in LMICs may be appropriate, measures to shift birth weight upward across the range may be inappropriate, because factors that cause both low and high birth weight (if related to maternal diabetes or obesity) are associated with an increased risk of later cardiometabolic disease.

Timing of Interventions

The associations between maternal obesity and adverse cardiometabolic outcomes in children and between rapid childhood weight gain and increased cardiometabolic risk in adulthood have led to concerns about trade-offs. For example, promoting better childhood nutrition to reduce child mortality and improve neurocognitive development may lead to excess childhood weight gain and increase the risk of cardiometabolic disease in adulthood. This line of argument suggests that, to escape undernutrition, LMICs will inevitably pay a price of chronic disease epidemics.

Analyses by the Consortium of Health-Orientated Research in Transitioning Societies collaboration, using data from five birth cohorts in LMICs, allay these fears to some extent. Higher birth weight and faster weight gain and linear growth in the first two years of life were associated with better human capital in adult life, as measured by attained schooling, income, height, and next-generation birth weight (Adair and others 2013; Victora and others 2008). These factors were associated with higher adult BMI, but with lean body mass more than fat mass, and were not associated with increased risk of adult hypertension or diabetes (Adair and others 2013). In contrast, faster weight gain after age two years was clearly associated with an increase in adult obesity, hypertension, and impaired fasting glucose. These data support the concept that intervening to improve nutrition in the first 1,000 days from conception until age two years offers the best chance of preventing the faltering of growth and neurocognitive development that occurs in LMICs (Victora and others 2010), while avoiding the trade-off of more cardiometabolic disease in later life. This concept has yet to be proven. Moreover, it does not preclude interventions at other ages; it does highlight the need to design interventions that avoid weight gain at the expense of linear growth in children and excessive weight gain in young and pregnant women.

A review of evidence-based interventions to improve maternal and child nutrition demonstrated a clear need to introduce evidence-based interventions in adolescence and before conception, especially in countries with a high burden of undernutrition and low age of first pregnancy (Bhutta and others 2013). The review recommended maternal micronutrient and balanced protein-energy supplementation, appropriate breastfeeding and complementary feeding strategies in infants, and micronutrient supplementation in infants and children under age five years as having clear short-term benefits. These interventions were delivered most equitably and cost-effectively in community-based settings. They have not been proven to have long-term benefits on cardiometabolic health. A holistic approach is recommended for interventions in adolescents and women in LMICs, where large gaps exist in knowledge about reproduction and parenting and where accessing optimal pregnancy care is difficult, but only on the basis of short-term benefits.

The field of DOHaD has moved to preconceptional intervention studies involving food-based and tablet-based micronutrient supplementation of women before and during pregnancy. If successful, these studies will offer, for the first time, a primordial preventive approach to reducing and eventually halting the epidemic of cardiovascular disease. The trials offer an opportunity to investigate the effects of maternal supplementation on offspring health as well as to examine mechanisms such as epigenetic changes in offspring. A preconceptional micronutrient food-based intervention in Mumbai, India, found an absolute risk reduction of 7 percent for low birth weight and approximately 6 percent for gestational diabetes (Potdar and others 2014; Sahariah and others 2016). These findings translate into numbers needed to treat of 15 for low birth weight and 17 for gestational diabetes. The daily cost of the intervention was US$0.09, which translates into US$675 to prevent one low birth weight by supplementing 15 women for nine months before conception and throughout pregnancy and US$765 to prevent one case of gestational diabetes. Given the perinatal and neonatal care required for low–birth weight infants, these costs would seem justifiable even apart from the potential reduced risk of future cardiovascular disease.

An analysis from the World Bank concluded that the economic benefit from reducing low birth weight in low-income countries was approximately US$580 per infant moved from low to normal birth weight categories (Alderman and Behrman 2004). The interventions considered ranged from provision of micronutrient and food supplements to social interventions to optimize birth spacing and marriage timing. The main economic benefits occurred from improved labor productivity, followed by reduced infant mortality and morbidity, with much smaller gains from reducing chronic disease. The latter outcome was partly due to discounting because gains occur many years after the intervention. However, evidence is limited; better estimates of costs and effects are necessary to obtain more accurate figures. Also, because discounting rates vary, the benefits may also be altered. In conclusion, preconceptional interventions have significant public health potential, not only for health-effectiveness but also for cost-effectiveness.

CONCLUSIONS

Key Policy Issues

Birth weight is not an exposure per se but rather a crude marker of a number of exposures influencing fetal nutrition. Policies to modify birth weight may not be the solution; however, it is reasonable to attempt to reduce the incidence of low birth weight (less than 2,500 grams) in undernourished mothers and of fetal macrosomia resulting from maternal obesity and gestational diabetes.

A holistic approach before and during pregnancy to improve the lifestyles of young women and mothers—incorporating good-quality nutritious diets that have adequate but not excessive calories, moderate physical activity, and measures to reduce smoking—deserves consideration. Although undernutrition is the main issue for most LMICs, rates of overweight and obesity are rising, accompanied by increases in gestational diabetes.

Considerable gaps exist in evidence sufficient to establish causal links between early life exposures and disease outcomes in later life and to develop interventions in early life to prevent disease. It is important that research planners take a long-term view and enable the follow-up of high-quality cohorts and intervention trials for long enough to obtain information on hard disease outcomes in later life. In addition, better surrogate markers of adverse early life programming at younger ages need to be identified; the field of epigenetics offers the potential to develop better biomarkers in the future. Further work is also needed on optimum growth patterns in fetal life, infancy, and childhood so that interventions can be targeted appropriately; these patterns may differ between populations. Longitudinal studies to investigate patterns of linear growth and weight gain and incorporate measurements of body composition and relate them to cardiovascular outcomes should be encouraged. Interventions to reduce childhood obesity should be more nuanced and consider upward crossing of centiles rather than focusing exclusively on obese children.

Main Platforms for Implementation

At the national level, policy makers can revisit recommendations on micronutrients given before and during pregnancy to address common deficiencies in their populations. At the community level, interventions to promote maternal and child health can be developed, implemented, and delivered. Schools can complement curricula with programs to promote healthy lifestyles. To maximize equity, governments should provide funding, at least during the initial stages.

Limitations of the Economic Analysis

The cost-effectiveness data are limited and were not collected explicitly for comprehensive analysis. Appropriate economic data need to be collected to enable cost-effectiveness analyses.

NOTES

World Bank Income Classifications as of July 2014 are as follows, based on estimates of gross national income (GNI) per capita for 2013:

- Low-income countries (LICs) = US$1,045 or less
- Middle-income countries (MICs) are subdivided:
  (a) lower-middle-income = US$1,046 to US$4,125
  (b) upper-middle-income (UMICs) = US$4,126 to US$12,745
- High-income countries (HICs) = US$12,746 or more.

1. Based on United Nations Children's Fund data; see http://data.unicef.org/nutrition/low-birthweight.
2. Based on data from the International Diabetes Federation Diabetes Atlas 2015 (http://www.diabetesatlas.org).
3. See also Centers for Disease Control and Prevention, National Center for Health Statistics, http://www.cdc.gov/growthcharts.
4. See World Health Organization, http://www.who.int/dietphysicalactivity/childhood/en/.

REFERENCES

Adair, L. S., C. Fall, C. Osmond, A. Stein, R. Martorell, and others. 2013. "Disentangling How Relative Weight Gain and Linear Growth during Early Life Relate to Adult Health and Human Capital in Low and Middle Income Countries: Findings from Five Birth Cohort Studies." *The Lancet* 382 (9891): 525–34.

Alastalo, H., K. Räikkönen, A. Pesonen, C. Osmond, D. Barker, and others. 2012. "Cardiovascular Morbidity and Mortality in Finnish Men and Women Separated Temporarily from Their Parents in Childhood: A Life Course Study." *Psychosomatic Medicine* 74 (6): 583–87.

———. 2013. "Early Life Stress and Blood Pressure Levels in Late Adulthood." *Journal of Human Hypertension* 27 (2): 90–94.

Alderman, H., and J. Behrman. 2004. "Estimated Economic Benefits of Reducing Low Birth Weight in Low-Income Countries." Health, Nutrition, and Population Policy Paper, World Bank, Washington, DC.

Andersen, A. M., and M. Osler. 2004. "Birth Dimensions, Parental Mortality, and Mortality in Early Adult Age: A Cohort Study of Danish Men Born in 1953." *International Journal of Epidemiology* 33 (1): 92–99.

Andersen, L. G., L. Angquist, J. Eriksson, T. Forsen, M. Gamborg, and others. 2010. "Birth Weight, Childhood Body Mass Index, and Risk of Coronary Heart Disease in Adults: Combined Historical Cohort Studies." *PLoS One* 5 (11): e14126.

Barker, D. J. P. 1998. *Mothers, Babies, and Health in Later Life.* London: Churchill Livingstone.

Barker, D. J. P., J. Eriksson, T. Forsen, and C. Osmond. 2002. "Fetal Origins of Adult Disease: Strength of Effects and Biological Basis." *International Journal of Epidemiology* 31 (6): 1235–39.

Barker, D. J. P., T. Forsen, A. Uutela, C. Osmond, and J. G. Eriksson. 2001. "Size at Birth and Resilience to Effects of Poor Living Conditions in Adult Life: Longitudinal Study." *BMJ* 323 (7324): 1273–76.

Barker, D. J. P., P. Gluckman, K. Godfrey, J. Harding, J. Owens, and others. 1993. "Fetal Nutrition and Cardiovascular Disease in Adult Life." *The Lancet* 341 (8850): 938–41.

Barker, D. J. P., T. Meade, C. Fall, A. Lee, C. Osmond, and others. 1992. "Relation of Fetal and Infant Growth to Plasma Fibrinogen and Factor VII Concentrations in Adult Life." *BMJ* 304 (6820): 148–52.

Barker, D. J. P., and C. Osmond. 1986. "Infant Mortality, Childhood Nutrition, and Ischaemic Heart Disease in England and Wales." *The Lancet* 1 (8489): 1077–81.

Barker, D. J. P., P. Winter, B. Margetts, and S. Simmonds. 1989. "Weight in Infancy and Death from Ischaemic Heart Disease." *The Lancet* 2 (8663): 577–80.

Bavdekar, A., C. Yajnik, C. Fall, S. Bapat, A. Pandit, and others. 1999. "The Insulin Resistance Syndrome (IRS) in Eight-Year-Old Indian Children: Small at Birth, Big at 8 Years or Both?" *Diabetes* 48 (12): 2422–29.

Ben-Shlomo, Y. 2001. "Commentary: Are Birth Weight and Cardiovascular Associations Due to Fetal Programming?" *International Journal of Epidemiology* 30 (4): 862–63.

Bhargava, S. K., H. Sachdev, C. Fall, C. Osmond, R. Lakshmy, and others. 2004. "Relation of Serial Changes in Childhood Body Mass Index to Impaired Glucose Tolerance in Young Adulthood." *New England Journal of Medicine* 350 (9): 865–75.

Bhutta, Z. A., J. Das, A. Rizvi, M. Gaffey, N. Walker, and others. 2013. "Evidence-Based Interventions for Improvement of Maternal and Child Nutrition: What Can Be Done and at What Cost?" *The Lancet* 382 (9890): 452–77.

Boney, C. M., A. Verma, R. Tucker, and B. R. Vohr. 2005. "Metabolic Syndrome in Childhood: Association with Birth Weight, Maternal Obesity, and Gestational Diabetes Mellitus." *Pediatrics* 115 (3): e290–96.

Boyko, E. J. 2000. "Proportion of Type 2 Diabetes Cases Resulting from Impaired Fetal Growth." *Diabetes Care* 23 (9): 1260–64.

Catalano, P. M., L. Presley, J. Minium, and S. Hauguel-de Mouzon. 2009. "Fetuses of Obese Mothers Develop Insulin Resistance In Utero." *Diabetes Care* 32 (6): 1076–80.

Conlisk, A. J., H. Barnhart, R. Martorell, R. Grajeda, and A. Stein. 2004. "Maternal and Child Nutritional Supplementation Are Inversely Associated with Fasting Plasma Glucose Concentration in Young Guatemalan Adults." *Journal of Nutrition* 134 (4): 890–97.

Dabelea, D., and D. Pettitt. 2001. "Intrauterine Diabetic Environment Confers Risks for Type 2 Diabetes Mellitus and Obesity in the Offspring, in Addition to Genetic Susceptibility." *Journal of Pediatric Endocrinology and Metabolism* 14 (8): 1085–91.

Dabelea, D., R. Hanson, R. Lindsay, D. Pettitt, G. Imperatore, and others. 2000. "Intrauterine Exposure to Diabetes Conveys Risks for Type 2 Diabetes and Obesity: A Study of Discordant Sibships." *Diabetes* 49 (12): 2208–11.

Devakumar, D., S. S. Chaube, J. C. Wells, N. M. Saville, J. G. Ayres, and others. 2014. "Effect of Antenatal Multiple Micronutrient Supplementation on Anthropometry and Blood Pressure in Mid-Childhood in Nepal: Follow-up of a Double-Blind Randomised Controlled Trial." *The Lancet Global Health* 2 (11): e654–63.

Duque-Guimaraes, D. E., and S. E. Ozanne. 2013. "Nutritional Programming of Insulin Resistance: Causes and Consequences." *Endocrinology and Metabolism* 24 (10): 525–35.

Eriksson, J. G., T. Forsen, J. Tuomilehto, and D. Barker. 2001. "Early Growth and Coronary Heart Disease in Later Life: Longitudinal Study." *BMJ* 322 (7292): 949–53.

Eriksson, J. G., T. Forsen, J. Tuomilehto, C. Osmond, and D. Barker. 2003. "Early Adiposity Rebound in Childhood and Risk of Type 2 Diabetes in Adult Life." *Diabetologia* 46 (2): 190–94.

Eriksson, J. G., T. Forsen, J. Tuomilehto, P. Winter, C. Osmond, and others. 1999. "Catch-up Growth in Childhood and Death from Coronary Heart Disease: Longitudinal Study." *BMJ* 318 (7181): 427–31.

Eriksson, M., M. A. Wallander, I. Krakau, H. Wedel, and K. Svardsudd. 2004. "The Impact of Birth Weight on Coronary Heart Disease Morbidity and Mortality in a Birth Cohort Followed up for 85 Years: A Population-Based Study of Men Born in 1913." *Journal of Internal Medicine* 256 (6): 472–81.

Fall, C. H. D. 2011. "Evidence for the Intra-Uterine Programming of Adiposity in Later Life." *Annals of Human Biology* 38 (4): 410–28.

Fall, C. H. D., J. Borja, C. Osmond, L. Richter, S. Bhargava, and others. 2011. "Infant-Feeding Patterns and Cardiovascular Risk Factors in Young Adulthood: Data from Five Cohorts in Low- and Middle-Income Countries." *International Journal of Epidemiology* 40 (1): 47–62.

Fall, C. H. D., C. Osmond, D. Barker, P. Clark, C. Hales, and others. 1995. "Fetal and Infant Growth and Cardiovascular Risk Factors in Women." *BMJ* 310 (6977): 428–32.

Fewtrell, M. S. 2011. "Breast Feeding and Later Risk of CVD and Obesity: Evidence from Randomised Trials." *Proceedings of the Nutrition Society* 70 (4): 472–77.

Forsdahl, A. 1977. "Are Poor Living Conditions in Childhood and Adolescence an Important Risk Factor for Arteriosclerotic Disease?" *British Journal of Preventive and Social Medicine* 31 (2): 91–95.

Forsen, T., J. Eriksson, J. Tuomilehto, C. Osmond, and D. Barker. 1999. "Growth In Utero and during Childhood among Women Who Develop Coronary Heart Disease: Longitudinal Study." *BMJ* 319 (7222): 1403–7.

Frankel, S., P. Elwood, P. Sweetnam, J. Yarnell, and G. Davey Smith. 1996. "Birth Weight, Body Mass Index, and Incident Coronary Heart Disease." *The Lancet* 348 (9040): 1478–80.

Fraser, A., K. Tilling, C. Macdonald-Wallis, N. Sattar, M. J. Brion, and others. 2010. "Association of Maternal Weight Gain in Pregnancy with Offspring Obesity and

Metabolic and Vascular Traits in Childhood." *Circulation* 121 (23): 2557–64.

Freinkel, N. 1980. "Of Pregnancy and Progeny. Banting Lecture." *Diabetes* 29 (12): 1023–35.

Gage, S. H., M. R. Munafo, and G. Davey Smith. 2016. "Causal Inference in Developmental Origins of Health and Disease (DOHaD) Research." *Annual Review of Psychology* 67 (January): 567–85.

Gillman, M. W., H. Oakley, P. Baghurst, R. Volkmer, J. Robinson, and others. 2010. "Effect of Treatment of Gestational Diabetes Mellitus on Obesity in the Next Generation." *Diabetes Care* 33 (5): 964–86.

Gunnarsdottir, I., B. E. Birghisdottir, I. Thorsdottir, V. Gudnason, and R. Benediktsson. 2002. "Size at Birth and Coronary Artery Disease in a Population with High Birth Weight." *American Journal of Clinical Nutrition* 76 (6): 1290–94.

Gunnell, D. 2001. "Commentary: Early Insights into Height, Leg Length, Proportionate Growth and Health." *International Journal of Epidemiology* 30 (2): 221–22.

Hales, C. N., D. Barker, P. Clark, L. Cox, C. Fall, and others. 1991. "Fetal and Infant Growth and Impaired Glucose Tolerance at Age 64." *BMJ* 303 (6809): 1019–22.

Han, S., C. Crowther, and P. Middleton. 2012. "Interventions for Pregnant Women with Hyperglycaemia Not Meeting Gestational Diabetes and Type 2 Diabetes Diagnostic Criteria." *Cochrane Database of Systematic Reviews* 1 (January): CD009037.

Han, S., P. Middleton, and C. Crowther. 2012. "Exercise for Pregnant Women for Preventing Gestational Diabetes Mellitus." *Cochrane Database of Systematic Reviews* 7 (July): CD009021.

Hattersley, A. T., and J. Tooke. 1999. "The Fetal Insulin Hypothesis: An Alternative Explanation of the Association of Low Birth Weight with Diabetes and Vascular Disease." *The Lancet* 1353 (9166): 1789–92.

Hawkesworth, S. 2009. "Conference on Multidisciplinary Approaches to Nutritional Problems. Postgraduate Symposium. Exploiting Dietary Supplementation Trials to Assess the Impact of the Prenatal Environment on CVD Risk." *Proceedings of the Nutrition Society* 68 (1): 78–88.

Hawkesworth, S., A. Prentice, A. Fulford, and S. Moore. 2008. "Dietary Supplementation of Rural Gambian Women during Pregnancy Does Not Affect Body Composition in Offspring at 11–17 Years of Age." *Journal of Nutrition* 138 (12): 2468–73.

———. 2009. "Maternal Protein-Energy Supplementation Does Not Affect Adolescent Blood Pressure in The Gambia." *International Journal of Epidemiology* 38 (1): 119–27.

Hawkesworth, S., Y. Wagatsuma, A. Kahn, M. Hawlader, A. Fulford, and others. 2013. "Combined Food and Micronutrient Supplements during Pregnancy Have Limited Impact on Child Blood Pressure and Kidney Function in Rural Bangladesh." *Journal of Nutrition* 143 (5): 728–34.

Hawkesworth, S., C. Walker, Y. Sawo, A. Fulford, L. Jarjou, and others. 2011. "Nutritional Supplementation during Pregnancy and Offspring Cardiovascular Disease Risk in The Gambia." *American Journal of Clinical Nutrition* 94 (6 Suppl): S1853–60.

Heindel, J. J., R. Newbold, and T. T. Schug. 2015. "Endocrine Disruptors and Obesity." *Nature Reviews Endocrinology* 11 (September): 653–61.

Hill, J. C., G. Krishnaveni, I. Annamma, S. Leary, and C. Fall. 2005. "Glucose Tolerance in Pregnancy in South India: Relationships to Neonatal Anthropometry." *Acta Obstetrica et Gynecologica Scandinavica* 84 (2): 159–65.

Horikoshi, M., H. Yaghootkar, D. Mook-Kanamori, U. Sovio, H. Taaland, and others. 2013. "New Loci Associated with Birth Weight Identify Genetic Links between Intrauterine Growth and Adult Height and Metabolism." *Nature Genetics* 45 (1): 76–82.

Huda, S. S., L. E. Brodie, and N. Sattar. 2010. "Obesity in Pregnancy: Prevalence and Metabolic Consequences." *Fetal and Neonatal Medicine* 15 (2): 70–76.

Huxley, R., A. Neil, and R. Collins. 2002. "Unravelling the Fetal Origins Hypothesis: Is There Really an Inverse Association between Birth Weight and Subsequent Blood Pressure?" *The Lancet* 360 (9334): 659–65.

Huxley, R., C. G. Owen, P. H. Whincup, D. G. Cook, J. Rich-Edwards, and others. 2007. "Is Birth Weight a Risk Factor for Ischemic Heart Disease in Later Life?" *American Journal of Clinical Nutrition* 85 (5): 1244–50.

Huxley, R., A. Shiell, and C. Law. 2000. "The Role of Size at Birth and Postnatal Catch-up Growth in Determining Systolic Blood Pressure: A Systematic Review of the Literature." *Journal of Hypertension* 18 (7): 815–31.

Joseph, K. S., and M. Kramer. 1997. "Should We Intervene to Improve Fetal Growth?" In *A Lifecourse Approach to Chronic Disease Epidemiology*, edited by D. Kuh and Y. Ben-Shlomo. Oxford: Oxford University Press.

Khan, A. I., S. Hawkesworth, E. C. Ekström, S. Arifeen, S. E. Moore, and others. 2013. "Effects of Exclusive Breastfeeding Intervention on Child Growth and Body Composition: The MINIMat Trial, Bangladesh." *Acta Paediatrica* 102 (8): 815–23.

Khan, A. I., I. Kabir, S. Hawkesworth, E. Ekström, S. Arifeen, and others. 2012. "Early Invitation to Food and/or Multiple Micronutrient Supplementation in Pregnancy Does Not Affect Body Composition in Offspring at 54 Months: Follow-up of the MINIMat Randomised Trial, Bangladesh." *Maternal and Child Nutrition* 11 (3): 385–97.

Kinra, S., K. V. Radha Krishna, H. Kuper, K. V. Rameshwar Sarma, P. Prabhakaran, and others. 2014. ''Cohort Profile: Andhra Pradesh Children and Parents Study (APCAPS).'' *International Journal of Epidemiology* 43 (5): 1417–24. doi:10.1093/ije/dyt128.

Kinra, S., K. Sarma, Ghafoorunissa, V. Mendu, R. Ravikumar, and others. 2008. "Effect of Integration of Supplemental Nutrition with Public Health Programmes in Pregnancy and Early Childhood on Cardiovascular Risk in Rural Indian Adolescents: Long Term Follow-up of Hyderabad Nutrition Trial." *BMJ* 337 (July 25): a605.

Kramer, M. S., L. Matush, I. Vanilovich, R. Platt, N. Bogdanovich, and others. 2007. "Effects of Prolonged and Exclusive Breastfeeding on Child Height, Weight, Adiposity, and Blood Pressure at Age 6.5 Y: Evidence from a Large Randomized Trial." *American Journal of Clinical Nutrition* 86 (6): 1717–21.

————. 2009. "Randomized Breast-Feeding Promotion Intervention Did Not Reduce Child Obesity in Belarus." *Journal of Nutrition* 139 (2): S417–21.

Krishnaveni, G. V., S. Veena, J. Hill, S. Kehoe, S. Karat, and others. 2010. "Intra-Uterine Exposure to Maternal Diabetes Is Associated with Higher Adiposity and Insulin Resistance and Clustering of Cardiovascular Risk Markers in Indian Children." *Diabetes Care* 33 (November): 402–24.

Kulkarni, B., H. Kuper, K. Radhakrishna, A. Hills, N. Byrne, and others. 2014. "The Association of Early Life Supplemental Nutrition with Lean Body Mass and Grip Strength in Adulthood: Evidence from APCAPS." *American Journal of Epidemiology* 179 (6): 700–9.

Kumaran, K., C. Fall, C. Martyn, M. Vijayakumar, C. Stein, and others. 2000. "Blood Pressure, Left Ventricular Mass, and Arterial Compliance: No Relation to Small Size at Birth in South Indian Adults." *Heart* 83 (3): 272–77.

Lamont, D., L. Parker, M. White, N. Unwin, S. Bennett, and others. 2000. "Risk of Cardiovascular Disease Measured by Carotid Intima-Media Thickness at Age 49–51: Lifecourse Study." *BMJ* 320 (7230): 273–78.

Lauren, L., M. Jarvelin, P. Elliott, U. Sovio, A. Spellman, and others. 2003. "EURO-BLCS Study Group: Relationship between Birth Weight and Blood Lipid Concentrations in Later Life: Evidence from the Existing Literature." *International Journal of Epidemiology* 32 (5): 862–76.

Law, C. M., and A. Shiell. 1996. "Is Blood Pressure Inversely Related to Birth Weight? The Strength of Evidence from a Systematic Review of the Literature." *Journal of Hypertension* 14 (8): 935–41.

Lawlor, D. A., G. Davey Smith, and S. Ebrahim. 2004. "Birth Weight Is Inversely Associated with Coronary Heart Disease in Post-Menopausal Women: Findings from the British Women's Heart and Health Study." *Journal of Epidemiology and Community Health* 58 (2): 120–5.

Lawlor, D. A., S. Ebrahim, and G. Davey Smith. 2002. "The Association between Components of Adult Height and Type II Diabetes and Insulin Resistance: The British Women's Heart and Health Study." *Diabetologia* 45 (8): 1097–106.

Lawlor, D. A., G. Ronalds, H. Clark, G. Davey Smith, and D. A. Leon. 2005. "Birthweight Is Inversely Associated with Incident Coronary Heart Disease and Stroke among Individuals Born in the 1950s: Findings from the Aberdeen Children of the 1950s Prospective Cohort Study." *Circulation* 112 (10): 1414–18.

Lawlor, D. A., M. Taylor, G. Davey Smith, D. Gunnell, and S. Ebrahim. 2004. "Associations of Components of Adult Height with Coronary Heart Disease in Postmenopausal Women: The British Women's Heart and Health Study." *Heart* 90 (7): 745–49.

Leon, D. A., I. Koupilova, H. Lithell, L. Berglund, R. Mohsen, and others. 1996. "Failure to Realise Growth Potential In Utero and Adult Obesity in Relation to Blood Pressure in 50 Year Old Swedish Men." *BMJ* 312 (7028): 410–16.

Leon, D. A., H. Lithell, D. Vagero, I. Koupilova, R. Mohsen, and others. 1998. "Reduced Fetal Growth Rate and Increased Risk of Death from Ischaemic Heart Disease: Cohort Study of 15,000 Swedish Men and Women Born 1915–29." *BMJ* 317 (7153): 241–45.

Lucas, A., M. Fewtrell, and T. Cole. 1999. "Fetal Origins of Adult Disease: The Hypothesis Revisited." *BMJ* 319 (7204): 245–49.

Lumley, J., C. Chamberlain, T. Dowswell, S. Oliver, L. Oakley, and others. 2013. "Interventions for Promoting Smoking Cessation during Pregnancy." *Cochrane Database of Systematic Reviews* 10 (July 8): CD001055.

Luyckx, V. A., J. F. Bertram, B. M. Brenner, C. H. Fall, W. E. Hoy, and others. 2013. "Effect of Fetal and Child Health on Kidney Development and Long-Term Risk of Hypertension and Kidney Disease." *The Lancet* 382 (9888): 273–83.

Malik, V. S., and F. B. Hu. 2017. "Obesity Prevention." In *Disease Control Priorities* (third edition): Volume 5, *Cardiovascular, Respiratory, and Related Disorders*, edited by D. Prabhakaran, S. Anand, T. A. Gaziano, J.-C. Mbanya, Y. Wu, and R. Nugent. Washington, DC: World Bank.

Martin, R. M., D. Gunnell, and G. Davey Smith. 2005. "Breast Feeding in Infancy and Blood Pressure in Later Life: Systematic Review and Meta-Analysis." *American Journal of Epidemiology* 161 (1): 15–26.

Martin, R. M., D. Gunnell, J. Pemberton, S. Frankel, and G. Davey Smith. 2005. "Cohort Profile: The Boyd Orr Cohort–An Historical Cohort Study Based on the 65 Year Follow-Up of the Carnegie Survey of Diet and Health (1937–39)." *International Journal of Epidemiology* 34: 742–49.

Martin, R. M., R. Patel, M. Kramer, K. Vilchuck, N. Bogdanovich, and others. 2014. "Effects of Promoting Longer-Term and Exclusive Breastfeeding on Cardiometabolic Risk Factors at Age 11.5 Years: A Cluster-Randomized, Controlled Trial." *Circulation* 129 (3): 321–29.

Martyn, C. N., D. Barker, S. Jespersen, S. Greenwald, C. Osmond, and others. 1995. "Growth In Utero, Adult Blood Pressure, and Arterial Compliance." *British Heart Journal* 73 (2): 116–21.

Mogren, I., U. Hogberg, B. Stegmayr, L. Lindahl, and H. Stenlund. 2001. "Fetal Exposure, Heredity, and Risk Indicators for Cardiovascular Disease in a Swedish Welfare Cohort." *International Journal of Epidemiology* 30 (4): 853–62.

Mu, M., S. Wang, J. Sheng, Y. Zhao, H. Li, and others. 2012. "Birth Weight and Subsequent Blood Pressure: A Meta-Analysis." *Archives of Cardiovascular Disease* 105 (2): 99–113.

Norman, M. 2008. "Low Birth Weight and the Developing Vascular Tree: A Systematic Review." *Acta Paediatrica* 97 (9): 1165–72.

Oken, E. 2009. "Maternal and Child Obesity: The Causal Link." *Obstetrics and Gynecology Clinics of North America* 36 (2): 361–77.

Oken, E., E. Levitan, and M. Gillman. 2008. "Maternal Smoking during Pregnancy and Child Overweight: Systematic Review and Meta-Analysis." *International Journal of Obesity* 32 (2): 201–10.

Oostdam, N., M. van Poppel, M. Wouters, and W. van Mechelen. 2011. "Interventions for Preventing Gestational Diabetes Mellitus: A Systematic Review and Meta-Analysis." *Journal of Women's Health* 20 (10): 1551–63.

Osmond, C., D. Barker, P. Winter, C. Fall, and S. Simmonds. 1993. "Early Growth and Death from Cardiovascular Disease in Women." *BMJ* 307 (6918): 1519–24.

Owen, C. G., P. H. Whincup, S. J. Kaye, R. M. Martin, G. D. Smith, and others. 2008. "Does Initial Breastfeeding Lead to Lower Blood Cholesterol in Adult Life? A Quantitative Review of the Evidence." *American Journal of Clinical Nutrition* 88 (2): 305–14.

Owen, C. G., R. Martin, P. Whincup, G. Davey Smith, and D. Cook. 2006. "Does Breast Feeding Influence Risk of Type 2 Diabetes in Later Life? A Quantitative Analysis of Published Evidence." *American Journal of Clinical Nutrition* 84 (5): 1043–54.

Owen, C. G., R. Martin, P. Whincup, G. Davey Smith, M. W. Gillman, and others. 2005. "The Effect of Breast Feeding on Mean Body Mass Index throughout Life: A Quantitative Review of Published and Unpublished Observational Evidence." *American Journal of Clinical Nutrition* 82 (6): 1298–307.

Owen, C. G., P. Whincup, and D. Cook. 2011. "Breast Feeding and Cardiovascular Risk Factors and Outcomes in Later Life: Evidence from Epidemiological Studies." *Proceedings of the Nutrition Society* 70 (4): 478–84.

Pedersen, J. 1954. "Weight and Length at Birth of Infants of Diabetes Mothers." *Acta Endocrinologica* 16 (4): 330–42.

Phillips, D. I. W. 1995. "Relation of Fetal Growth to Adult Muscle Mass and Glucose Tolerance." *Diabetic Medicine* 12 (8): 686–90.

Poston, L., R. Bell, H. Croker, A. C. Flynn, K. M. Godfrey, and others. 2015. "Effect of a Behavioural Intervention in Obese Pregnant Women (the UPBEAT Study): A Multicentre, Randomised Controlled Trial." *The Lancet Diabetes and Endocrinology* 3 (10): 767–77.

Potdar, R. D., S. Sahariah, M. Gandhi, S. Kehoe, N. Brown, and others. 2014. "Improving Women's Diet Quality Preconceptionally and during Gestation: Effects on Birth Weight and Prevalence of Low Birth Weight—A Randomized Controlled Efficacy Trial in India (Mumbai Maternal Nutrition Project)." *American Journal of Clinical Nutrition* 100 (5): 1257–68.

Reynolds, R. M., K. Allan, E. Raja, S. Bhattacharya, G. McNeill, and others. 2013. "Maternal Obesity during Pregnancy and Premature Mortality from Cardiovascular Event in Adult Offspring: Follow-Up of 1,323,275 Person-Years." *BMJ* 347 (August 13): F4539.

Rich-Edwards, J. W., K. Kleinman, K. B. Michels, M. J. Stampfer, J. E. Manson, and others. 2005. "Longitudinal Study of Birthweight and Adult Body Mass Index in Predicting Risk of Coronary Heart Disease and Stroke in Women." *BMJ* 330 (7500): 1115.

Richmond, R. C., A. Al-Amin, G. Davey Smith, and C. L. Relton. 2014. "Approaches for Drawing Causal Inferences from Epidemiological Birth Cohorts: A Review." *Early Human Development* 90 (11): 769–80.

Roseboom, T. J., J. H. van der Meulen, C. Osmond, D. J. Barker, A. C. Ravelli, and others. 2000. "Coronary Heart Disease after Prenatal Exposure to the Dutch Famine, 1944–45." *Heart* 84: 595–98.

Sahariah, S. A., R. D. Potdar, M. Gandhi, S. H. Kehoe, N. Brown, and others. 2016. "A Daily Snack Containing Green Leafy Vegetables, Fruit and Milk before and during Pregnancy Prevented Gestational Diabetes in a Randomized Controlled Trial in Mumbai, India." *Journal of Nutrition* 146 (7): 1453S–60S.

Schooling, C. M., C. Jiang, T. Lam, N. Thomas, M. Heys, and others. 2007. "Height, Its Components, and Cardiovascular Risk among Older Chinese: A Cross-Sectional Analysis of the Guangzhou Biobank Cohort Study." *American Journal of Public Health* 97 (10): 1834–41.

Seshiah, V., V. Balaji, M. S. Balaji, C. B. Sanjeevi, and A. Green. 2004. "Gestational Diabetes Mellitus in India." *Journal of the Association of Physicians of India* 52 (September): 707–11.

Skouteris, H., H. Morris, C. Nagle, and A. Nankervis. 2014. "Behavior Modification Techniques Used to Prevent Gestational Diabetes: A Systematic Review of the Literature." *Current Diabetes Reports* 14 (4): 480.

Stein, A. D., M. Wang, M. Ramirez-Zea, R. Flores, R. Grajeda, and others. 2006. "Exposure to a Nutrition Supplementation Intervention in Early Childhood and Risk Factors for Cardiovascular Disease in Adulthood: Evidence from Guatemala." *American Journal of Epidemiology* 164 (12): 1160–70.

Stein, C. E., C. Fall, K. Kumaran, C. Osmond, V. Cox, and others. 1996. "Fetal Growth and Coronary Heart Disease in South India." *The Lancet* 348 (9037): 1269–73.

Stewart, C. P., P. Christian, S. Leclerq, K. P. West Jr., and S. K. Khatry. 2009. "Antenatal Supplementation with Folic Acid + Iron + Zinc Improves Linear Growth and Reduces Peripheral Adiposity in School-Age Children in Rural Nepal." *American Journal of Clinical Nutrition* 90 (1): 132–40.

Stewart, C. P., P. Christian, K. Schulze, S. Leclerq, K. West Jr., and others. 2009. "Antenatal Micronutrient Supplementation Reduces Metabolic Syndrome in 6- to 8-Year-Old Children in Rural Nepal." *Journal of Nutrition* 139 (8): 1575–81.

Swanson, J. M., S. Etringer, C. Buss, and P. Wadhwa. 2009. "Developmental Origins of Health and Disease: Environmental Exposures." *Seminars in Reproductive Medicine* 27 (5): 391–402.

Tanvig, M., C. A. Vinter, J. S. Jørgensen, S. Wehberg, O. G. Ovesen, and others. 2014. "Anthropometrics and Body Composition by Dual Energy X-Ray in Children of Obese Women: A Follow-Up of a Randomized Controlled Trial (the Lifestyle in Pregnancy and Offspring [LiPO] Study)." *PLoS One* 9 (2): e89590.

———. 2015. "Effects of Lifestyle Intervention in Pregnancy and Anthropometrics at Birth on Offspring Metabolic Profile at 2.8 Years: Results from the Lifestyle in Pregnancy and Offspring (LiPO) Study." *Journal of Clinical Endocrinology and Metabolism* 100 (1): 175–83.

Tarry-Adkins, J. L., and S. Ozanne. 2011. "Mechanisms of Early Life Programming: Current Knowledge and Future Directions." *American Journal of Clinical Nutrition* 94 (Suppl 6): S1765–71.

Tu, Y. K., R. West, G. Ellison, and M. Gilthorpe. 2005. "Why Evidence for the Fetal Origins of Adult Disease Might Be a Statistical Artefact: The 'Reversal Paradox' for the Relation between Birth Weight and Blood Pressure in Later Life." *American Journal of Epidemiology* 161 (1): 27–32.

Vafeiadi, M., T. Roumeliotaki, A. Myridakis, G. Chalkiadaki, E. Fthenou, and others. 2016. "Association of Early Life Exposure to Bisphenol A with Obesity and Cardiometabolic Traits in Childhood." *Environmental Research* 146 (April): 379–87.

Vaidya, A., N. Saville, B. Shrestha, A. Costello, D. Manandhar, and others. 2008. "Effects of Antenatal Multiple Micronutrient Supplementation on Children's Weight and Size at 2 Years of Age in Nepal: Follow-Up of a Double-Blind Randomised Controlled Trial." *The Lancet* 371 (9611): 492–99.

Victora, C. G., L. Adair, C. Fall, P. Hallal, R. Martorell, and others. 2008. "Maternal and Child Undernutrition: Consequences for Adult Health and Human Capital." *The Lancet* 371 (9609): 340–57.

Victora, C. G., M. de Onis, P. Hallal, M. Blossner, and R. Shrimpton. 2010. "Worldwide Timing of Growth Faltering: Revisiting Implications for Interventions." *Pediatrics* 125 (3): E473–80.

Vijayakumar, M., C. Fall, C. Osmond, and D. Barker. 1995. "Birth Weight, Weight at 1 Year, and Left Ventricular Mass in Adult Life." *British Heart Journal* 73 (4): 363–67.

Wadsworth, M. E., J. R. Hardy, A. Paul, S. Marshall, and T. Cole. 2002. "Leg and Trunk Length at 43 Years in Relation to Childhood Health, Diet and Family Circumstances: Evidence from the 1946 Cohort." *International Journal of Epidemiology* 31 (2): 383–90.

Wadsworth, M. E., and D. J. Kuh. 1997. "Childhood Influences on Adult Health: A Review of Recent Work from the British 1946 National Birth Cohort Study, the MRC National Survey of Health and Development." *Paediatric and Perinatal Epidemiology* 11 (1): 2–20.

Waters, E., A. De Silva-Sanigorski, B. Burford, T. Brown, K. Campbell, and others. 2011. "Interventions for Preventing Obesity in Children." *Cochrane Database of Systematic Reviews* 12 (December 7): CD001871.

Webb, A. L., A. Conlisk, H. Barnhart, R. Martorell, R. Grajeda, and others. 2005. "Maternal and Childhood Nutrition and Later Blood Pressure Levels in Young Guatemalan Adults." *International Journal of Epidemiology* 34 (4): 898–904.

Wells, J. C., S. Chomtho, and M. Fewtrell. 2007. "Programming of Body Composition by Early Growth and Nutrition." *Proceedings of the Nutrition Society* 66 (3): 423–34.

Whincup, P. H., S. Kaye, C. Owen, R. Huxley, D. Cook, and others. 2008. "Birth Weight and Risk of Type 2 Diabetes: A Quantitative Systematic Review of Published Evidence." *Journal of the American Medical Association* 300 (24): 2885–97.

Chapter 4

Tobacco and Cardiovascular Disease: A Summary of Evidence

Ambuj Roy, Ishita Rawal, Samer Jabbour, and
Dorairaj Prabhakaran

INTRODUCTION

Current and Projected Burden of Tobacco and Cardiovascular Diseases

Tobacco use is a leading global cause of death, accounting for more than 6 million deaths annually or at least 12 percent of deaths among people age 30 years and older (16 percent for men, 7 percent for women) (WHO 2012, 2013). It is the single most preventable cause of cardiovascular diseases (CVDs), which comprise a large number of conditions and are the leading cause of death globally, accounting for an estimated 17.3 million to 17.5 million deaths yearly (Naghavi and others 2015; WHO 2015a). Tobacco is also the leading cause of premature death from CVD (deaths before age 70 years), accounting for an estimated 5.9 million premature deaths in 2013 (Roth, Nguyen, and others 2015). Such deaths deprive families of productive members, and communities and economies of a productive workforce (Rigotti and Clair 2013). Tobacco use also causes substantial morbidity and results in tremendous health care costs related to CVD. Although tobacco use affects all countries regardless of their level of economic or health system development, the impact is most profound in low- and middle-income countries (LMICs), which shoulder the largest share of total and premature deaths from CVD globally (WHO 2015a). Future projections

are alarming, with LMICs accounting for much of the future global burden of tobacco use and related CVD mortality and morbidity (Ezzati and Lopez 2003). China (with 301 million tobacco users) and India have the highest burden of tobacco use in the world (WHO n.d.).

Generally, high rates of tobacco use mean a higher burden of CVD. This association is compounded by population growth and aging, both of which are major contributors to the absolute number of CVD sufferers (Roth, Nguyen, and others 2015).

Reducing tobacco use is thus crucial to averting tobacco deaths, which are projected to increase to 10 million annually by 2030 if current trends continue (WHO 2013, 2015a). Premature deaths from CVDs are also projected to increase to 7.8 million in 2025 if business as usual continues, including in the approach to controlling tobacco use and preventing noncommunicable diseases (Roth, Nguyen, and others 2015). Urgent action is needed to halt and reverse this course.

Mandate and Opportunity for Action

The global mandate for reducing tobacco use is stronger than ever, with the World Health Assembly's adoption of a 30 percent global target for relative reduction of tobacco use by 2025. This goal is one among several targets to reduce premature mortality from four noncommunicable

Corresponding author: Dorairaj Prabhakaran, Centre for Chronic Disease Control, Public Health Foundation of India, Gurgaon, India; dprabhakaran@ccdcindia.org.

diseases, including CVD, by 25 percent by 2025 (the 25×25 target). Unfortunately, many countries are not on course to meet this target (Bilano and others 2015).

Studies clearly show that reducing tobacco use is key to achieving these targets (Kontis and others 2014; Kontis and others 2015). Reducing tobacco use would offset some of the increase in the absolute number of cardiovascular deaths caused by population growth and aging, especially in LMICs (Roth, Forouzanfar, and others 2015). Indeed, several studies demonstrate the need to achieve more ambitious targets for reducing tobacco use (50 percent relative to 2010) if countries are to reach the 25×25 target (Kontis and others 2014; Kontis and others 2015; Roth, Nguyen, and others 2015).

This chapter reviews the literature to synthesize key knowledge on the links between tobacco use and CVD. The introduction on burden of CVD attributable to tobacco is followed by a brief review of the main pathophysiological mechanisms by which tobacco use causes CVD. The third section highlights the role of tobacco and other CVD risk factors, and the fourth reviews tobacco-related CVDs that are most important from a public health and health systems perspective. The focus is on cigarette smoking, but other forms are also discussed in the fifth section. This is followed by a section on the socioeconomic dimensions of tobacco use. The seventh section highlights the cardiovascular health benefits of stopping tobacco use. The concluding section calls for enhanced engagement and cooperation of public health and health care providers to stem the rise of tobacco-related CVDs, especially in LMICs.

TOBACCO USE AND CARDIOVASCULAR DISEASE: PATHOPHYSIOLOGY AND MECHANISMS

Tobacco use has myriad effects on the cardiovascular system that contribute to CVD pathophysiology. Box 4.1 reviews some of the terms used to explain the mechanisms by which tobacco use can cause CVD. The effects of cigarette smoking and exposure to secondhand smoke have been studied most, but many of the effects are common to other forms of use, including smokeless tobacco.

Burning tobacco products produce two forms of smoke: mainstream and sidestream. Mainstream smoke is inhaled and exhaled by the smoker, whereas sidestream smoke comes from the burning end of the cigarette (Ambrose and Barua 2004) and is even more toxic than mainstream smoke (Schick and Glantz 2005). Among the more than 7,000 chemicals in cigarette smoke, many components are known to mediate the pathophysiology of CVD (Borgerding and Klus 2005). Toxic chemicals such as carbon monoxide, polycyclic aromatic hydrocarbons, nicotine, and heavy metals and their oxides have profound effects on vascular endothelium (cells lining the blood vessels), blood lipids (fats), and clotting (thrombotic) factors causing atherosclerosis (plaque buildup). The latter affects arteries (vessels carrying oxygenated blood to organs across various vascular beds). These effects can lead to adverse cardiovascular events such as myocardial infarction (heart attack), stroke (brain attack), and aortic dissection (rupture of the aorta, the main artery emanating

---

Box 4.1

Glossary of Terms

- *Atherosclerosis.* Development of atherosclerotic plaque, which is filled with lipids (fats) and inflammatory substances
- *Atherothrombosis.* Disruption of atherosclerotic plaque with superimposed thrombus formation
- *Coronary vasoconstriction.* Narrowing of the lumen of vessels supplying the heart as a result of contraction of muscular layer
- *Endothelial dysfunction.* Imbalance between dilating and constricting characteristics of the inner lining of the vessel wall that can affect clotting and blood flow
- *Inflammation.* Response of vascular tissues to harmful stimuli in order to remove the cause and initiate repair

- *Myocardial ischemia.* Reduced oxygen supply to the muscles of the heart
- *Oxidative stress.* Disruption of normal cellular structure resulting from damage caused to DNA, proteins, and lipids by reactive oxygen species
- *Prothrombotic state.* The hypercoagulable state, induced by vessel injury and other changes in the blood, that affects the clotting mechanism
- *Sympathetic stimulation.* Stimulation mediated by a sympathetic nervous system and the release of catecholamines to increase the rate and force of contraction.

from the heart). Figure 4.1 illustrates the pathophysiological mechanisms implicated in tobacco-associated atherosclerosis.

The mechanisms by which cigarette smoking induces and promotes atherogenesis and, consequently, atherosclerosis and atherothrombosis are complex and interconnected. The key pathways are inflammation, endothelial dysfunction, prothrombosis, altered lipid metabolism, insulin resistance, and increased demand for but diminished supply of myocardial oxygen and blood (demand-supply mismatch) (U.S. Department of Health and Human Services 2014). Smoking is also known to be responsible for increased release of catecholamines, which exert cardiovascular effects such as increased heart rate, vasoconstriction, and increased cardiac output (Cryer and others 1976). Figure 4.2 displays the key constituents involved in some of these mechanisms.

Briefly, atherogenesis starts when smoking-activated inflammatory cells adhere to the inner vessel wall (endothelium) that has been damaged by smoking and accumulate under the vessel surface (subendothelium), causing chronic inflammation. This and other mechanisms contribute to endothelial dysfunction. Subendothelial inflammatory cells secrete substances that promote the development and growth of plaque through the accumulation of cholesterol-rich cells. Continued inflammation destabilizes and ruptures some of these plaques, causing vasoconstriction (acute narrowing of arteries) and

Figure 4.1 Pathophysiological Mechanisms of Tobacco-Associated Atherosclerosis

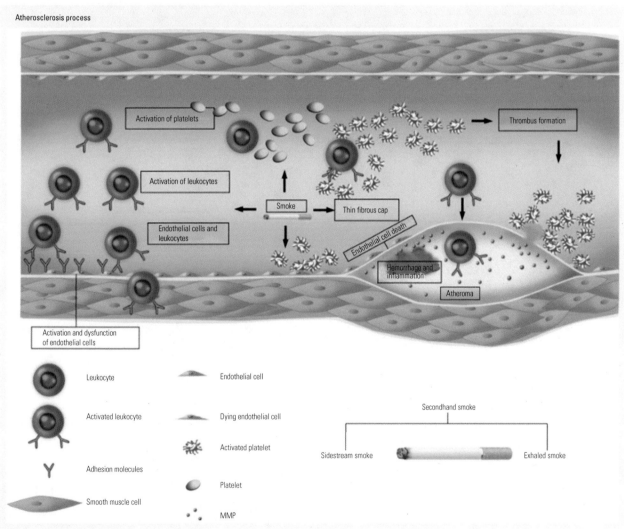

Source: Morris and others 2015.
Note: MMP = matrix metalloproteinase.

Figure 4.2 Overview of Pathophysiological Mechanisms of Tobacco in the Development of Cardiovascular Disease

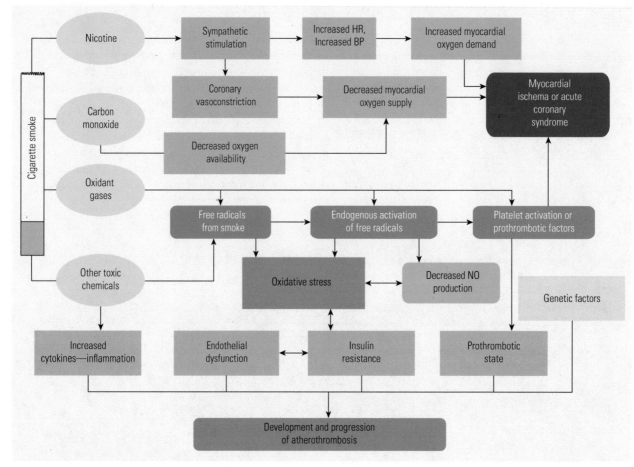

Source: Salahuddin, Prabhakaran, and Roy 2012.
Note: BP = blood pressure; HR = heart rate; NO = nitric oxide.

thrombosis (clots, which are made up mainly of platelets, or thrombocytes, which are components of blood responsible for stopping bleeding). This process can lead to occlusion of blood vessels, causing cardiovascular events such as heart or brain attacks.

Endothelial Dysfunction

A healthy vascular endothelium is crucial to cardiovascular functioning and health. The blood vessels normally dilate in response to external or internal stress and increased demands for flow caused by the endothelium's production and release of nitric oxide (a vessel relaxant), thus maintaining blood flow. A healthy endothelium also fights thrombosis and inflammation. Smoking undermines all of these functions, making endothelial dysfunction (decreased dilatation and ability to fight thrombosis and inflammation) a central mechanism in CVD pathophysiology.

Nicotine, oxidants, and free radicals in smoke—and free radicals generated by endothelial cells themselves in response to smoke—reduce the availability of nitric oxide; thus, there is either no response to stress or vasoconstriction (Barua and others 2001; Ichiki and others 1996; Kugiyama and others 1996; Salahuddin, Prabhakaran, and Roy 2012; U.S. Department of Health and Human Services 2014; Wolf and Baynes 2007). Vasoconstriction can, in turn, increase the prothrombotic (clotting) response, although this is not the only mechanism for thrombosis. Smoking-induced damage to the endothelium also alters the interaction with flowing blood cells, thus increasing the chances that inflammatory substances and platelets will stick to the vessel wall. In addition, this damage decreases the ability of the endothelium to regulate the local levels of clot-forming versus clot-dissolving substances in favor of clotting (Nowak and others 1987; U.S. Department of Health and Human Services 2014). Smoking also reduces the elasticity of arteries, resulting in stiffening and trauma to their walls and reducing coronary flow reserve (Celermajer and others 1993; Celermajer and others 1996; Stefanadis and others 1997).

Other components are also implicated in endothelial dysfunction, including heavy metals such as lead, arsenic, and mercury, which catalyze the oxidation of cellular proteins and may lead to structural cellular damage and endothelial dysfunction. In addition to free radicals and oxidants, further endothelial dysfunction may be mediated by polycyclic aromatic hydrocarbons (Salahuddin, Prabhakaran, and Roy 2012; Wolf and Baynes 2007). These compounds also enhance oxidation of low-density lipoprotein (LDL), as discussed later in this chapter.

The adverse effects of smoking on endothelial function occur early, with recent studies showing that even brief exposure (one hour or less) to smoke, including secondhand smoke, results in endothelial damage and can potentially be long lasting (Juonala and others 2012). Fortunately, quitting smoking is associated with improved endothelial function (Johnson and others 2010).

Prothrombotic Effects of Smoking

Smoking promotes thrombosis through two mechanisms strongly implicated in adverse cardiovascular events: (1) activation and aggregation (clumping together) of platelets and (2) activation of the coagulation (clotting) system (U.S. Department of Health and Human Services 2014). Although the latter mechanism is important and occurs through increased production of thrombosis factors—such as thrombin, fibrinogen, and von Willebrand factor—and decreased dissolution of blood clots (fibrinolysis), the former is especially critical in CVD pathophysiology. This mechanism is largely responsible for thrombi that form in coronary arteries following plaque rupture and cause heart attacks by blocking arterial blood supply to the myocardium.

Several mechanisms explain the platelet-activating effects of smoking. These mechanisms include elevated levels of platelet-activating substance, which are partly caused by oxidation of phospholipids; impaired release of nitric oxide, which inhibits platelet activation, caused by oxidative stress and endothelial dysfunction (Owens and Mackman 2010; Ruggeri 2000); and increased production of substances that promote platelet aggregation (U.S. Department of Health and Human Services 2014). Fibrinogen levels are known to vary with the number of cigarettes smoked, as do high red blood cell count and blood viscosity (Glantz and Parmley 1991; Kannel, D'Agostino, and Belanger 1987; Powell 1998; Smith and Fischer 2001; Smith and others 1997). Smoking also leads to more binding of platelets to white blood cells, a process that is both proinflammatory and prothrombotic and changes the structure of platelets to make them more susceptible to aggregation.

Lipid Oxidation and Insulin Resistance

Although smoking can enhance the endothelial dysfunction caused directly by elevated cholesterol, smoking produces its major impact through lipid oxidation. Cigarette smoking enhances oxidation of plasma LDL cholesterol, the "bad cholesterol" that is proatherogenic and known to impair endothelial function (Frei and others 1991; Heitzer and others 1996; Pech-Amsellem and others 1996). Evidence from animal models supports smoking-induced atherosclerosis through oxidized LDL products (Yamaguchi and others 2000). Simultaneously, the release of neuromodulators such as catecholamines may result in lipolysis, producing free fatty acids in the blood stream (Muscat and others 1991). These modified lipid products are rapidly engulfed by circulating macrophages to form foam cells. These foam cells are an integral part of the atherosclerosis plaque.

Another product of lipid peroxidation (caused by tobacco) is acrolein, an aldehyde that reacts with lipoproteins in high-density lipoprotein (HDL), the "good cholesterol," and modifies them, making them unavailable to remove cholesterol from cells lining the vessels (Shao and others 2005). This process undermines a key mechanism that the body uses to fight atherosclerosis.

Smoking is also associated with increased insulin resistance and hyperinsulinemia, which has been implicated in the link with diabetes and the acceleration of atherosclerosis. Insulin resistance often co-occurs with derangement in lipid metabolism. Chronic smoking influences the accumulation of visceral fat, which further aggravates insulin resistance (Chiolero and others 2008). Insulin secretion may also be affected by the direct action of nicotine on beta cells, which secrete insulin (Bruin and others 2008; Stadler and others 2014; Yoshikawa, Hellström-Lindahl, and Grill 2005). Tobacco smoke dysregulates and imbalances other endocrine secretions (catecholamines, growth hormone) that counter the effect of insulin (Kapoor and Jones 2005).

Proinflammatory Effects of Smoking

CVD is now understood to be an inflammatory condition, with inflammation playing a major role in the initiation and progression of atherosclerosis and the development of cardiovascular events. Inflammatory markers are a harbinger of damage to blood vessels and contribute to all of the pathways already mentioned (Kannel, D'Agostino, and Belanger 1987; Matetzky and others 2000; Newby and others 1999).

Large, well-conducted population studies demonstrate that markers of inflammation, including white blood cells, fibrinogens, interleukin-6, and other proteins, are elevated in smokers (Bermudez and others 2002; Smith and Fischer 2001; Tracy and others 1997). Such markers return to normal baseline levels within five years of quitting smoking, as demonstrated in the Northwick Park Heart Study and the Monitoring of Trends and Determinants in Cardiovascular Disease study (Dobson and others 1991; Meade, Imeson, and Stirling 1987). Using data from 15,489 individuals who participated in the third National Health and Nutrition Examination Survey, Bakhru and Erlinger (2005) demonstrated that inflammatory markers—including C-reactive protein, fibrinogen, white cell count, and albumin—have a dose-dependent, temporal relationship to smoking and smoking cessation, with the markers returning to baseline levels five years after smoking cessation. This finding suggests that the inflammatory pathway of smoking-related CVD may be reversible with smoking cessation and reduced exposure to secondhand smoke.

Oxygen Supply-Demand Mismatch

Nicotine and carbon monoxide, among other components of tobacco smoke, also contribute to CVD by affecting the myocardial (heart muscle) oxygen demand-supply balance (the first two pathways in figure 4.2). Nicotine exerts its cardiometabolic effects through sympathetic stimulation (the adrenaline system) (U.S. Department of Health and Human Services 1988). It increases myocardial oxygen demand by increasing heart rate, blood pressure, and myocardial contractility (pumping), while reducing myocardial blood supply through vasoconstriction and endothelial dysfunction (Salahuddin, Prabhakaran, and Roy 2012). At the same time, stiffness of peripheral arteries and the effect mediated by catecholamines lead to increased myocardial workload. This process results in ischemia (reduced blood and oxygen supply, which, when symptomatic, can produce angina or heart attacks). Carbon monoxide also produces ischemia because it competes with oxygen to combine with hemoglobin, the blood component responsible for carrying oxygen to tissues. Carbon monoxide binds more tightly to hemoglobin and compromises the availability of oxygen to the myocardium (Aronow 1974; Glantz and Parmley 1991).

Role of Genes

Most of the harmful CVD effects of smoking are attributed to the poisonous substances in cigarette smoke.

However, genes also influence the impact of smoking, altering the metabolism of the by-products of smoke and playing an intermediate role in other pathophysiologic pathways leading to CVD (Winkelmann, von Holt, and Unverdorben 2009). While genes may play a marginal role in the addiction to smoking and the relationship to CVD, the epigenetic modification of genes may play a larger role in increasing the risk of CVD. Epigenetic modifications by tobacco smoke of several cells of the body lead to damage of the vessel wall, increasing the tendency toward clotting and inflammation, all of which contribute to CVD (Ambrose and Barua 2004; Breitling 2013; Freson, Izzi, and Van Geet 2012; Schleithoff and others 2012; Vinci, Polvani, and Pesce 2013).

In summary, the interplay of alterations in coronary vasoconstriction, endothelial dysfunction, and altered lipids stimulates a cascade of events leading to atherothrombosis and, subsequently, cardiovascular events such as heart attacks.

TOBACCO USE AND CARDIOVASCULAR DISEASE RISK FACTORS

Smoking and Dyslipidemia

Compared with nonsmokers, smokers have higher levels of bad cholesterol (LDL) and lower serum concentrations of good cholesterol (HDL). Smokers have 3 percent more cholesterol, 9 percent more triglycerides, and 5.7 percent less HDL (Craig, Palomaki, and Haddow 1989). A clinical trial showed that stopping smoking improved total HDL and the amount of large HDL particles, but that it did not affect LDL cholesterol levels or LDL size (Gepner and others 2011). The combination of smoking and dyslipidemia significantly increases the risk of coronary atherosclerotic disease.

Smoking and Hypertension

Smoking unequivocally increases the cardiovascular risks associated with hypertension. However, the role of smoking in altering blood pressure itself remains unclear, given that observational studies in diverse populations, mostly in high-income countries (HICs), have found no association between smoking and blood pressure (Brummett and others 2011; Green, Jucha, and Luz 1986). Blood pressure rises abruptly after smoking starts, but it returns to presmoking levels within a few hours (Tachmes, Fernandez, and Sackner 1978). Age may modify the link between smoking and blood pressure. A large cross-sectional study from a nationally representative sample of adults in the United Kingdom reported higher systolic blood pressure among older male smokers after adjusting for covariates. This was not the same for young smokers, however, or for diastolic blood pressure levels (Primatesta and others 2001). Ambulatory daytime diastolic blood pressure was also significantly higher, by 5 millimeters of mercury (mmHg, a measure of pressure) among tobacco users over "never-users" age 45 years and older. When daytime heart rates of tobacco users and nonusers were compared, those of the former were significantly higher. The increase in heart rate associated with smoking may be the key factor in the added cardiovascular risk associated with smoking in people with high blood pressure.

Smoking and Diabetes

Smokers have more insulin resistance and are more hyperinsulinemic (higher levels of insulin are postulated to be a precursor of type 2 diabetes) compared with nonsmokers (Facchini and others 1992). Cigarette smoking is a risk factor for the development of type 2 diabetes through two pathways (Eliasson 2003). The first is mediated directly through hyperinsulinemia and insulin resistance. The second is mediated through the accumulation of visceral fat, and the effect is confounded by low physical activity and unhealthy diet (Chiolero and others 2008). Evidence is increasing that smoking causes greater accumulation of visceral fat. Several cross-sectional studies indicate that the waist-to-hip ratio is higher in smokers than in nonsmokers (Bamia and others 2004; Canoy and others 2005). Smokers with diabetes have higher hemoglobin A1c levels (glycated hemoglobin, which indicates long-term control of blood sugar), require more insulin, and have increased risk of vascular complications of diabetes such as kidney disease, blindness, and CVD (Zhu and others 2011).

Insulin resistance, central obesity, and dyslipidemia caused by smoking increase the risk of metabolic syndrome—a constellation of metabolic abnormalities that includes high waist circumference, high blood pressure, abnormal blood sugar, and high lipid levels. The mechanistic link between cigarette smoking and insulin resistance has not been fully established, but evidence exists of a role for nicotine. Sympathetic activation and release of corticosteroids and growth hormone by nicotine may contribute to insulin resistance. A systematic review comprehensively investigated the association between smoking and diabetes using compiled results from 88 prospective studies with more than 5 million participants. The pooled relative risk (RR) of diabetes was 1.37 (95 percent confidence interval [CI] 1.33–1.42) among current active smokers and

1.22 (95 percent CI 1.10–1.35) among passive smokers. The study also highlighted the long-term benefits of cessation in reducing diabetes risk to the same level as that of nonsmokers after 10 or more years of abstinence (RR 1.11, 95 percent CI 1.02–1.20) (Pan and others 2015).

Will and others (2001) found a positive association between frequency of smoking and incidence of diabetes in a large cohort study, the Cancer Prevention Study I. The adjusted incidence density ratio (the ratio of the incidence rate among exposed to the incidence rate among unexposed) increased as the number of packs per day increased, from 1.05 for persons smoking less than one pack a day (95 percent CI 0.98–1.12) to 1.45 for persons smoking two or more packs a day (95 percent CI 1.34–1.57). Results of similar magnitude were reported among women. The risk reversed with an increase in the duration of cessation.

Smoking multiplies the risk of CVD in the presence of each of the three main risk factors. For example, the presence of both high blood pressure and smoking results in a striking 15-fold higher risk of stroke. This relationship is graded and consistent across all levels of blood pressure (Neaton and others 1993). Similar effects have been observed for noncigarette and smokeless forms of tobacco use (Boffetta and Straif 2009; Gupta and Asma 2008; Yusuf and others 2004).

CARDIOVASCULAR DISEASE OUTCOMES AND MANIFESTATIONS OF TOBACCO USE

This review focuses on the major CVDs caused by tobacco use, primarily through atherosclerosis of various vessel beds (figure 4.3). The latter include the aorta and vessels originating from it: the coronary arteries (supplying blood to the heart muscle), the carotid and cerebral arteries (supplying blood to the head and brain), and the renal and peripheral arteries (supplying blood to the kidneys and limbs, respectively). Box 4.2 lists the main CVDs and their complications (Ambrose and Barua 2004; Aronow 1974; Borgerding and Klus 2005; Glantz and Parmley 1991; Salahuddin, Prabhakaran, and Roy 2012; U.S. Department of Health and Human Services 1988).

Concerns about the harmful effects of smoking initially centered on lung diseases, but vascular diseases occur earlier in life and contribute to a substantial number of deaths (Lopez, Collishaw, and Piha 1994; U.S. Department of Health and Human Services 1983). Cigarette smoking is known to increase the risk of CVD, just as it is known to increase the risk of hypertension, hypercholesterolemia, and diabetes (U.S. Department of Health and Human Services 1983).

Figure 4.3 Diagram Representing Cardiovascular Manifestations of Tobacco Use

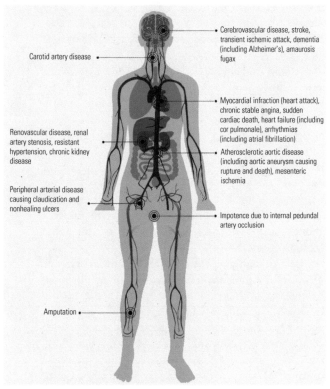

Carotid artery disease

Cerebrovascular disease, stroke, transient ischemic attack, dementia (including Alzheimer's), amaurosis fugax

Myocardial infraction (heart attack), chronic stable angina, sudden cardiac death, heart failure (including cor pulmonale), arrhythmias (including atrial fibrillation)

Renovascular disease, renal artery stenosis, resistant hypertension, chronic kidney disease

Atherosclerotic aortic disease (including aortic aneurysm causing rupture and death), mesenteric ischemia

Peripheral arterial disease causing claudication and nonhealing ulcers

Impotence due to internal pedundal artery occlusion

Amputation

Source: Jana Chams, American University of Beirut.

Smoking and Cardiovascular Mortality

Cigarette smoking increases the rates of all-cause and CVD death (Brummett and others 2011; Qiao and others 2000). The risk of 35-year all-cause mortality and 35-year heart disease mortality is nearly 60 percent higher in smokers than in nonsmokers (Qiao and others 2000). Smoking is an even stronger independent predictor of all-cause and cardiovascular mortality in older adults. Pooled data on more than 500,000 older adults (older than age 60 years) from 25 cohort studies indicate more than a doubling of risk for current smokers and a 37 percent increased risk for former smokers compared with never-smokers (Mons and others 2015).

The seminal work of Doll and others (2004) on the relationship between smoking and cardiovascular mortality followed a large cohort of doctors from 1951 until 2001 to monitor cause-specific mortality and attributed 25 percent of excess risk of death to coronary heart disease (in that cohort). Similarly, in a large cohort of construction workers, age-adjusted coronary heart disease mortality was higher among smokers than nonsmokers and highest among heavy smokers, with almost a doubling of risk (Bolinder and others 1994). Young smokers (younger than age 50 years) were found to have five to six times higher death rates than nonsmokers (Parish and others 1995).

Box 4.2

Major Cardiovascular Diseases Caused by Tobacco Use

- *Coronary (ischemic) heart disease*, including myocardial infarction (heart attacks) and unstable or stable angina (chest pain resulting from blockage in the arteries supplying the heart)
- *Cerebrovascular diseases*, including stroke (brain attack), transient ischemic attacks (mini or transient stroke), and dementia (such as Alzheimer's disease)
- *Arrhythmias* (electrical disturbances of the heart), including sudden death
- *Heart failure*, including left and right heart dysfunction, including cor pulmonale (bad lungs leading to strain on the heart and fluid retention)
- *Aortic disease*, including aneurysm (ballooning of the largest blood vessel in the thorax or abdomen, which can lead to rupture and possibly death)
- *Kidney disease*, including renal artery stenosis (narrowing of arteries to kidneys that leads to reduced blood flow), leading to resistant hypertension and progressive renal failure (potentially leading to dialysis)
- *Peripheral arterial disease* (narrowing of arteries to limbs), causing claudication or pain in walking, limiting mobility, and possibly leading to gangrene and leg amputation
- *Impotence*, including internal pudendal and penile atherosclerosis.

Smoking and Coronary Heart Disease

Coronary (ischemic) heart disease is the most common form of atherosclerotic CVD and is responsible for the largest share of cardiovascular morbidity and mortality. It is also associated with increased risk of sudden death (Aronow 1974; Bolinder and others 1994). Cigarette smoking has been consistently and causally linked to coronary heart disease in prospective studies (Njølstad, Arnesen, and Lund-Larsen 1996; Prescott and others 1998; U.S. Department of Health and Human Services 2010). The INTERHEART study (Yusuf and others 2004), a large international case-control study, showed that smoking tripled the risk of heart attack. The risk was highest among younger patients, in whom tobacco use increased risk more than sevenfold. The risk had a dose-response relationship, increasing linearly with an increase in the number of cigarettes smoked per day and duration of use (Yusuf and others 2004). In addition, women using tobacco lose the gender protection against heart disease noted among women younger than age 50 years (U.S. Department of Health and Human Services 2001). In the Nurses' Health Study (Kawachi and others 1994), heart disease increased more than fourfold (RR 4.23, 95 percent CI 3.6–4.96) among female nurse smokers over never-smokers. This risk was greatest among those who started smoking before age 15 years (Kawachi and others 1994). In a pooled analysis of more than 2.4 million people, female smokers were 25 percent more likely to develop coronary heart disease than male smokers (RR 1.25, 95 percent CI 1.12–1.39) (King 2011).

Smoking and Heart Failure

Heart failure is a rising global public health challenge. It is associated with either reduced myocardial relaxation (stiffness resulting from ischemia or uncontrolled hypertension) or reduced myocardial pumping (because of previous heart attacks). It may also be associated with smoking-related lung conditions, such as chronic obstructive pulmonary disease. Heart failure is often characterized by dyspnea, fluid retention, weight gain, and peripheral edema. Coronary (ischemic) heart disease, in which smoking plays a major part, is among the most common causes of heart failure. Heart failure is especially prevalent in the elderly and is associated with significant mortality and morbidity, requiring repeated hospitalization. It ranks among the top causes of health care costs in HICs. This portends trouble for LMICs currently experiencing a rise in cardiovascular risk factors and diseases known to increase the risk of heart failure.

A systematic review found that smoking is associated with a 60 percent increased risk of incident heart failure (Yang and others 2015). A similar association was found among older people, with the highest risk among current smokers and a dose-effect association among former smokers. The risk of heart failure increases with the number of cigarettes smoked. Men who smoked more than 15 cigarettes a day were at 2.5 times the risk of heart failure compared with never-smokers (odds ratio 2.31, 95 percent CI 1.58–3.37) (Wilhelmsen and others 2008). Continued cigarette smoking is also associated with increased risk of recurrent heart failure. A study retrospectively charting the admission status in a U.S. Veterans Administration facility found that noncompliance with smoking cessation interventions was a significant predictor of multiple readmissions for heart failure, with 80 percent excess risk (Evangelista, Doering, and Dracup 2000).

Smoking and Carotid and Cerebrovascular Diseases

Similar to its association with heart attack, cigarette smoking is causally associated with stroke (Ambrose and Barua 2004; U.S. Department of Health and Human Services 2014). The INTERSTROKE study—a study involving 3,000 cases and controls in 22 countries and designed to establish associations between various risk factors and stroke—revealed that the odds of having ischemic stroke (resulting from occlusion of blood supply to the brain) was 2.3 (99 percent CI 1.9–2.8) and that of having hemorrhagic stroke (bleeding into the brain) was 1.4 (99 percent CI 1.1–1.9) times higher among smokers than among nonsmokers (O'Donnell and others 2010).

Smoking in conjunction with hypertension was the main risk factor identified for stroke, and a dose-response relationship exists with the number of cigarettes smoked per day. A meta-analysis using 32 cohorts and case-control studies involving more than 11,000 stroke events showed a 50 percent overall increase in risk of stroke in smokers. This risk appears to be higher among women, young smokers, and heavy smokers (Shinton and Beevers 1989). Smoking is also strongly implicated in transient ischemic attacks, a transient and milder form of stroke with symptoms typically resolving within 24 hours. Smoking has also been shown to increase the risk of dementia, another increasing global health challenge, including dementia caused by Alzheimer's disease (Cataldo, Prochaska, and Glantz 2010; WHO 2015b).

Smoking and Arrhythmia

Although substantial evidence exists on the role of tobacco in the initiation and progression of atherosclerosis, its role in arrhythmias is less defined and likely to be complex (D'Alessandro and others 2011). Two of the most common conditions associated with smoking—coronary heart disease and chronic lung disease—are both strongly associated with arrhythmias, making it difficult to tease out the direct pro-arrhythmic effects of smoking and its components. Nonetheless, D'Alessandro and others (2011) argue strongly that smoking has direct and acute toxic pro-arrhythmia effects. They propose several mechanisms that mediate the risk: nicotine-induced catecholamine release; myocardial profibrotic effects of nicotine, which can increase susceptibility to catecholamine; oxidative stress; and ischemia or hypoxia, especially associated with carbon monoxide (D'Alessandro and others 2011).

We have alluded to the increased risk of sudden cardiac death in smokers. Smoking has been linked in several studies to ventricular arrhythmia (lethal heart rhythm disorder arising from the lower chambers of the heart) in people with coronary heart disease (Engström and others 1999; Goldenberg and others 2006; Vlietstra and others 1986). Smoking is also associated with increasing risk of supraventricular arrhythmia (often benign fast heart rhythm from the upper chambers of the heart), as documented in a study of the Multicenter Automated Defibrillator Implantation Trial (Goldenberg and others 2006). In addition, smoking is associated with atrial fibrillation, the most common form of supraventricular arrhythmia, with a review suggesting a doubling of risk of atrial fibrillation in smokers (Morris and others 2015). Both the Atherosclerosis Risk in Communities Study (Chamberlain and others 2011), with 15,000 participants, and the Rotterdam Study (Heeringa and others 2008), with 5,668 subjects, showed increased incidence of atrial fibrillation in current smokers (RR 2.05, 95 percent CI 1.71–2.47 and RR 1.51, 95 percent CI 1.07–2.12) and former smokers (RR 1.32, 95 percent CI 1.10–1.57 and RR 1.49, 95 percent CI 1.14–1.97) (Chamberlain and others 2011; Heeringa and others 2008). The risk was dose dependent. The risk also increased in the Manitoba Follow-up Study (Krahn and others 1995). Limitations in older studies may have masked the association between smoking and atrial fibrillation (D'Alessandro and others 2011). Evidence for the link between smoking and arrhythmias also exists in studies showing less arrhythmia in persons who stop smoking (Kinoshita and others 2009; Peters and others 1995).

Smoking and Aortic and Peripheral Artery Disease

It is well established that various risk factors differ in their association with atherosclerosis. Studies confirm that smoking is associated more strongly with aortic disease—particularly abdominal aortic and peripheral arterial disease—than any other risk factor and that the association of smoking with abdominal aortic aneurysm and peripheral arterial disease is much stronger than its association with any other CVD. The EPIC-Norfolk prospective population study, with 21,798 participants, quantified the magnitude of association: smoking increased risk of abdominal aortic aneurysm more than sevenfold (RR 7.66, 95 percent CI 4.50–13.04) and peripheral arterial disease more than fourfold (RR 4.66, 95 percent CI 3.29–6.61) (Stoekenbroek and others 2015). In a large study in the United Kingdom involving 1,937,360 people, the corresponding relative risks were 5.18 (95 percent CI 4.61–5.82) for abdominal aortic aneurysm and 5.16 (95 percent CI 4.80–5.54) for peripheral arterial disease (Pujades-Rodriguez and others 2015). These results are consistent with the findings of a meta-analysis of smoking and peripheral arterial disease involving 55 studies (Lu, Mackay, and Pell 2014). In countries with a high proportion of smokers, nearly 50 percent of peripheral arterial disease can be attributed to smoking (Willigendael and others 2004). Smoking is also strongly associated with the risk of expansion and rupture of an abdominal aortic aneurysm, suggesting that screening for abdominal aortic aneurysm should be restricted to smokers (Howard and others 2015; Sweeting and others 2012). Former smokers have a lower risk of both abdominal aortic aneurysm and peripheral arterial disease.

Smoking and Chronic Kidney Disease

Chronic kidney disease, a condition associated with increased mortality, morbidity, and health care costs, is a growing global public health concern. It is strongly linked to CVD and its risk factors, including smoking. Smokers have a higher risk of macroalbuminuria (elevated urinary albumin excretion) (Halimi and others 2000; Pinto-Sietsma and others 2000). Halimi and colleagues found that renal function, estimated by creatinine clearance, was reduced among smokers. Chronic smoking may result in proteinuria and irreversible kidney damage: the adjusted relative risk was 3.26 (95 percent CI 1.66–6.80) and 2.69 (95 percent CI 1.24–5.99), respectively, among current and former smokers (Halimi and others 2000). Several factors affect the association between smoking and chronic kidney disease, including hemodynamic mechanisms such as cardiorenal syndrome in people with heart failure, and increase in blood pressure, which is known to promote progression of chronic kidney disease (Orth 2004). A large population-based cohort with a median follow-up of 10.3 years demonstrated that smokers younger than age 70 years were at fourfold higher risk of chronic kidney disease than never-smokers (Hallan and Orth 2011). Similarly, in a large population study in Japan, the risk of developing chronic kidney disease was greater among smokers (Yamagata and others 2007). Current male and female smokers had a relative risk of 1.26 (95 percent CI 1.14–1.41) and 1.40 (95 percent CI, 1.16–1.69), respectively, for developing chronic kidney disease over nonsmokers. Persons with preexisting chronic kidney disease have a substantial risk of CVD mortality. In the Cardiovascular Health Study, the group of elderly persons (older than age 65 years) with chronic kidney disease had a CVD risk rate of 32 deaths per 1,000 person-years, compared with 16 per 1,000 person-years in the group without chronic kidney disease, with smoking a major predictor of the same (Shlipak and others 2005).

CARDIOVASCULAR DISEASE ASSOCIATED WITH OTHER FORMS OF TOBACCO USE

Other aspects of cigarette smoking, such as secondhand smoke, also have harmful cardiovascular effects. As detailed in table 4.1, tobacco is consumed worldwide in many forms other than cigarettes, both smoked and smokeless (Saleheen, Zhao, and Rasheed 2014). Although most other forms have been documented to affect cardiovascular health, differences exist in their magnitude and nature of cardiovascular impact (Katsiki and others 2013).

Secondhand Smoke

Also known as environmental tobacco smoke, secondhand smoke has physiological effects similar to those of active smoke: oxidized lipids, increased arterial thickening, and decreased coronary flow velocity (Howard and others 1998; Otsuka and others 2001). Detrimental cardiovascular effects are even demonstrated in exposed children (Raghuveer and other 2016). Many studies have examined the association of secondhand smoke with CVD outcomes and results. An influential meta-analysis of 10 cohort studies and 8 case-control studies showed a 25 percent higher risk (RR 1.25, 95 percent CI 1.17–1.32) of coronary heart disease among nonsmokers exposed to secondhand smoke with a dose-response relationship (He and others 1999). An updated meta-analysis came to a similar conclusion, finding a 27 percent increased risk (RR 1.27, 95 percent CI 1.10–1.48) (Fischer and Kraemer 2015). Similarly, the INTERHEART study, which was not included in the updated meta-analysis, found a 24 percent to 62 percent increased risk with secondhand smoke, depending on the dose of exposure (Teo and others 2006). In focusing on LMICs, Olasky, Levy, and Moran (2012) found a high prevalence of secondhand smoke and increased risk of both ischemic heart disease and stroke. The consistency of these findings after taking account of other (confounding) factors suggests that the association is causal and definitive (Glantz and Parmley 1991). The ill effects of secondhand smoke can be confirmed by the presence of physiological markers of tobacco smoke. Compared with men not exposed to secondhand smoke, those exposed had higher levels of carbon monoxide and lower pulmonary function (Svendsen and others 1987). Biomarkers of CVD, such as C-reactive protein, homocysteine, fibrinogen, and white cell count, were assessed among never-smoking adults participating in the third National Health and Nutrition Examination Survey. It was found that the levels of fibrinogen (mean difference 14.39 milligrams per deciliter, 95 percent CI 5.7–23.1, $p = 0.002$) and homocysteine (mean difference 1.02 micromoles per liter, 95 percent CI 0.6–1.4, $p < 0.001$) were significantly raised among passive smokers with higher cotinine levels when compared with those with no cotinine levels (Venn and Britton 2007).

Thirdhand Smoke

The lasting or residual tobacco smoke contamination that persists after the cigarette is extinguished is referred to as

Table 4.1 Forms of Tobacco Use

Smoked forms of tobacco	Smokeless forms of tobacco
Rolled products: Cigarettes, bidis, kreteks, cheroot, cigars	*Tobacco chewing:* Paan, gutika, mawa, qiwam (khiwam), zarda, khaini
Piped tobacco: Chillum, pipes	*Tobacco sucking:* Naswar (nass), chimo, tommbak, snus, dipping tobacco (moist snuff)
Waterpipes: Sheesha, hookah, goza, narghile (arghileh)	
	Tobacco dentifrice: Masheri (mishri), gul (gudakhu), creamy snuff
	Tobacco sniffing: Dry snuff (tapkeer)

Source: Saleheen, Zhao, and Rasheed 2014.

thirdhand smoke (Winickoff and others 2009). It reflects the contamination of surfaces with tobacco smoke. Surface-mediated reactions of tobacco smoke products (hydrogen cyanide, butane, toluene, polonium-201, and others) may form carcinogenic compounds that accumulate over time to become progressively toxic (Petrick and Dubowski 2011; Sleiman and others 2010). Animal studies have found thirdhand smoke to be associated with increased lipid levels, inflammatory cytokine production, and collagen stimulation, all of which potentially contribute to CVD (Martins-Green and others 2014). Although preliminary research suggests that thirdhand smoke may be associated with a risk of heart disease, the magnitude of risk needs further research.

Other Forms of Tobacco Smoking

Bidi, Cigar, and Pipe

Bidi smoking is practiced in India and other countries in South Asia. Bidi smoking is more common among low-socioeconomic-status groups, raising equity issues related to its use and health effects. Tobacco is wrapped in leaves that are then thinly rolled and secured with threads. Bidi rolling is an unregulated business that includes households, small workshops, and cooperatives that evade regulations and taxes (Gupta and Asma 2008). Bidis have concentrations of nicotine, tar, and other toxic ingredients equal to or greater than those in cigarettes. Given the increased risk of CVD at a young age among the Indian population, the adverse effects of this and other forms of tobacco use have large population-level health impacts. The INTERHEART study revealed that, in addition to cigarette smoking, use of other forms of tobacco such as bidi and chewing tobacco (also common in South Asian countries) was associated with a significantly higher risk of heart attack. The risk with bidi use was as high as the risk with cigarettes, but that of chewed tobacco was slightly lower. However, the risk was highest (fourfold compared with those who never smoked) in individuals who used both smoked and smokeless forms of tobacco (Teo and others 2006). Another hospital-based case-control study confirmed nine times greater risk (RR 9.1, 95 percent CI 4.7–17.7) of myocardial infarction among those who smoked more than 10 bidis a day compared with nonsmokers; the risk was slightly less for persons smoking an equal number of cigarettes per day (RR 7.3, 95 percent CI 3.9–13.8) (Rastogi and others 2005).

Cigars and pipes for smoking tobacco are also associated with risk of CVD. Cigars, tightly rolled bundles of dried and fermented tobacco leaves, are commonly smoked in Brazil, Cameroon, Mexico, and Africa. The relative risk of coronary heart disease among cigar smokers when compared with nonsmokers was 1.27 (95 percent CI 1.12–1.45) (Iribarren and others 1999). The risk was of similar magnitude among British men who smoked either pipes or cigars. The relative risk was 1.59 for coronary heart disease (95 percent CI 1.05–2.39) and 1.83 for stroke (95 percent CI 0.98–3.42) among pipe or cigar smokers when compared with never-smokers (Shaper 2003). Therefore, it is an underestimation to count cigarettes as the only form of tobacco smoking.

Waterpipe Tobacco

Waterpipe (hookah, shisha, or narghile) smoking has been popular among Asians, Arabs, and in other Middle Eastern and some African countries for a long time. This mode of tobacco use has seen a global resurgence recently, especially among youth (Maziak and others 2004). Waterpipe smoking varies widely across the globe. Among men, the prevalence is highest in Vietnam (13 percent) followed by the Arab Republic of Egypt (6.2 percent); among women, it is the highest in the Russian Federation (3.2 percent) (Morton and others 2014). A common misconception is that the smoke gets filtered and becomes less toxic after passing through a water receptacle (Kandela 2000; Varsano and others 2003). Waterpipe smokers engage in longer smoking sessions, which exposes them to more smoke (Shihadeh 2003). Although the health risks associated with waterpipe smoking have not been fully determined, the cardiovascular effects are clear and range from increased heart rate, higher blood pressure, and increased serum fibrinogen to ischemic heart disease, angina, aneurysms, and stroke (El-Zaatari, Chami, and Zaatari 2015). Cumulative exposure to waterpipe smoking is also significantly associated with coronary artery disease. Exposure as high as 40 waterpipe-years (reflecting both duration and dose) was associated with almost a threefold increase in the risk of obstructive coronary disease compared with nonsmokers (Sibai and others 2014). A dose-response relationship exists between heart disease and waterpipe smoking. Among more than 50,000 residents of Golestan, the Islamic Republic of Iran, heavy waterpipe smokers had significantly greater risk of heart disease than nonsmokers (Islami and others 2013).

Smokeless Tobacco

Commonly used in South and Southeast Asia, Sub-Saharan Africa, and Northern Europe, smokeless tobacco has been associated with CVD (Gupta, Gupta, and Khedar 2013). A pooled analysis of both cohort and case-control studies estimated a 13 percent higher risk of fatal heart attack and 40 percent higher risk of fatal stroke among users compared with nonusers, with evidence of a dose-response relationship. The increased risk of fatal myocardial infarction in this meta-analysis appears to be small, but the effect is large at the population level, especially given the consistency of results and robust study designs and analysis (Boffetta and Straif 2009). This finding has prompted strong calls for discouraging the use of smokeless tobacco (Gupta, Gupta, and Khedar 2013; Piano and others 2010).

Electronic Nicotine Delivery Systems (Electronic Cigarettes)

Electronic cigarettes typically involve converting liquid into an aerosol, facilitated by a battery circuit. The liquid contents include nicotine, propylene glycol, flavoring agents, and other substances. Growing awareness and use of electronic cigarettes has been observed among the young and high-income groups, and popularity is growing through advertising (Adkison and others 2013; Regan and others 2013). Electronic cigarettes do not fall under the ambit of regulatory authorities in most countries. Although some have advocated electronic cigarettes as a smoking cessation aid, many public health experts have spoken strongly against popularizing e-cigarettes. This is not only because of concerns about limited evidence of e-cigarettes' aiding cessation; it is also because of evidence of e-cigarettes' toxicity and of their potential to induce smoking in nonsmokers, especially youth, and to perpetuate nicotine addiction among users, thereby jeopardizing users' attempts to quit smoking. The research on the chemical constituents and toxicity of e-cigarettes is growing. This toxicity is particularly concerning in people with CVD (Benowitz and Burbank 2016). This and other reviews (Morris and others 2015) document the many negative cardiovascular effects of e-cigarettes. Furthering the results of chemical and toxicological studies, preclinical research shows that compared with cigarettes, e-cigerettes also have detrimental effects on vascular function, specifically oxidative stress and endothelial function (Carnevale and others 2016). Clinical studies of the chronic cardiovascular effects of e-cigarettes are forthcoming.

SOCIOECONOMIC DIMENSIONS OF TOBACCO-USE-RELATED CARDIOVASCULAR DISEASES

Many socioeconomic variables modify the relationship between tobacco use and CVD. We have alluded to some of these and their interactions, for example, age (young male smokers are at higher risk of sudden death), gender (women have more risk for coronary heart disease), and ethnicity (South Asians face greater risks) (Huxley and Woodward 2011). However, it is crucial to consider many other socioeconomic dimensions, such as the impact of heterogeneous macroeconomic and human development, income inequality, and socioeconomic status. The tobacco industry quickly takes advantage of the opportunities provided by urbanization and improved social standards. Their ubiquitous packaging and advertisements reach out to all segments of society, making tobacco products available and accessible (Bhan and others 2016). In most settings, strong socioeconomic gradients have persisted, with smoking being more prevalent among the poor and disadvantaged groups. This outcome can be explained by lack of knowledge, inadequate penetration of behavioral interventions, and inability to choose healthy options (Laaksonen and others 2005). The expenses associated with smoking often divert the resources of vulnerable groups from basic necessities. Although the links between each of these variables and either tobacco use or CVD have been well researched, their complex interactions as modifiers of the link between tobacco use and CVD have been less studied, especially in LMICs. This is an important agenda for future research. It is critical to understand the effects of these factors because they determine temporal patterns, quit attempts, and inequalities in morbidity and mortality, and to direct specific interventions to target groups.

CARDIOVASCULAR BENEFITS OF TOBACCO USE CESSATION

The profound cardiovascular harm of tobacco use and its global toll, especially in LMICs, indicates that prevention of tobacco initiation and lifelong avoidance of all tobacco products are the best strategies. The link has prompted calls for a tobacco-free world (Beaglehole and others 2015). The evidence for the cardiovascular benefits of tobacco cessation, particularly cigarette smoking, is compelling (box 4.3). Smoking cessation benefits all users, irrespective of form, duration, and age. Cardiovascular benefits are consistent and set in early after tobacco cessation (Bakhru and Erlinger 2005; Gratziou 2009; Hatsukami and others 2005).

In general population studies, smoking cessation has clearly been shown to prolong life, especially when it occurs early in life. For example, in a cohort of doctors followed for 50 years, smokers who continued to smoke lost, on average, 10 years of life (Doll and others 2004). The years of life gained were three, six, and nine for those who stopped at ages 60, 50, and 40, respectively. However, this relationship does not set a threshold age for quitting, and age should not be a refraining factor for quitting—even the elderly benefit from smoking cessation (Burns 2000).

Time to Cardiovascular Benefit of Smoking Cessation after Last Cigarette

- *Within 20 minutes.* Blood pressure decreases and body temperature and pulse rate return to normal.
- *Within 24 hours.* Risk of myocardial infarction decreases.
- *Within 1 year.* Excess risk of coronary heart disease is half that of a person who smokes.
- *At 5 years.* Stroke risk is reduced to that of someone who has never smoked.
- *Within 15 years.* Coronary heart disease risk is the same as a person who has never smoked.

In people diagnosed with CVD, persistent smoking is associated with a significant increase in cardiovascular events and mortality (Buckley and others 2009; Simpson and others 2011). Tobacco cessation is a key intervention for preventing further cardiovascular events, particularly heart attacks, and for prolonging survival. A meta-analysis of 12 cohort studies reported a reduction in mortality, irrespective of gender, duration of follow-up, or time of assessment of smoking status after the cardiovascular event. The overall reduction in mortality after a mean follow-up of 4.8 years was nearly 50 percent (odds ratio 0.54, 95 percent CI 0.46–0.62) (Wilson and others 2000). The systematic review by Critchley and Capewell (2003) of 20 cohort studies of patients with coronary heart disease, with at least two years of follow-up, estimated that one-third of CVD outcomes—such as coronary artery bypass surgery, angioplasty, and recurrent heart attacks— can be prevented by quitting smoking (Critchley and Capewell 2003). Unfortunately, numerous studies in diverse populations (HICs and LMICs) have documented persistent smoking in people who have been diagnosed with CVD, including those who have suffered heart attacks. Several barriers are described in the literature, including lack of support to quit, lack of resources to quit, cultural norms, and stressful living conditions (Rosenthal and others 2013; Twyman and others 2014). In addition to the barriers perceived by the smokers, physicians perceive an additional set of barriers, including their own disbelief in the effectiveness of lifestyle intervention, lack of adequate counseling skills, and scarcity of time during their practice (Ockene and Miller 1997). These barriers indicate a tremendous missed opportunity for secondary prevention, especially among patients with CVD. Because strong advice by health care providers, particularly physicians, leads to more quitting, there have been calls for cardiovascular specialists to pay greater attention to smoking cessation (Jabbour and others 2002). Patient-centered advice does not take much time and helps the patient gain confidence to attempt and maintain cessation.

Although interventions targeted at individual smokers are important, policy interventions, particularly for persons at high risk of or with existing CVD, are also crucial for reducing overall rates of tobacco use at the population level. The World Health Organization (WHO) Framework Convention on Tobacco Control is a comprehensive, binding convention that provides member countries, now numbering 180, with measures and corresponding guidelines to reduce both demand and supply (see Jha and others [2015] for a more detailed discussion of strategies of tobacco control). The cardiovascular impact of implementing various policy measures in the framework has been studied, with smoke-free legislation and policies banning smoking in public spaces receiving the most attention. A meta-analysis of 31 studies of cardiovascular impact in 47 locations showed a 12 percent reduction in hospitalization for acute coronary events (RR 0.88, 95 percent CI 0.85–0.90). At places where the reduction in smoking prevalence was more than the mean (2.1 percent reduction) there was a 14 percent reduction in events after the enforcement of legislation (Jones and others 2014). This impact translates into large benefits at the population level. Although it is difficult to know with certainty what proportion of the benefit comes from reduced exposure to secondhand smoke in nonsmokers as opposed to reduced consumption or more quitting among smokers, evidence suggests that both smokers and nonsmokers benefit (Seo and Torabi 2007).

CONCLUSIONS

Robust evidence indicates that tobacco use causes atherosclerotic CVD. The link is strong with various forms of tobacco use, and the magnitude is substantial and consistent across all cardiovascular manifestations.

Tobacco use acts both independently of and synergistically with other risk factors common to CVD. Complex mechanisms underlie the pathophysiology of tobacco-attributed CVD. The risk appears to be higher among younger age groups who are smoking more cigarettes a day, among women than among men, and in certain ethnicities such as South Asians.

The most common manifestations of tobacco-related CVD include myocardial infarction, angina, stroke, aortic aneurysm, and peripheral artery disease. However, heart failure, chronic kidney disease, and atrial fibrillation are emerging as global health issues. These manifestations lead to morbidity, premature mortality, loss of productive years of life, and tremendous health care costs, burdening already stretched health systems, especially in LMICs.

Tobacco cessation protects against CVD at all ages and adds years to life. Population- and individual-level interventions to reduce the number of people starting to smoke and getting more people to quit have great promise, especially for those with or at high risk of CVD. Implementation of the full provisions of the Framework Convention on Tobacco Control provides a clear path toward a world free of tobacco use and where tobacco-related CVD becomes a thing of the past.

NOTES

Professor Dorairaj Prabhakaran is supported through a research grant from the Wellcome Trust and the National Heart, Lung, and Blood Institute of the United States (Contract no. HHSN268200900026C).

World Bank Income Classifications as of July 2014 are as follows, based on estimates of gross national income per capita for 2013:

- Low-income countries = US$1,045 or less
- Middle-income countries are subdivided:
  (a) lower-middle-income = US$1,046 to US$4,125
  (b) upper-middle-income = US$4,126 to US$12,745
- High-income countries = US$12,746 or more.

REFERENCES

Adkison, S. E., R. J. O'Connor, M. Bansal-Travers, A. Hyland, R. Borland, and others. 2013. "Electronic Nicotine Delivery Systems: International Tobacco Control Four-Country Survey." *American Journal of Preventive Medicine* 44 (3): 207–15.

Ambrose, J. A., and R. S. Barua. 2004. "The Pathophysiology of Cigarette Smoking and Cardiovascular Disease: An Update." *Journal of the American College of Cardiology* 43 (10): 1731–37.

Aronow, W. S. 1974. "Tobacco and the Heart." *JAMA* 229 (13): 1799–800.

Bakhru, A., and T. P. Erlinger. 2005. "Smoking Cessation and Cardiovascular Disease Risk Factors: Results from the Third National Health and Nutrition Examination Survey." *PLoS Medicine* 2 (6): e160.

Bamia, C., A. Trichopoulou, D. Lenas, and D. Trichopoulos. 2004. "Tobacco Smoking in Relation to Body Fat Mass and Distribution in a General Population Sample." *International Journal of Obesity and Related Metabolic Disorders* 28 (8): 1091–96.

Barua, R. S., J. A. Ambrose, L.-J. Eales-Reynolds, M. C. DeVoe, J. G. Zervas, and D. C. Saha. 2001. "Dysfunctional Endothelial Nitric Oxide Biosynthesis in Healthy Smokers with Impaired Endothelium-Dependent Vasodilatation." *Circulation* 104 (16): 1905–10.

Beaglehole, R., R. Bonita, D. Yach, J. Mackay, and K. S. Reddy. 2015. "A Tobacco-Free World: A Call to Action to Phase Out the Sale of Tobacco Products by 2040." *The Lancet* 385 (9972): 1011–18.

Benowitz, N. L., and A. D. Burbank. 2016. "Cardiovascular Toxicity of Nicotine: Implications for Electronic Cigarette Use." *Trends in Cardiovascular Medicine* 26 (6): 515–23.

Bermudez, E. A., N. Rifai, J. E. Buring, J. E. Manson, and P. M. Ridker. 2002. "Relation between Markers of Systemic Vascular Inflammation and Smoking in Women." *American Journal of Cardiology* 89 (9): 1117–19.

Bhan, N., A. Karan, S. Srivastava, S. Selvaraj, S. V. Subramanian, and others. 2016. "Have Socioeconomic Inequalities in Tobacco Use in India Increased over Time? Trends from the National Sample Surveys (2000–2012)." *Nicotine and Tobacco Research* (April): ii.

Bilano, V., S. Gilmour, T. Moffiet, E. T. d'Espaignet, and G. A. Stevens. 2015. "Global Trends and Projections for Tobacco Use, 1990–2025: An Analysis of Smoking Indicators from the WHO Comprehensive Information Systems for Tobacco Control." *The Lancet* 385 (9972): 966–76.

Boffetta, P., and K. Straif. 2009. "Use of Smokeless Tobacco and Risk of Myocardial Infarction and Stroke: Systematic Review with Meta-Analysis." *BMJ* 339 (August): 1–6.

Bolinder, G., L. Alfredsson, A. Englund, and U. de Faire. 1994. "Smokeless Tobacco Use and Increased Cardiovascular Mortality among Swedish Construction Workers." *American Journal of Public Health* 84 (3): 399–404.

Borgerding, M., and H. Klus. 2005. "Analysis of Complex Mixtures—Cigarette Smoke." *Experimental and Toxicologic Pathology* 57 (Suppl 1): 43–73.

Breitling, L. P. 2013. "Current Genetics and Epigenetics of Smoking/Tobacco-Related Cardiovascular Disease." *Arteriosclerosis, Thrombosis, and Vascular Biology* 33 (7): 1468–72.

Bruin, J. E., H. C. Gerstein, K. M. Morrison, and A. C. Holloway. 2008. "Increased Pancreatic Beta-Cell Apoptosis Following Fetal and Neonatal Exposure to Nicotine Is Mediated via the Mitochondria." *Toxicological Sciences* 103 (2): 362–70.

Brummett, B. H., M. A. Babyak, I. C. Siegler, M. Shanahan, K. M. Harris, and others. 2011. "Systolic Blood Pressure, Socioeconomic Status, and Biobehavioral Risk Factors in a Nationally Representative U.S. Young Adult Sample." *Hypertension* 58 (2): 161–66.

Buckley, B. S., C. R. Simpson, D. J. McLernon, A. W. Murphy, and P. C. Hannaford. 2009. "Five-Year Prognosis in Patients with Angina Identified in Primary Care: Incident Cohort Study." *BMJ* 339 (August): b3058.

Burns, D. M. 2000. "Cigarette Smoking among the Elderly: Disease Consequences and the Benefits of Cessation." *American Journal of Health Promotion* 14 (6): 357–61.

Canoy, D., N. Wareham, R. Luben, A. Welch, S. Bingham, and others. 2005. "Cigarette Smoking and Fat Distribution in 21,828 British Men and Women: A Population-Based Study." *Obesity Research* 13 (8): 1466–75.

Carnevale, R., S. Sciarretta, F. Violi, C. Nocella, L. Loffredo, and others. 2016. "Acute Impact of Tobacco vs Electronic Cigarette Smoking on Oxidative Stress and Vascular Function." *Chest* 150 (3): 606–12

Cataldo, J. K., J. J. Prochaska, and S. A. Glantz. 2010. "Cigarette Smoking Is a Risk Factor for Alzheimer's Disease: An Analysis Controlling for Tobacco Industry Affiliation." *Journal of Alzheimer's Disease* 19 (2): 465–80.

Celermajer, D. S., M. R. Adams, P. Clarkson, J. Robinson, R. McCredie, and others. 1996. "Passive Smoking and Impaired Endothelium-Dependent Arterial Dilatation in Healthy Young Adults." *New England Journal of Medicine* 334 (3): 150–54.

Celermajer, D. S., K. E. Sorensen, D. Georgakopoulos, C. Bull, O. Thomas, and others. 1993. "Cigarette Smoking Is Associated with Dose-Related and Potentially Reversible Impairment of Endothelium-Dependent Dilation in Healthy Young Adults." *Circulation* 88 (5): 2149–55.

Chamberlain, A. M., S. K. Agarwal, A. R. Folsom, S. Duval, E. Z. Soliman, and others. 2011. "Smoking and Incidence of Atrial Fibrillation: Results from the Atherosclerosis Risk in Communities Study." *Heart Rhythm* 8 (8): 1160–66.

Chiolero, A., D. Faeh, F. Paccaud, and J. Cornuz. 2008. "Consequences of Smoking for Body Weight, Body Fat Distribution, and Insulin Resistance." *American Journal of Clinical Nutrition* 87 (4): 801–9.

Craig, W. Y., G. E. Palomaki, and J. E. Haddow. 1989. "Cigarette Smoking and Serum Lipid and Lipoprotein Concentrations: An Analysis of Published Data." *BMJ* 298 (6676): 784–88.

Critchley, J. A., and S. Capewell. 2003. "Mortality Risk Reduction Associated with Smoking Cessation in Patients with Coronary Heart Disease: A Systematic Review." *JAMA* 290 (1): 86–97.

Cryer, P. E., M. W. Haymond, J. V. Santiago, and S. D. Shah. 1976. "Norepinephrine and Epinephrine Release and Adrenergic Mediation of Smoking-Associated Hemodynamic and Metabolic Events." *New England Journal of Medicine* 295 (11): 573–77.

D'Alessandro, A., I. Boeckelmann, M. Hammwhoner, and A. Goette. 2011. "Nicotine, Cigarette Smoking, and Cardiac Arrhythmia: An Overview." *European Journal of Preventive Cardiology* 19 (3): 297–305.

Dobson, A. J., H. M. Alexander, R. F. Heller, and D. M. Lloyd. 1991. "How Soon after Quitting Smoking Does Risk of Heart Attack Decline?" *Journal of Clinical Epidemiology* 44 (11): 1247–53.

Doll, R., R. Peto, J. Boreham, and I. Sutherland. 2004. "Mortality in Relation to Smoking: 50 Years' Observations on Male British Doctors." *BMJ* 328 (7455): 1519.

Eliasson, B. 2003. "Cigarette Smoking and Diabetes." *Progress in Cardiovascular Diseases* 45 (5): 405–13.

El-Zaatari, Z. M., H. A. Chami, and G. S. Zaatari. 2015. "Health Effects Associated with Waterpipe Smoking." *Tobacco Control* 24 (Suppl 1): i31–43.

Engström, G., B. Hedblad, L. Janzon, and S. Juul-Möller. 1999. "Ventricular Arrhythmias during 24-H Ambulatory ECG Recording: Incidence, Risk Factors, and Prognosis in Men with and without a History of Cardiovascular Disease." *Journal of Internal Medicine* 246 (4): 363–72.

Evangelista, L. S., L. V. Doering, and K. Dracup. 2000. "Usefulness of a History of Tobacco and Alcohol Use in Predicting Multiple Heart Failure Readmissions among Veterans." *American Journal of Cardiology* 86 (12): 1339–42.

Ezzati, M., and A. D. Lopez. 2003. "Estimates of Global Mortality Attributable to Smoking in 2000." *The Lancet* 362 (9387): 847–52.

Facchini, F. S., C. B. Hollenbeck, J. Jeppesen, Y. D. Chen, and G. M. Reaven. 1992. "Insulin Resistance and Cigarette Smoking." *The Lancet* 339 (8802) 1128–30.

Fischer, F., and A. Kraemer. 2015. "Meta-Analysis of the Association between Second-Hand Smoke Exposure and Ischaemic Heart Diseases, COPD, and Stroke." *BMC Public Health* 15 (December): 1202.

Frei, B., T. M. Forte, B. N. Ames, and C. E. Cross. 1991. "Gas Phase Oxidants of Cigarette Smoke Induce Lipid Peroxidation and Changes in Lipoprotein Properties in Human Blood Plasma: Protective Effects of Ascorbic Acid." *Biochemical Journal* 277 (Pt 1): 133–38.

Freson, K., B. Izzi, and C. Van Geet. 2012. "From Genetics to Epigenetics in Platelet Research." *Thrombosis Research* 129 (3): 325–29.

Gepner, A. D., M. E. Piper, H. M. Johnson, M. C. Fiore, T. B. Baker, and others. 2011. "Effects of Smoking and Smoking Cessation on Lipids and Lipoproteins: Outcomes from a Randomized Clinical Trial." *American Heart Journal* 161 (1): 145–51.

Glantz, S. A., and W. W. Parmley. 1991. "Passive Smoking and Heart Disease. Epidemiology, Physiology, and Biochemistry." *Circulation* 83 (1): 1–12.

Goldenberg, I., A. J. Moss, S. McNitt, W. Zareba, J. P. Daubert, and others. 2006. "Cigarette Smoking and the Risk of Supraventricular and Ventricular Tachyarrhythmias in High-Risk Cardiac Patients with Implantable Cardioverter Defibrillators." *Journal of Cardiovascular Electrophysiology* 17 (9): 931–36.

Gratziou, C. 2009. "Respiratory, Cardiovascular, and Other Physiological Consequences of Smoking Cessation." *Current Medical Research and Opinion* 25 (2): 535–45.

Green, M. S., E. Jucha, and Y. Luz. 1986. "Blood Pressure in Smokers and Nonsmokers: Epidemiologic Findings." *American Heart Journal* 111 (5): 932–40.

Gupta, P. C., and S. Asma, eds. 2008. *Bidi Smoking and Public Health*. New Delhi: Ministry of Health and Family Welfare, Government of India.

Gupta, R., N. Gupta, and R. S. Khedar. 2013. "Smokeless Tobacco and Cardiovascular Disease in Low- and Middle-Income Countries." *Indian Heart Journal* 65 (4): 369–77.

Halimi, J. M., B. Giraudeau, S. Vol, E. Cacès, H. Nivet, and others. 2000. "Effects of Current Smoking and Smoking Discontinuation on Renal Function and Proteinuria in the General Population." *Kidney International* 58 (3): 1285–92.

Hallan, S. I., and S. R. Orth. 2011. "Smoking Is a Risk Factor in the Progression to Kidney Failure." *Kidney International* 80 (5): 516–523.

Hatsukami, D. K., M. Kotlyar, S. Allen, J. Jensen, S. Li, and others. 2005. "Effects of Cigarette Reduction on Cardiovascular Risk Factors and Subjective Measures." *Chest* 128 (4): 2528–37.

He, J., S. Vupputuri, K. Allen, M. R. Prerost, J. Hughes, and others. 1999. "Passive Smoking and the Risk of Coronary Heart Disease: A Meta-Analysis of Epidemiologic Studies." *New England Journal of Medicine* 340 (12): 920–26.

Heeringa, J., J. A. Kors, A. Hofman, F. J. A. van Rooij, and J. C. M. Witteman. 2008. "Cigarette Smoking and Risk of Atrial Fibrillation: The Rotterdam Study." *American Heart Journal* 156 (6): 1163–69.

Heitzer, T., S. Ylä-Herttuala, J. Luoma, S. Kurz, T. Münzel, and others. 1996. "Cigarette Smoking Potentiates Endothelial Dysfunction of Forearm Resistance Vessels in Patients with Hypercholesterolemia: Role of Oxidized LDL." *Circulation* 93 (7): 1346–53.

Howard, D. P. J., A. Banerjee, J. F. Fairhead, A. Handa, L. E. Silver, and others. 2015. "Population-Based Study of Incidence of Acute Abdominal Aortic Aneurysms with Projected Impact of Screening Strategy." *Journal of the American Heart Association* 4 (8): e001926.

Howard, G., L. E. Wagenknecht, G. L. Burke, A. Diez-Roux, G. W. Evans, and others. 1998. "Cigarette Smoking and Progression of Atherosclerosis: The Atherosclerosis Risk in Communities Study." *Journal of the American Medical Association* 279 (2): 119–24.

Huxley, R. R., and M. Woodward. 2011. "Cigarette Smoking as a Risk Factor for Coronary Heart Disease in Women Compared with Men: A Systematic Review and Meta-Analysis of Prospective Cohort Studies." *The Lancet* 378 (9799): 1297–305.

Ichiki, K., H. Ikeda, N. Haramaki, T. Ueno, and T. Imaizumi. 1996. "Long-Term Smoking Impairs Platelet-Derived Nitric Oxide Release." *Circulation* 94 (12): 3109–14.

Iribarren, C., I. S. Tekawa, S. Sidney, and G. D. Friedman. 1999. "Effect of Cigar Smoking on the Risk of Cardiovascular Disease, Chronic Obstructive Pulmonary Disease, and Cancer in Men." *New England Journal of Medicine* 340 (23): 1773–80.

Islami, F., A. Pourshams, R. Vedanthan, H. Poustchi, F. Kamangar, and others. 2013. "Smoking Water-Pipe, Chewing Nass, and Prevalence of Heart Disease: A Cross-Sectional Analysis of Baseline Data from the Golestan Cohort Study, Iran." *Heart* 99 (4): 272–78.

Jabbour, S., K. S. Reddy, W. F. T. Muna, and A. Achutti. 2002. "Cardiovascular Disease and the Global Tobacco Epidemic: A Wake-Up Call for Cardiologists." *International Journal of Cardiology* 86 (2–3): 185–92.

Jha, P., M. MacLennan, F. J. Chaloupka, A. Yureki, C. Ramasundarahettige, and others. 2015. "Global Hazards of Tobacco and the Benefits of Smoking Cessation and Tobacco Taxes." In *Disease Control Priorities* (third edition): Volume 3, *Cancer*, edited by H. Gelband, P. Jha, R. Sankaranarayanan, and S. Horton. Washington, DC: World Bank.

Johnson, H. M., L. K. Gossett, M. E. Piper, S. E. Aeschlimann, C. E. Korcarz, and others. 2010. "Effects of Smoking and Smoking Cessation on Endothelial Function: 1-Year Outcomes from a Randomized Clinical Trial." *Journal of the American College of Cardiology* 55 (18): 1988–95.

Jones, M. R., J. Barnoya, S. Stranges, L. Losonczy, and A. Navas-Acien. 2014. "Cardiovascular Events Following Smoke-Free Legislations: An Updated Systematic Review and Meta-Analysis." *Current Environmental Health Reports* 1 (3): 239–49.

Juonala, M., C. G. Magnussen, A. Venn, S. Gall, M. Kähönen, and others. 2012. "Parental Smoking in Childhood and Brachial Artery Flow-Mediated Dilatation in Young Adults: The Cardiovascular Risk in Young Finns Study and the Childhood Determinants of Adult Health Study." *Arteriosclerosis, Thrombosis, and Vascular Biology* 32 (4): 1024–31.

Kandela, P. 2000. "Nargile Smoking Keeps Arabs in Wonderland." *The Lancet* 356 (9236): 1175.

Kannel, W. B., R. B. D'Agostino, and A. J. Belanger. 1987. "Fibrinogen, Cigarette Smoking, and Risk of Cardiovascular Disease: Insights from the Framingham Study." *American Heart Journal* 113 (4): 1006–10.

Kapoor, D., and T. H. Jones. 2005. "Smoking and Hormones in Health and Endocrine Disorders." *European Journal of Endocrinology* 152 (4): 491–99.

Katsiki, N., S. K. Papadopoulou, A. I. Fachantidou, and D. P. Mikhailidis. 2013. "Smoking and Vascular Risk: Are All Forms of Smoking Harmful to All Types of Vascular Disease?" *Public Health* 127 (5): 435–41.

Kawachi, I., G. A. Colditz, M. J. Stampfer, W. C. Willett, J. E. Manson, and others. 1994. "Smoking Cessation and Time Course of Decreased Risks of Coronary Heart Disease in Middle-Aged Women." *Archives of Internal Medicine* 154 (2): 169–75.

King, A. 2011. "Risk Factors: Cigarette Smoking Increases the Risk of Coronary Heart Disease in Women More than in Men." *Nature Reviews Cardiology* 8 (November): 612.

Kinoshita, M., R. M. Herges, D. O. Hodge, L. Friedman, N. M. Ammash, and others. 2009. "Role of Smoking in the Recurrence of Atrial Arrhythmias after Cardioversion." *American Journal of Cardiology* 104 (5): 678–82.

Kontis, V., C. D. Mathers, R. Bonita, G. A. Stevens, J. Rehm, and others. 2015. "Regional Contributions of Six Preventable Risk Factors to Achieving the 25×25 Non-Communicable Disease Mortality Reduction Target: A Modelling Study." *The Lancet Global Health* 3 (12): e746–57.

Kontis, V., C. D. Mathers, J. Rehm, G. A. Stevens, K. D. Shield, and others. 2014. "Contribution of Six Risk Factors to Achieving the 25×25 Non-Communicable Disease Mortality Reduction Target: A Modelling Study." *The Lancet* 384 (9941): 427–37.

Krahn, A. D., J. Manfreda, R. B. Tate, F. A. Mathewson, and T. E. Cuddy. 1995. "The Natural History of Atrial Fibrillation: Incidence, Risk Factors, and Prognosis in the Manitoba Follow-Up Study." *American Journal of Medicine* 98 (5): 476–84.

Kugiyama, K., H. Yasue, M. Ohgushi, T. Motoyama, H. Kawano, and others. 1996. "Deficiency in Nitric Oxide Bioactivity in Epicardial Coronary Arteries of Cigarette Smokers." *Journal of the American College of Cardiology* 28 (5): 1161–67.

Laaksonen, M., O. Rahkonen, S. Karvonen, and E. Lahelma. 2005. "Socioeconomic Status and Smoking: Analysing Inequalities with Multiple Indicators." *European Journal of Public Health* 15 (3): 262–69.

Lopez, A. D., N. E. Collishaw, and T. Piha. 1994. "A Descriptive Model of the Cigarette Epidemic in Developed Countries." *Tobacco Control* 3 (3): 242–47.

Lu, L., D. F. Mackay, and J. P. Pell. 2014. "Meta-Analysis of the Association between Cigarette Smoking and Peripheral Arterial Disease." *Heart* 100 (5): 414–23.

Martins-Green, M., N. Adhami, M. Frankos, M. Valdez, B. Goodwin, and others. 2014. "Cigarette Smoke Toxins Deposited on Surfaces: Implications for Human Health." *PLoS One* 9 (1): e86391.

Matetzky, S., S. Tani, S. Kangavari, P. Dimayuga, J. Yano, and others. 2000. "Smoking Increases Tissue Factor Expression in Atherosclerotic Plaques: Implications for Plaque Thrombogenicity." *Circulation* 102 (6): 602–04.

Maziak, W., K. D. Ward, R. A. Afifi Soweid, and T. Eissenberg. 2004. "Tobacco Smoking Using a Waterpipe: A Re-Emerging Strain in a Global Epidemic." *Tobacco Control* 13 (4): 327–33.

Meade, T. W., J. Imeson, and Y. Stirling. 1987. "Effects of Changes in Smoking and Other Characteristics on Clotting Factors and the Risk of Ischaemic Heart Disease." *The Lancet* 2 (8566): 986–88.

Mons, U., A. Müezzinler, C. Gellert, B. Schöttker, C. C. Abnet, and others. 2015. "Impact of Smoking and Smoking Cessation on Cardiovascular Events and Mortality among Older Adults: Meta-Analysis of Individual Participant Data from Prospective Cohort Studies of the Chances Consortium." *BMJ* 350 (April): h1551.

Morris, P. B., B. A. Ference, E. Jahangir, D. N. Feldman, J. J. Ryan, and others. 2015. "Cardiovascular Effects of Exposure to Cigarette Smoke and Electronic Cigarettes." *Journal of the American College of Cardiology* 66 (12): 1378–91.

Morton, J., Y. Song, H. Fouad, F. El Awa, R. Abou El Naga, and others. 2014. "Cross-Country Comparison of Waterpipe Use: Nationally Representative Data from 13 Low- and Middle-Income Countries from the Global Adult Tobacco Survey (GATS)." *Tobacco Control* 23 (5): 419–27.

Muscat, J. E., R. E. Harris, N. J. Haley, and E. L. Wynder. 1991. "Cigarette Smoking and Plasma Cholesterol." *American Heart Journal* 121 (1, Pt 1): 141–47.

Naghavi, M., H. Wang, R. Lozano, A. Davis, X. Liang, and others. 2015. "Global, Regional, and National Age-Sex Specific All-Cause and Cause-Specific Mortality for 240 Causes of Death, 1990–2013: A Systematic Analysis for the Global Burden of Disease Study 2013." *The Lancet* 385 (9963): 117–71.

Neaton, J. D., D. N. Wentworth, J. Cutler, J. Stamler, and L. Kuller. 1993. "Risk Factors for Death from Different Types of Stroke." *Annals of Epidemiology* 3 (5): 493–99.

Newby, D. E., R. A. Wright, C. Labinjoh, C. A. Ludlam, K. A. Fox, and others. 1999. "Endothelial Dysfunction, Impaired Endogenous Fibrinolysis, and Cigarette Smoking: A Mechanism for Arterial Thrombosis and Myocardial Infarction." *Circulation* 99 (11): 1411–15.

Njølstad, I., E. Arnesen, and P. G. Lund-Larsen. 1996. "Smoking, Serum Lipids, Blood Pressure, and Sex Differences in Myocardial Infarction. A 12-Year Follow-Up of the Finnmark Study." *Circulation* 93 (3): 450–56.

Nowak, J., J. J. Murray, J. A. Oates, and G. A. Fitzgerald. 1987. "Biochemical Evidence of a Chronic Abnormality in Platelet and Vascular Function in Healthy Individuals Who Smoke Cigarettes." *Circulation* 76 (1): 6–14.

Ockene, I. S., and N. H. Miller. 1997. "Cigarette Smoking, Cardiovascular Disease, and Stroke: A Statement for Healthcare Professionals from the American Heart Association." *Circulation* 96 (9): 3243–47.

O'Donnell, M. J., D. Xavier, L. Liu, H. Zhang, S. L. Chin, and others. 2010. "Risk Factors for Ischaemic and Intracerebral Haemorrhagic Stroke in 22 Countries (the INTERSTROKE Study): A Case-Control Study." *The Lancet* 376 (9735): 112–23.

Olasky, S. J., D. Levy, and A. Moran. 2012. "Second-Hand Smoke and Cardiovascular Disease in Low- and Middle-Income Countries: A Case for Action." *Global Heart* 7 (2): 151–60.e5.

Orth, S. R. 2004. "Effects of Smoking on Systemic and Intrarenal Hemodynamics: Influence on Renal Function." *Journal of the American Society of Nephrology* 15 (1): S58–63.

Otsuka, R., H. Watanabe, K. Hirata, K. Tokai, T. Muro, and others. 2001. "Acute Effects of Passive Smoking on the Coronary Circulation in Healthy Young Adults." *JAMA* 286 (4): 436–41.

Owens, A. P., and N. Mackman. 2010. "Tissue Factor and Thrombosis: The Clot Starts Here." *Thrombosis and Haemostasis* 104 (3): 432–39.

Pan, A., Y. Wang, M. Talaei, F. B. Hu, and T. Wu. 2015. "Relation of Active, Passive, and Quitting Smoking with Incident Type 2 Diabetes: A Systematic Review and Meta-Analysis." *The Lancet Diabetes and Endocrinology* 3 (12): 958–67.

Parish, S., R. Collins, R. Peto, L. Youngman, J. Barton, and others. 1995. "Cigarette Smoking, Tar Yields, and Non-Fatal Myocardial Infarction: 14,000 Cases and 32,000 Controls in the United Kingdom; the International Studies of Infarct Survival (ISIS) Collaborators." *BMJ* 311 (7003): 471–77.

Pech-Amsellem, M. A., I. Myara, M. Storogenko, K. Demuth, A. Proust, and others. 1996. "Enhanced Modifications of Low-Density Lipoproteins (LDL) by Endothelial Cells from Smokers: A Possible Mechanism of Smoking-Related Atherosclerosis." *Cardiovascular Research* 31 (6): 975–83.

Peters, R. W., M. M. Brooks, L. Todd, P. R. Liebson, and L. Wilhelmsen. 1995. "Smoking Cessation and Arrhythmic Death: The CAST Experience." *Journal of the American College of Cardiology* 26 (5): 1287–92.

Petrick, L. M., and Y. Dubowski. 2011. "Thirdhand Smoke: Heterogeneous Oxidation of Nicotine and Secondary Aerosol Formation in the Indoor Environment." *Environmental Science and Technology* 45 (1): 328–33.

Piano, M. R., N. L. Benowitz, G. A. Fitzgerald, S. Corbridge, J. Heath, and others. 2010. "Impact of Smokeless Tobacco Products on Cardiovascular Disease: Implications for Policy, Prevention, and Treatment: A Policy Statement from the American Heart Association." *Circulation* 122 (15): 1520–44.

Pinto-Sietsma, S. J., J. Mulder, W. M. Janssen, H. L. Hillege, D. de Zeeuw, and others. 2000. "Smoking Is Related to

Albuminuria and Abnormal Renal Function in Nondiabetic Persons." *Annals of Internal Medicine* 133 (8): 585–91.

Powell, J. T. 1998. "Vascular Damage from Smoking: Disease Mechanisms at the Arterial Wall." *Vascular Medicine* 3 (1): 21–28.

Prescott, E., M. Hippe, P. Schnohr, H. O. Hein, and J. Vestbo. 1998. "Smoking and Risk of Myocardial Infarction in Women and Men: Longitudinal Population Study." *BMJ* 316 (7137): 1043–47.

Primatesta, P., E. Falaschetti, S. Gupta, M. G. Marmot, and N. R. Poulter. 2001. "Association between Smoking and Blood Pressure: Evidence from the Health Survey for England." *Hypertension* 37 (2): 187–93.

Pujades-Rodriguez, M., J. George, A. D. Shah, E. Rapsomaniki, S. Denaxas, and others. 2015. "Heterogeneous Associations between Smoking and a Wide Range of Initial Presentations of Cardiovascular Disease in 1 937 360 People in England: Lifetime Risks and Implications for Risk Prediction." *International Journal of Epidemiology* 44 (1): 129–41.

Qiao, Q., M. Tervahauta, A. Nissinen, and J. Tuomilehto. 2000. "Mortality from All Causes and from Coronary Heart Disease Related to Smoking and Changes in Smoking during a 35-Year Follow-Up of Middle-Aged Finnish Men." *European Heart Journal* 21 (19): 1621–26.

Raghuveer, G., D. A. White, L. L. Hayman, J. G. Woo, J. Villafane, and others. 2016. "Cardiovascular Consequences of Childhood Secondhand Tobacco Smoke Exposure: Prevailing Evidence, Burden, and Racial and Socioeconomic Disparities—A Scientific Statement From the American Heart Association." *Circulation* 134 (13). http://dx.doi.org/10.1161/CIR.0000000000000443.

Rastogi, T., P. Jha, K. S. Reddy, D. Prabhakaran, D. Spiegelman, and others. 2005. "Bidi and Cigarette Smoking and Risk of Acute Myocardial Infarction among Males in Urban India." *Tobacco Control* 14 (5): 356–58.

Regan, A. K., G. Promoff, S. R. Dube, and R. Arrazola. 2013. "Electronic Nicotine Delivery Systems: Adult Use and Awareness of the 'E-Cigarette' in the USA." *Tobacco Control* 22 (1): 19–23.

Rigotti, N. A., and C. Clair. 2013. "Managing Tobacco Use: The Neglected Cardiovascular Disease Risk Factor." *European Heart Journal* 34 (42): 3259–67.

Rosenthal, L., A. Carroll-Scott, V. A. Earnshaw, N. Sackey, S. S. O'Malley, and others. 2013. "Targeting Cessation: Understanding Barriers and Motivations to Quitting among Urban Adult Daily Tobacco Smokers." *Addictive Behaviors* 38 (3): 1639–42.

Roth, G. A., M. H. Forouzanfar, A. E. Moran, R. Barber, G. Nguyen, and others. 2015. "Demographic and Epidemiologic Drivers of Global Cardiovascular Mortality." *New England Journal of Medicine* 372 (14): 1333–41.

Roth, G. A., G. Nguyen, M. H. Forouzanfar, A. H. Mokdad, M. Naghavi, and others. 2015. "Estimates of Global and Regional Premature Cardiovascular Mortality in 2025." *Circulation* 132 (13): 1270–82.

Ruggeri, Z. M. 2000. "Old Concepts and New Developments in the Study of Platelet Aggregation." *Journal of Clinical Investigation* 105 (6): 699–701.

Salahuddin, S., D. Prabhakaran, and A. Roy. 2012. "Pathophysiological Mechanisms of Tobacco-Related CVD." *Global Heart* 7 (2): 113–20.

Saleheen, D., W. Zhao, and A. Rasheed. 2014. "Epidemiology and Public Health Policy of Tobacco Use and Cardiovascular Disorders in Low- and Middle-Income Countries." *Arteriosclerosis, Thrombosis, and Vascular Biology* 34 (9): 1811–19.

Schick, S., and S. Glantz. 2005. "Philip Morris Toxicological Experiments with Fresh Sidestream Smoke: More Toxic than Mainstream Smoke." *Tobacco Control* 14 (6): 396–404.

Schleithoff, C., S. Voelter-Mahlknecht, I. N. Dahmke, and U. Mahlknecht. 2012. "On the Epigenetics of Vascular Regulation and Disease." *Clinical Epigenetics* 4 (May): 7.

Seo, D.-C., and M. R. Torabi. 2007. "Reduced Admissions for Acute Myocardial Infarction Associated with a Public Smoking Ban: Matched Controlled Study." *Journal of Drug Education* 37 (3): 217–26.

Shao, B., K. D. O'Brien, T. O. McDonald, X. Fu, J. F. Oram, and others. 2005. "Acrolein Modifies Apolipoprotein A-I in the Human Artery Wall." *Annals of the New York Academy of Sciences* 1043 (June): 396–403.

Shaper, A. 2003. "Pipe and Cigar Smoking and Major Cardiovascular Events, Cancer Incidence, and All-Cause Mortality in Middle-Aged British Men." *International Journal of Epidemiology* 32 (5): 802–8.

Shihadeh, A. 2003. "Investigation of Mainstream Smoke Aerosol of the Argileh Water Pipe." *Food and Chemical Toxicology* 41 (1): 143–52.

Shinton, R., and G. Beevers. 1989. "Meta-Analysis of Relation between Cigarette Smoking and Stroke." *BMJ* 298 (6676): 789–94.

Shlipak, M. G., L. F. Fried, M. Cushman, T. A. Manolio, D. Peterson, and others. 2005. "Cardiovascular Mortality Risk in Chronic Kidney Disease." *JAMA* 293 (14): 1737.

Sibai, A. M., R. A. Tohme, M. M. Almedawar, T. Itani, S. I. Yassine, and others. 2014. "Lifetime Cumulative Exposure to Waterpipe Smoking Is Associated with Coronary Artery Disease." *Atherosclerosis* 234 (2): 454–60.

Simpson, C. R., B. S. Buckley, D. J. McLernon, A. Sheikh, A. Murphy, and others. 2011. "Five-Year Prognosis in an Incident Cohort of People Presenting with Acute Myocardial Infarction." *PLoS One* 6 (1): e26573.

Sleiman, M., L. A. Gundel, J. F. Pankow, P. Jacob, B. C. Singer, and others. 2010. "Formation of Carcinogens Indoors by Surface-Mediated Reactions of Nicotine with Nitrous Acid, Leading to Potential Thirdhand Smoke Hazards." *Proceedings of the National Academy of Sciences of the United States of America* 107 (15): 6576–81.

Smith, C. J., and T. H. Fischer 2001. "Particulate and Vapor Phase Constituents of Cigarette Mainstream Smoke and Risk of Myocardial Infarction." *Atherosclerosis* 158 (2): 257–67.

Smith, F. B., A. J. Lee, F. G. Fowkes, J. F. Price, A. Rumley, and others. 1997. "Hemostatic Factors as Predictors of Ischemic Heart Disease and Stroke in the Edinburgh Artery Study." *Arteriosclerosis, Thrombosis, and Vascular Biology* 17 (11): 3321–25.

Stadler, M., L. Tomann, A. Storka, M. Wolzt, S. Peric, and others. 2014. "Effects of Smoking Cessation on B-Cell Function, Insulin Sensitivity, Body Weight, and Appetite." *European Journal of Endocrinology* 170 (2): 219–27.

Stefanadis, C., E. Fischer, C. Vlachopoulos, C. Stratos, and K. Toutouzas. 1997. "Unfavorable Effect of Smoking on the Elastic Properties of the Human Aorta." *Circulation* 95 (1): 31–38.

Stoekenbroek, R. M., S. M. Boekholdt, R. Luben, G. K. Hovingh, A. H. Zwinderman, and others. 2015. "Heterogeneous Impact of Classic Atherosclerotic Risk Factors on Different Arterial Territories: The EPIC-Norfolk Prospective Population Study." *European Heart Journal* 37 (11): 880–90.

Svendsen, K. H., L. H. Kuller, M. J. Martin, and J. K. Ockene. 1987. "Effects of Passive Smoking in the Multiple Risk Factor Intervention Trial." *American Journal of Epidemiology* 126 (5): 783–95.

Sweeting, M. J., S. G. Thompson, L. C. Brown, J. T. Powell, and RESCAN Collaborators. 2012. "Meta-Analysis of Individual Patient Data to Examine Factors Affecting Growth and Rupture of Small Abdominal Aortic Aneurysms." *British Journal of Surgery* 99 (5): 655–65.

Tachmes, L., R. J. Fernandez, and M. A. Sackner. 1978. "Hemodynamic Effects of Smoking Cigarettes of High and Low Nicotine Content." *Chest* 74 (3): 243–46.

Teo, K. K., S. Ounpuu, S. Hawken, M. R. Pandey, V. Valentin, and others. 2006. "Tobacco Use and Risk of Myocardial Infarction in 52 Countries in the INTERHEART Study: A Case-Control Study." *The Lancet* 368 (9536): 647–58.

Tracy, R. P., B. M. Psaty, E. Macy, E. G. Bovill, M. Cushman, and others. 1997. "Lifetime Smoking Exposure Affects the Association of C-reactive Protein with Cardiovascular Disease Risk Factors and Subclinical Disease in Healthy Elderly Subjects." *Arteriosclerosis, Thrombosis, and Vascular Biology* 17 (10): 2167–76.

Twyman, L., B. Bonevski, C. Paul, and J. Bryant. 2014. "Perceived Barriers to Smoking Cessation in Selected Vulnerable Groups: A Systematic Review of the Qualitative and Quantitative Literature." *BMJ Open* 4 (12): e006414.

U.S. Department of Health and Human Services. 1983. *The Health Consequences of Smoking: Cardiovascular Disease. A Report of the Surgeon General*. Washington, DC: U.S. Department of Health and Human Services.

———. 1988. *The Health Consequences of Smoking: Nicotine Addiction. A Report of the Surgeon General*. Washington, DC: U.S. Department of Health and Human Services.

———. 2001. *Women and Smoking. A Report of the Surgeon General*. Atlanta, GA: U.S. Surgeon General.

———. 2010. *How Tobacco Smoke Causes Disease: The Biology and Behavioral Basis for Smoking-Attributable Disease. A Report of the Surgeon General*. Atlanta, GA: U.S. Surgeon General.

———. 2014. *The Health Consequences of Smoking—50 Years of Progress. A Report of the Surgeon General: Executive Summary*. Washington, DC: U.S. Department of Health and Human Services.

Varsano, S., I. Ganz, N. Eldor, and M. Garenkin. 2003. "Water-Pipe Tobacco Smoking among School Children in Israel: Frequencies, Habits, and Attitudes." *Harefuah* 142 (11): 736–41, 807.

Venn, A., and J. Britton. 2007. "Exposure to Secondhand Smoke and Biomarkers of Cardiovascular Disease Risk in Never-Smoking Adults." *Circulation* 115 (8): 990–95.

Vinci, M. C., G. Polvani, and M. Pesce. 2013. "Epigenetic Programming and Risk: The Birthplace of Cardiovascular Disease?" *Stem Cell Reviews and Reports* 9 (3): 241–53.

Vlietstra, R. E., R. A. Kronmal, A. Oberman, R. L. Frye, and T. Killip. 1986. "Effect of Cigarette Smoking on Survival of Patients with Angiographically Documented Coronary Artery Disease. Report from the CASS Registry." *JAMA* 255 (8): 1023–27.

WHO (World Health Organization). 2012. *WHO Global Report: Mortality Attributable to Tobacco*. Geneva: WHO.

———. 2013. *WHO Report on the Global Tobacco Epidemic: Enforcing Bans on Advertising, Promotion, and Sponsorship*. Geneva: WHO.

———. 2015a. "Cardiovascular Diseases: Fact Sheet." WHO, Geneva.

———. 2015b. *Tobacco and Dementia*. Geneva: WHO Tobacco Knowledge Summaries, WHO. http://802quits.org/wordpress/wp-content/uploads/2015/04/WHO-Tobacco-and-Dementia.pdf.

———. n.d. "Global Adult Tobacco Survey." Tobacco Free Initiative, WHO, Geneva. http://www.who.int/tobacco/surveillance/survey/gats/en/.

Wilhelmsen, L., A. Rosengren, H. Eriksson, and G. Lappas. 2008. "Heart Failure in the General Population of Men: Morbidity, Risk Factors, and Prognosis." *Journal of Internal Medicine* 249 (3): 253–61.

Will, J. C., D. A. Galuska, E. S. Ford, A. Mokdad, and E. E. Calle. 2001. "Cigarette Smoking and Diabetes Mellitus: Evidence of a Positive Association from a Large Prospective Cohort Study." *International Journal of Epidemiology* 30 (3): 540–46.

Willigendael, E. M., J. A. W. Teijink, M.-L. Bartelink, B. W. Kuiken, J. Boiten, and others. 2004. "Influence of Smoking on Incidence and Prevalence of Peripheral Arterial Disease." *Journal of Vascular Surgery* 40 (6): 1158–65.

Wilson, K., N. Gibson, A. Willan, and D. Cook. 2000. "Effect of Smoking Cessation on Mortality after Myocardial Infarction: Meta-Analysis of Cohort Studies." *Archives of Internal Medicine* 160 (7): 939–44.

Winickoff, J. P., J. Friebely, S. E. Tanski, C. Sherrod, G. E. Matt, and others. 2009. "Beliefs about the Health Effects of 'Thirdhand' Smoke and Home Smoking Bans." *Pediatrics* 123 (1): e74–79.

Winkelmann, B. R., K. von Holt, and M. Unverdorben. 2009. "Smoking and Atherosclerotic Cardiovascular Disease: Part I: Atherosclerotic Disease Process." *Biomarkers in Medicine* 3 (4): 411–28.

Wolf, M. B., and J. W. Baynes. 2007. "Cadmium and Mercury Cause an Oxidative Stress-Induced Endothelial Dysfunction." *Biometals* 20 (1): 73–81.

Yamagata, K., K. Ishida, T. Sairenchi, H. Takahashi, S. Ohba, and others. 2007. "Risk Factors for Chronic Kidney Disease in a Community-Based Population: A 10-Year Follow-Up Study." *Kidney International* 71 (2): 159–66.

Yamaguchi, Y., S. Kagota, J. Haginaka, and M. Kunitomo. 2000. "Evidence of Modified LDL in the Plasma of Hypercholesterolemic WHHL Rabbits Injected with Aqueous Extracts of Cigarette Smoke." *Environmental Toxicology and Pharmacology* 8 (4): 255–60.

Yang, H., K. Negishi, P. Otahal, and T. H. Marwick. 2015. "Clinical Prediction of Incident Heart Failure Risk: A Systematic Review and Meta-Analysis." *Open Heart* 2 (1): e000222.

Yoshikawa, H., E. Hellström-Lindahl, and V. Grill. 2005. "Evidence for Functional Nicotinic Receptors on Pancreatic Beta Cells." *Metabolism: Clinical and Experimental* 54 (2): 247–54.

Yusuf, S., S. Hawken, S. Ounpuu, T. Dans, A. Avezum, and others. 2004. "Effect of Potentially Modifiable Risk Factors Associated with Myocardial Infarction in 52 Countries (the INTERHEART Study): Case-Control Study." *The Lancet* 364 (9438): 937–52.

Zhu, Y., M. Zhang, X. Hou, J. Lu, L. Peng, and others. 2011. "Cigarette Smoking Increases Risk for Incident Metabolic Syndrome in Chinese Men—Shanghai Diabetes Study." *Biomedical and Environmental Sciences* 24 (5): 475–82.

Chapter 5

Physical Activity for the Prevention of Cardiometabolic Disease

Fiona Bull, Shifalika Goenka, Vicki Lambert, and Michael Pratt

INTRODUCTION

Increased mechanization, urbanization, and technological advances are changing how and where we work, travel, and recreate. People sit for increasingly long hours at computers, and emails dominate work and communications. Social and recreational activities include using a wide variety of screen-based devices, such as televisions, smartphones, and tablets. In many countries, cars dominate transportation, creating congestion and gridlock. One-way commutes of two hours are common in cities like Bangkok, Delhi, and São Paulo. The global decline in levels of physical activity and increase in time spent in sedentary activities have contributed to major shifts in the landscape of diseases (Archer and others 2013; Barnett and others 2008; Bhurosy and Jeewon 2014; Church and others 2011; Hallal and others 2014; Lozano and others 2012; Ng, Norton, and Popkin 2009; Ng and Popkin 2012).

In 2014, two of every three deaths globally—38 million total—were due to noncommunicable diseases (NCDs) (WHO 2014a). Physical inactivity is an established risk factor for NCDs and specifically for cardiometabolic diseases. Being inactive contributes significantly to unhealthy weight gain and obesity, high cholesterol, and elevated blood pressure and blood glucose levels, all of which heighten the risk of developing cardiometabolic diseases (WHO 2010a).

Physical activity includes different types of activities that can be done in different types of settings, including sports, recreation, play, and transport-related walking and cycling, as well as general movement undertaken as part of daily living, such as shopping, cleaning, or climbing stairs (box 5.1). Physical activities may be undertaken with different degrees of effort and for different durations. Because of this breadth in type, duration, frequency, and even location, measuring, monitoring, and understanding physical activity is complex. Nevertheless, a significant body of knowledge has accumulated on physical activity, its role in primary and secondary prevention of leading NCDs (Physical Activity Guidelines Advisory Committee 2008a), and the causes of participation and nonparticipation in different populations. This evidence forms a strong base for informing current practice and policy in health care and other fields of public policy.

This chapter provides an overview of the potential of public health action aimed at increasing population levels of physical activity and contributing directly and indirectly to reducing cardiometabolic diseases. It begins by providing data on global and regional levels of physical activity and the burden of disease attributable to inactivity. It then provides an overview of the epidemiological evidence on the protective effects of physical activity and emerging evidence on the risks of sitting and sedentary activities, dubbed the new smoking (Berry 2013); summarizes the available evidence on the cost of physical inactivity to the health sector; and presents the most promising policy and

Corresponding author: Fiona Bull, Department for Prevention of Noncommunicable Diseases, World Health Organization, Geneva; Switzerland; bullf@who.int.

program actions across seven key settings to increase population-level physical activity and, where available, evidence on their cost-effectiveness. It concludes by reviewing the opportunities for action through global, regional, and national policy initiatives and by identifying some of the challenges and barriers to implementation.

Box 5.1

Definition of Physical Activity

Physical activity can incorporate a wide range of lifestyle, sport, and exercise activities (Caspersen, Powell, and Christenson 1985; WHO 2015).

For children and young people, physical activity includes play, games, sports, walking to school, cycling, and physical education or planned exercise such as dance classes.

For adults, physical activity includes recreational or leisure-time physical activity, active transport (walking or cycling), work-related activity, household chores, play, games, sports, or planned exercise such as fitness classes.

PREVALENCE AND BURDEN OF PHYSICAL INACTIVITY

Worldwide, 23 percent of the adult population is insufficiently active, defined as not achieving at least 150 minutes of moderate-intensity or 75 minutes of vigorous-intensity activity or an equivalent combination per week (WHO 2014a). Gender differences are notable in many countries. Globally, men, in general, are more active than women (prevalence of inactivity globally of 20 percent in men and 27 percent in women). Regional differences are also notable, with proportions of insufficiently active adults ranging from 17 percent in South-East Asia to about 36 percent in the Americas and 38 percent in the Eastern Mediterranean (WHO 2014a) (figure 5.1).

A concerning trend is that levels of inactivity increase with economic development. Adults are less active in high-income countries (HICs) than in low- and middle-income countries (LMICs), a pattern suggesting that inactivity will rise as middle-income countries develop economically. For example, evidence indicates that, in India, urban populations are less active than rural populations (Gupta and others 2008); this is due, in part, to rapid globalization and increasing mechanization leading to less occupational activity and, when coupled with increased affluence, an increase in the use of motor vehicles for transport. These societal changes are well underway in many LMICs; without mitigation,

Figure 5.1 Age-Standardized Prevalence of Insufficient Physical Activity in Adults, by Gender and WHO Regions and World Bank Income Groups, 2014

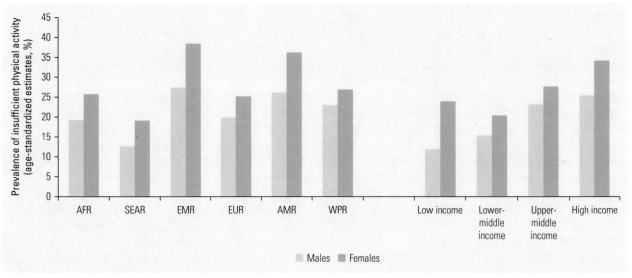

Source: WHO 2014a.
Note: AFR = African Region, AMR = Region of the Americas; SEAR = South-East Asia Region; EUR = European Region; EMR = Eastern Mediterranean Region; WHO = World Health Organization; WPR = Western Pacific Region.

they will likely lead to further decreases in levels of physical activity.

Considerable progress has been made in population-level monitoring of physical inactivity since 2004. In 2000, fewer than 50 countries had any population-level data on physical activity, and many of these were of poor quality and limited reliability (Bull and others 2004). Following the development of the International Physical Activity Questionnaire (Craig and others 2003) and the Global Physical Activity Questionnaire (Armstrong and Bull 2006), many countries began monitoring physical activity, with more than 140 countries reporting population data on physical activity in 2014 (WHO 2014a). These data enable comparisons to be made within and between countries. Furthermore, a growing number of countries have established or committed to establishing surveillance systems for monitoring physical activity to track trends within and between subpopulations and countries.

Less progress has been made in the population-level assessment of physical activity in young people. Few countries have surveillance systems covering ages 5–18 years. Some countries have participated in the Global School-Based Student Health Survey, a large, well-established survey that includes items on physical activity (WHO 2016). However, the survey only covers ages 11–17 years and only reports the proportion not meeting the minimum recommended 60 minutes of moderate-to-vigorous activity per day. These data show that more than 75 percent of adolescents do not meet the global recommendation and that adolescent girls are less active than adolescent boys (Guthold and others 2010; WHO 2010b). The use of objective measures for assessing physical activity in children is preferred and strongly recommended given the complexities of having this age group recall their physical activity behaviors (Wijndaele and others 2015).

Time spent in sedentary (sitting) behaviors is emerging as an independent risk for cardiometabolic disease. Self-reported measures of sedentary behaviors were included in both the International Physical Activity Questionnaire and the Global Physical Activity Questionnaire and provide some of the first population data on prevalence (Hallal and others 2012). Less than half (41 percent) of the adult population globally spends more than four hours a day sitting (figure 5.2). Notably, older adults (older than age 60 years) are more sedentary than younger adults, but the data show little difference by gender. There are, however, regional differences, with the highest prevalence of sedentary activity in the Middle East (64 percent) and the lowest in South-East Asia (24 percent) (data not shown). These data may underestimate how much populations sit because self-reported measures are poorly suited to measuring time spent in diverse sedentary behaviors across a day.

Figure 5.2 Proportion of Individuals Reporting Sitting for Four or More Hours a Day

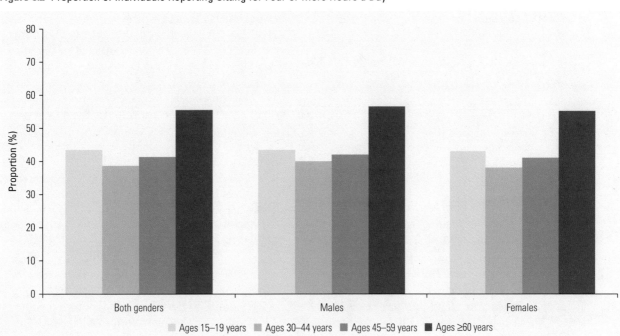

Source: Hallal and others 2012.

Increasing levels of inactivity in both HICs and LMICs is cause for concern (Barnett and others 2008; Bhurosy and Jeewon 2014; Hallal and others 2014; Ng, Norton, and Popkin 2009). In the United States, studies have demonstrated an 8 percent to 10 percent decline in occupation-related and 3 percent to 42 percent decline in household-related physical activity during the past four decades (Church and others 2011). Using time-use surveys, Ng and Popkin (2012) modeled changes in physical activity–related energy expenditure and sedentary time for 1991 to 2030 based on current trends in Brazil, China, India, and the United Kingdom. In these four countries, energy expenditure related to physical activity is expected to decline about 50 percent over four decades. It is therefore necessary to identify and intervene with effective mitigating strategies that provide safe and equitable opportunities for physical activity.

Physical inactivity causes an estimated 9 percent of premature mortality from all causes, or between 3.1 million (Lim and others 2013) and 5.3 million (Lee and others 2012) premature deaths worldwide in 2010. Inactivity accounts for 6 percent of coronary artery disease, 7 percent of type 2 diabetes, 10 percent of breast cancers, and 10 percent of colon cancers (Lee and others 2012). Although eliminating physical inactivity would have the largest effect on colon cancer (due to a higher hazards ratio), it would avert the largest number of cases of coronary artery disease (due to higher incidence). These estimates are viewed as conservative because of the limitations of using self-reported measures of exposure.

PHYSICAL INACTIVITY AND CARDIOMETABOLIC RISK

The value of physical activity has long been recognized (Agarwal 2012; Kokkinos 2012), but during the past 60 years scientists have intensified efforts to measure and specify the optimal type, frequency, and duration of physical activity required for different health benefits. The 1996 landmark report by the U.S. Surgeon General, *Physical Activity and Health*, shifted the focus away from training regimes involving shorter bouts of high-intensity exercise and toward the benefits of accumulating regular, sustained amounts of moderate-intensity activity, such as walking (U.S. Department of Health and Human Services 1996). The report recommended that all adults should accumulate at least 30 minutes of moderate-intensity activity, through bouts of no less than 10 minutes, at least five times a week; this same volume of energy expenditure could be achieved in three 20-minute bouts

of vigorous-intensity activity (Pate and others 1995; U.S. Department of Health and Human Services 1996). The recommended minimum threshold of physical activity reflected the curvilinear dose-response relationship identified in epidemiological studies.

More recent reviews confirm that physical activity has a wide range of benefits, including reducing all-cause mortality risk, preventing cardiovascular disease (CVD) and diabetes, improving lipid levels, lowering hypertension, reducing the risks of breast and colon cancer, and improving functional status (Aune and others 2015; Physical Activity Guidelines Advisory Committee 2008b; World Cancer Research Fund 2007). Evidence from epidemiological and clinical studies has identified positive neurological health outcomes showing that physical activity can improve cognition in people without dementia, reduce the incidence of dementia, and improve health among people with dementia (Blondell, Hammersley-Mather, and Veerman 2014).

The following sections provide a brief overview of scientific findings on the relationship between physical activity and specific cardiometabolic health outcomes, including heart disease, stroke, and diabetes, as well as selected key metabolic risk factors.

Physical Activity and Coronary Heart Disease

Regular moderate- or vigorous-intensity physical activity, especially leisure-time physical activity, significantly lowers mortality from coronary heart disease (CHD) (Karjalainen and others 2015; Kodama and others 2009; Lee and others 2012). In a meta-analysis of epidemiological studies investigating physical activity and primary prevention of CHD, individuals engaging in the equivalent of 150 minutes of moderate-intensity leisure-time physical activity per week had a 14 percent lower risk of CHD than individuals reporting no leisure-time physical activity (Sattelmair and others 2011). The dose-response relationship clearly showed that undertaking some physical activity is better than none and that additional benefits occur with more physical activity (Sattelmair and others 2011). Persons engaging in the equivalent of 300 minutes of moderate-intensity leisure-time physical activity per week had a 20 percent lower risk than persons not engaging in any leisure-time physical activity (figure 5.3). These results are consistent with the systematic review–level evidence (Physical Activity Guidelines Advisory Committee 2008b) and recent consensus statements (Swift and others 2013), which concluded that there is a strong inverse relationship between the amount of habitual physical activity performed and CHD morbidity or mortality in men and women at middle age or older. Furthermore, these results may underestimate risk reduction because multivariate models in many studies include adjustments for hypertension, dyslipidemia, and glucose tolerance, conditions that may represent biological intermediates in the causal pathway (Physical Activity Guidelines Advisory Committee 2008b).

Of particular importance is that the protective effects of physical activity (as measured by cardiorespiratory fitness) on CVD and CHD are independent of levels of overweight and obesity, as measured by body mass index (BMI) (Barry and others 2014; Blair and others 1989; Kodama and others 2009). A meta-analysis confirmed that fit individuals who are overweight or obese are not automatically at higher risk for all-cause mortality and that low-fit individuals have twice the risk of death regardless of BMI (Barry and others 2014). Such findings are important for all individuals, including those unable to lose weight or maintain weight loss, because significant health benefits can be attained by maintaining a moderate level of cardiorespiratory fitness through regular physical activity (Barry and others 2014).

To date, few studies have assessed the potential for differential risk reduction from physical activity undertaken in different domains, with the majority of studies assessing either total physical activity or only leisure-time activity. A meta-analysis of 21 prospective cohort studies assessed the separate protective effects of occupation and leisure-time physical activity on CHD and stroke outcomes (Li and Siegrist 2012). This analysis of 650,000 adults (with 20,000 incident cases) showed that both moderate and high levels of leisure-time activity and moderate levels of occupational physical activity have protective effects in both men and women. The pooled analyses (men and women) showed an overall 18 percent reduction in risk of CVD (relative risk [RR] 0.82, 95 percent confidence interval [CI] 0.67–0.88, $p < 0.001$) compared with the reference group with low leisure-time physical activity, while a high level of leisure-time physical activity reduced the overall risk of CVD by 27 percent (RR 0.73, 95 percent CI 0.68–0.78, $p < 0.001$) (Li and Siegrist 2012).

Exercise-based cardiac rehabilitation is the cornerstone of secondary prevention of CVD and should include baseline patient assessment, nutritional and physical activity counseling, and exercise training (Balady and others 2007). Results from a recent Cochrane Review of 63 studies, with median follow-up of 12 months, showed a reduction in cardiovascular mortality (RR 0.74, 95 percent CI 0.64–0.86) and risk of hospital admissions (RR 0.82, 95 percent CI 0.70–0.96) (Anderson and others 2016). Furthermore, the majority of studies (14 of 20) showed higher levels of health-related quality of life in one or more domains following exercise-based cardiac rehabilitation compared with control subjects.

Figure 5.3 Dose-Response between Leisure-Time Physical Activity and Risk of Coronary Heart Disease

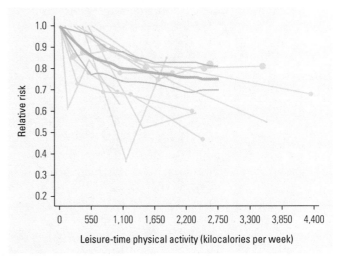

Source: Sattelmair and others 2011.

Participation in exercise-based cardiac rehabilitation programs has also been found to be associated with reduced angina symptoms and depression, improved exercise capacity, and enhanced health-related quality of life (Taylor and others 2004).

Overall, strong evidence supports the role of physical activity in primary and secondary prevention of CHD. Strategies to integrate physical activity counseling and referral within care pathways for patients with, or at risk of, CHD are needed (Swift and others 2013).

Physical Activity and Stroke

Evidence regarding the protective effect of physical activity on stroke has shown mixed results, with some studies showing positive, inverse, and even U-shaped associations (Diep and others 2010). Yet, on balance, systematic review–level evidence does conclude that physical activity has a favorable impact on stroke end points. In 2008 a systematic review conducted for the U.S. Physical Activity Guidelines concluded that physical activity can reduce the risk of both ischemic and hemorrhagic stroke, although noting that the data on stroke subtypes were limited (Physical Activity Guidelines Advisory Committee 2008b). Diep and others (2010) conducted a meta-analysis of 13 cohort studies and found that, compared with low levels of physical activity, moderate levels of activity were associated with an 11 percent reduction in the risk of stroke (RR 0.89, 95 percent CI 0.86–0.93, $p < 0.01$), and high levels of activity were associated with a 19 percent reduction (RR 0.81, 95 percent CI 0.77–0.84, $p < 0.01$).

Although similar results were seen in men and women for higher levels of activity, only in men was there a significant association between moderate levels of activity and reduced risk of stroke (Diep and others 2010). This review suggested that high levels of activity may be required in women, but it did not specify what that dose (intensity, frequency, or duration) might be.

Another review involving 21 studies assessed the associations between occupation and leisure-time physical activity and stroke (Li and Siegrist 2012) and reported that both types of activity were protective in both men and women. Although more research is needed to understand the causal pathways and to confirm the amount of physical activity required, there is a general consensus that participation in physical activity consistent with global recommendations for adults and older adults should be stressed as part of an overall stroke prevention strategy (Howard and McDonnell 2015).

Figure 5.4 Moderate-Intensity Physical Activity and Rate Ratio of Type 2 Diabetes for Individual Cohort Studies and All Studies Combined

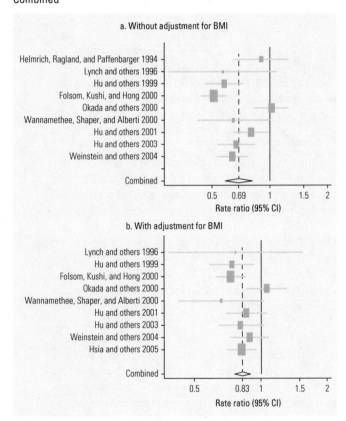

Source: Jeon and others 2007.
Note: BMI = body mass index; CI = confidence interval.

Physical Activity and Type 2 Diabetes

Physical activity has a strong and inverse association with type 2 diabetes. In both cohort studies and randomized controlled intervention trials, physical activity has been shown to lower the overall risk for type 2 diabetes between 30 percent and 60 percent (Ishida, Ito, and Murakami 2005; Knowler and others 2002; Li and others 2008; Ramachandran and others 2006). A systematic review (Jeon and others 2007) of 10 prospective cohort studies of moderate-intensity physical activity and type 2 diabetes, involving 301,221 participants and 9,367 incident cases of diabetes, found that the relative risk of developing type 2 diabetes was 31 percent lower in persons who participated regularly in physical activity than in those who had a sedentary lifestyle (figure 5.4). The results remained significant even after adjusting for BMI. Among these studies, five investigated the role of walking (Helmrich, Ragland, and Paffenbarger 1994; Hu and others 1999; Hu and others 2001; Hu and others 2003; Weinstein and others 2004); results showed that regular brisk walking of 2.5 hours per week decreased the risk of diabetes by 30 percent compared with no walking (figure 5.5). These results included adjustments for age, family history, educational status, smoking, alcohol, cholesterol level, BMI, and, in some instances, waist-to-hip ratio (Lindstrom and others 2006). These are important findings given the popularity and ease of walking as a form of daily physical activity and thus support potential population-based walking interventions targeting middle- and older-age adults.

Physical activity is also beneficial for patients with impaired glucose tolerance (IGT) (Mohan and others 2006; Ramachandran and others 2006). Two landmark clinical trials—the Diabetes Prevention Program (Knowler and others 2002) and the Finnish Diabetes Prevention Trial (Folsom, Kushi, and Hong 2000; Weinstein and others 2004)—established that physical activity combined with dietary modulation can lower the risk of diabetes in individuals with impaired fasting glucose or with IGT. Some studies have shown that these beneficial effects can persist for 10 years or more (Perreault and others 2009; Weinstein and others 2004).

Figueira and others (2014) conducted a meta-analysis of 30 randomized controlled clinical trials of structured training programs (2,217 patients) and 21 studies of the effectiveness of providing advice on physical activity (7,323 patients). They assessed the effect on blood pressure in patients with type 2 diabetes of different structured exercise programs (aerobic, resistance, or combined) compared with advice alone. The results showed that structured exercise was associated with significant reductions in the weighted mean difference of −4.22 millimeter of mercury (mmHg, a measure of pressure) (95 percent CI −5.89 to −2.56) for systolic and −2.07 mmHg (95 percent CI −3.03 to −1.11) for diastolic blood pressure versus controls. Higher levels of structured exercise (more than 150 minutes per week) were associated with even greater reductions in blood pressure (Figueira and others 2014).

These studies provide strong evidence that behavioral interventions aimed at encouraging regular physical activity can be effective for tackling diabetes at the population level, including in LMICs (American Diabetes Association 2014; Goenka 2008; Goenka and others 2009). More than 77 percent of the 316 million people with IGT worldwide live in LMICs and are ages 20–39 years (Li and others 2008). Given that the conversion to diabetes is more rapid in India and South-East Asian countries than globally (Mohan and others 2006; Ramachandran and others 2006), the assessment of and referral to physical activity programs should be integrated into primary health care pathways for patients at risk of diabetes (Adler and others 2000; Alberti, Zimmet, and Shaw 2007; Chobanian and others 2003; Stamler and others 1993; U.K. Prospective Diabetes Study Group 1998).

Physical Activity and Cardiometabolic Disease Risk Factors

Physical activity has been shown to be effective in improving key risk factors of cardiometabolic disease. Regular physical activity can decrease systolic and diastolic blood pressure (Fagard 2005), with evidence supporting the benefits achieved from moderate-intensity activity (such as walking) as well as vigorous activity. Results from the Coronary Artery Risk Development in Young Adults Study suggest that approximately 34 percent of hypertension could be prevented if adults would increase their physical activity and fitness (Carnethon and others 2010; Pereira and others 1999). Adjustment for fasting insulin level and waist circumference attenuated the results, indicating that the association between activity and incident hypertension may be mediated by obesity and the metabolic syndrome. However, both insulin levels and waist circumference are part of the causal pathway, and adjusting for them therefore results in overadjustment.

In a study of 7,400 older adults ages 45–65 years (Atherosclerosis Risk in Communities), white men in the highest quartile of the sport and leisure indexes had significant reductions in the odds of developing hypertension of 23 percent and 34 percent, respectively, compared with men in the lowest quartiles (Pereira and others 1999). A similar magnitude of risk reduction was

Figure 5.5 Walking and Rate Ratio of Type 2 Diabetes for Individual Cohort Studies and All Studies Combined

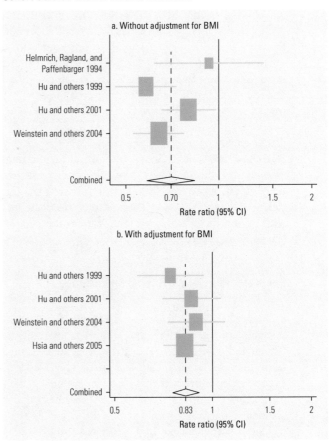

Source: Jeon and others 2007.
Note: BMI = body mass index; CI = confidence interval.

reported in the Henry Ford Exercise Testing Project, which observed the associations across strata of age, gender, race, obesity, resting blood pressure, and diabetes (Juraschek and others 2014).

Physical activity can directly and indirectly reduce the effects of excess cholesterol and other atherosclerotic agents (Durstine, Haskell, and Holloszy 1994; Farrell, Finley, and Grundy 2012; Pedersen and Saltin 2015). A review article of 13 studies and two review articles concluded that both aerobic and resistance exercise and the combination of aerobic and resistance training have an impact on cholesterol levels and blood lipids (Mann, Beedie, and Jimenez 2014). Participation in both moderate- and higher-intensity physical activity was shown to provide beneficial improvements in cholesterol levels, specifically increasing good (high-density lipoprotein) cholesterol, while maintaining and theoretically offsetting increases in bad (low-density lipoprotein) cholesterol and triglycerides (Kokkinos 2012; Mann, Beedie, and Jimenez 2014).

Regular physical activity in overweight and obese adults can have positive effects on waist circumference and body weight, both of which are risk factors for cardiometabolic disease. Results from a Cochrane Review show that physical activity combined with a restricted diet and dietary counseling is effective and more effective than physical activity alone (Shaw and others 2006). Physical training combined with a restricted diet and dietary counseling reduces body weight slightly, but significantly more than a restricted diet or dietary counseling alone (Shaw and others 2006). Studies of physical training without dietary change showed that high-intensity physical training reduced body weight more than low-intensity physical training (Shaw and others 2006). These results are consistent with other meta-analyses (Johns and others 2014; Wu and others 2009).

Sedentary Activity and Sitting: An Emerging Risk Factor

Sedentary behavior is emerging as a new and potentially independent risk factor for cardiometabolic disease (Owen and others 2010). Sedentary behavior is distinct from physical activity and comprises very low-level energy expenditure activities such as sitting or lying down. There is now good evidence that time spent in prolonged, particularly uninterrupted, "sitting" is a risk factor for cardiovascular and associated comorbidities, including higher waist circumference and obesity, IGT and insulin resistance, systemic inflammation, and elevated blood pressure, even after adjusting for levels of moderate-to-vigorous physical activity (de Heer and others 2012; Dunstan and others 2010; Dunstan, Thorp, and Healy 2011; Healy and others 2008).

Patel and others (2010) assessed the relationship between sitting and physical activity and total mortality in a large prospective study of U.S. adults. Results showed time spent sitting (six or more versus fewer than three hours a day) was associated with mortality in both women (RR 1.34, 95 percent CI 1.25–1.44) and men (RR 1.17, 95 percent CI 1.11–1.24), after adjustment for smoking, BMI, and other factors. These associations were strongest for CVD mortality. Interrupting or breaking up the time spent sitting with short bouts of physical activity has been shown to be associated with lower blood pressure, two-hour plasma glucose, triglycerides, waist circumference, and BMI (Dunstan and others 2012; Healy and others 2008; Larsen and others 2014).

Other studies using objective measures of sedentary time (such as accelerometers) have also reported increased risks associated with sedentary behavior for long durations and the benefits of breaking up sitting

time by brief periods of standing or light activity (Chau and others 2013; Parsons and others 2016). Collectively this emerging body of evidence suggests that public health action is warranted both to increase physical activity and to reduce time spent sitting. Although global guidelines on how much sitting is too much are not yet available, some countries have already reviewed the evidence and developed national recommendations, particularly for children and youth (Tremblay and others 2011).

Summary of the Evidence

Physical activity has well-established benefits for the prevention and management of cardiometabolic diseases. In addition, regular physical activity can provide numerous other health and social benefits, such as preventing and treating depression and anxiety (Warburton, Nicol, and Bredin 2006), preventing cognitive decline and dementia (Scholz and others 2009), preventing falls and promoting independent living in older adults (Sherrington and others 2008), and preventing osteoporosis by generating and maintaining peak bone mass (Bielemann, Martinez-Mesa, and Gigante 2014; Kemmler and others 2015). Regular participation in physical activity is important across the life span. For young children, regular active play and active recreation promote healthy growth and development, fitness, and healthy weight and can improve cognitive development and academic performance (Singh and others 2012). Physical activity is independently associated with prevention of CHD, stroke, and diabetes and can modify other metabolic risk factors such as hypertension, hyperlipidemia, and overweight and obesity. Walking and other forms of moderate-intensity physical activity can provide protective effects, and emerging evidence now suggests the importance of efforts to reduce time spent in prolonged sedentary behaviors for optimal health outcomes.

ECONOMIC COSTS OF PHYSICAL INACTIVITY

Before the 1990s, virtually no published data addressing the costs of inactivity were available. However, with the development of better measures of exposure and increasing availability of data on disease-specific health care costs, studies have now been conducted to assess the direct costs of inactivity to national health care systems in more than a dozen countries, mostly HICs.

Online annex 5A provides a summary of recent studies using the cost-of-illness approach and reporting estimates of the direct health care costs attributable to physical inactivity.

Pratt and others (2014) synthesized 11 published estimates from six HICs and, despite heterogeneity between studies and health systems, found consistent results attributing between 1.0 percent and 2.6 percent of total health care costs (for the selected health outcomes) to inactivity. Higher estimates were explained by the inclusion of additional health outcomes over and above CHD, stroke, diabetes, and cancer—for example, osteoporosis, musculoskeletal conditions (that is, hip fractures and falls), and mental health issues such as depression (Colditz 1999; Katzmarzyk, Gledhill, and Shephard 2000). Including these additional conditions can yield estimates of direct health care costs of well over 1 billion in national currencies. These estimates may appear high, but given the substantial evidence on the role of physical activity in the prevention and treatment of other health outcomes, estimates that exclude these conditions are generally viewed as conservative. Although desirable, inclusion of these other conditions is frequently hampered by a lack of reliable data, especially in LMICs.

Studies from LMICs, such as Brazil (São Paulo) and Colombia (Bogotá), provide similar estimates of total direct health care costs from physical inactivity (3.3 percent and 2.5 percent, respectively). In Eastern Europe, an analysis from the Czech Republic reported that physical inactivity caused an estimated 2,442 deaths, or 2.3 percent of all deaths, 1.2 percent of all disability-adjusted life years, and almost CZK 700 million (US$29 million), or 0.4 percent, of total health care costs for public insurance companies (Maresova 2014). In China, Popkin and others (2006) reported estimates of US$1 billion in direct medical costs of physical inactivity for 2001 and projected that these costs will reach 8.7 percent of total health care costs by 2025.

Most of the economic evidence to date has estimated direct health care costs. However, the *indirect* costs of inactivity include the value of economic output lost because of illness (productivity lost due to sickness and absenteeism), injury-related work disability, or premature death before retirement, as well as privately incurred health care costs and informal care for persons with NCDs. Furthermore, a complete analysis should also include the costs of being active (equipment) and the costs of the consequences of activity (such as injuries and lost productivity due to injuries). Few scholars have taken such a comprehensive approach, although Katzmarzyk and Janssen (2004) estimated the total economic burden of physical inactivity in Canada in 2001 to be Can$5.3 billion (US$4 billion), of which Can$1.6 billion (US$1.2 billion) was direct costs and Can$3.7 billion (US$2.8 billion) was indirect costs.

Another example is from the United Kingdom, where Game Plan, the national policy on sports and physical activity, reported that inactivity cost almost £2 billion (US$2.8 billion) a year, of which £0.3 billion (US$0.4 billion) was direct costs to the national health system, £0.8 billion (US$1.1 billion) was due to absence from work, and £0.8 billion (US$1.1 billion) was due to premature mortality (Department of Culture, Media, and Sports 2002; Scarborough and others 2011). Modeling of total costs using higher levels of inactivity and a wider range of health outcomes (including lower back pain) produced estimates up to £8 billion (US$11.5 billion) a year, although some challenge these estimates because of the lack of transparency of methods (Allender and others 2007). Nonetheless, Game Plan takes a more sophisticated approach to incorporating all costs and benefits of inactivity in a model.

Several countries have undertaken economic modeling of change in level of activity. In Northern Ireland, reducing inactivity from 20 percent to 15 percent could save £0.62 million (US$0.89 million) in avoidable health care costs. This estimate was considered conservative because it excluded adults older than age 75 years. In New Zealand, reducing inactivity from 31 percent to 21 percent could potentially save $NZ 48 (US$32 million) a year, while in Australia a 10 percent reduction could save 25,000 of the 174,000 attributable disability-adjusted life years and save the health care sector $A 96 million (US$72.6 million)—about 14 percent of annual health sector costs (Cadilhac and others 2011).

To date the economic arguments for savings in health care costs are not used extensively, at least at the global level, which may reflect the heterogeneity of current evidence and suggests a need for greater international collaboration to develop capacity in this field. Gaps in evidence include more estimates from LMICs; estimates of total costs (including wider societal impacts); and estimates of cost savings for specific subpopulations, particularly women, high-risk patients, and older adults. The efforts to develop extensive global, regional, and national datasets on the burden of disease are providing a strong foundation and good research opportunities to support the rapid maturation of this field over the next three to five years.

INTERVENTIONS TO INCREASE POPULATION-LEVEL PHYSICAL ACTIVITY

Demand is growing for clear policy direction on how to increase population-level participation in physical activity supported by robust evidence on the effectiveness of strategies that are transferable to diverse settings and contexts globally. To date, research undertaken in HICs (notably Australia, Europe, and North America) dominates the published literature; however, evidence from LMICs is accumulating and now includes some systematic reviews (Barbosa Filho and others 2016; Hoehner and others 2013).

National governments have periodically reviewed the evidence to produce guidance for policy development; notable examples are in the United Kingdom and the United States (see online annex 5B for references). However, to date few globally relevant resources provide easily accessible, evidence-based information with wider applicability on what works to increase physical activity. To fill this gap, the Global Advocacy for Physical Activity Initiative developed a "blueprint" for a settings-based, population approach to increasing physical activity (GAPA 2012). The resulting document, "NCD Prevention: Seven Investments That Work for Physical Activity," provides a framework for national action that is applicable to all countries:

- *Whole-of-school programs*, including regular, quality opportunities for physical education and activity for all children before, during, and after the school day
- *Primary health care* that promotes and integrates physical activity in patient risk assessment systems and primary and secondary care pathways
- *Public education campaigns* that raise health awareness of physical activity and create positive social norms
- *Transport and urban design policies, regulations, and infrastructure* that prioritize and support safe, accessible walking and cycling; use of public transport; and safe access to recreational and sporting opportunities
- *Sports systems and programs* that promote sports for development or sports for all and encourage participation across the life span
- *Community-based programs* that provide spaces and programs tailored to the community's cultures and traditions.

The latest evidence and best practice support the importance of each of these seven areas. Schools and primary health care are well-established settings for primary prevention and health promotion, including physical activity. Community-wide public education strategies also can and should address physical inactivity. Recent evidence has reinforced the importance of transport and urban design in shaping activity levels because these sectors provide the supportive infrastructure and environments for physical activity, such as on- and off-road cycle paths, footpaths and pedestrian networks, sporting and recreational facilities, and public open spaces.

This following sections summarize programs in these settings and identifies key barriers to scaling up action and implementation.

Whole-of-School Programs

Substantial evidence indicates that undertaking whole-of-school programs can promote physical activity. This approach should ensure that physical education takes place regularly and that classes provide opportunities for all students to be highly active (Kemmler and others 2015). Schools should also provide supportive environments, within the limitations of their resources, to support both structured and unstructured play and physical activity by children throughout the school day. Approaches should include promoting of walking and cycling to school, where safe and appropriate, and an enabling policy environment with engagement of parents, teachers, students, and members of surrounding communities (GAPA 2012).

The key principles of a whole-of-school approach have been shown to be effective in high-income as well as resource-constrained contexts, such as in Latin America (Barbosa Filho and others 2016; Ribeiro and others 2010). However, although good examples exist, to date, very few countries have implemented a comprehensive school strategy on a national scale, partially because of competing priorities, inadequate resources, and weak enforcement of the legislative and policy structures.

Primary Health Care

There is a well-established evidence base, albeit largely from HICs, supporting the effectiveness of having health care professionals counsel patients on physical inactivity as part of primary and secondary prevention care pathways. A typical approach includes a brief assessment of patients' level of physical activity as a vital sign for NCD prevention and provision of brief advice by the health care professional with referral to community -based opportunities and programs (Arena, Harrington, and Després 2015). Often called *exercise referral* or *exercise by prescription*, these approaches have been integrated, in varying degrees, into the primary health care systems of countries such as New Zealand and the United Kingdom as well as those of some health care providers in the United States. For example, as described in online annex 5C, New Zealand's Green Prescription has been scaled up to a national level through a partnership between general practitioner groups and the Ministry of Sport and Recreation and with funding from the Ministry of Health (Elley and others 2003). Such initiatives can also be found in Sweden (Kallings and others 2008), the United Kingdom (Boehler and others 2011), and elsewhere (Sørensen, Skovgaard, and Puggaard 2006). The American College of Sports Medicine has initiated a global initiative, Exercise Is Medicine (Lobelo, Stoutenberg, and Hutber 2014), to expand this concept to more countries. However, more research is needed to assess the effectiveness and feasibility of this approach in LMICs in which the system and resource context of primary health and other competing priorities present significant challenges.

Public Education Campaigns

Public education through mass media campaigns can provide an effective way to transmit consistent and clear messages about the benefits of physical activity to large populations. It can include paid advertisements and non-paid news coverage across a variety of media platforms and aim to raise awareness, increase knowledge, shift community norms, and motivate populations to be more active (Cavill and Bauman 2004). Public education campaigns should ideally involve multiple channels (print, audio, and electronic media; outdoor billboards; and posters) as well as new media (text messaging, social networking, and other uses of the Internet) in coordination with other community-based activities to form a comprehensive strategy. Combinations of these approaches, sustained over time (usually years), is most effective, and there are published examples from high- and some middle-income countries of the effectiveness of this approach (Hoehner and others 2013; Leavy and others 2011). Although public education campaigns were identified as a best buy by the World Health Organization (WHO) (2014b), and it is recommended that countries scale up implementation, education strategies alone are insufficient to achieve population-level change in physical activity; coordinated strategies across other settings are needed (Leavy and others 2011).

Transport and Urban Design Policies, Regulations, and Infrastructure

The need for supportive policy, programs, and systems within the transport and urban design sector was highlighted nearly two decades ago (Sallis, Bauman, and Pratt 1998), and there is now an impressive body of evidence reporting the strong and consistent impacts of urban and transport design on levels of physical activity in both HICs and LMICs (Adams and others 2013; Sallis and others 2016). Interventions that provide relevant infrastructure aimed at promoting safe walking and cycling ("active transport") are practical, sustainable ways to increase daily physical activity in whole populations.

They also provide benefits to other sectors by reducing traffic congestion, noise and air pollution, and carbon dioxide emissions. Supportive policy frameworks in transport and planning are needed that reorient and reprioritize land use allocation and infrastructure provision to encourage walking, cycling, and public transport. When combined with effective promotional programs, supportive policies can shift the chosen mode of transport away from personal motorized vehicles and toward physical activity (Ogilvie and others 2016).

Such approaches are beginning to gain traction, particularly in cities where the cost of urban sprawl and levels of congestion and pollution have supported a reappraisal of regional, city, and neighborhood urban planning. Cities such as Amsterdam, Copenhagen, and New York as well as Bogotá and Recife provide good examples of how changes in design and infrastructure can lead to significantly higher levels of walking and cycling for short trips and overall physical activity (New York State Government 2010; Paez and others 2015; Pratt, Perez, and others 2015; Pucher, Dill, and Handy 2010). In Bogotá, Colombia (Torres and others 2013), and Recife, Brazil (Reis and others 2010), the provision of off-road cycle and footpaths and the closure of roads to motorized vehicles provided improved access to safe and enjoyable places to be active and made cycling and walking safe and convenient forms of transport for short trips (box 5.2). Robust longitudinal evidence is now available from studies evaluating new urban planning policies that prioritize design elements that support active transport and outdoor recreation (Goodman, Sahlqvist, and Ogilvie 2014; Hooper and others 2015; Ogilvie and others 2016), although more examples, particularly from longitudinal evaluations of city redesign in LMICs, are needed to demonstrate this feasible population-based approach to promoting physical activity (Goenka and others 2007; Goenka and others 2009) (boxes 5.2 and 5.3).

Sports Systems and Programs

Potential synergies exist between sports and the promotion of physical activity given that sports, by definition, involve physical activity. However, sports programs do not necessarily encourage mass participation because they often focus on supporting the talented, encouraging high performance and elite competitions. Yet, population levels of physical activity could be increased through greater engagement with community-based sports programs, particularly those using the Sport for All principles (International Olympic Committee 2014). Building on the universal appeal of sports, a comprehensive and inclusive national sports policy and system should

Box 5.2

Community-Based Programs in Brazil

Academia da Cidade was initiated in the city of Recife, a state capital in northeast Brazil. The program provides free daily physical activity classes in early mornings and late afternoons led by trained physical educators. Restructuring and reengineering of public parks and plazas, often in poor and dangerous neighborhoods, increased provision of safe public spaces in the community for physical activity along with good equipment and supervision. Strong connections with the public primary health care system allowed for easy referrals for prevention and treatment of non-communicable diseases. Program evaluation showed positive results, and it has been adapted and expanded to more than 400 cities that are delivering community classes and improving infrastructure to support physical activity (Simoes and others 2009).

Agita São Paulo (Move São Paulo) aims to increase knowledge of the benefits of and levels of physical activity in the general population. The program name itself, *Agita*, is a strong idiomatic expression that means much more than just move your body, it also means move your mind, move your citizenship, be ready for change (Matsudo and others 2002). It focuses on students, workplaces, and the community and applies an ecological model with strategies aimed at addressing the intrapersonal, social, and physical-environment factors that influence physical activity (Matsudo and others 2004). Evaluation showed high levels of program awareness, an increase in physical activity, and reductions in sitting time. Agita São Paulo was led and coordinated by the Studies Center of the Physical Fitness Research Laboratory of São Caetano do Sul.

Key success factors include the following:

- A clear message promoting at least 30 minutes of physical activity per day
- Use of social marketing and a successful program logo and group of mascots
- Strong intersectoral and intrasectoral partnerships involving government, nongovernmental organizations, and the private sector
- Targeting of subpopulations with tailored messages and exploiting cultural links
- Combining permanent actions with large events (for example, Agita Galera involves almost 6 million students from more than 6,000 schools)
- Maximal use of unpaid mass media for promotion
- Capacity building across 17 regional departments of health covering 645 cities.

Box 5.3

Community-Based Programs in Colombia

In Colombia, a number of city programs began in the 1990s, eventually forming a national physical activity network in 2002. In 2008, an intersectoral government commission for physical activity was created, and in 2009, the Congress of Colombia passed a national obesity law that included strategies for improving environments, policies, and programs for physical activity. The National Development Plan 2010–14 included physical activity promotion as a priority, with specific 10-year plans for sports, recreation, physical education, and public health. Stimulated by both supportive policies and local programs, the national sports institute (Coldeportes) launched a national physical activity program focused on training public health and physical activity professionals across Colombia to deliver community-based programs modeled on Muévete Bogotá (Gámez and others 2006) and the *ciclovías* of Bogotá, Medellin, and Cali (where it is referred to as open streets programs) (Sarmiento and others 2010). Free physical activity classes in public parks, plazas, and community centers similar to those in Brazil and a network of 67 open streets programs (Vías Activas y Saludables) are key components of the national program.

include the provision of sporting opportunities to match the interests, skills, and capabilities of men, women, girls, and boys of all ages. The Sport for All initiative focuses on the democratization of, and mass participation in, sports and recreation with the aim of improving health and social inclusion through sports, particularly for vulnerable groups such as the poor, the elderly, and women (Cousineau, Collins, and Cooper 1998). With a strong focus on enjoyment, Sport for All programs are usually community based, culturally adapted, and inclusive, and they build on partnerships between local sporting clubs, municipal sports and recreational authorities, and national sports organizations (Cousineau, Collins, and Coopeer 1998; Marlier and others 2015).

One example of a successful sports-based program is Football Fans in Training, which has incorporated attributes of community-wide programs and the health-through-sport conceptual model. It targets hard-to-reach men from low-income communities in Scotland and provides weekly physical activity sessions at a professional soccer club along with nutritional information and follow-up. The results have included significant weight loss; reduction in waist circumference, body fat, and blood pressure; as well as improvements in physical activity compared with the control group (who received information only) (Hunt and others 2014). Furthermore, there has been minimal loss at follow-up, and the approach has been shown to be cost-effective and capable of attracting and retaining men at risk of cardiometabolic diseases (Hunt and others 2014). Sport for All programs can also address gender inequalities (see box 5.4).

Promotion of physical activity is aligned with the United Nations Sport for Development and Peace Initiative (United Nations 2016). This program focuses on promoting the benefits of sports participation and social outcomes such as increasing social capital, providing diversionary activities, changing social norms, and addressing selected health issues. Grassroots Soccer is a well-known initiative typically practiced in low-income settings. It has increased awareness of and lowered the stigma regarding human immunodeficiency virus/acquired immune deficiency syndrome (HIV/AIDS) and contributed significantly to achieving the recommended guidelines for moderate-to-vigorous activity for youth (Fenton, Duda, and Barrett 2014).

Community-Based Programs

Community-based programs are programs run outside of schools and the health care system, including programs offering exercise classes in worksite, faith-based, and other community venues and public spaces. This is a diverse area of research, but it has shown some positive results, particularly in low-income settings. Boxes 5.2 and 5.3 discuss examples of programs run in the community and changes to the use of road infrastrcture to support safe walking and cycling. Other examples of community-based programs include exercise equipment and programs provided in urban parks, often free of charge for community use.

COST-EFFECTIVENESS OF PHYSICAL ACTIVITY INTERVENTIONS

Several reviews provide estimates of the cost-effectiveness of population-level physical activity interventions (Laine and others 2014; Roux and others 2008). Roux and others (2008) conducted a lifetime cost-effectiveness analysis using a societal perspective to estimate the costs, health gains, and cost-effectiveness (dollars per quality-adjusted life year [QALY] gained) of seven public health

---

Box 5.4

Gender Issues and Physical Activity

In many cultures, girls and women have fewer opportunities to participate in physical activities than boys and men. For example, customs and cultural norms related to women's clothing may make it difficult for women and girls to be physically active, and societal values may prohibit women from being active in public. These barriers can be overcome by providing women-only, culturally acceptable opportunities and facilities, although resources are scarce and not always available for separate facilities and programs.

The recently agreed-on Sustainable Development Goals (United Nations 2015) address gender inequalities, with several targets related to equitable educational environments and opportunities for women and girls.

interventions recommended by the U.S. Guide to Community Preventive Services. The interventions tested were community-wide campaigns; individually adapted health behavior change; social support interventions; and creation or enhancement of access to information on, and opportunities for, physical activity. Each intervention was compared with the alternative of no intervention. Cost-effectiveness ratios ranged between US$14,000 and US$69,000 per QALY gained. Results were sensitive to intervention-related costs and effect size.

Laine and others (2014) developed methods to convert the costs of interventions into costs per person per day in 2012 U.S. dollars and calculated the physical activity results as the metabolic equivalent of task hours (MET-h) gained per person per day. The results showed that population-based interventions such as providing opportunities for biking and cycling were cost-effective (US$0.006 per MET-h), as were school-based education programs (US$0.056 per MET-h), point-of-decision prompts to promote stair use (US$0.07 per MET-h), and the use of pedometers (US$0.014 per MET-h) (Laine and others 2014). Interventions that sought to affect the behavior of individuals were the least cost-effective but had the largest effects (Wu and others 2011). In primary care settings, Garrett and others (2011) estimated the cost to move one person to the "active" category at 12 months to be between €331 and €3,673 (between US$369 and US$4,095). The estimated cost-utility varied across nine studies from €348 (US$388) to €86,877 (US$96,865) per QALY.

Further research is needed to assess the cost-effectiveness of different interventions across different settings and resource contexts. Although this research has been called for before (Kohl and others 2012), inadequate progress has been made toward strengthening this evidence base.

GLOBAL PROGRESS IN PUBLIC POLICY

The 2004 Global Strategy on Diet, Physical Activity and Health (WHO 2004) provided consensus on the importance of physical activity for NCD prevention and detailed the recommended national actions required to increase physical activity and decrease sedentary activity globally. The 2011 United Nations Declaration (United Nations 2011) and the 2014 WHO Global Action Plan for the Prevention and Control of NCDs 2013–2020 (WHO 2013) provide an updated framework for physical activity in national NCD policies. The NCD monitoring and evaluation framework requested by the United Nations and led by the WHO resulted in the first global target on physical activity—namely, to reduce inactivity by 10 percent by 2025 (WHO 2013).

Collectively, these documents provide the global policy framework for population-based action on physical activity within all countries.

Although many Northern and Western European countries began by developing national policies on physical activity in the late 1990s, the global target and United Nations Declaration provide a new stimulus to all countries, particularly to LMICs. Recent reviews of current national policy approaches have identified areas that need strengthening (Bull and others 2014; Bull and others 2015; Daugbjerg and others 2009). Policy documents often state no measurable, time-bound targets for physical activity; many countries have no systematic population surveillance system in place to track trends; policy implementation is weak and inadequately resourced; and relevant sectors have limited capacity (Bull and Bauman 2011).

In LMICs, progress on national physical activity policies and actions has been much slower, although global policy frameworks have stimulated a notable increase in recent years. Indeed, the proportion of countries with policies on physical activity has risen from 29 percent in 2005 to 73 percent in 2010 and to 80 percent in 2013 (Sallis and others 2016; WHO 2015). However, ensuring and monitoring policy implementation are now a priority area. Although 80 percent of countries reported policies on physical activity in 2013, only 56 percent of these policies were operational—that is, the policy was "active and funded" (WHO 2015). This highlights a significant gap in country capacity to implement actions on physical activity, even when a policy priority is established.

Other civil society reporting systems (Pratt, Ramirez, and others 2015; Tremblay and others 2014) are providing useful data and reports assessing individual country progress. Such report cards vary in their content, level of detail, and intended audience. Other tools support countries undertaking comprehensive situational analyses of physical activity policy. Use of the Policy Audit Tool (Bull and others 2015) in the Middle East (WHO 2014b) has provided a regional overview as well as between-country comparison of policy and program initiatives, which can help guide decision making and selection of areas for investment.

Examples of country action are useful for sharing lessons of what did and did not work. Recent work assessing programs in Brazil, Canada, Colombia, and Finland provides an interesting contrast. Both Brazil and Colombia developed their national programs from a base of well-evaluated city-scale programs, while Canada implemented a sustained national mass media campaign (ParticipACTION) over decades to promote the benefits of physical activity and establish strong and enduring awareness in the community (Pratt, Perez, and others 2015). Finland benefited from the strong cultural value placed on physical activity combined with a steady flow of supportive programs, local government grants, and other initiatives coordinated by a national steering committee. Both Canada and Finland had good preexisting infrastructure, public open spaces, and an urban environment conducive to physical activity in daily living, as well as a lower density of population and greater socioeconomic equity than Brazil and Colombia. Despite differences in context and approaches, these countries have experienced success because they cultivated political support, secured sustained leadership from key agencies, and made large-scale efforts to obtain community engagement.

CONCLUSIONS

A strong body of evidence supports the benefits of promoting physical activity to reduce cardiometabolic disease. Economic analyses conducted in a variety of countries indicate that between 3 percent and 6 percent of national health care costs are attributable to physical inactivity. Good evidence suggests that effective interventions can increase population-level physical activity by encouraging activity in daily living and providing opportunities for sports and recreational activity. National policy recommendations include implementing population-based strategies to provide the supportive environments that make physical activity possible, accessible, and desirable, combined with interventions and programs that enhance the knowledge and social value of physical activity, particularly in countries where physical activity is not yet socially or culturally viewed as desirable. Although there is a strong global policy framework and consensus-based recommendations on physical activity, in most countries, particularly LMICs, a significant disconnect exists between the scientific evidence, public health need, and implementation. The challenge is to find ways to translate evidence into effective public health action within the context of rising levels of inactivity at work, during transport, and during recreation.

National policy makers need to identify and address the gaps in implementation. Examples of successful implementation show how physical activity can be increased through sustained multisectoral policy actions. Key elements of success are engaging stakeholders and working in partnership across ministries and portfolios. Establishing and maintaining such partnerships are challenging for all governments. However, many of the determinants of active living lie outside of the health sector, and such partnerships are essential for sustained success in

increasing national levels of physical activity. Individually targeted behavior change programs will be unsuccessful or short lived without changes to the physical environment to support active lifestyles. Site-specific interventions can improve schools, worksites, and even primary health care settings to provide significant benefits.

National strategies to promote physical activity should include policies and programs across multiple settings, and these approaches need to be adapted to the country context and culture. Strong political leadership is needed to raise the priority given to physical activity as part of the NCD-prevention agenda, and cross-sector engagement using participatory approaches and community engagement is critical to success.

ANNEXES

The annexes to this chapter are as follows. They are available at http://www.dcp-3.org/CVRD.

- Annex 5A. Summary of Results on Direct Costs of Inactivity from 18 Studies between 1980–2014
- Annex 5B. Tabulation of the Population Strategies and Interventions to Increase Physical Activity Levels at Multiple Levels of Interventions
- Annex 5C. New Zealand's Green Prescription (GRx)

NOTES

The authors wish to acknowledge the contributions of Victor Matsudo.

World Bank Income Classifications as of July 2014 are as follows, based on estimates of gross national income (GNI) per capita for 2013:

- Low-income countries (LICs) = US$1,045 or less
- Middle-income countries (MICs) are subdivided:
  (a) lower-middle-income = US$1,046 to US$4,125
  (b) upper-middle-income (UMICs) = US$4,126 to US$12,745
- High-income countries (HICs) = US$12,746 or more.

REFERENCES

Adams, M. A., D. Ding, J. F. Sallis, H. R. Bowles, B. E. Ainsworth, and others. 2013. "Patterns of Neighborhood Environment Attributes Related to Physical Activity across 11 Countries: A Latent Class Analysis." *International Journal of Behavioral Nutrition and Physical Activity* 10: 34.

Adler, A. I., I. M. Stratton, H. A. W. Neil, J. S. Yudkin, D. R. Matthews, and others. 2000. "Association of Systolic Blood Pressure with Macrovascular and Microvascular Complications of Type 2 Diabetes (UKPDS 36): Prospective Observational Study." *BMJ* 321 (7258): 412–19.

Agarwal, S. K. 2012. "Cardiovascular Benefits of Exercise." *International Journal of General Medicine* 5 (June): 541–45.

Alberti, K. G. M., P. Zimmet, and J. Shaw. 2007. "International Diabetes Federation: A Consensus on Type 2 Diabetes Prevention." *Diabetic Medicine* 24 (5): 451–63.

Allender, S., C. Foster, P. Scarborough, and M. Rayner. 2007. "The Burden of Physical Activity–Related Ill Health in the UK." *Journal of Epidemiology and Community Health* 61 (4): 344–48.

American Diabetes Association. 2014. "Position Statement: Standards of Medical Care in Diabetes: 2014." *Diabetes Care* 37 (Suppl 1): S14–80.

Anderson, L., N. Oldridge, D. R. Thompson, A.-D. Zwisler, K. Rees, and others. 2016. "Exercise-Based Cardiac Rehabilitation for Coronary Heart Disease: Cochrane Systematic Rand Meta-Analysis." *Journal of the American College of Cardiology* 67 (1): 1–12.

Archer, E., R. P. Shook, D. M. Thomas, T. S. Church, P. T. Katzmarzyk, and others. 2013. "45-Year Trends in Women's Use of Time and Household Management Energy Expenditure." *PLoS One* 8 (2): e56620.

Arena, R., R. A. Harrington, and J.-P. Després. 2015. "A Message from Modern-Day Healthcare to Physical Activity and Fitness: Welcome Home!" *Progress in Cardiovascular Diseases* 57 (4): 293–95.

Armstrong, T., and F. Bull. 2006. "Development of the World Health Organization Global Physical Activity Questionnaire (GPAQ)." *Journal of Public Health* 14 (2): 66–70.

Aune, D., T. Norat, M. Leitzmann, S. Tonstad, and L. Vatten. 2015. "Physical Activity and the Risk of Type 2 Diabetes: A Systematic Review and Dose-Response Meta-Analysis." *European Journal of Epidemiology* 30 (7): 529–42.

Balady, G. J., M. A. Williams, P. A. Ades, V. Bittner, P. Comoss, and others. 2007. "Core Components of Cardiac Rehabilitation/Secondary Prevention Programs: 2007 Update." *Circulation* 115 (20): 2675–82.

Barbosa Filho, V. C., G. Minatto, J. Mota, K. S. Silva, W. de Campos, and others. 2016. "Promoting Physical Activity for Children and Adolescents in Low- and Middle-Income Countries: An Umbrella Systematic Review: A Review on Promoting Physical Activity in LMIC." *Preventive Medicine* 88 (July): 115–26.

Barnett, T. A., L. Gauvin, C. L. Craig, and P. T. Katzmarzyk. 2008. "Distinct Trajectories of Leisure Time Physical Activity and Predictors of Trajectory Class Membership: A 22-Year Cohort Study." *International Journal of Behavioral Nutrition and Physical Activity* 5 (1): 57.

Barry, V. W., M. Baruth, M. W. Beets, J. L. Durstine, J. Liu, and others. 2014. "Fitness vs. Fatness on All-Cause Mortality: A Meta-Analysis." *Progress in Cardiovascular Diseases* 56 (4): 382–90.

Berry, S. 2013. "Sitting Is the New Smoking." *Sydney Morning Herald,* May 30.

Bhurosy, T., and R. Jeewon. 2014. "Overweight and Obesity Epidemic in Developing Countries: A Problem with Diet, Physical Activity, or Socioeconomic Status?" *Scientific World Journal* 2014 (October): 964236.

Bielemann, R. M., J. Martinez-Mesa, and D. P. Gigante. 2014. "Physical Activity during Life Course and Bone Mass: A Systematic Review of Methods and Findings from Cohort Studies with Young Adults." *BMC Musculoskeletal Disorders* 14 (March): 77.

Blair, S. N., H. W. Kohl, R. S. Paffenbarger, D. G. Clark, K. H. Cooper, and others. 1989. "Physical Fitness and All-Cause Mortality: A Prospective Study of Healthy Men and Women." *Journal of the American Medical Association* 262 (17): 2395–401.

Blondell, S. J., R. Hammersley-Mather, and J. L. Veerman. 2014. "Does Physical Activity Prevent Cognitive Decline and Dementia? A Systematic Review and Meta-Analysis of Longitudinal Studies." *BMC Public Health* 14 (May): 510.

Boehler, C. E., K. E. Milton, F. C. Bull, and J. A. Fox-Rushby. 2011. "The Cost of Changing Physical Activity Behaviour: Evidence from a 'Physical Activity Pathway' in the Primary Care Setting." *BMC Public Health* 11 (1): 1.

Bull, F. C., T. P. Armstrong, T. Dixon, S. Ham, A. Neiman, and others. 2004. "Physical Inactivity." In *Global and Regional Burden of Disease Attributable to Selected Major Risk Factors*, edited by M. Ezzati, A. Lopez, J. Rogers, and C. J. Murray. Geneva: World Health Organization.

Bull, F. C., and A. E. Bauman. 2011. "Physical Inactivity: The 'Cinderella' Risk Factor for Noncommunicable Disease Prevention." *Journal of Health Communication* 16 (Suppl 2): 13–26.

Bull, F. C., K. Milton, S. Kahlmeier, A. Arlotti, A. B. Juričan, and others. 2015. "Turning the Tide: National Policy Approaches to Increasing Physical Activity in Seven European Countries." *British Journal of Sports Medicine* 49 (11): 749–56.

Bull, F. C., K. Milton, S. Kahlmeier, H. E. Brown, N. Burton, and others. 2014. "National Policy on Physical Activity: The Development of a Policy Audit Tool." *Journal of Physical Activity and Health* 11 (2): 233–40.

Cadilhac, D. A., T. B. Cumming, L. Sheppard, D. C. Pearce, R. Carter, and others. 2011. "The Economic Benefits of Reducing Physical Inactivity: An Australian Example." *International Journal of Behavioral Nutrition and Physical Activity* 8 (1): 99.

Carnethon, M. R., N. S. Evans, T. S. Church, C. E. Lewis, P. J. Schreiner, and others. 2010. "Joint Associations of Physical Activity and Aerobic Fitness on the Development of Incident Hypertension Coronary Artery Risk Development in Young Adults." *Hypertension* 56 (1): 49–55.

Caspersen, C. J., K. E. Powell, and G. M. Christenson. 1985. "Physical Activity, Exercise, and Physical Fitness: Definitions and Distinctions for Health-Related Research." *Public Health Reports* 100 (2): 126–31.

Cavill, N., and A. Bauman. 2004. "Changing the Way People Think about Health-Enhancing Physical Activity: Do Mass Media Campaigns Have a Role?" *Journal of Sports Sciences* 22 (8): 771–90.

Chau, J. Y., A. C. Grunseit, T. Chey, E. Stamatakis, W. J. Brown, and others. 2013. "Daily Sitting Time and All-Cause Mortality: A Meta-Analysis." *PLoS One* 8 (11): e80000.

Chobanian, A. V., G. L. Bakris, H. R. Black, W. C. Cushman, L. A. Green, and others. 2003. "The Seventh Report of the

Joint National Committee on Prevention, Detection, Evaluation, and Treatment of High Blood Pressure: The JNC 7 Report." *Journal of the American Medical Association* 289 (19): 2560–71.

Church, T. S., D. M. Thomas, C. Tudor-Locke, P. T. Katzmarzyk, C. P. Earnest, and others. 2011. "Trends over 5 Decades in US Occupation-Related Physical Activity and Their Associations with Obesity." *PLoS One* 6 (5): e19657.

Colditz, G. A. 1999. "Economic Costs of Obesity and Inactivity." *Medicine and Science in Sports and Exercise* 31 (11 Suppl): S663–67.

Cousineau, C., M. Collins, and I. Cooper. 1998. "Leisure and Recreation and the 'Sport for All' Policy in Developing Countries: Critical Analysis." In *Leisure Management: Issues and Applications*, edited by M. F. Collins, and I. S. Cooper, 29–48. Wallingford, U.K.: Centre for Agriculture and Biosciences International.

Craig, C. L., A. L. Marshall, M. Sjostrom, A. E. Bauman, M. L. Booth, and others. 2003. "International Physical Activity Questionnaire: 12-Country Reliability and Validity." *Medicine and Science in Sports and Exercise* 35 (8): 1381–95.

Daugbjerg, S. B., S. Kahlmeier, F. Racioppi, E. Martin-Diener, B. Martin, and others. 2009. "Promotion of Physical Activity in the European Region: Content Analysis of 27 National Policy Documents." *Journal of Physical Activity and Health* 6 (6): 805.

de Heer, H. D., A. V. Wilkinson, L. L. Strong, M. L. Bondy, and L. M. Koehly. 2012. "Sitting Time and Health Outcomes among Mexican-Origin Adults: Obesity as a Mediator." *BMC Public Health* 12 (1): 1.

Department of Culture, Media, and Sports. 2002. *Game Plan: A Strategy for Delivering Government's Sport and Physical Activity Objectives.* London: Government Cabinet Office.

Diep, L., J. Kwagyan, J. Kurantsin-Mills, R. Weir, and A. Jayam-Trouth. 2010. "Association of Physical Activity Level and Stroke Outcomes in Men and Women: A Meta-Analysis." *Journal of Women's Health* 19 (10): 1815–22.

Dunstan, D. W., E. Barr, G. Healy, J. Salmon, J. Shaw, and others. 2010. "Television Viewing Time and Mortality: The Australian Diabetes, Obesity, and Lifestyle Study (AusDiab)." *Circulation* 121 (3): 384–91.

Dunstan, D. W., B. A. Kingwell, R. Larsen, G. N. Healy, E. Cerin, and others. 2012. "Breaking Up Prolonged Sitting Reduces Postprandial Glucose and Insulin Responses." *Diabetes Care* 35 (5): 976–83.

Dunstan, D. W., A. A. Thorp, and G. N. Healy. 2011. "Prolonged Sitting: Is It a Distinct Coronary Heart Disease Risk Factor?" *Current Opinion in Cardiology* 26 (5): 412–19.

Durstine, J., W. Haskell, and J. Holloszy. 1994. "Effects of Exercise Training on Plasma Lipids and Lipoprotein." *Exercise and Sports Sciences Reviews* 22: 477–521.

Elley, C. R., N. Kerse, B. Arroll, and E. Robinson. 2003. "Effectiveness of Counselling Patients on Physical Activity in General Practice: Cluster Randomised Controlled Trial." *BMJ* 326 (7393): 793.

Fagard, R. H. 2005. "Physical Activity, Physical Fitness, and the Incidence of Hypertension." *Journal of Hypertension* 23 (2): 265–67.

Farrell, S. W., C. E. Finley, and S. M. Grundy. 2012. "Cardiorespiratory Fitness, LDL Cholesterol, and CHD Mortality in Men." *Medicine and Science in Sports and Exercise* 44 (11): 2132–37.

Fenton, S. A., J. L. Duda, and T. Barrett. 2014. "The Contribution of Youth Sport Football to Weekend Physical Activity for Males Aged 9 to 16 Years: Variability Related to Age and Playing Position." *Pediatric Exercise Science* 27 (2): 208–18.

Figueira, F. R., D. Umpierre, F. V. Cureau, A. T. Zucatti, M. B. Dalzochio, and others. 2014. "Association between Physical Activity Advice Only or Structured Exercise Training with Blood Pressure Levels in Patients with Type 2 Diabetes: A Systematic Review and Meta-Analysis." *Sports Medicine* 44 (11): 1557–72.

Folsom, A. R., L. H. Kushi, and C.-P. Hong. 2000. "Physical Activity and Incident Diabetes Mellitus in Postmenopausal Women." *American Journal of Public Health* 90 (1): 134–38.

Gámez, R., D. Parra, M. Pratt, and T. Schmid. 2006. "Muévete Bogotá: Promoting Physical Activity with a Network of Partner Companies." *Promotion and Education* 13 (2): 138–43.

GAPA (Global Advocacy for Physical Activity). 2012. "NCD Prevention: Seven Investments that Work for Physical Activity." *British Journal of Sports Medicine* 46 (10): 709–12.

Garrett, S., C. R. Elley, S. B. Rose, D. O'Dea, B. A. Lawton, and others. 2011. "Are Physical Activity Interventions in Primary Care and the Community Cost-Effective? A Systematic Review of the Evidence." *British Journal of General Practice* 61 (584): e125–33.

Goenka, S. 2008. "Preventing Diabetes in Bangladeshi People in Britain." *BMJ* 337 (November): a2010.

Goenka, S., V. S. Ajay, P. Jeemon, D. Prabhakaran, C. Varghese, and K. S. Reddy. 2007. "Powering India's Growth." World Health Organization and IC Health Scientific Secretariat, New Delhi, India.

Goenka, S., D. Prabhakaran, V. S. Ajay, and K. S. Reddy. 2009. "Preventing Cardiovascular Disease in India: Translating Evidence to Action." *Current Science* 97 (3): 367–77.

Goodman, A., S. Sahlqvist, and D. Ogilvie. 2014. "New Walking and Cycling Routes and Increased Physical Activity: One- and 2-Year Findings from the UK iConnect Study." *American Journal of Public Health* 104 (9): e38–46.

Gupta, R., P. Joshi, V. Mohan, K. S. Reddy, and S. Yusuf. 2008. "Epidemiology and Causation of Coronary Heart Disease and Stroke in India." *Heart* 94 (1): 16–26

Guthold, R., M. J. Cowan, C. S. Autenrieth, L. Kann, and L. M. Riley. 2010. "Physical Activity and Sedentary Behavior among Schoolchildren: A 34-Country Comparison." *Journal of Pediatrics* 157 (1): 43–49.e1.

Hallal, P. C., L. B. Andersen, F. C. Bull, R. Guthold, W. Haskell, and others. 2012. "Global Physical Activity Levels: Surveillance Progress, Pitfalls, and Prospects." *The Lancet* 380 (9838): 247–57.

Hallal, P. C., K. Cordeira, A. G. Knuth, G. I. Mielke, and C. G. Victora. 2014. "Ten-Year Trends in Total Physical Activity Practice in Brazilian Adults: 2002–2012." *Journal of Physical Activity and Health* 11 (8): 1525–30.

Healy, G. N., D. W. Dunstan, J. Salmon, E. Cerin, J. E. Shaw, and others. 2008. "Breaks in Sedentary Time: Beneficial Associations with Metabolic Risk." *Diabetes Care* 31 (4): 661–66.

Helmrich, S., D. Ragland, and R. Paffenbarger. 1994. "Prevention of Non-Insulin-Dependent Diabetes Mellitus with Physical Activity." *Medicine and Science in Sports and Exercise* 26 (7): 824–30.

Hoehner, C. M., I. C. Ribeiro, D. C. Parra, R. S. Reis, M. R. Azevedo, and others. 2013. "Physical Activity Interventions in Latin America: Expanding and Classifying the Evidence." *American Journal of Preventive Medicine* 44 (3): e31–40.

Hooper, P., M. Knuiman, F. Bull, E. Jones, and B. Giles-Corti. 2015. "Are We Developing Walkable Suburbs through Urban Planning Policy? Identifying the Mix of Design Requirements to Optimise Walking Outcomes from the 'Liveable Neighbourhoods' Planning Policy in Perth, Western Australia." *International Journal of Behavioral Nutrition and Physical Activity* 12 (May): 63.

Howard, V. J., and M. N. McDonnell. 2015. "Physical Activity in Primary Stroke Prevention: Just Do It!" *Stroke* 46 (6): 1735–39.

Hsia, J., L. Wu, C. Allen, A. Oberman, W. E. Lawson, and others. 2005. "Physical Activity and Diabetes Risk in Postmenopausal Women." *American Journal of Preventive Medicine* 28 (1): 19–25.

Hu, F. B., M. F. Leitzmann, M. J. Stampfer, G. A. Colditz, W. C. Willett, and others. 2001. "Physical Activity and Television Watching in Relation to Risk for Type 2 Diabetes Mellitus in Men." *Archives of Internal Medicine* 161 (12): 1542–48.

Hu, F. B., R. J. Sigal, J. W. Rich-Edwards, G. A. Colditz, C. G. Solomon, and others. 1999. "Walking Compared with Vigorous Physical Activity and Risk of Type 2 Diabetes in Women: A Prospective Study." *Journal of the American Medical Association* 282 (15): 1433–39.

Hu, G., Q. Qiao, K. Silventoinen, J. G. Eriksson, P. Jousilahti, and others. 2003. "Occupational, Commuting, and Leisure-Time Physical Activity in Relation to Risk for Type 2 Diabetes in Middle-Aged Finnish Men and Women." *Diabetologia* 46 (3): 322–29.

Hunt, K., S. Wyke, C. M. Gray, A. S. Anderson, A. Brady, and others. 2014. "A Gender-Sensitised Weight Loss and Healthy Living Programme for Overweight and Obese Men Delivered by Scottish Premier League Football Clubs (FFIT): A Pragmatic Randomised Controlled Trial." *The Lancet* 383 (9924): 1211–21.

International Olympic Committee. 2014. *Get Moving! The IOC Guide to Managing Sport for All Programmes.* Lausanne, Switzerland: International Olympic Committee.

Ishida, S., C. Ito, and F. Murakami. 2005. "Prevention of Type 2 Diabetes Mellitus by Changing Life-Styles among High Risk Persons: The Diabetes Prevention Program in Hiroshima (DPPH)." *Nihon Rinsho [Japanese Journal of Clinical Medicine]* 63 (Suppl 2): 578–81.

Jeon, C. Y., R. P. Lokken, F. B. Hu, and R. M. Van Dam. 2007. "Physical Activity of Moderate Intensity and Risk of Type 2 Diabetes: A Systematic Review." *Diabetes Care* 30 (3): 744–52.

Johns, D. J., J. Hartmann-Boyce, S. A. Jebb, P. Aveyard, and Behavioral Weight Management Research Group. 2014. "Diet or Exercise Interventions vs. Combined Behavioral Weight Management Programs: A Systematic Review and Meta-Analysis of Direct Comparisons." *Journal of the Academy of Nutrition and Dietetics* 114 (10): 1557–68.

Juraschek, S. P., M. J. Blaha, S. P. Whelton, R. Blumenthal, S. R. Jones, and others. 2014. "Physical Fitness and Hypertension in a Population at Risk for Cardiovascular Disease: The Henry Ford Exercise Testing (FIT) Project." *Journal of the American Heart Association* 3 (6): e001268.

Kallings, L., M. Leijon, M. L. Hellénius, and A. Ståhle. 2008. "Physical Activity on Prescription in Primary Health Care: A Follow-Up of Physical Activity Level and Quality of Life." *Scandinavian Journal of Medicine and Science in Sports* 18 (2): 154–61.

Karjalainen, J. J., A. M. Kiviniemi, A. J. Hautala, O.-P. Piira, E. S. Lepojärvi, and others. 2015. "Effects of Physical Activity and Exercise Training on Cardiovascular Risk in Coronary Artery Disease Patients with and without Type 2 Diabetes." *Diabetes Care* 38 (4): 706–15.

Katzmarzyk, P. T., N. Gledhill, and R. J. Shephard. 2000. "The Economic Burden of Physical Inactivity in Canada." *Canadian Medical Association Journal* 163 (11): 1435–40.

Katzmarzyk, P. T., and I. Janssen. 2004. "The Economic Costs Associated with Physical Inactivity and Obesity in Canada: An Update." *Canadian Journal of Applied Physiology* 29 (1): 90–115.

Kemmler, W., M. Bebenek, S. von Stengel, and J. Bauer. 2015. "Peak-Bone-Mass Development in Young Adults: Effects of Study Program Related Levels of Occupational and Leisure Time Physical Activity and Exercise: A Prospective 5-Year Study." *Osteoporosis International* 26 (2): 653–62.

Knowler, W. C., E. Barrett-Connor, S. E. Fowler, R. F. Hamman, J. M. Lachin, and others. 2002. "Reduction in the Incidence of Type 2 Diabetes with Lifestyle Intervention or Metformin." *New England Journal of Medicine* 346 (6): 393–403.

Kodama, S., K. Saito, S. Tanaka, M. Maki, Y. Yachi, and others. 2009. "Cardiorespiratory Fitness as a Quantitative Predictor of All-Cause Mortality and Cardiovascular Events in Healthy Men and Women: A Meta-Analysis." *Journal of the American Medical Association* 301 (19): 2024.

Kohl, H. W., C. L. Craig, E. V. Lambert, S. Inoue, J. R. Alkandari, and others. 2012. "The Pandemic of Physical Inactivity: Global Action for Public Health." *The Lancet* 380 (9838): 294–305.

Kokkinos, P. 2012. "Physical Activity, Health Benefits, and Mortality Risk." *ISRN Cardiology* 2012 (October): 718789.

Laine, J., V. Kuvaja-Köllner, E. Pietilä, M. Koivuneva, H. Valtonen, and others. 2014. "Cost-Effectiveness of Population-Level Physical Activity Interventions: A Systematic Review." *American Journal of Health Promotion* 29 (2): 71–80.

Larsen, R., B. Kingwell, P. Sethi, E. Cerin, N. Owen, and others. 2014. "Breaking Up Prolonged Sitting Reduces Resting Blood Pressure in Overweight/Obese Adults." *Nutrition, Metabolism, and Cardiovascular Diseases* 24 (9): 976–82.

Leavy, J. E., F. C. Bull, M. Rosenberg, and A. Bauman. 2011. "Physical Activity Mass Media Campaigns and Their Evaluation: A Systematic Review of the Literature 2003–2010." *Health Education Research* 26 (6): 1060–85.

Lee, I.-M., E. J. Shiroma, F. Lobelo, P. Puska, S. N. Blair, and others. 2012. "Effect of Physical Inactivity on Major Non-Communicable Diseases Worldwide: An Analysis of Burden of Disease and Life Expectancy." *The Lancet* 380 (9838): 219–29.

Li, G., P. Zhang, J. Wang, E. W. Gregg, W. Yang, and others. 2008. "The Long-Term Effect of Lifestyle Interventions to Prevent Diabetes in the China Da Qing Diabetes Prevention Study: A 20-Year Follow-Up Study." *The Lancet* 371 (9626): 1783–89.

Li, J., and J. Siegrist. 2012. "Physical Activity and Risk of Cardiovascular Disease: A Meta-Analysis of Prospective Cohort Studies." *International Journal of Environmental Research and Public Health* 9 (2): 391–407.

Lim, S. S., T. Vos, A. D. Flaxman, G. Danaei, K. Shibuya, and others. 2013. "A Comparative Risk Assessment of Burden of Disease and Injury Attributable to 67 Risk Factors and Risk Factor Clusters in 21 Regions, 1990–2010: A Systematic Analysis for the Global Burden of Disease Study 2010." *The Lancet* 380 (9859): 2224–60.

Lindstrom, J., P. Ilanne-Parikka, M. Peltonen, S. Aunola, J. G. Eriksson, and others. 2006. "Sustained Reduction in the Incidence of Type 2 Diabetes by Lifestyle Intervention: Follow-Up of the Finnish Diabetes Prevention Study." *The Lancet* 368 (9548): 1673–79.

Lobelo, F., M. Stoutenberg, and A. Hutber. 2014. "The Exercise Is Medicine Global Health Initiative: A 2014 Update." *British Journal of Sports Medicine* 48 (22): 1627–33.

Lozano, R., M. Naghavi, K. Foreman, S. Lim, K. Shibuya, and others. 2012. "Global and Regional Mortality from 235 Causes of Death for 20 Age Groups in 1990 and 2010: A Systematic Analysis for the Global Burden of Disease Study 2010." *The Lancet* 380 (9859): 2095–128.

Lynch, J., S. P. Helmrich, T. A. Lakka, G. A. Kaplan, R. D. Cohen, and others. 1996. "Moderately Intense Physical Activities and High Levels of Cardiorespiratory Fitness Reduce the Risk of Non-Insulin-Dependent Diabetes Mellitus in Middle-Aged Men." *Archives of Internal Medicine* 156 (12): 1307–14.

Mann, S., C. Beedie, and A. Jimenez. 2014. "Differential Effects of Aerobic Exercise, Resistance Training, and Combined Exercise Modalities on Cholesterol and the Lipid Profile: Review, Synthesis, and Recommendations." *Sports Medicine* 44 (2): 211–21.

Maresova, K. 2014. "The Costs of Physical Inactivity in the Czech Republic in 2008." *Journal of Physical Activity and Health* 11 (3): 489–94.

Marlier, M., D. Van Dyck, G. Cardon, I. De Bourdeaudhuij, K. Babiak, and others. 2015. "Interrelation of Sport Participation, Physical Activity, Social Capital, and Mental Health in Disadvantaged Communities: A SEM-Analysis." *PLoS One* 10 (10): e0140196.

Matsudo, S., V. Matsudo, D. Andrade, T. Araújo, E. Andrade, and others. 2004. "Physical Activity Promotion: Experiences and Evaluation of the Agita São Paulo Program Using the Ecological Mobile Model." *Journal of Physical Activity and Health* 1 (2): 81–97.

Matsudo, V., S. Matsudo, D. Andrade, T. Araujo, E. Andrade, and others. 2002. "Promotion of Physical Activity in a Developing Country: The Agita São Paulo Experience." *Public Health Nutrition* 5 (1A): 253–61.

Mohan, V., M. Deepa, R. Deepa, C. Shanthirani, S. Farooq, and others. 2006. "Secular Trends in the Prevalence of Diabetes and Impaired Glucose Tolerance in Urban South India: The Chennai Urban Rural Epidemiology Study (CURES-17)." *Diabetologia* 49 (6): 1175–78.

New York State Government. 2010. *Active Design Guidelines: Promoting Physical Activity and Health in Design.* New York: New York State Government.

Ng, S. W., E. C. Norton, and B. M. Popkin. 2009. "Why Have Physical Activity Levels Declined among Chinese Adults? Findings from the 1991–2006 China Health and Nutrition Surveys." *Social Science and Medicine* 68 (7): 1305–14.

Ng, S. W., and B. M. Popkin. 2012. "Time Use and Physical Activity: A Shift away from Movement across the Globe." *Obesity Reviews* 13 (8): 659–80.

Ogilvie, D., J. Panter, C. Guell, A. Jones, R. Mackett, and others. 2016. "Health Impacts of the Cambridgeshire Guided Busway: A Natural Experimental Study." *Public Health Research* 4 (1).

Okada, K., T. Hayashi, K. Tsumura, C. Suematsu, G. Endo, and S. Fujii. 2000. "Leisure-Time Physical Activity at Weekends and the Risk of Type 2 Diabetes Mellitus in Japanese Men: The Osaka Health Survey." *Diabetic Medicine* 17 (1): 53–58.

Owen, N., G. N. Healy, C. E. Matthews, and D. W. Dunstan. 2010. "Too Much Sitting: The Population-Health Science of Sedentary Behavior." *Exercise and Sport Sciences Reviews* 38 (3): 105–13

Paez, D. C., R. S. Reis, D. C. Parra, C. M. Hoehner, O. L. Sarmiento, and others. 2015. "Bridging the Gap between Research and Practice: An Assessment of External Validity of Community-Based Physical Activity Programs in Bogotá, Colombia, and Recife, Brazil." *Translational Behavioral Medicine* 5 (1): 1–11.

Parsons, T. J., C. Sartini, E. A. Ellins, J. P. J. Halcox, K. E. Smith, and others. 2016. "Objectively Measured Physical Activity and Sedentary Behaviour and Ankle Brachial Index: Cross-Sectional and Longitudinal Associations in Older Men." *Atherosclerosis* 247 (April): 28–34.

Pate, R. R., M. Pratt, S. N. Blair, W. L. Haskell, C. A. Macera, and others. 1995. "Physical Activity and Public Health: A Recommendation from the Centers for Disease Control and Prevention and the American College of Sports Medicine." *Journal of the American Medical Association* 273 (5): 402–7.

Patel, A. V., L. Bernstein, A. Deka, H. S. Feigelson, P. T. Campbell, and others. 2010. "Leisure Time Spent Sitting in Relation to Total Mortality in a Prospective Cohort of U.S. Adults." *American Journal of Epidemiology* 172 (4): 419–29.

Pedersen, B., and B. Saltin. 2015. "Exercise as Medicine: Evidence for Prescribing Exercise as Therapy in 26 Different Chronic Diseases." *Scandinavian Journal of Medicine and Science in Sports* 25 (Suppl 3): 1–72.

Pereira, M. A., A. R. Folsom, P. G. McGovern, M. Carpenter, D. K. Arnett, and others. 1999. "Physical Activity and Incident Hypertension in Black and White Adults: The Atherosclerosis Risk in Communities Study." *Preventive Medicine* 28 (3): 304–12.

Perreault, L., S. E. Kahn, C. A. Christophi, W. C. Knowler, R. F. Hamman, and others. 2009. "Regression from Pre-Diabetes to Normal Glucose Regulation in the Diabetes Prevention Program." *Diabetes Care* 32 (9): 1583–88.

Physical Activity Guidelines Advisory Committee. 2008a. *Physical Activity Guidelines Advisory Committee Report 2008.* Washington, DC: U.S. Department of Health and Human Services.

———. 2008b. *Physical Activity Guidelines Report.* Washington, DC: U.S. Department of Health and Human Services, Office of Disease Prevention and Health Promotion.

Popkin, B. M., S. Kim, E. R. Rusev, S. Du, and C. Zizza. 2006. "Measuring the Full Economic Costs of Diet, Physical Activity, and Obesity-Related Chronic Diseases." *Obesity Reviews* 7 (3): 271–93.

Pratt, M., J. Norris, F. Lobelo, L. Roux, and G. Wang. 2014. "The Cost of Physical Inactivity: Moving into the 21st Century." *British Journal of Sports Medicine* 48 (3): 171–73.

Pratt, M., L. G. Perez, S. Goenka, R. C. Brownson, A. Bauman, and others. 2015. "Can Population Levels of Physical Activity Be Increased? Global Evidence and Experience." *Progress in Cardiovascular Diseases* 57 (4): 356–67.

Pratt, M., A. Ramirez, R. Martins, A. Bauman, G. Heath, and others. 2015. "127 Steps toward a More Active World." *Journal of Physical Activity and Health* 12 (9): 1193–94.

Pucher, J., J. Dill, and S. Handy. 2010. "Infrastructure, Programs, and Policies to Increase Bicycling: An International Review." *Preventive Medicine* 50 (Suppl): S106–25.

Ramachandran, A., C. Snehalatha, S. Mary, B. Mukesh, A. D. Bhaskar, and others. 2006. "The Indian Diabetes Prevention Programme Shows that Lifestyle Modification and Metformin Prevent Type 2 Diabetes in Asian Indian Subjects with Impaired Glucose Tolerance (IDPP-1)." *Diabetologia* 49 (2): 289–97.

Reis, R. S., P. C. Hallal, D. C. Parra, I. C. Ribeiro, R. C. Brownson, and others. 2010. "Promoting Physical Activity through Community-Wide Policies and Planning: Findings from Curitiba, Brazil." *Journal of Physical Activity and Health* 7 (Suppl 2): S137–45.

Ribeiro, I. C., D. C. Parra, C. M. Hoehner, J. Soares, A. Torres, and others. 2010. "School-Based Physical Education Programs: Evidence-Based Physical Activity Interventions for Youth in Latin America." *Global Health Promotion* 17 (2): 5–15.

Roux, L., M. Pratt, T. O. Tengs, M. M. Yore, T. L. Yanagawa, and others. 2008. "Cost-Effectiveness of Community-Based Physical Activity Interventions." *American Journal of Preventive Medicine* 35 (6): 578–88.

Sallis, J. F., A. Bauman, and M. Pratt. 1998. "Environmental and Policy Interventions to Promote Physical Activity." *American Journal of Preventive Medicine* 15 (4): 379–97.

Sallis, J. F., F. Bull, R. Guthold, G. M. Heath, S. Inoue, and others. 2016. "Progress in Physical Activity over the Olympic Quadrennium." *The Lancet* 38 (10051): 1325–36. doi:10.1016/S0140-6736(16)30581-5.

Sarmiento, O., A. Torres, E. Jacoby, M. Pratt, T. L. Schmid, and G. Stierling. 2010. "The Ciclovía-Recreativa: A Mass-Recreational Program with Public Health Potential." *Journal of Physical Activity and Health* 7 (2): S163.

Sattelmair, J., J. Pertman, E. L. Ding, H. W. Kohl, W. Haskell, and others. 2011. "Dose Response between Physical Activity and Risk of Coronary Heart Disease: A Meta-Analysis." *Circulation* 124 (7): 789–95.

Scarborough, P., P. Bhatnagar, K. K. Wickramasinghe, S. Allender, C. Foster, and others. 2011. "The Economic Burden of Ill Health due to Diet, Physical Inactivity, Smoking, Alcohol, and Obesity in the UK: An Update to 2006–07 NHS Costs." *Journal of Public Health* 33 (4): 527–35.

Scholz, J., M. C. Klein, T. E. Behrens, and H. Johansen-Berg. 2009. "Training Induces Changes in White-Matter Architecture." *Nature Neuroscience* 12 (11): 1370–71.

Shaw, K. A., H. C. Gennat, P. O'Rourke, and C. Del Mar. 2006. "Exercise for Overweight or Obesity." *Cochrane Database of Systematic Reviews* 4 (October): CD003817.

Sherrington, C., J. C. Whitney, S. R. Lord, R. D. Herbert, R. G. Cumming, and others. 2008. "Effective Exercise for the Prevention of Falls: A Systematic Review and Meta-Analysis." *Journal of the American Geriatrics Society* 56 (12): 2234–43.

Simoes, E. J., P. Hallal, M. Pratt, L. Ramos, M. Munk, and others. 2009. "Effects of a Community-Based, Professionally Supervised Intervention on Physical Activity Levels among Residents of Recife, Brazil." *American Journal of Public Health* 99 (1): 68–75.

Singh, A., L. Uijtdewilligen, J. W. Twisk, W. Van Mechelen, and M. J. Chinapaw. 2012. "Physical Activity and Performance at School: A Systematic Review of the Literature Including a Methodological Quality Assessment." *Archives of Pediatrics and Adolescent Medicine* 166 (1): 49–55.

Sørensen, J. B., T. Skovgaard, and L. Puggaard. 2006. "Exercise on Prescription in General Practice: A Systematic Review." *Scandinavian Journal of Primary Health Care* 24 (2): 69–74.

Stamler, J., O. Vaccaro, J. D. Neaton, D. Wentworth, and Multiple Risk Factor Intervention Trial Research Group. 1993. "Diabetes, Other Risk Factors, and 12-Yr Cardiovascular Mortality for Men Screened in the Multiple Risk Factor Intervention Trial." *Diabetes Care* 16 (2): 434–44.

Swift, D. L., C. J. Lavie, N. M. Johannsen, R. Arena, C. P. Earnest, and others. 2013. "Physical Activity, Cardiorespiratory Fitness, and Exercise Training in Primary and Secondary Coronary Prevention." *Circulation* 77 (2): 281–92.

Taylor, R. S., A. Brown, S. Ebrahim, J. Jolliffe, H. Noorani, and others. 2004. "Exercise-Based Rehabilitation for Patients with Coronary Heart Disease: Systematic Review and Meta-Analysis of Randomized Controlled Trials." *American Journal of Medicine* 116 (10): 682–92.

Torres, A., O. L. Sarmiento, C. Stauber, and R. Zarama. 2013. "The Ciclovia and Cicloruta Programs: Promising Interventions to Promote Physical Activity and Social Capital in Bogotá, Colombia." *American Journal of Public Health* 103 (2): e23–30.

Tremblay, M. S., C. E. Gray, K. K. Akinroye, D. M. Harrington, P. T. Katzmarzyk, and others. 2014. "Physical Activity of Children: A Global Matrix of Grades Comparing 15 Countries." *Journal of Physical Activity and Health* 11 (Supp 1): 113–25.

Tremblay, M. S., A. G. LeBlanc, I. Janssen, M. E. Kho, A. Hicks, and others. 2011. "Canadian Sedentary Behaviour Guidelines for Children and Youth." *Applied Physiology, Nutrition, and Metabolism* 36 (1): 59–64.

U.K. Prospective Diabetes Study Group. 1998. "Tight Blood Pressure Control and Risk of Macrovascular and Microvascular Complications in Type 2 Diabetes (UKPDS 38)." *BMJ* 317 (September): 703–13.

United Nations. 2011. *Political Declaration of the High-level Meeting of the General Assembly on the Prevention and Control of Non-communicable Diseases (A/Res/66/2).* New York: United Nations.

———. 2015. *Sustainable Development Goals 2030.* New York: United Nations.

———. 2016. *Sport for Development and Peace.* New York: United Nations. http://www.un.org/wcm/content/site/sport/home.

U.S. Department of Health and Human Services. 1996. *Physical Activity and Health: A Report of the Surgeon General.* Washington, DC: Diane Publishing.

Wannamethee, S. G., A. G. Shaper, and K. G. Alberti. 2000. "Physical Activity, Metabolic Factors, and the Incidence of Coronary Heart Disease and Type 2 Diabetes." *Archives of Internal Medicine* 160 (14): 2108–16.

Warburton, D. E., C. W. Nicol, and S. S. Bredin. 2006. "Health Benefits of Physical Activity: The Evidence." *Canadian Medical Association Journal* 174 (6): 801–9.

Weinstein, A. R., H. D. Sesso, I. M. Lee, N. R. Cook, J. E. Manson, and others. 2004. "Relationship of Physical Activity vs. Body Mass Index with Type 2 Diabetes in Women." *Journal of the American Medical Association* 292 (10): 1188–94.

WHO (World Health Organization). 2004. *Global Strategy on Diet, Physical Activity, and Health.* Geneva: WHO.

———. 2010a. *Global Recommendations on Physical Activity for Health.* Geneva: WHO.

———. 2010b. *Assessing National Capacity for the Prevention and Control of Noncommunicable Diseases.* Geneva: WHO.

———. 2013. *Global Action Plan for the Prevention and Control of Noncommunicable Diseases 2013-2020.* Geneva: WHO.

———. 2014a. *Global Status Report on Non-Communicable Diseases 2014.* Geneva: WHO.http://www.who.int/nmh/publications/ncd-status-report-2014/en/.

———. 2014b. *Promoting Physical Activity in the Eastern Mediterranean Region through a Life-Course Approach.* Cairo: WHO Regional Office for the Eastern Mediterranean.

———. 2015. *Assessing National Capacity for the Prevention and Control of Noncommunicable Diseases.* Geneva: WHO.

———. 2016. *Global School-Based Student Health Survey.* Geneva: WHO.

Wijndaele, K., K. Westgate, S. K. Stephens, S. N. Blair, F. C. Bull, and others. 2015. "Utilization and Harmonization of Adult Accelerometry Data: Review and Expert Consensus." *Medicine and Science in Sports and Exercise* 47 (10): 2129–39.

World Cancer Research Fund. 2007. *Food, Nutrition, Physical Activity, and the Prevention of Cancer: A Global Perspective.* Vol. 1. Washington, DC: American Institute for Cancer Research.

Wu, S., D. Cohen, Y. Shi, M. Pearson, and R. Sturm. 2011. "Economic Analysis of Physical Activity Interventions." *American Journal of Preventive Medicine* 40 (2): 149–58.

Wu, T., X. Gao, M. Chen, and R. Van Dam. 2009. "Long-Term Effectiveness of Diet-Plus-Exercise Interventions vs. Diet-Only Interventions for Weight Loss: A Meta-Analysis." *Obesity Reviews* 10 (3): 313–23.

Chapter 6

Effectiveness of Dietary Policies to Reduce Noncommunicable Diseases

Ashkan Afshin, Renata Micha, Michael Webb, Simon Capewell,
Laurie Whitsel, Adolfo Rubinstein, Dorairaj Prabhakaran,
Marc Suhrcke, and Dariush Mozaffarian

INTRODUCTION

In nearly every region, suboptimal diet is the leading risk factor for poor health; hunger and malnutrition result in substantial burdens and contribute to the incidence and prevalence of noncommunicable diseases (NCDs) (Forouzanfar and others 2015; Lim and others 2012). Improving individual and population dietary habits needs to become a health system and public health priority (IFPRI 2015). In recent years, interventions have been evaluated to improve dietary habits, including individual-level interventions in the health system (for example, nutrition counseling); population-level interventions; and novel, technology-based interventions (for example, Internet- and mobile-based programs). A detailed discussion of these interventions is beyond the scope of this chapter. Here, we focus on dietary priorities and policies for global NCDs, including key dietary targets, current distributions of consumption, and ensuing health burdens. We summarize the evidence for effective population-level interventions to improve diet quality, and we discuss data gaps and needs for assessing cost-effectiveness.

The global effects of hunger and nutrient deficiencies have been recognized for more than a century, but the emergence of poor diet as a major cause of NCDs has been documented only in recent decades (Forouzanfar and others 2015; Lim and others 2012). Optimal responses to this global challenge have been slowed by several factors, including the relatively recent attention given to the science of diet and NCDs; a historical focus on isolated nutrients rather than foods and diet patterns; and an emphasis on diet-induced obesity (WHO 2012). These factors have led to the neglect of the far larger burdens of NCDs owing to nonobesity-related pathways. Modern nutritional science, originating in the early 20th century, focused on nutrient deficiency diseases, such as scurvy, pellagra, and rickets. The initial recognition in the late twentieth century of the additional major effect of diet on NCDs led to nutrient deficiency paradigms being extended to the study of chronic diseases (Mozaffarian and Ludwig 2010). Nutrient deficiency diseases, however, are explicitly caused and can be prevented or treated by single nutrients. In contrast, NCDs arise from complex perturbations of food intakes and overall dietary patterns, including insufficiencies of specific healthful foods and excesses of unhealthful foods (Afshin and others 2014; Chen and others 2013; de Munter and others 2007; Imamura and others 2015; Kaluza, Wolk, and Larsson 2012; Micha, Wallace, and Mozaffarian 2010; Mozaffarian and Rimm 2006; Mozaffarian and others 2006).

Corresponding author: Ashkan Afshin, Acting Assistant Professor of Global Health, Institute for Health Metrics and Evaluation, University of Washington, Seattle, Washington, United States; aafshin@uw.edu.

The global obesity epidemic has appropriately focused attention on diet. However, adiposity is only one pathway of effect of diet on NCDs. Diet quality has an enormous effect on NCDs, in particular, cardiovascular diseases, independent of body weight or obesity. Although *undernutrition* is an appropriate term for caloric and nutrient deficiency, *overnutrition* is an incorrect corollary for NCDs and even obesity. The term fails to capture the complexity of poor food habits that cause NCDs: (1) inadequate ingestion of healthful foods; and (2) ingestion of foods created by suboptimal processing (for example, those rich in refined grains, starches, and sugars), foods prepared by modern methods (for example, high temperature commercial cooking), and foods containing additives such as trans fats and sodium. Accordingly, the appropriate term for the global epidemic of diet-induced NCDs is not *overnutrition*, but *malnutrition*: poor dietary quality or composition.

DIETARY RISK FACTORS FOR NONCOMMUNICABLE DISEASES

Understanding the key dietary factors that have the strongest evidence of effect on NCDs, and the effective and cost-effective policies to address these factors, is essential to help guide public health planning and interventions. The Global Burden of Disease Study (GBD) of 2010 and 2013 systematically evaluated the evidence for effects of key foods, beverages, and nutrients on NCDs, including causal effects, optimal consumption levels for lowering risk, and current distributions of intakes worldwide (Forouzanfar and others 2015; Lim and others 2012; Micha and others 2012; Micha and others 2014; Micha and others 2015; Powles and others 2013; Singh, Micha, Khatibzadeh, Lim, and others 2015; Singh, Micha, Khatibzadeh, Shi, and others 2015).

Overall, consumption levels were suboptimal for each evaluated dietary risk factor on a global scale, but substantial diversity in consumption existed across regions and even neighboring countries (Micha and others 2104; Micha and others 2015; Mozaffarian and others 2014; Singh, Micha, Khatibzadeh, Lim, and others 2015; Singh, Micha, Khatibzadeh, Shi, and others 2015). For most dietary factors, the proportion of nations with average consumption levels meeting optimal intakes was low, typically representing less than 20 percent of the global adult population. Based on the 2010 GBD analysis, the five leading dietary contributors to death were as follows:

- Low fruits (4.9 million attributable deaths per year)
- High sodium (3.1 million)
- Low nuts and seeds (2.5 million)
- Low vegetables (1.8 million)
- Low whole grains (1.7 million).

In comparison, high sugar-sweetened beverage (SSB), low milk, and high red meat intakes had lower estimated mortality burdens at 184,000; 101,000; and 38,000 attributable deaths per year, respectively. These findings highlight the particular relevance of malnutrition rather than overnutrition. This evidence contrasts with conventional dietary priorities to reduce NCDs, which have traditionally focused on unhealthful factors such as saturated fat, sodium, red meats, SSBs, and added sugars. Reductions in these factors are important. However, such reductions would have a relatively small effect on overall NCD burdens compared with a coordinated strategy that increases intakes of healthful foods.

The 2010 and 2013 GBD studies focused not only on foods, beverages, and nutrients with probable or convincing evidence of effect on NCDs, but also on available global evidence on their consumption levels (table 6.1). Because of a lack of available global data, certain dietary factors such as refined carbohydrates and dairy foods beyond milk could not be included. Refined carbohydrates include white rice, bread, most breakfast cereals, added sugars, and starches such as white potatoes. Refined carbohydrates are clearly relevant for NCDs, with clear links to greater weight gain (Mozaffarian and others 2011; Te Morenga, Mallard, and Mann 2013), diabetes, and coronary heart disease (CHD) (Mozaffarian 2014). Recent global policy efforts focus on added sugars, especially SSBs. SSBs are clearly adverse for weight gain and cardiometabolic health (Mozaffarian and others 2011; Pan and Hu 2011) and are particularly heavily consumed by youth and younger adults. A general focus on reducing all refined carbohydrates—not only added sugars—is warranted because of their adverse health effects (Dietary Guidelines Advisory Committee 2015).

Dairy foods are a major component of many diets; they are particularly relevant for sufficient protein, nutrients, and calories among the poorest populations. Their cardiometabolic effects, relevant bioactive characteristics (for example, fatty acids, probiotics, and fermentation), and potential effects by subtype (for example, milk, cheese, and yogurt) remain understudied. Current evidence supports guidelines for modest dairy consumption of two to three servings a day, in particular, yogurt and cheese (Aune and others 2013; Chen and others 2014). Conventional recommendations to select fat-reduced, rather than whole-fat, dairy are not strongly evidence based; according to current data, both appear to be reasonable choices (Mozaffarian 2014).

Table 6.1 Global Consumption and Optimal Levels, Deaths, and Disability-Adjusted Life Years Attributable to Dietary Habits with Largest Public Health Effect, 2010

Dietary factor[a]	Global consumption, 2010 (mean, 95% UIs)[b]	Optimal consumption[c]	Global adult population meeting optimal levels (%)	Related NCD outcomes at increased intakes	Global deaths, 2010 (mean, 95% UIs)[d]	Global DALYs, 2010 (mean, 95% UIs)[d]
Foods						
Fruits	81.3 g/d (78.9–83.7)	300 ± 30 g/d	0.4	↓ CHD; ↓ stroke; ↓ mouth, pharynx, larynx, esophagus, lung cancers	4,902,242 (3,818,356–5,881,561)	104,095 (81,833–124,169)
Vegetables	208.8 g/d (203.4–214.3)	400 ± 40 g/d	7.8	↓ CHD; ↓ stroke; ↓ mouth, pharynx, larynx, esophagus cancers	1,797,254 (1,205,059–2,394,366)	38,559 (26,006–51,658)
Nuts and seeds	8.9 g/d (8.3–9.5)	4 (28.35 g = 1 oz) ± 0.4 servings/wk	9.6	↓ CHD	2,471,823 (1,559,603–3,226,994)	51,289 (33,482–65,959)
Whole grains	38.4 g/d (35.5–41.7)	2.5 (50 g) ± 0.25 servings/d	7.6	↓ CHD; ↓ stroke; ↓ DM	1,725,812 (1,342,896–2,067,224)	40,762 (32,112–48,486)
Red meats	41.8 g/d (40.8–42.8)	1 (100 g) ± 0.1 serving/wk	20.3	↑ DM; ↑ colorectal cancer	38,092 (10,749–65,727)	1,853 (870–2,946)
Processed meats	13.7 g/d (13.2–14.3)	0	0	↑ CHD; ↑ DM; ↑ colorectal cancer	840,857 (188,952–1,460,279)	20,939 (6,982–33,468)
Milk	81.7 g/d (79.7–83.9)	2 (226.8 g = 8 oz) ± 0.2 servings/d	0	↓ Colorectal cancer	100,951 (29,728–171,340)	2,101 (619–3,544)
SSBs	101.4 g/d (94.9–109.1)	0	0	↑ BMI-mediated effects[e]; ↑ DM	210,780 (136,271–299,863)	5,250 (3,052–7,402)

table continues next page

Table 6.1 Global Consumption and Optimal Levels, Deaths, and Disability-Adjusted Life Years Attributable to Dietary Habits with Largest Public Health Effect, 2010 (continued)

Dietary factor[a]	Global consumption, 2010 (mean, 95% UIs)[b]	Optimal consumption[c]	Global adult population meeting optimal levels (%)	Related NCD outcomes at increased intakes	Global deaths, 2010 (mean, 95% UIs)[d]	Global DALYs, 2010 (mean, 95% UIs)[d]
Nutrients						
PUFA in place of SFA	n-6 PUFA: 5.9 %E (5.7–6.1); SFA: 9.4 %E (9.2–9.5)	12 ± 1.2 %E[f]	n-6 PUFA: 0.1; SFA: 61.8[f]	↓ CHD	533,603 (245,096–820,854)	11,680 (5,360–17,798)
Seafood omega-3 fats	163 mg/d (154–172)	250 ± 25 mg/d	18.9	↓ CHD	1,389,896 (1,010,300–1,781,401)	28,199 (20,624–35,974)
Trans fats	1.4 %E (1.36–1.44)	0.5 ± 0.05 %E	0.6	↑ CHD	515,260 (371,081–649,451)	11,592 (8,395–14,623)
Sodium	3,953.6 mg/d (3,885.4–4,014.0)	1,000 ± 100 mg/d	0	↑ SBP-mediated effects[g]; ↑ stomach cancer	3,104,308 (2,016,734–4,105,019)	61,231 (40,124–80,342)

Source: Lim and others 2012.

Note: BMI = body mass index; CHD = coronary heart disease; d = day; DALYs = disability-adjusted life years; DM = diabetes mellitus; %E = percent energy; g = gram; mg = milligram; NCD = noncommunicable disease; oz = ounce; PUFA = polyunsaturated fatty acid; SBP = systolic blood pressure; SFA = saturated fatty acid; SSBs = sugar-sweetened beverages; UIs = uncertainty intervals; wk = week.

a. These are dietary risk factors for which we identified probable or convincing evidence of etiologic effects on chronic diseases, including CHD, stroke, type 2 DM, BMI, SBP, or cancers. Using available evidence, we identified etiologic effects on CHD, stroke, or DM by fruits, vegetables, nuts and seeds, whole grains, red meats, processed meats, SSBs, PUFAs as a replacement for SFAs, trans fats, and dietary sodium. For cancers, we based our assessments on World Cancer Research Fund and American Institute for Cancer Research (2007) and subsequent updates (World Cancer Research Fund International 2016).

b. Optimal metrics for each dietary factor were defined to be consistent with definitions used in epidemiological studies that provided evidence of etiologic effects on chronic diseases, and optimal units were applied to match those of studies used to evaluate relationships with disease risk as well as major dietary guidelines (Micha and others 2012). Dietary factors were evaluated as percent energy, or %E (PUFA, SFA, trans fats), or were standardized using the residual method (Willett 1998) to 2,000 kilocalories per day (fruits, vegetables, nuts and seeds, whole grains, red meats, processed meats, milk, SSBs, seafood omega-3 fats, dietary sodium). We performed systematic searches for individual-level dietary surveys in all countries (187 worldwide). The results of our search strategy by dietary factor, time, and region have been reported (Khatibzadeh and others 2012). We identified a total of 266 surveys of adults representing 113 of 187 countries and 82 percent of the global population. Measurement comparability and consistency across surveys was maximized by (1) using a standardized data analysis approach, which accounted for sampling strategies within the survey by including sampling weights; the average of all days of dietary assessment to quantify mean dietary intakes; a corrected population standard deviation (SD) to account for within- versus between-person variation; and standardized dietary metrics and units of measure across surveys and (2) adjusting for total energy to reduce measurement error and also account for differences in body size, metabolic efficiency, and physical activity (Willett 1998). To address missing data, imperfect estimates, incomparability, and related effects on uncertainty of dietary estimates, we developed an age-integrating Bayesian hierarchical imputation model, which has been described in detail (Lim and others 2012). Using simulation (Monte Carlo) analyses, we drew 1,000 times from the posterior distribution of each exposure for each age-sex-country-year stratum; computed the mean exposure from the 1,000 draws; and used the 95 percent UIs as the 2.5th and 97.5th percentiles of the 1,000 draws.

c. For each dietary factor, the optimal consumption level was identified on the basis of both the observed levels at which lowest disease risk occurs and the observed mean consumption levels in at least two to three countries. We considered whether such identified levels were consistent with major dietary guidelines (FAO 2010; U.S. Department of Health and Human Services and U.S. Department of Agriculture 2010). Because not all individuals within a population can have precisely the same exposure level, the plausible SD of optimal consumption was calculated from the average SD for all metabolic risk factors in the Global Burden of Disease Study 2010 (10 percent of the mean).

d. We estimated the burden (mortality and morbidity) attributable to dietary risk factors by comparing the present distribution of exposure to the optimal exposure distribution. Attributable mortality was estimated using the diet-disease population-attributable fraction (PAF) (Lim and others 2012). The number of deaths attributable to each dietary factor was calculated by multiplying the estimated PAF by the observed number of disease-specific deaths. The proportion of total DALYs was similarly estimated. Mean deaths and DALYs were computed from the 1,000 draws of probabilistic simulation analyses, and the 95 percent UIs were used as the 2.5th and 97.5th percentiles of the 1,000 draws, further incorporating uncertainty in dietary exposure data and etiologic relative risks by age and sex. These comparative risk assessment analyses do not account for joint effects of multiple risk factors (multi-causality). Given potential for joint distributions and interactions, the effects of multiple dietary factors should not simply be summed to determine total effects (Lim and others 2012).

e. The effects of high intake of SSBs on CHD, stroke, other cardiovascular diseases, DM, and other related diseases; other NCDs; and cancers were estimated through their measured effects on BMI (Renehan and others 2008; Singh and others 2013). Direct effects on BMI and (independent of this) additional direct effects on DM were included.

f. Optimal consumption was based on increasing PUFA to 12%E as a replacement for SFA, in accordance with evidence that this specific nutrient replacement reduces risk (Jakobsen and others 2009; Mozaffarian, Micha, and Wallace 2010). To estimate the percentage of global adult population meeting optimal levels for SFA only, we based recommended intake levels of less than 10%E or a 2,000 kilocalorie per day diet on the U.S. Department of Agriculture and United Nations Food and Agriculture Organization guidelines (U.S. Department of Health and Human Services and U.S. Department of Agriculture 2010).

g. The effects of high intake of dietary sodium on CHD, stroke, and other cardiovascular diseases were estimated through their measured effects on SBP (Singh and others 2013).

GBD 2010 and 2013 also did not systematically assess the cardiometabolic effects of flavonoid-rich foods, including cocoa, berries, apples, and tea. Although these appear potentially beneficial, the heterogeneity of specific phenolics, the variability of dietary sources, and fewer studies that evaluate clinical endpoints limit strong conclusions (Hooper and others 2012; Shrime and others 2011) but provide a strong basis for further investigation.

EFFECTIVENESS OF POPULATION INTERVENTIONS TO IMPROVE DIET

Because of current and projected disease burdens, identifying and implementing effective interventions to improve diet quality needs to be a health system priority and public health priority for all regions. Behavior change interventions that target individuals with individualized nutrition counseling within the health system can be effective. However, these often have limited coverage, can be more costly, and may have limited sustainability (Artinian and others 2010; Rose 1985). In comparison, population-based interventions can have broader effect, lower cost, and greater sustainability, as

well as the potential to reduce disparities (McGill and others 2015; Mozaffarian and others 2012). Such interventions include those implemented at health system, organizational (for example, schools and workplaces), community, state, and national levels. The evidence of effectiveness of such interventions has been systematically reviewed, including for education and mass media campaigns, food labeling and consumer information, food pricing and economic incentives, school and worksite interventions, and direct restrictions and mandates (Afshin, Penalvo, and others 2015; Mozaffarian and others 2012). Several effective policy strategies are listed in table 6.2.

Mass Media Campaigns

Mass media campaigns, alone or as a part of multicomponent interventions, can improve diet when focused on specific dietary targets. Supportive evidence includes quasi-experimental studies of the "5 A Day For Better Health!" and "Fruits & Veggies—More Matters" campaigns in the United States and multicomponent strategies in Finland (Pekka, Pirjo, and Ulla 2002; Puska and Stahl 2010), Singapore (Bhalla and others 2006), and

Table 6.2 Evidence-Based Population Interventions to Improve Diet[a]

Population area	Intervention
Media and education	• Sustained, focused media and education campaigns (using multiple modes) for increasing consumption of specific healthful foods or reducing consumption of specific less healthful foods or beverages, either alone (class IIa B) or as part of multicomponent strategies (class I B)[b,c,d]
	• On-site supermarket and grocery store educational programs to support the purchase of healthier foods (class IIa B)[b]
Labeling and information	• Mandated nutrition facts panels or front-of-pack labels or icons as a means to influence industry behavior and product formulations (class IIa B)[b,e]
Economic incentives	• Subsidy strategies to lower prices of more healthful foods and beverages (class I A)[b]
	• Tax strategies to increase prices of less healthful foods and beverages (class IIa B)[b]
	• Changes in both agricultural subsidies and other related policies to create infrastructure that facilitates production, transportation, and marketing of healthier foods, sustained over several decades (class IIa B)[b]
Schools	• Multicomponent interventions focused on improving both diet and physical activity, including specialized educational curricula, trained teachers, supportive school policies, formal physical education programs, serving of healthier food and beverage options, and parental or family component (class I A)[b]
	• School garden programs, including nutrition and gardening education and hands-on gardening experiences (class IIa A)[b]
	• Fresh fruit and vegetable programs that provide free fruits and vegetables to students during the school day (class IIa A)[b]
Workplaces	• Comprehensive worksite wellness programs with nutrition, physical activity, and tobacco cessation or prevention components (class IIa A)[b]
	• Increased availability of healthier food and beverage options and strong nutrition standards for foods and beverages served, in combination with vending machine prompts, labels, or icons to select healthier choices (class IIa B)[b]
Local environment	• Increased availability of supermarkets near homes (class IIa B)[b,c,f]

table continues next page

Table 6.2 Evidence-Based Population Interventions to Improve Diet[a] (continued)

Population area	Intervention
Restrictions and mandates	• Restrictions on television advertisements for less healthful foods or beverages advertised to children (class I B)[b] • Restrictions on advertising and marketing of less healthful foods or beverages near schools and public places frequented by youths (class IIa B)[b] • General nutrition standards for foods and beverages marketed and advertised to children in any fashion, including on-package promotion (class IIa B)[b] • Regulatory policies to reduce specific nutrients in foods (for example, trans fats, salt, certain fats) (class I B)[b,d]
Agricultural	• Fiscal, trade, and regulatory instruments where feasible and proven effective to improve production, storage, and distribution of healthful foods (for example, fruits and vegetables) • Development of mutual metrics that can be used to measure and evaluate the contributions of each relevant sector to improving diet

Source: Adapted from Mozaffarian and others 2012.

a. The specific population interventions listed here are those that achieved either a class I or a class IIa recommendation, together with an evidence grade of either A or B. The American Heart Association evidence grading system is as follows:

• **Class I:** Evidence or general agreement exists that the intervention is beneficial, useful, and effective; the intervention should be performed.
• **Class II:** There is conflicting evidence or a divergence of opinion about the usefulness or efficacy of the intervention.
• **Class IIa:** Weight of evidence or opinion is in favor of usefulness or efficacy; performing the intervention is reasonable.
• **Class IIb:** Usefulness or efficacy is less well established by evidence or opinion; the intervention may be considered.
• **Class III:** There is evidence or general agreement that the intervention is not useful or effective and in some cases may be harmful.

The weight of evidence in support of the recommendation is classified as follows:

• **Level of Evidence A:** Data are derived from multiple randomized clinical trials or, given the nature of population interventions, from well-designed quasi-experimental studies combined with supportive evidence from several other types of studies.
• **Level of Evidence B:** Data are derived from a single randomized trial or nonrandomized studies.
• **Level of Evidence C:** Evidence consists of only consensus opinion of experts, case studies, or standard-of-care. For brevity, we have not cited all of the more than 500 individual studies reviewed in that American Heart Association Scientific Statement.

b. At least some evidence is found in studies conducted in high-income western regions and countries, for example, North America, Europe, Australia, and New Zealand.
c. At least some evidence is found in studies conducted in high-income nonwestern regions and economies, for example, Hong Kong SAR, China; Japan; the Republic of Korea; and Singapore.
d. At least some evidence is found in studies conducted in low- and middle-income regions and countries, for example, Africa, China, India, and Pakistan.
e. Such labeling strategies alone have limited effect if not complemented with environmental changes.
f. Based on cross-sectional studies only; only two longitudinal studies have been performed, with no significant relations seen.

Mauritius (Dowse and others 1995) that included mass media. The effect size of mass media campaigns appears to vary depending on the population (for example, generally more effectiveness in more educated and higher-income groups) and the features of the campaign (for example, coverage, duration, modes of delivery and communication, and presence or absence of additional intervention components). The cost-effectiveness of such strategies, which can require relatively high resources, has not been formally evaluated.

We recently systematically reviewed and synthesized the evidence of effectiveness of mass media campaigns to improve diet (Afshin and others 2013; Afshin, Penalvo, and others 2015). We identified eight studies of a mass media campaign in isolation and six of a mass media campaign as part of multicomponent national programs. The campaigns were implemented nationally (four studies), regionally (two studies), and locally (eight studies). They used a variety of mediums: audiocassette tapes (Connell, Goldberg, and Folta 2001); television, radio, and print advertising (Pollard and others 2008;

Stables and others 2002); logos and branding (Ashfield-Watt 2006; Stables and others 2002); newspapers (Nishtar and others 2004); and booklets and brochures (Marcus and others 2001). The duration of campaigns varied from one month to 30 years. The number of participants in these studies totaled approximately 60,000 adults and children (n = 700 to 32,500 in individual studies). Women constituted the majority of study participants in each study (range, 52–94 percent). The populations covered a wide range of income and socioeconomic levels, and most were Caucasian. Pooling the results of five studies evaluating mass media campaigns in isolation, we identified a 0.2-serving-per-day increase in fruit and vegetable consumption. Among national multicomponent interventions that included a prominent mass media campaign (n = 3), we found lower prevalence of hypertension (15 percent less, 95 percent confidence interval 10–21) and hypercholesterolemia (61 percent less, 95 percent confidence interval 40–75).

In contrast with focused media campaigns, passive provision of consumer information appears to have little effect on behavior (Afshin, Penalvo, and others 2015). Evidence from both observational and quasi-experimental studies demonstrates that providing nutrition information on food packages, on restaurant menus, or at the point of purchase is generally ineffective for altering consumer behavior (Shangguan and others 2015). Anecdotal evidence suggests that mandating such information might in some cases influence food industry reformulations, but further investigation of this approach is required.

In sum, these findings support effectiveness of mass media campaigns for improving diet. However, more studies are needed to confirm and expand these findings.

Fiscal Policies

Fiscal measures, including taxation and subsidies, are among the most promising dietary policies. These measures are recommended in the American Heart Association Scientific Statement on population interventions; by the United Nations Political Declaration on NCDs; and by the World Health Organization's (WHO) Global Strategy on Diet, Physical Activity and Health (Mozaffarian and others 2012; UN 2011; WHO 2004). Cross-sectional price-elasticity analyses of demand (Andreyeva, Long, and Brownell 2009; Green and others 2013), evidence from prospective studies (Thow, Downs, and Jan 2014), and evidence from intervention studies (An 2013) demonstrate consistent efficacy of changes in food pricing, including subsidies to increase healthful foods and taxes to decrease unhealthful foods and drinks. The magnitude of the effect is proportional to the price change; larger changes of 10–50 percent have greater effect. Although small taxes are not expected to have a major effect on population consumption levels, such taxes are more politically feasible and can generate large amounts of revenue for other prevention programs. Fiscal approaches also have larger effects in low-income countries and on lower socioeconomic groups, the populations who are at highest risk and have the most to gain from improved diets (Green and others 2013).

Evidence from cross-sectional analyses of price elasticity of demand suggests that each 10 percent change in the price of foods and beverages is associated with a 4 percent to 8 percent change in consumption (table 6.3). Several factors may influence the magnitude of this effect, including the specific dietary target and national and individual socioeconomic status.

We systematically evaluated and quantified the prospective effect of price changes on dietary consumption in 23 interventional and seven observational studies (Afshin, Del Gobbo, and others 2015). The interventional studies were conducted in five countries (France, the

Table 6.3 Change in Demand for Major Food Groups per 10 Percent Change in Price of the Food Groups in Low-, Middle-, and High-Income Countries, 1990–2011

percent

Food group	Countries		
	Low income	Middle income	High income
Fruits and vegetables	7.2 (6.6–7.7)	6.5 (5.9–7.1)	5.3 (4.8–5.9)
Meat	7.8 (7.3–8.3)	7.2 (6.6–7.8)	6.0 (5.4–6.6)
Fish	8.0 (7.4–8.5)	7.3 (6.7–7.9)	6.1 (5.5–6.7)
Dairy	7.8 (7.3–8.4)	7.2 (6.6–7.8)	6.0 (5.4–6.6)
Eggs	5.4 (4.2–6.7)	4.8 (3.5–6.1)	3.6 (2.3–4.9)
Cereals	6.1 (5.6–6.6)	5.5 (4.9–6.1)	4.3 (3.6–4.8)
Fats and oils	6.0 (5.4–6.5)	5.4 (4.7–6.0)	4.2 (3.5–4.8)
Sweets, confectioneries, and SSBs	7.4 (6.5–8.2)	6.8 (5.9–7.7)	5.6 (4.8–6.5)
All food groups combined	7.4 (6.9–7.9)	6.8 (6.2–7.3)	5.6 (5.0–6.1)

Source: Based on Green and others 2013.
Note: SSBs = sugar-sweetened beverages.

Netherlands, New Zealand, South Africa, and the United States), and the observational studies were conducted in the United States. Pooling all studies, we found that each 10 percent price decrease was associated with a 14 percent (95 percent confidence interval 11–17) increase in consumption of fruits and vegetables and a 16 percent (95 percent confidence interval 10–23) increase in consumption of other healthful foods. A 10 percent price increase was associated with 7 percent (95 percent confidence interval 3–10) lower consumption of SSBs and 3 percent (95 percent confidence interval 1–5) lower consumption of fast foods. The study also found that lower prices of fruits and vegetables were associated with lower body mass index (0.04 kilogram per square meter [kg/m^2] per 10 percent price decrease [95 percent confidence interval 0.00–0.08 kg/m^2]). Thus, price changes clearly influence consumption significantly. The effect on health can be modified by other factors, such as alternative choices (for example, a consumer's selection of substitutes in response to reducing purchases of a taxed food or increasing purchases of a subsidized food) and food industry responses (for example, use of internal pricing strategies to reduce the effect of taxation).

Organizational Settings

In accordance with randomized controlled trials and quasi-experimental studies, both schools and workplaces represent effective settings for improving diet and diet-related risk factors (Afshin, Penalvo, and others 2015;

Micha and others 2016). Isolated interventions have limited effects, but more comprehensive, multicomponent programs are effective. Interventions are most effective if they include formal educational curricula; supportive school or worksite policies; environmental changes, such as healthier vending machine and cafeteria options; and family and parental or peer-support components.

Local Food Environment

Differences in neighborhood food environments, such as supermarkets, grocery stores, fast food outlets, and other restaurants, have come under investigation as determinants of diet (Mozaffarian and others 2012). The low availability of supermarkets, termed *food deserts*, has been considered a potential risk factor for poor diet (Cummins and Macintyre 2002). Yet, the evidence for the effect of neighborhood food environments on consumption has generally been mixed and inconclusive. Across numerous studies, differences in proximity and density of grocery stores, convenience stores, fast food outlets, and other restaurants each inconsistently relate to either dietary intakes or diet-related risk factors, such as adiposity (Afshin, Penalvo, and others 2015). Positive associations of the availability of supermarkets with healthier diets (in particular, intakes of fruits and vegetables) and lower adiposity have been the most consistent. However, nearly all the investigations of neighborhood food environments have been cross-sectional, greatly limiting inference on either temporality or causality. Insufficient evidence exists to draw strong conclusions on the dietary effects of altering the availability or density of different types of food establishments.

Examples of Successful National Policies to Improve Diet

Trans Fats Restrictions

Denmark was the first country to pass legislation to limit the trans fat content of foods (Leth and others 2006). Danish Order No. 160 of March 11, 2003, stipulated a maximum of 2 percent of industrially produced trans fats in oils and fats (2 grams per 100 grams of fat). Evidence from a series of assessments of the trans fat content in a broad range of foods sold in Denmark conducted from the end of 2002 to early 2003 (253 samples preregulation) and again at the end of 2004 to early 2005 (148 samples postregulation) indicated this policy was highly effective in reducing the trans fat content of foods to the targeted levels. The legislation represented a final key step after a decade of intermittent, industry-specific voluntary attempts to reduce the consumption of trans fat in the country (Bech-Larsen and Aschemann-Witzel

2012; Leth and others 2006). Subsequently, several other European countries, including Austria, Hungary, Iceland, Norway, Sweden, and Switzerland, also banned trans fat at the national level (WHO 2015). The United States recently indicated that partially hydrogenated oils (the major source of industrial trans fat) would no longer be generally recognized as safe, effectively eliminating their use in the food supply (Downs, Thow, and Leeder 2013; U.S. Food and Drug Administration 2015). Among low- and middle-income countries (LMICs), Argentina is the first to restrict industrial trans fat content of vegetable oils and margarines to 2 percent of total fat (Rubinstein and others 2015).

Taxation of Unhealthy Beverages or Foods

Several countries have introduced specific taxes on unhealthy foods and beverages (Mytton, Clarke, and Rayner 2012). Evidence from legislative documents and political debates, as well as the size of the implemented taxes, suggests that, in addition to the aim of improving diets, revenue generation has been a major driving force behind most of the implemented taxes (Bodker and others 2015; Vallgarda, Holm, and Jensen 2015).

In 2011, Hungary introduced a tax on specific packaged foods and beverages with a high content of sugar, salt, or caffeine, such as SSBs, energy drinks, confectionery products, salted snacks, condiments, flavored alcohol, and fruit jams. This tax now generates more than US$75 million per year, but its size and target food categories have changed since implementation. In 2012, France introduced a tax on nonalcoholic beverages with added sugars and artificial sweeteners (US$0.03 per can), which has generated nearly US$300 million per year. In 2014, Mexico implemented a tax of 10 percent per liter of soda. A preliminary analysis in Mexico demonstrates significant reductions in SSB consumption at one year, with an average national decline of 6 percent, and partial replacement with noncaloric beverages (Colchero and others 2016). SSB reductions were largest in lower-income groups (average decline of 9 percent), strongly suggesting a causal effect of the tax rather than population trends as a result of public awareness or education. Mexico's tax also targeted many processed snack foods, generating substantial national revenue that was intended to help increase access to water in public schools.

In October 2011, Denmark implemented a national "fat tax" that was based on the saturated fat content of foods (Bodker and others 2015; Vallgarda, Holm, and Jensen 2015). The tax (US$2.30 per kg of saturated fat) was introduced on all foods containing more than 2.3 percent saturated fat, including meats, dairy, and many cooking oils). The result was price increases ranging from 7 percent for one liter of olive oil to 30 percent for a package of butter. This tax was anticipated to generate more than US$200 million per year and reduce saturated fat consumption by 4–10 percent. However, after only 15 months, the tax was repealed mainly because of sustained industry opposition and lobbying alleging economic harms that include administrative costs, job losses, and consumer reactions (Bodker and others 2015; Vallgarda, Holm, and Jensen 2015). The weak evidence for prioritizing fat or even saturated fat alone as a metric (Mozaffarian 2015; Mozaffarian and Ludwig 2015) may also have contributed to the failure of this proposal.

Based on these experiences, national taxes can be effective to both generate revenue and improve dietary habits when they are focused on strong evidence-based priorities that also resonate with the public, such as reduction of SSBs. Optimally, revenue from such taxes should be used to improve population diet further, for example, by means of policies that reduce the prices of more healthful food choices.

Multicomponent Interventions
In 1987, Mauritius instituted a five-year national, multicomponent intervention to reduce NCD risk factors (Uusitalo and others 1996). Approaches included a mass media campaign; fiscal and legislative changes; education; and a regulatory policy that mandated replacement of palm oil—the most common cooking oil—with 100 percent soybean oil, which is high in n-6 and n-3 polyunsaturated fats. National cross-sectional surveys in 1987 and 1992 demonstrated reductions in saturated fat intake (by 3.5 percent energy) and increases in intake of polyunsaturated fat intake (by approximately 5.5 percent energy) over that period. In addition, mean population total blood cholesterol levels fell significantly, with absolute reductions of 0.80 millimoles per liter. In accordance with established effects of dietary fats on blood cholesterol, the changes in cooking oil were estimated to account for about 50 percent of this improvement. The prevalence of hypercholesterolemia decreased by 80 percent.

Other targeted lifestyle factors also improved, including decreased smoking (from 58 percent to 47 percent in men and 7 percent to 4 percent in women), increased moderate leisure activity (from 17 percent to 22 percent in men and 1 percent to 3 percent in women), and decreased frequent alcohol intake (from 18 percent to 14 percent in men). The prevalence of all hypertension and borderline hypertension tended to decrease (Dowse and others 1995). In contrast, during this same period, the prevalence of overweight and obesity increased (in men, from 23 percent to 30 percent and from 3 percent

to 5 percent, respectively; in women, from 28 percent to 33 percent and from 10 percent to 15 percent, respectively). However, the prevalence of diabetes and impaired glucose tolerance remained stable. Because overweight and obesity increased in all nations globally during this period, whether these increases in Mauritius might have been even worse without the national interventions is unclear.

Overall, these findings, together with similar experiences in Finland, indicate that multicomponent national dietary policies, including mandates to increase healthier foods, can have major positive effects on NCD risk factors.

COST-EFFECTIVENESS OF POPULATION INTERVENTIONS TO IMPROVE DIET

Cost is a key potential barrier to implementation and sustainability of any evidence-based intervention. Although based on the first principles that many population-level dietary interventions may be highly cost-effective or even cost saving, formal cost-effectiveness analyses in this area are limited (Cobiac, Veerman, and Vos 2013). Historically, this paucity of data results from lack of reliable data on dietary habits in many populations, insufficient systematically determined effect sizes of population-level interventions to improve diet, controversy over causal effects of dietary changes, and little systematically collected data on costs of such interventions. In recent years, efforts have been made to address these gaps. The 2010 and 2013 GBDs assess global consumption levels of a range of dietary factors by age and gender in 187 countries and the best evidence for their etiologic effects on NCDs. The WHO NCD Costing Tool provides data on health care costs in many countries, as well as resource ingredient needs and corresponding costs of selected policy interventions such as mass media campaigns and alcohol taxation (Evans and others 2005; Murray and others 2000; WHO 2003). For most policies, acquiring the data needed to estimate the cost of the intervention remains a challenge. Chapter 20 in this volume (Watkins, Nugent, and Verguet 2017) offers a detailed review of cost-effectiveness studies of dietary policies.

The early evidence that has emerged from evaluations of actual policies is mixed. In a short-term evaluation of the first city-level tax on SSBs in the United States, Cawley and Frisvold (2015) found relatively little pass through of the Berkeley, California, SSB tax to consumers; retail prices rose by less than half of the amount of the tax. The direct effect on consumption and obesity is likely to be smaller than expected in much of the literature that found or assumed full shifting or even overshifting of taxes. In light of the uncertainty about the effectiveness of diet-related fiscal policies, the examination of their cost-effectiveness by only a minority of studies is not surprising, particularly in LMICs. Cecchini and others' (2010) article was the only published paper to model obesity prevention policies in LMICs, covering Brazil, China, India, Mexico, and South Africa. Their results indicate that fiscal measures (including increasing the price of unhealthy food content or reducing the cost of healthful foods rich in fiber) were less expensive per person than were regulatory or individual interventions; they were the only measures considered that were cost saving for all LMICs at both 20- and 50-year time horizons. In addition, they were cost saving by a magnitude of twice the other interventions considered. Price interventions and regulation appear to produce the largest health gains in the shortest time frame.

As one of the earlier, fairly wide-ranging applications of the modeling approach based on the WHO Choosing Interventions that are Cost-Effective (WHO-CHOICE), Murray and others (2003) modeled salt reduction, mass media health education, and individual treatment, as well as various combinations of different interventions, in two lower-income regions (South-East Asia, with high rates of adult and child mortality, and Latin America, with low adult and child mortality) and one high-income region (Europe, with very low adult and child mortality). Their findings indicate that the nonpersonal interventions have a lower, more favorable cost-effectiveness ratio than do the personalized health service interventions. Voluntary agreements to reduce salt are less cost-effective than legislative measures; salt reduction legislation is estimated to buy one DALY for as little as US$3.74 in South-East Asia and US$2.60 in Latin America. Combinations of salt legislation and mass media programs on healthy behavior have the potential to lower the cost-effectiveness ratio even further. However, the most cost-effective set of interventions is a mix of population-level interventions, preventive interventions, and personalized treatments.

Two follow-up studies to Murray and others (2003) have attempted to provide global or at least multiregional estimates of the cost-effectiveness of salt regulation (as well as other interventions). Asaria and others (2007) modeled the cost and effects of shifts in the distribution of risk factors associated with salt intake and tobacco use on chronic disease mortality for 23 countries that account for 80 percent of chronic disease burden in LMICs. They showed that, over 10 years (2006–15), 13.8 million deaths could have been averted by implementation of these interventions, at a cost of less than US$0.40 per person per year in low-income countries and lower-middle-income countries and US$0.50–US$1.00 per person per year in upper-middle-income countries, as of 2005. Ortegon and others (2012) provide updated evidence on broadly similar interventions in Africa and South-East Asia. In the salt domain, they model the cost-effectiveness of salt reduction in processed foods via voluntary agreements with industry and salt reduction in processed foods via legislation. Rubinstein and others used a more geographically focused application of the WHO-CHOICE approach in two closely related papers, one focusing on Buenos Aires (Rubinstein and others 2009) and the other on Argentina as a whole (Rubinstein and others 2010). The interventions modeled in both studies are similar, including lowering salt intake in the population through voluntary agreements to reduce the levels of salt in bread and providing mass education programs and individual treatment options (Murray and others 2003). The findings in Argentina indicate that any salt reduction would be cost saving; the Buenos Aires–related study suggests that a salt reduction policy would cost very little and would be more cost-effective than a mass media campaign.

Ferrante and others (2012) also looked at salt reduction in Argentina using a simulation model not based on WHO-CHOICE. They analyzed the costs and expected effects of a slightly different salt-related intervention entailing a salt content reduction by 5–25 percent, not only in bread but also in a wider range of food groups that contribute a significant percentage of the salt consumed in the normal diet (for example, bread products, meat products, canned foods, soups, and dressings). Results suggested that this intervention was cost saving and produced substantial benefits to population-wide, diet-related health outcomes. The expectation that salt reduction may be cost saving, applied on its own or in combination with other interventions, has been supported by evidence from four countries in the eastern Mediterranean region (Mason and others 2014). This study evaluated three policies to reduce dietary salt intake, alone and in combination: a health promotion campaign, labeling of food packaging, and mandatory reformulation of salt content in processed food.

In light of the scarcity of evidence of policy effect in high-income countries as well, cost-effectiveness estimates of trans fat policies are difficult to obtain. A recent exception is a much-discussed contested modeling study by Allen and others (2015) that simulated costs and effects of three options for further restricting trans fat consumption in England: a ban of trans fatty acids in processed foods, improved labeling of trans fatty acids, and a restaurant ban of trans fatty acids. The researchers had a specific interest in examining the distributional effects of the various approaches across different socio-economic groups. The reported findings suggest that the expected health effects of a total ban, as well as policies to improve labeling or simply remove trans fatty acids from restaurants and fast food stores, would lead to a considerable reduction in coronary heart disease mortality. Moreover, these benefits would be larger among lower socioeconomic groups—a rare example of an intervention that may increase average population health and health equity. In addition, the study predicts large cost savings from these policies. However, through inclusion of informal care costs and productivity costs, the cost categories in the analysis of cost-effectiveness reach far beyond the types of costs commonly included in health economic evaluations. Nevertheless, the study is critical of the health and economic effects of a continued reliance on industry to voluntarily reformulate products.

CONCLUSIONS

Suboptimal diet is the single-largest risk factor for poor health globally. Specific population interventions, including taxation and subsidies, food regulations, mass media campaigns, and school and workplace interventions, appear effective in improving diet. Many such interventions may be highly cost-effective (efficient health gained per dollar spent) or even cost saving (health gains with reduced overall spending). These interventions are highly attractive and complement the preventive health system strategies promoted in high-, middle-, and low-income countries. Selected policy interventions may also reduce health disparities.

Specific knowledge gaps remain in quantitative effectiveness and cost-effectiveness of several dietary policies in different settings and within different population subgroups. These gaps highlight the urgent need for governments, foundations, advocacy groups, and private industry to prioritize relevant implementation and evaluation of these approaches.

NOTE

World Bank Income Classifications as of July 2014 are as follows, based on estimates of gross national income (GNI) per capita for 2013:

- Low-income countries (LICs) = US$1,045 or less
- Middle-income countries (MICs) are subdivided:
  (a) lower-middle-income = US$1,046 to US$4,125
  (b) upper-middle-income (UMICs) = US$4,126 to US$12,745
- High-income countries (HICs) = US$12,746 or more.

REFERENCES

Afshin, A., A. I. Abioye, O. N. Ajala, A. B. Nguyen, K. C. See, and others. 2013. "Abstract P087: Effectiveness of Mass Media Campaigns for Improving Dietary Behaviors: A Systematic Review and Meta-Analysis." *Circulation* 127 (Suppl 12): AP087.

Afshin, A., L. Del Gobbo, J. Silva, M. Michaelson, M. O'Flaherty, and others. 2015. "The Prospective Impact of Food Pricing on Improving Dietary Consumption: A Systematic Review and Meta-Analysis." Manuscript submitted for publication.

Afshin, A., R. Micha, S. Khatibzadeh, and D. Mozaffarian. 2014. "Consumption of Nuts and Legumes and Risk of Incident Ischemic Heart Disease, Stroke, and Diabetes: A Systematic Review and Meta-Analysis." *American Journal of Clinical Nutrition* 100 (1): 278–88. doi:10.3945/ajcn.113.076901.

Afshin, A., J. Penalvo, L. Del Gobbo, M. Kashaf, R. Micha, and others. 2015. "CVD Prevention through Policy: A Review of Mass Media, Food/Menu Labeling, Taxation/Subsidies, Built Environment, School Procurement, Worksite Wellness, and Marketing Standards to Improve Diet." *Current Cardiology Reports* 17 (11): 98. doi:10.1007/s11886-015-0658-9.

Allen, K., J. Pearson-Stuttard, W. Hooton, P. Diggle, S. Capewell, and M. O'Flaherty. 2015. "Potential of Trans Fats Policies to Reduce Socioeconomic Inequalities in Mortality from Coronary Heart Disease in England: Cost Effectiveness Modelling Study." *BMJ* 351: h4583. doi:10.1136/bmj.h4583.

An, R. 2013. "Effectiveness of Subsidies in Promoting Healthy Food Purchases and Consumption: A Review of Field Experiments." *Public Health Nutrition* 16 (7): 1215–28. doi:10.1017/S1368980012004715.

Andreyeva, T., M. W. Long, and K. D. Brownell. 2009. "The Impact of Food Prices on Consumption: A Systematic Review of Research on the Price Elasticity of Demand for Food." *American Journal of Public Health* 100 (2): 216–22. doi:10.2105/ajph.2008.151415.

Artinian, N. T., G. F. Fletcher, D. Mozaffarian, P. Kris-Etherton, L. Van Horn, and others. 2010. "Interventions to Promote Physical Activity and Dietary Lifestyle Changes for Cardiovascular Risk Factor Reduction in Adults: A Scientific Statement from the American Heart Association." *Circulation* 122 (4): 406–41.

Asaria, P., D. Chisholm, C. Mathers, M. Ezzati, and R. Beaglehole. 2007. "Chronic Disease Prevention: Health Effects and Financial Costs of Strategies to Reduce Salt Intake and Control Tobacco Use." *The Lancet* 370 (9604): 2044–53. doi:10.1016/S0140-6736(07)61698-5.

Ashfield-Watt, P. A. 2006. "Fruits and Vegetables, 5+ a Day: Are We Getting the Message Across?" *Asia Pacific Journal of Clinical Nutrition* 15 (2): 245–52.

Aune, D., T. Norat, P. Romundstad, and L. J. Vatten. 2013. "Dairy Products and the Risk of Type 2 Diabetes: A Systematic Review and Dose-Response Meta-Analysis of Cohort Studies." *American Journal of Clinical Nutrition* 98 (4): 1066–83. doi:10.3945/ajcn.113.059030.

Bech-Larsen, T., and J. A. Aschemann-Witzel. 2012. "A Macromarketing Perspective on Food Safety Regulation:

The Danish Ban on Trans-Fatty Acids." *Journal of Macromarketing* (32): 208–19.

Bhalla, V., C. W. Fong, S. K. Chew, and K. Satku. 2006. "Changes in the Levels of Major Cardiovascular Risk Factors in the Multi-Ethnic Population in Singapore after 12 Years of a National Non-Communicable Disease Intervention Programme." *Singapore Medical Journal* 47 (10): 841–50.

Bodker, M., C. Pisinger, U. Toft, and T. Jorgensen. 2015. "The Rise and Fall of the World's First Fat Tax." *Health Policy* 119 (6): 737–42. doi:10.1016/j.healthpol.2015.03.003.

Cawley, J., and D. Frisvold. 2015. "The Incidence of Taxes on Sugar-Sweetened Beverages: The Case of Berkeley, California." NBER Working Paper 21465, Cambridge, MA, National Bureau of Economic Research. http://www.nber.org/papers/w21465.

Cecchini, M., F. Sassi, J. A. Lauer, Y. Y. Lee, V. Guajardo-Barron, and D. Chisholm. 2010. "Tackling of Unhealthy Diets, Physical Inactivity, and Obesity: Health Effects and Cost-Effectiveness." *The Lancet* 376 (9754): 17759–84. doi:10.1016/S0140-6736(10)61514-0.

Chen, G. C., D. B. Lv, Z. Pang, and Q. F. Liu. 2013. "Red and Processed Meat Consumption and Risk of Stroke: A Meta-Analysis of Prospective Cohort Studies." *European Journal of Clinical Nutrition* 67 (1): 91–95. doi:10.1038/ejcn.2012.180.

Chen, M., Q. Sun, E. Giovannucci, D. Mozaffarian, J. E. Manson, and others. 2014. "Dairy Consumption and Risk of Type 2 Diabetes: 3 Cohorts of US Adults and an Updated Meta-Analysis." *BMC Medicine* 12: 215. doi:10.1186/s12916-014-0215-1.

Cobiac, L. J., L. Veerman, and T. Vos. 2013. "The Role of Cost-Effectiveness Analysis in Developing Nutrition Policy." *Annual Review of Nutrition* 33: 373–93. doi:10.1146/annurev-nutr-071812-161133.

Colchero, M. A., B. M. Popkin, J. A. Rivera, and S. W. Ng. 2016. "Beverage Purchases from Stores in Mexico under the Excise Tax on Sugar Sweetened Beverages: Observational Study." *BMJ* 352: h6704. doi:10.1136/bmj.h6704.

Connell, D., J. P. Goldberg, and S. C. Folta. 2001. "An Intervention to Increase Fruit and Vegetable Consumption Using Audio Communications: In-Store Public Service Announcements and Audiotapes." *Journal of Health Communication* 6 (1): 31–43.

Cummins, S., and S. Macintyre. 2002. "'Food Deserts'—Evidence and Assumption in Health Policy Making." *BMJ* 325 (7361): 436–38.

de Munter, J. S., F. B. Hu, D. Spiegelman, M. Franz, and R. M. van Dam. 2007. "Whole Grain, Bran, and Germ Intake and Risk of Type 2 Diabetes: A Prospective Cohort Study and Systematic Review." *PLoS Medicine* 4 (8): e261.

Dietary Guidelines Advisory Committee. 2015. *Scientific Report of the 2015 Dietary Guidelines Advisory Committee.* Washington, DC: U.S. Department of Health and Human Services, U.S. Department of Agriculture.

Downs, S. M., A. M. Thow, and S. R. Leeder. 2013. "The Effectiveness of Policies for Reducing Dietary Trans Fat: A Systematic Review of the Evidence." *Bulletin of the World Health Organization* 91 (4): 262–9H. doi:10.2471/BLT.12.111468.

Dowse, G. K., H. Gareeboo, K. G. Alberti, P. Zimmet, J. Tuomilehto, and others. 1995. "Changes in Population Cholesterol Concentrations and Other Cardiovascular Risk Factor Levels after Five Years of the Non-Communicable Disease Intervention Programme in Mauritius. Mauritius Non-Communicable Disease Study Group." *BMJ* 311 (7015): 1255–59.

Evans, D. B., T. T. Edejer, T. Adam, and S. S. Lim. 2005. "Methods to Assess the Costs and Health Effects of Interventions for Improving Health in Developing Countries." *BMJ* 331 (7525): 1137–40. doi:10.1136/bmj.331.7525.1137.

FAO (Food and Agriculture Organization of the United Nations). 2010. *Fats and Fatty Acids in Human Nutrition: Report of an Expert Consultation.* Rome: FAO.

Ferrante, D., J. Konfino, R. Mejia, P. Coxson, A. Moran, and others. 2012. "The Cost-Utility Ratio of Reducing Salt Intake and Its Impact on the Incidence of Cardiovascular Disease in Argentina." *Rev Panam Salud Publica* 32 (4): 274–80.

Forouzanfar, M. H., L. Alexander, H. R. Anderson, V. F. Bachman, S. Biryukov, and others. 2015. "Global, Regional, and National Comparative Risk Assessment of 79 Behavioural, Environmental and Occupational, and Metabolic Risks or Clusters of Risks in 188 Countries, 1990–2013: A Systematic Analysis for the Global Burden of Disease Study 2013." *The Lancet* 386 (10010): 2287–323. doi:10.1016/S0140-6736(15)00128-2.

Green, R., L. Cornelsen, A. D. Dangour, R. Turner, B. Shankar, and others. 2013. "The Effect of Rising Food Prices on Food Consumption: Systematic Review with Meta-Regression." *BMJ* 346: f3703. doi:10.1136/bmj.f3703.

Hooper, L., C. Kay, A. Abdelhamid, P. A. Kroon, J. S. Cohn, and others. 2012. "Effects of Chocolate, Cocoa, and Flavan-3-Ols on Cardiovascular Health: A Systematic Review and Meta-Analysis of Randomized Trials." *American Journal of Clinical Nutrition* 95 (3): 740–51. doi:10.3945/ajcn.111.023457.

IFPRI (International Food Policy Research Institute). 2015. *Global Nutrition Report 2015: Actions and Accountability to Advance Nutrition and Sustainable Development.* Washington, DC: IFPRI.

Imamura, F., L. O'Connor, Z. Ye, J. Mursu, Y. Hayashino, and others. 2015. "Consumption of Sugar Sweetened Beverages, Artificially Sweetened Beverages, and Fruit Juice and Incidence of Type 2 Diabetes: Systematic Review, Meta-Analysis, and Estimation of Population Attributable Fraction." *BMJ* 351: h3576. doi:10.1136/bmj.h3576.

Jakobsen, M. U., E. J. O'Reilly, B. L. Heitmann, M. A. Pereira, K. Balter, and others. 2009. "Major Types of Dietary Fat and Risk of Coronary Heart Disease: A Pooled Analysis of 11 Cohort Studies." *American Journal of Clinical Nutrition* 89 (5): 1425–32.

Kaluza, J., A. Wolk, and S. C. Larsson. 2012. "Red Meat Consumption and Risk of Stroke: A Meta-Analysis of Prospective Studies." *Stroke* 43 (10): 2556–60. doi:10.1161/strokeaha.112.663286.

Khatibzadeh, S., R. Micha, I. Elmadfa, S. Kalantarian, J. Powles, and others. 2012. "Available Data on Food and Nutrient

Intake around the World: Global Burden of Nutrition and Chronic Disease Expert Group." Abstract P141, American Heart Association/American Stroke Association EPI/NPAM Final Program and Abstracts, San Diego, CA.

Leth, T., H. G. Jensen, A. A. Mikkelsen, and A. Bysted. 2006. "The Effect of the Regulation on Trans Fatty Acid Content in Danish Food." *Atherosclerosis* (Suppl) 7 (2): 53–56. doi:10.1016/j.atherosclerosissup.2006.04.019.

Lim, S. S., T. Vos, A. D. Flaxman, G. Danaei, K. Shibuya, and others. 2012. "A Comparative Risk Assessment of Burden of Disease and Injury Attributable to 67 Risk Factors and Risk Factor Clusters in 21 Regions, 1990–2010: A Systematic Analysis for the Global Burden of Disease Study 2010." *The Lancet* 380 (9859): 2224–60. doi:10.1016/S0140-6736(12)61766-8.

Marcus, A. C., J. Heimendinger, P. Wolfe, D. Fairclough, B. K. Rimer, and others. 2001. "A Randomized Trial of a Brief Intervention to Increase Fruit and Vegetable Intake: A Replication Study among Callers to the CIS." *Preventive Medicine* 33 (3): 204–16.

Mason, H., A. Shoaibi, R. Ghandour, M. O'Flaherty, S. Capewell, and others. 2014. "A Cost Effectiveness Analysis of Salt Reduction Policies to Reduce Coronary Heart Disease in Four Eastern Mediterranean Countries." *PLoS One* 9 (1): e84445. doi:10.1371/journal.pone.0084445.

McGill, R., E. Anwar, L. Orton, H. Bromley, F. Lloyd-Williams, and others. 2015. "Are Interventions to Promote Healthy Eating Equally Effective for All? Systematic Review of Socioeconomic Inequalities in Impact." *BMC Public Health* 15: 457. doi:10.1186/s12889-015-1781-7.

Micha, R., I. Bakogianni, D. Karageorgou, E. Trichia, M. L. Shulkin, and others. 2016. "Abstract MP89: Effectiveness of School Procurement Policies for Improving Dietary Behaviors: A Systematic Review and Meta-analysis." *Circulation* 133 (Suppl 1): AMP89–89.

Micha, R., S. Kalantarian, P. Wirojratana, T. Byers, G. Danaei, and others. 2012. "Estimating the Global and Regional Burden of Suboptimal Nutrition on Chronic Disease: Methods and Inputs to the Analysis." *European Journal of Clinical Nutrition* 66 (1): 119–29.

Micha, R., S. Khatibzadeh, P. Shi, K. G. Andrews, R. E. Engell, and others. 2015. "Global, Regional and National Consumption of Major Food Groups in 1990 and 2010: A Systematic Analysis Including 266 Country-Specific Nutrition Surveys Worldwide." *BMJ Open* 5 (9): e008705. doi:10.1136/bmjopen-2015-008705.

Micha, R., S. Khatibzadeh, P. Shi, S. Fahimi, S. Lim, and others. 2014. "Global, Regional, and National Consumption Levels of Dietary Fats and Oils in 1990 and 2010: A Systematic Analysis Including 266 Country-Specific Nutrition Surveys." *BMJ* 348: g2272. doi:10.1136/bmj.g2272.

Micha, R., S. K. Wallace, and D. Mozaffarian. 2010. "Red and Processed Meat Consumption and Risk of Incident Coronary Heart Disease, Stroke, and Diabetes Mellitus: A Systematic Review and Meta-Analysis." *Circulation* 121 (21): 2271–83.

Mozaffarian, D. 2014. "Chapter 46. Nutrition and Cardiovascular Disease and Metabolic Diseases." In *Braunwald's Heart Disease: A Textbook of Cardiovascular Medicine*, edited by D. L. Mann, D. P. Zipes, P. Libby, and R. O. Bonow. Philadelphia: Elsevier/Saunders.

———. 2015. "Diverging Global Trends in Heart Disease and Type 2 Diabetes: The Role of Carbohydrates and Saturated Fats." *The Lancet Diabetes Endocrinology* 3 (8): 586–88. doi:10.1016/S2213-8587(15)00208-9.

Mozaffarian, D., A. Afshin, N. L. Benowitz, V. Bittner, S. R. Daniels, and others. 2012. "Population Approaches to Improve Diet, Physical Activity, and Smoking Habits: A Scientific Statement from the American Heart Association." *Circulation* 126 (12): 1514–63. doi:10.1161/CIR.0b013e318260a20b.

Mozaffarian, D., S. Fahimi, G. M. Singh, R. Micha, S. Khatibzadeh, and others. 2014. "Global Sodium Consumption and Death from Cardiovascular Causes." *New England Journal of Medicine* 371 (7): 624–34. doi:10.1056/NEJMoa1304127.

Mozaffarian, D., T. Hao, E. B. Rimm, W. C. Willett, and F. B. Hu. 2011. "Changes in Diet and Lifestyle and Long-Term Weight Gain in Women and Men." *New England Journal of Medicine* 364 (25): 2392–404.

Mozaffarian, D., M. B. Katan, A. Ascherio, M. J. Stampfer, and W. C. Willett. 2006. "Trans Fatty Acids and Cardiovascular Disease." *New England Journal of Medicine* 354 (15): 1601–13.

Mozaffarian, D., and D. S. Ludwig. 2010. "Dietary Guidelines in the 21st Century: A Time for Food." *Journal of the American Medical Association* 304 (6): 681–82. doi:10.1001/jama.2010.1116.

———. 2015. "The 2015 US Dietary Guidelines: Lifting the Ban on Total Dietary Fat." *Journal of the American Medical Association* 313 (24): 2421–22. doi:10.1001/jama.2015.5941.

Mozaffarian, D., R. Micha, and S. Wallace. 2010. "Effects on Coronary Heart Disease of Increasing Polyunsaturated Fat in Place of Saturated Fat: A Systematic Review and Meta-Analysis of Randomized Controlled Trials." *PLoS Medicine* 7 (3): e1000252. doi:10.1371/journal.pmed.1000252.

Mozaffarian, D., and E. B. Rimm. 2006. "Fish Intake, Contaminants, and Human Health: Evaluating the Risks and the Benefits." *Journal of the American Medical Association* 296 (15): 1885–99.

Murray, C. J., D. B. Evans, A. Acharya, and R. M. Baltussen. 2000. "Development of WHO Guidelines on Generalized Cost-Effectiveness Analysis." *Health Economics* 9 (3): 235–51.

Murray, C. J., J. A. Lauer, R. C. Hutubessy, L. Niessen, N. Tomijima, and others. 2003. "Effectiveness and Costs of Interventions to Lower Systolic Blood Pressure and Cholesterol: A Global and Regional Analysis on Reduction of Cardiovascular-Disease Risk." *The Lancet* 361 (9359): 717–25. doi:10.1016/S0140-6736(03)12655-4.

Mytton, O. T., D. Clarke, and M. Rayner. 2012. "Taxing Unhealthy Food and Drinks to Improve Health." *BMJ* 344: e2931. doi:10.1136/bmj.e2931.

Nishtar, S., Y. A. Mirza, S. Jehan, Y. Hadi, A. Badar, and others. 2004. "Newspaper Articles as a Tool for Cardiovascular Prevention Programs in a Developing Country." *Journal of Health Communication* 9 (4): 355–69.

Ortegon, M., S. Lim, D. Chisholm, and S. Mendis. 2012. "Cost Effectiveness of Strategies to Combat Cardiovascular Disease, Diabetes, and Tobacco Use in Sub-Saharan Africa and South East Asia: A Mathematical Modelling Study." *BMJ* 344: e607. doi:10.1136/bmj.e607.

Pan, A., and F. B. Hu. 2011. "Effects of Carbohydrates on Satiety: Differences between Liquid and Solid Food." *Current Opinions in Clinical Nutrition and Metabolic Care* 14 (4): 385–90. doi:10.1097/MCO.0b013e328346df36.

Pekka, P., P. Pirjo, and U. Ulla. 2002. "Influencing Public Nutrition for Non-Communicable Disease Prevention: From Community Intervention to National Programme— Experiences from Finland." *Public Health Nutrition* 5 (1A): 245–51.

Pollard, C. M., M. R. Miller, A. M. Daly, K. E. Crouchley, K. J. O'Donoghue, and others. 2008. "Increasing Fruit and Vegetable Consumption: Success of the Western Australian Go for 2&5 Campaign." *Public Health Nutrition* 11 (3): 314–20.

Powles, J., S. Fahimi, R. Micha, S. Khatibzadeh, P. Shi, and others. 2013. "Global, Regional and National Sodium Intakes in 1990 and 2010: A Systematic Analysis of 24 h Urinary Sodium Excretion and Dietary Surveys Worldwide." *BMJ Open* 3 (12): e003733. doi:10.1136/bmjopen-2013-003733.

Puska, P., and T. Stahl. 2010. "Health in All Policies: The Finnish Initiative—Background, Principles, and Current Issues." *Annual Reviews of Public Health* 31: 315–828. doi:10.1146/annurev.publhealth.012809.103658.

Renehan, A. G., M. Tyson, M. Egger, R. F. Heller, and M. Zwahlen. 2008. "Body-Mass Index and Incidence of Cancer: A Systematic Review and Meta-Analysis of Prospective Observational Studies." *The Lancet* 371 (9612): 569–78. doi:10.1016/s0140-6736(08)60269-x.

Rose, G. 1985. "Sick Individuals and Sick Populations." *International Journal of Epidemiology* 14 (1): 32–38.

Rubinstein, A., L. Colantonio, A. Bardach, J. Caporale, S. G. Marti, and others. 2010. "Estimation of the Burden of Cardiovascular Disease Attributable to Modifiable Risk Factors and Cost-Effectiveness Analysis of Preventative Interventions to Reduce This Burden in Argentina." *BMC Public Health* 10: 627. doi:10.1186/1471-2458-10-627.

Rubinstein, A., N. Elorriaga, O. U. Garay, R. Poggio, J. Caporale, and others. 2015. "Eliminating Artificial Trans Fatty Acids in Argentina: Estimated Effects on the Burden of Coronary Heart Disease and Costs." *Bulletin of the World Health Organization* 93 (9): 614–22. doi:10.2471/BLT.14.150516.

Rubinstein, A., S. Garcia Marti, A. Souto, D. Ferrante, and F. Augustovski. 2009. "Generalized Cost-Effectiveness Analysis of a Package of Interventions to Reduce Cardiovascular Disease in Buenos Aires, Argentina." *Cost Effectivenesss and Resource Allocation* 7: 10. doi:10.1186/1478-7547-7-10.

Shangguan, S., J. Smith, W. Ma, L. Tanz, A. Afshin, and others. 2015. "Abstract P323: Effectiveness of Point-of-Purchase Labeling on Dietary Behaviors and Nutrient Contents of Foods—A Systemic Review and Meta-Analysis." *Circulation* 131 (Suppl 1): AP323.

Shrime, M. G., S. R. Bauer, A. C. McDonald, N. H. Chowdhury, C. E. Coltart, and others. 2011. "Flavonoid-Rich Cocoa Consumption Affects Multiple Cardiovascular Risk Factors in a Meta-Analysis of Short-Term Studies." *Journal of Nutrition* 141 (11): 1982–88. doi:10.3945/jn.111.145482.

Singh, G. M., G. Danaei, F. Farzadfar, G. A. Stevens, M. Woodward, and others. 2013. "The Age-Specific Quantitative Effects of Metabolic Risk Factors on Cardiovascular Diseases and Diabetes: A Pooled Analysis." *PloS One* 8 (7): e65174. doi:10.1371/journal.pone.0065174.

Singh, G. M., R. Micha, S. Khatibzadeh, S. Lim, M. Ezzati, and others. 2015. "Estimated Global, Regional, and National Disease Burdens Related to Sugar-Sweetened Beverage Consumption in 2010." *Circulation* 132 (8): 639–66. doi:10.1161/CIRCULATIONAHA.114.010636.

Singh, G. M., R. Micha, S. Khatibzadeh, P. Shi, S. Lim, and others. 2015. "Global, Regional, and National Consumption of Sugar-Sweetened Beverages, Fruit Juices, and Milk: A Systematic Assessment of Beverage Intake in 187 Countries." *PLoS One* 10 (8): e0124845. doi:10.1371/journal.pone.0124845.

Stables, G. J., A. F. Subar, B. H. Patterson, K. Dodd, J. Heimendinger, and others. 2002. "Changes in Vegetable and Fruit Consumption and Awareness among US Adults: Results of the 1991 and 1997 5-A-Day for Better Health Program Surveys." *Journal of the American Dietetic Association* 102 (6): 809–17.

Te Morenga, L., S. Mallard, and J. Mann. 2013. "Dietary Sugars and Body Weight: Systematic Review and Meta-Analyses of Randomised Controlled Trials and Cohort Studies." *BMJ* 346: e7492. doi:10.1136/bmj.e7492.

Thow, A. M., S. Downs, and S. Jan. 2014. "A Systematic Review of the Effectiveness of Food Taxes and Subsidies to Improve Diets: Understanding the Recent Evidence." *Nutrition Reviews* 72 (9): 551–65. doi:10.1111/nure.12123.

UN (United Nations). 2011. "Political Declaration of the High-Level Meeting of the General Assembly on the Prevention and Control of Non-Communicable Diseases." UN, New York.

U.S. Department of Health and Human Services and U.S. Department of Agriculture 2010. *Dietary Guidelines for Americans 2010.* Washington, DC: U.S. Government Printing Office. http://www.cnpp.usda.gov/DGAs2010 -PolicyDocument.htm.

U.S. Food and Drug Administration. 2015. "FDA Cuts *Trans* Fat in Processed Foods." http://www.fda.gov/ForConsumers /ConsumerUpdates/ucm372915.htm.

Uusitalo, U., E. J. Feskens, J. Tuomilehto, G. Dowse, U. Haw, and others. 1996. "Fall in Total Cholesterol Concentration Over Five Years in Association with Changes in Fatty Acid Composition of Cooking Oil in Mauritius: Cross-Sectional Survey." *BMJ* 313 (7064): 1044–46.

Vallgarda, S., L. Holm, and J. D. Jensen. 2015. "The Danish Tax on Saturated Fat: Why It Did Not Survive." *European Journal of Clinical Nutrition* 69 (2): 223–26. doi:10.1038 /ejcn.2014.224.

Watkins, D. A., R. Nugent, and S. Verguet. 2017. "Extended Cost-Effectiveness Analyses of Cardiovascular Risk Factor Reduction Policies." In *Disease Control Priorities* (third edition): Volume 5, *Cardiovascular, Respiratory, and Related Disorders,* edited by D. Prabhakaran, S. Anand,

T. A. Gaziano, J.-C. Mbanya, Y. Wu, and R. Nugent. Washington, DC: World Bank.

Willett, W. C. 1998. *Nutritional Epidemiology*. 2nd ed. New York: Oxford University Press.

WHO (World Health Organization). 2003. *Making Choices in Health: WHO Guide to Cost-Effectiveness Analysis*. Geneva: WHO.

———. 2004. "Global Strategy on Diet, Physical Activity and Health." http://www.who.int/dietphysicalactivity/en/.

———. 2012. "Nutrition: Global Targets 2025." http://www.who.int/nutrition/global-target-2025/en/.

———. 2015. Eliminating *Trans* Fats in Europe: A Policy Brief." Regional Office for Europe, WHO, Copenhagen. http://www.euro.who.int/__data/assets/pdf_file/0010/288442/Eliminating-trans-fats-in-Europe-A-policy-brief.pdf.

World Cancer Research Fund International. 2016. "Continuous Update Project (CUP)." http://wcrf.org/int/research-we-fund/continuous-update-project-cup.

World Cancer Research Fund and American Institute for Cancer Research. 2007. *Food, Nutrition, Physical Activity, and the Prevention of Cancer: A Global Perspective*. Washington, DC: American Institute for Cancer Research.

Chapter 7

Obesity Prevention

Vasanti S. Malik and Frank B. Hu

INTRODUCTION

Once considered a problem only in high-income countries (HICs), obesity has become a major contributor to the global disease burden (Finucane and others 2011; Misra and Khurana 2008). Excess adiposity, particularly around the visceral abdominal region, is an important risk factor for morbidity and mortality from type 2 diabetes, cardiovascular diseases, and some cancers (Danaei and others 2009; Whitlock and others 2009; WHO 2009). Although some studies have suggested lower mortality among overweight or obese persons than among healthy-weight persons (Carnethon and others 2012), this outcome has not been observed in studies that properly account for the confounding effects of smoking, preexisting chronic conditions, and other biases (Global BMI Mortality Collaboration 2016; Tobias, Pan, and Hu 2014). The costs of obesity and comorbid conditions are staggering as measured by both health care expenditures and quality of life, underscoring the importance of implementing obesity prevention strategies and treatment strategies on a global scale.

The changes needed to reverse global trends in obesity will likely require numerous interventions and policy recommendations that target diet, lifestyle, access to care, and environmental risk factors. In this chapter, we summarize the global burden of obesity and the impact of a spectrum of obesity risk factors, ranging from sociopolitical and economic forces that are largely beyond an individual's control to modifiable lifestyle factors, and discuss genetic and epigenetic risks. We also review the effectiveness of population-based interventions and policies for preventing obesity, some individual-level treatment options across various platforms, and the cost-effectiveness of select interventions.

GLOBAL BURDEN OF OBESITY

Obesity arises as the result of an energy imbalance between calories consumed and calories expended, creating an energy surplus resulting in excess body weight. In adults, overweight and obesity are typically defined as having a body mass index (BMI), measured as weight in kilograms divided by height in meters squared, equal to or greater than 25 and 30, respectively. These values are based on associations with chronic disease risk (WHO 1995, 2000). However, since Asian populations develop type 2 diabetes and metabolic risk at a younger age and lower BMI than Western populations, the World Health Organization (WHO) has proposed lower BMI action points of 23 and 28 for Asian adults (WHO Expert Consultation 2004). South Asian adults, in particular, also have a higher percentage of body fat and are more prone to developing abdominal obesity at a given BMI than Western adults, which may account for their high risk for type 2 diabetes (WHO Expert Consultation 2004). In children, obesity is generally defined as BMI equal to or greater than the 95th percentile age-for-sex BMI (Kuczmarski

Corresponding author: Vasanti Malik, Department of Nutrition, Harvard T. H. Chan School of Public Health, Boston, Massachusetts, United States; vmalik@hsph.harvard.edu.

and others 2000). However, obesity-related comorbid conditions may develop at values less than this threshold, and ethnic differences may exist in these processes. In a cross-sectional analysis of 662 rural Indian children, Indian boys had a higher percentage of body fat than white boys in the United Kingdom, despite lower BMI (Lakshmi and others 2012).

The WHO formally recognized the global impact of the obesity epidemic during a special obesity consultation in 1997. In the past 15 years, a large body of evidence has been accumulated illustrating temporal increases in the prevalence of obesity across the world. Globally, between 1980 and 2008, obesity prevalence rose to 9.8 percent from 4.8 percent in men and to 13.8 percent from 7.9 percent in women (Finucane and others 2011). Based on a more recent analysis of global data with longer follow-up, the prevalence of obesity increased from 3.2 percent in 1975 to 10.8 percent in 2014 in men, and from 6.4 percent to 14.9 percent in women; 2.3 percent of the world's men and 5.0 percent of women are classified as having severe obesity (BMI $\geq$35 kg/m^2) (NCD Risk Factor Collaboration 2016). For the first time in human history, more overweight than underweight individuals are living on the planet (NCD Risk Factor Collaboration 2016). Over the next two decades, the largest proportional increase in the number of adults who are overweight or obese is expected to occur in low- and middle-income countries (LMICs), where estimates range from increases of 62 percent to 205 percent for overweight and 71 percent to 263 percent for obesity (Kelly and others 2008). Of particular concern has been the rising prevalence of severe or morbid obesity (BMI greater than 40) in the United States, with rates increasing by 70 percent between 2000 and 2010 (Sturm and Hattori 2013). Clinically severe obesity results in more serious health consequences than moderate obesity (BMI greater than 30) for patients and creates additional challenges for health care.

Although the prevalence of obesity is higher in adults than in children, the incidence of obesity has risen more rapidly among children than among adults in some countries, such as Brazil, China, and the United States (Popkin and others 2006). The worldwide prevalence of childhood overweight and obesity among preschool children increased to 6.7 percent from 4.2 percent between 1990 and 2010 (de Onis, Blossner, and Borghi 2010). This increase means that an estimated 43 million children were overweight or obese in 2010, of whom 35 million live in LMICs. The total number of children worldwide who are overweight or obese is expected to reach 60 million (9.1 percent) by 2020 if current trends continue. As reported in a paper as part of the second *Lancet* obesity series, in the United States, the average weight of a child has risen by more than 5 kg within three decades, to a point where one-third of children in the United States are overweight or obese. Some LMICs have reported similar or more rapid rises in child obesity, despite continuing high levels of undernutrition (Lobstein and others 2015). When interpreting the data on obesity prevalence, it is important to note that for some LMICs, major challenges to documenting temporal trends have been both limited sources of data and limited access to high-quality data, due in part to lack of national-level surveillance. This is an important knowledge gap that requires future efforts.

In many LMICs, the percentage of people who are overweight already exceeds the percentage of people who are underweight. However, the percentage of the population who are underweight still remains a major concern in some populations. Undernutrition and obesity can exist side by side within a country, community, or household. Within a given country, obesity tends to be more prevalent in urban than in rural areas. Obesity correlates positively with economic growth and wealth in LMICs, but as a country becomes increasingly wealthy, low-income groups are at greater risk (Malik, Willett, and Hu 2013). Children younger than age five years are most vulnerable to undernutrition because of higher requirements during growth, which might explain the paradox of having overweight adults and underweight children within the same home. Cheap food that is high in energy and low in nutritional quality could adversely affect growth in young children while providing excess calories to older children and adults. Related to this is the increased obesity and metabolic risk observed among children born with low birthweight due to the interplay between in utero fetal programming and an obesogenic environment. Caloric sufficiency and adequate nutrition during pregnancy have been a major focus in many LMICs to ensure good health of both the mother and her offspring. However, excessive weight gain before and during pregnancy has been associated with gestational hyperglycemia and obesity in mothers as well as metabolic complications, such as insulin resistance in offspring (Bellamy and others 2009). These factors pose a particular challenge for implementing obesity prevention policies in many LMICs. Reducing obesity without exacerbating undernutrition, and vice versa, is critical.

RISK FACTORS FOR OBESITY

Energy imbalance is partially a result of the profound sociopolitical and economic changes, including global free trade, economic growth, and urbanization, that have been occurring in HICs since the early twentieth century but are now accelerating in LMICs. Although these "macrolevel" changes are largely beyond the control of the health sector, they influence and interact with numerous modifiable environmental and lifestyle risk factors. At the same time, not all individuals living in obesogenic environments experience the same risk of obesity. Heredity and particular socioeconomic and cultural milieus have also been shown to affect obesity risk even in ostensibly similar obesogenic environments. Body weight regulation is thus a complex interaction between many forces, and personal behaviors in response to these conditions continue to play a dominant role in obesity prevention (figure 7.1). Although the global obesity epidemic has many causes, in this section, we summarize the impact of global trade liberalization, economic growth, and urbanization on obesity risk; discuss global changes in major dietary risk factors, physical activity, and sociocultural norms; and consider genetic and epigenetic obesity factors.

Global Trade Liberalization

Between the 1970s and 1990s, many countries underwent economic structural adjustments, including implementation of more market-oriented or liberal agricultural trade policies (Hawkes 2006). These policies have altered the food supply and are thought to have had direct effects on the obesity epidemic, contributing to nutritional transition and changing food choice and availability. At the same time, however, some of these changes to the food system have led to improvements in quality of life and food security and to reductions in poverty. Trade liberalization can affect the availability of certain foods by enabling the trade of greater amounts and varieties of food, by removing barriers to foreign investment in food distribution, and by expanding multinational food companies and fast-food chains (Kearney 2010). For example, in 1998, transnational food companies based in the United States invested US$5.7 billion in establishing outlets globally (Harris and others 2002). Analysis shows that LMICs that enter free trade agreements with the United States have a 63.4 percent higher consumption of sugar-sweetened beverages per capita than those that do not, after adjusting for a given country's level of gross domestic product (GDP) per capita and urbanization (Stuckler and others 2012). Some scholars have suggested that implementation of the North American Free Trade Agreement has coincided with the burgeoning obesity epidemic in Mexico through increased sales of low-quality processed and fast foods (Clark and others 2012). The relationship between economic policies,

Figure 7.1 Determinants of Obesity

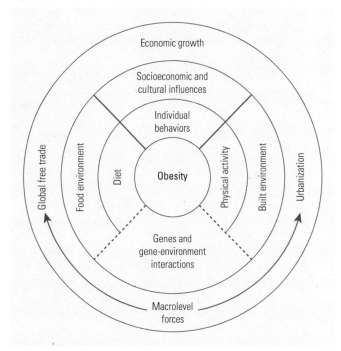

Source: Modified from Public Health Systems, Foresight Systems Map, 2007 (https://www.noo.org.uk/NOO_about_obesity/causes).
Note: Macrolevel forces are largely beyond our control, but they influence and interact with numerous modifiable environmental and population-level factors. These factors, in turn, can greatly influence diet, physical activity, and individual-level behaviors. Genetic factors that underlie susceptibility to obesity may be amplified in the presence of certain environmental factors. Together, these forces interact in a complex network leading to positive energy balance and obesity.

global trade agreements, and obesity should be investigated as points of intervention, given the potential scale of their impact.

Income and Socioeconomic Status

During the next three to four decades, global income per capita is projected to rise at a rate of more than 2 percent per year, with more rapid rates expected in LMICs (Kearney 2010). The prevalence of obesity correlates positively with the initial stages of economic growth and development, as populations of rapidly developing LMICs undergo nutritional and lifestyle transitions while having little access to health services and education. An analysis of global patterns of nutritional risks in relation to economic development in 100 countries showed that BMI increased rapidly in relation to national income (Ezzati and others 2005). This association declined as countries achieved upper-middle-income and high-income status, primarily as a result of improved access to health services and education as well as behavioral changes. As average income rises, habits associated with obesity are adopted, such as watching television, purchasing convenience foods at supermarkets, and consuming highly processed fast food. However, access to health care, education, healthy food, and recreational activities that support weight maintenance remain limited.

Within countries, obesity is related to socioeconomic status. In many LMICs, body weight is positively associated with socioeconomic status, which contrasts with general patterns observed in the United States and other HICs, where body weight tends to be inversely associated with socioeconomic status. The association between socioeconomic status and body weight is thought to depend on the level of economic development in the country. In a review of nationally representative surveys of women in 37 LMICs, the burden of obesity was shown to shift toward low-socioeconomic groups as the country's gross national product per capita increased to about US$2,500 (Monteiro and others 2004). Countries with gross national product per capita greater than US$2,500 include Brazil, Mexico, South Africa, and Turkey.

Urbanization

The proportion of the world's population living in urban areas has increased markedly, from 13 percent in 1900 to almost 50 percent in 2005 (Kearney 2010). This trend is expected to continue, primarily in countries where the vast majority of the population is currently rural. Low- to medium-density residential areas around urban centers have been associated with obesity in the United States (Hu 2008) and are starting to appear in some LMICs. Globally, 93 percent of urban growth is estimated to occur in LMICs, with 80 percent of that urban growth occurring in Africa and Asia (UN Population Fund 2007). In China, for example, more than 1 billion people are projected to be living in urban centers by 2050, which is nearly twice the size of China's current urban population (UN Department of Economic and Social Affairs 2009).

The consequences of urban living on the development of obesity are numerous and occur largely as a result of changes in the built living environment, range of available food options, and lifestyles related to technological advancement and mechanization. Collectively, these changes have played a role in lowering the quality of urban diets and the expenditure of energy. These trends of positive energy balance are expected to continue as urbanization continues. At the same time, urbanization facilitates greater access to health care and education, which have beneficial effects on obesity. However, many LMICs undergo urbanization at such a rapid pace that the development of essential infrastructure lags behind. It is also important to note that some inhabitants of rural areas have worse diet quality than those of urban areas, especially diet diversity, but it is unclear how this lower quality may affect obesity risk. One review noted that the relative annual change in weighted obesity prevalence is higher for rural (3.9 percent) than for urban (2.5 percent) women, suggesting that women in rural areas are catching up to their urban counterparts (Popkin, Adair, and Ng 2012). Overall, the trends likely differ between HICs and LMICs and are influenced by socioeconomic status (Darmon and Drewnowski 2008).

Physical Activity

Densely populated areas with little outdoor recreational space provide limited opportunities for walking and leisure-time physical activity. Physical activity, including walking and cycling, has modest benefits for weight, with more appreciable effects seen when lifestyle changes occur in combination with dietary intervention. The combination of increased caloric intake and reduced energy expenditure can have a significant impact on the development of obesity. Lower energy expenditure decreases energy requirements, allowing excess calories to accumulate faster. Current physical activity guidelines for preventing chronic diseases recommend 150 minutes per week of moderate-intensity aerobic activity or 75 minutes per week of vigorous-intensity activity or a combination thereof (U.S. DHHS 2008). A recent paper published as part of the *Lancet*'s second series on physical activity estimated that the prevalence of inactivity (defined as not meeting the physical activity guidelines above) among adult populations worldwide was 23.3 percent in 2016 (Sallis, Bull, and Guthold 2016). The trend data from the United States show that leisure-time physical activity has been relatively stable or increased slightly, while activities related to work, transportation, and household chores have declined dramatically and sedentary behaviors, such as television viewing and other activities involving digital devices, have increased substantially. These changes have led to an overall reduction in total physical activity (Brownson, Boehmer, and Luke 2005).

In many LMICs, a pronounced movement has occurred away from jobs with high energy expenditure, such as farming, mining, and forestry and toward jobs in the more sedentary sectors of manufacturing, services, and office-based work. This trend is typical of countries experiencing economic growth and urbanization, and these processes will determine the timeframe over which such movement takes place. In addition, computer technology, factories, and mechanization have become widespread in jobs that previously required high energy expenditure. In China, for example, the proportion of the population working in very light-activity jobs increased to 66 percent from 44 percent between 1989 and 2004 (Popkin 2009). Household chores also have become increasingly mechanized with the emergence of appliances, such as washing machines and vacuum cleaners. It was recently found that in contrast to evidence from HICs, urban (versus rural) residence was an inverse correlate of physical activity in LMICs; this finding is a concern, given global trends toward urbanization (Sallis, Bull, and Guthold 2016).

Leisure-time activities also have become more sedentary, shifting from outdoor play to indoor entertainment, such as television viewing, Internet use, and computer gaming. In China, a study published in 2005 showed that fewer than 25 percent of adults reported participating in at least 30 minutes of moderate physical activity per day, and television ownership increased from 38 sets per 1,000 persons in 1985 to 155 in 1990 and 270 in 1997 (Wang and others 2007). Data on television viewing and screen time in LMICs are sparse, but many epidemiological studies have shown a link between time spent watching television and weight gain in both children and adults, and reducing sedentary behavior has been shown to have beneficial effects on weight independent of exercise (Muntner and others 2005).

Changes to the built living environment include the construction of roads and highways and the implementation of motorized transportation systems that have created sprawl that limits the opportunities for walking or bicycling and provides less healthy alternatives. The proportion of journeys made on foot or by bicycle has declined from 37 percent and 26 percent, respectively, in cities with 100,000–250,000 inhabitants to 28 percent and 9 percent, respectively, in cities with more than 5 million inhabitants (Singh 2005). Another major shift affecting energy expenditure in LMICs is the displacement of human-propelled modes of transportation, such as bicycles, in favor of motorized transportation, including cars and mopeds. In India, the annual rate of motor vehicle ownership increased 11 percent between 1997 and 2008; in China, new car sales are increasing an estimated 30 percent per year (Kjellstrom, Hakansta, and Hogstedt 2007; Siegel, Narayan, and Kinra 2008).

Behavioral Change and Sociocultural Norms

Certain behavioral changes brought about by urban living could also contribute to the development of obesity in LMICs. Although not formally documented, urbanization is associated with a decrease in sleep duration, because noise pollution, street and domestic lighting, access to television and the Internet, shift work, and nighttime social activities are more common in urban than in rural areas. In epidemiological studies, short sleep duration has been associated with weight gain in both children and adults (Berkey, Rockett, and Colditz 2008; Patel and Hu 2008). Similar evidence is starting to emerge from various LMICs, including Brazil, Senegal, and Tunisia, as well as from Taiwan, China (Hu 2008). Stress, which has been associated with obesity (Hu 2008), may also be a risk factor in rapidly urbanizing LMICs because of occupational demands and lack of the kind of social support that is available in traditional villages.

Obesity can also be affected by cultural and social norms, with wide variation across LMICs. These norms include cultural food preferences, societal norms for body shape, cultural practices surrounding the use of leisure time and physical activity, gender norms, and academic expectations, all of which can interact with other risk factors to contribute to rising rates of obesity. For example, Polynesians, who have one of the highest rates of obesity in the world, equate large body size with power, beauty, and affluence (Brewis and others 1998), and in India and many LMICs, there is a general misconception that an obese child is a healthy child (Bhardwaj and others 2008). In contrast, in the United States and some other cultures, some demographics consider being underweight to be the epitome of beauty (Low and others 2003). Although cultural and social norms are embedded in society, they are not static. Globalization of the food supply, including through multinational supermarkets, fast-food chains, mass media, and marketing, has altered consumer preferences and behaviors in many LMICs in a relatively short period.

Diet

As many countries experience the rapid economic growth and urbanization that have changed the choice and availability of food, concomitant shifts in dietary structure or nutritional transitions occur that promote a positive energy balance. These transitions are also fueled by reductions in the price of low-quality foods that are high in energy and by increases in GDP, which leads to higher family income and enhanced purchasing power. Weight gain and obesity in free-living populations result from the cumulative effects of small changes in daily energy balance. A typical diet is composed of energy-bearing macronutrients, including carbohydrates, protein, and fat, as well as micronutrients, including vitamins and minerals. These dietary factors can directly or indirectly tip the balance in energy intake and expenditure and thus effect changes in body weight. Similar to noncommunicable diseases, weight gain and obesity are complex processes that are caused by perturbations of multiple dietary habits and behaviors rather than by changes in any single dietary factor. This course contrasts with deficiency syndromes, which can usually be ascribed to one or a few factors. While dietary patterns vary enormously between and within countries and limited data are available to document dietary shifts, some broad themes are apparent, such as the global decrease in diet quality—excess consumption of unhealthful and highly processed foods and inadequate consumption of healthful whole foods. Many of the dietary risk factors for weight gain and obesity are covered in chapter 6.

Another major shift contributing to poor diets has been an increase in the consumption of highly refined carbohydrates, such as polished white rice and refined wheat flour. Milling and processing of whole grains to produce refined grains remove the fiber and numerous micronutrients, which have a variety of health benefits. Fiber is largely responsible for the beneficial effects of whole grains on body weight, promoting satiety and leading to decreased energy intake. Given the number and variety of nutrients, whole grains can also be useful for addressing undernutrition. Temporal data from the United States show an association between intake of refined carbohydrates and risk of obesity and type 2 diabetes mellitus (Gross and others 2004). In urban South India, nearly half of an average individual's daily energy intake comes from refined grains, with polished white rice constituting more than 75 percent of refined grain intake (Mattei and others 2015). In China, white rice accounts for more than 30 percent of an average individual's daily caloric intake (Mattei and others 2015). A meta-analysis of prospective cohort studies in Asian and Western populations found that, for each increment of one serving per day of white rice, the risk of type 2 diabetes increased 11 percent (Hu and others 2012). Associations were stronger in Asian populations than in Western populations because Asian populations consume larger quantities of white rice. The adverse effects of refined grains tend to be more evident in individuals who are overweight or obese and generally more insulin resistant than individuals who are lean. This finding is of great concern because as obesity becomes more prevalent globally, more people will be susceptible to the adverse effects of diets high in refined carbohydrates. Although some refined carbohydrates, such as white rice, have been staples in countries such as China for hundreds of years, the negative health effects of refined grains were likely offset by high levels of physical activity.

In addition to the intake of specific foods, certain dietary habits have been associated with body weight. Regular consumption of breakfast has been widely recommended for preventing obesity. Skipping breakfast increases the production of appetite-stimulating hormones, which may lead to overeating throughout the day. In a randomized controlled trial (RCT), omitting breakfast led to increased energy intake and adverse effects on blood lipids and glycemic control (Farshchi, Taylor, and Macdonald 2005). Data on breakfast consumption and body weight are limited, but some prospective cohort studies have reported inverse associations between breakfast consumption and weight gain in European and U.S. populations (Hu 2008). Increased consumption of fast food is thought to be a major factor contributing to rising rates of obesity, and the intake of fast food is on the rise in many LMICs, as multinational chains seek large new markets. Epidemiological studies from Europe and the United States have shown positive associations between the consumption of fast food and weight gain and adverse metabolic outcomes (Rosenheck 2008). These associations are likely due to a combination of large portion sizes and high calorie content; high amounts of processed meat, refined carbohydrates, sugary beverages, and unhealthful fats; enhanced palatability; and low cost, resulting in overeating and positive energy balance.

From a public health point of view, identifying the dietary determinants of weight gain is critical for reducing the prevalence of obesity because once an individual develops obesity, it is metabolically difficult to lose weight and maintain weight loss. However, numerous short- and long-term studies across a variety of general and clinical populations have attempted to identify the optimal ratio of macronutrients for weight loss. Lowering the proportion of daily calories consumed from fat has been targeted for many reasons, including the high energy density of fat (that is, a single gram of fat contains more than twice the calories of a gram of carbohydrates or protein) and enhanced palatability of high-fat foods. Thus, prevailing guidelines for weight loss have recommended reducing the intake of fat, but studies have produced inconsistent findings regarding the benefits of restricting fat for weight loss. One reason is the reciprocal relationship between energy from fats and carbohydrates in most diets; in addition, as previously discussed, intake of refined carbohydrates has been positively associated with weight gain. Although the relative influence of macronutrients on body weight remains unclear, accumulating evidence suggests that low-carbohydrate and Mediterranean-style diets, which are rich in plant-based foods and have a moderate fat content, have benefits for weight loss (Tobias and others 2015). These regimens may be more sustainable than other strategies because of the greater diversity and palatability of foods.

Genetic Risk of Obesity

The search for human obesity genes began several decades ago with findings from studies of adopted twins suggesting that obesity and obesity-related traits have a substantial heritable component, although the exact degree of genetic heritability is still debatable. Because the prevalence of obesity in many countries has tripled during the past three decades, it is unlikely that genetics is the primary cause of obesity. Compelling evidence indicates that obesity is driven largely by changes in diet and lifestyle. However, ethnic differences in obesity rates cannot be explained by these factors alone. A more probable hypothesis is that obesity is the outcome of an adverse obesogenic environment interacting with a susceptibility genotype. Genetic factors that underlie susceptibility to obesity may be amplified in the presence of certain environmental factors or, given the same diet and lifestyle factors, some individuals may be genetically more prone to obesity than others. Epigenetic mechanisms, in which environmental factors cause changes in the expression of genes but do not involve changes in DNA (deoxyribonucleic acid) sequence, could also help explain the global increase in obesity prevalence.

Efforts to identify obesity genes have intensified in recent years with advances in genotyping technology and genetic epidemiologic methods. Several genetic factors responsible for rare monogenic forms of obesity have been identified; however, genes for common forms of obesity remain an active area of research. Unlike monogenic obesity, which results from an alteration in a single gene, the genetic profile of common or polygenic obesity is complex and likely results from the effects of several altered genes. Genome-wide association studies, which determine whether an association between a genetic variation and an obesity-related trait exists by surveying the entire genome for causal genetic variants in a comprehensive and unbiased manner, have identified more than 52 loci associated with obesity traits (Albuquerque and others 2015). Of all the currently identified loci, the fat mass and obesity-associated (FTO) gene has the largest effect on susceptibility to obesity (Albuquerque and others 2015). However, FTO polymorphism has a modest effect on BMI, explaining only 0.31 percent of the variation in BMI among individuals (Albuquerque and others 2015). These findings have been independently replicated and confirmed in several African, Asian, and European populations in both children and adults, although the functional mechanism underlying the role of FTO in obesity remains unknown.

Identification of gene-environment interactions related to obesity has been challenging because many genetic association studies lack detailed information on diet or other types of exposure. However, some recent observational studies and trials have evaluated gene-diet interactions. For example, the association between sugar-sweetened beverages and obesity was strengthened by an analysis examining whether consumption of sugar-sweetened beverages can modify the genetic risk of obesity, using a genetic predisposition score based on 32 obesity genes identified from genome-wide association studies (Qi and others 2012). Based on data from three large cohorts, greater consumption of sugar-sweetened beverages was associated with a more pronounced genetic effect on elevated BMI and an increased risk of obesity. Individuals who consumed one or more servings of sugar-sweetened beverages per day had genetic effects on BMI and obesity risk that were approximately twice as large as those who consumed less than one serving per month. These data suggest that regular consumers of sugar-sweetened beverages may be more susceptible to the genetic effects on obesity, implying that a genetic predisposition to obesity can be partly offset by healthier beverage choices. Alternatively, persons with a greater genetic predisposition to obesity may be more susceptible to the deleterious effects of sugar-sweetened drinks on BMI. These findings may partly explain individual differences in the metabolic response to sugar-sweetened beverages. A better understanding of gene-environment interactions and epigenetics could lead to more accurate estimates of the impact of environmental factors on genetically susceptible individuals and identify high-risk populations for targeted prevention and intervention.

INTERVENTIONS AND POLICIES FOR OBESITY PREVENTION AND TREATMENT

Population-based interventions have the potential to shift the distribution of risk factors and social norms of an entire population in a favorable direction, making them a cost-effective approach. Policy changes, in particular, have the potential to improve physical and social environments with long-lasting benefits for public health and quality of life. Continued surveillance of obesity and national health outcomes is also necessary to monitor and evaluate programs. In this section, we summarize evidence for the effectiveness of population-level interventions to improve diet and physical activity for preventing obesity in six domains: nutritional and agricultural policies, food labeling, food advertising, mass media campaigns, school and workplace interventions, and urban planning. Strategies to improve diet are also reviewed in chapter 6 (Afshin and others 2017) and reinforced here given the importance of dietary modification for preventing obesity. Because little data from LMICs are available, much of the evidence summarized is from HICs, with the understanding that findings can be translatable to LMICs with appropriate cultural adjustments. In contrast to clinical decision making, where the evidence base is dominated by RCTs, we also consider different types of evidence, such as observational studies, natural experiments, and policy changes. Despite the paucity of data and systematic reviews evaluating the effectiveness of some domains, these domains are discussed here because they have great potential for benefit and scalability and represent important knowledge gaps. Finally, we provide a brief summary of select individual-level interventions for weight loss. Although the emphasis is on preventing obesity, weight loss and obesity treatment can prevent or improve obesity-related comorbid conditions and reduce health care costs among overweight and obese individuals and may have a benefit for mortality.

Nutritional and Agricultural Policies

Combining incentives and deterrents can be an effective strategy for encouraging production and consumption of nutritionally beneficial foods and discouraging production and consumption of unhealthful foods. Some governments are considering taxing select foods and beverages, particularly sugar-sweetened beverages, as a means to improve consumer choice and generate revenue. Whether these programs will have the desired effect is yet to be determined. Some studies have suggested that, for such interventions to have an appreciable impact, tax increases of at least 10 percent are needed (Gortmaker and others 2011). The most relevant data currently available come from Mexico, where a peso-per-liter tax on sugar-sweetened beverages (roughly US$0.08 per liter, equivalent to a 10 percent tax increase) resulted in a 10 percent decline in purchases of taxed beverages in the first quarter of 2014, compared with the first quarter of 2013. These preliminary results also show roughly a 7 percent increase in purchases of untaxed beverages (such as diet sodas, sparkling and still plain water, 100 percent fruit juices, flavored water with noncaloric sweeteners, and milk without added sugar), including approximately a 13 percent increase in purchases of plain water.[1] A more recent evaluation found that purchases of taxed beverages decreased by an average of 6 percent 1 year after implementation of the tax. Purchases of untaxed beverages were 4 percent higher

over this period, mainly driven by an increase in purchases of bottled plain water (Colchero and others 2016). Removing subsidies on animal-based foods, unhealthful oils, and sugar in exchange for subsidies on fruits, vegetables, legumes, nuts, and whole grains could be an effective strategy for improving diet quality. In 2000, India produced 26.6 million tons of fruits and 96.5 million tons of vegetables (Siegel, Narayan, and Kinra 2008). However, inaccessibility and high costs prohibited consumption of these foods in all but affluent, urban populations. In China, subsidies on fruits, vegetables, and soybeans have increased the production and consumption of these products (Zhai and others 2002). Voluntary actions and regulations made by industry to reduce calories in the food supply are underway in the United Kingdom and the United States (Malik, Willett, and Hu 2013). Translating similar initiatives to other countries represents a promising long-term goal for preventing obesity.

Food Labeling

Nutritional labeling is emerging as a major global initiative, and some LMICs, including Brazil, Chile, China, India, Mexico, and South Africa, are also considering developing systems to identify nutritionally beneficial foods and beverages (Popkin, Adair, and Ng 2012). In comparison with nutritional facts panels, which consumers use to draw their own conclusions about how healthy a product is on the basis of the nutrient content of foods, these systems would identify foods that benefit health, such as whole grains, to help consumers make healthy choices. An increasingly popular strategy being considered by various jurisdictions is calorie labeling on restaurant menus. The U.S. Food and Drug Administration recently finalized two rules requiring that calorie information be listed on menus and menu boards in chain restaurants as well as in similar retail food establishments and vending machines. A systematic review and meta-analysis of 19 studies in the United States found that menu labeling was associated with a reduction of 18.13 kilocalories ordered per meal, but significant heterogeneity between studies limits interpretation of the results (Long and others 2015). Another small meta-analysis found that labeling menus with calories alone significantly reduced the amount of calories ordered by 31 kilocalories and the amount of calories consumed by 13 kilocalories (Sinclair, Cooper, and Mansfield 2014). In addition, it found that the use of interpretative nutritional information on menus assisted consumers in selecting and consuming foods with fewer calories, saving 67 kilocalories and 81 kilocalories, respectively.

To provide some context, one small apple provides approximately 55 kilocalories.

These initiatives hold promise for LMICs, where the increasing availability of processed and packaged foods and fast-food chains is accompanying increasing rates of urbanization. Educational campaigns must precede or accompany both food package and point-of-purchase nutrition labeling to raise awareness about these initiatives and provide context, so that individuals know to look for the labels and understand why they are important and how to interpret them. Other important caveats include the need to have consensus on the definition of specific healthy foods such as whole grains and, in the context of LMICs, a system in place to ensure accurate labeling.

Food Advertising

A growing body of evidence indicates that food marketing can influence food preferences and consumption habits, especially of children (Hawkes 2007). However, evidence from systematic reviews is lacking, and few studies have evaluated the impact of advertising on energy intake or body weight. A systematic review of seven RCTs aiming to assess the effect of television advertising on food intake of children ages 4–12 years concluded that there is a positive association between television and energy intake but that this association is based on a very limited number of trials lacking a solid ground of first-level evidence (Gregori and others 2014). Despite the lack of systematic evidence, regulation of advertising targeted toward children through television, the Internet, or other media is thought to be a potentially effective strategy that should be adopted globally to reduce the harmful effects of marketing unhealthful high-energy foods. In 2010, the WHO released a set of recommendations on the marketing of foods and nonalcoholic beverages high in fat, sugar, and salt to children in an effort to encourage healthy dietary choices and promote the maintenance of healthy weight (WHO 2010). To date, several countries, including Brazil, Chile, the Islamic Republic of Iran, Ireland, the Republic of Korea, Mexico, Peru, and the United Kingdom, as well as economies such as Taiwan, China, have taken steps to reduce such marketing (World Cancer Research Fund International 2016). Since 2007, France has banned the marketing of foods high in fat, sugar, and salt unless they are taxed and labeled with a health warning. In other countries, including Switzerland, Thailand, and the United States, industry has made voluntary pledges to restrict marketing to children. At the same time, governments can institute zoning laws, if available, that limit the number of fast-food restaurants in a given area.

Mass Media Campaigns

The mass media, including national-level social marketing and public service campaigns, have the potential to be very useful tools in delivering public health messages about healthy diets and lifestyles, either independently or as part of multicomponent interventions. Concurrently, these strategies should be carefully monitored and evaluated to gauge their effectiveness. However, very few studies have examined the impact of mass media campaigns on diets and lifestyle behaviors or on body weight. This is an important knowledge gap.

School and Workplace Interventions

School-based programs and policies to increase physical activity by requiring physical education classes or breaks and to improve diet by providing healthy school meals and heathier snack options in vending machines and cafeterias are effective strategies to address childhood obesity and should be part of the global obesity prevention agenda. These strategies are likely to be more effective if reinforced through curriculum-based education about healthy diets and active lifestyles and efforts to engage parents and families. A recent systematic review including 115 school-based interventions (mostly in the United States) concluded that moderately strong evidence supports the effectiveness of school-based interventions for preventing childhood obesity (Wang and others 2015). However, more evidence is needed to evaluate programs in other settings or with other types of design, especially interventions oriented toward providing environmental, policy, and consumer health information.

School meal programs, which provide low-cost or free meals to ensure nutritional adequacy among schoolchildren, provide a unique opportunity to encourage healthy eating habits while preventing undernutrition. WHO Europe has a food and nutrition policy, which can be adapted for use in schools in individual countries, that emphasizes the importance of breakfast clubs; intake of fruits, vegetables, and milk; access to water; and removal of vending machines containing snacks and beverages of poor nutritional quality (WHO Europe 2006).

Similar to the school setting, worksite-based interventions can overcome barriers to choosing a healthy lifestyle by providing resources and a socially supportive environment for change at a place where individuals spend much of their week and by offering programs at low or no cost. A meta-analysis of worksite-based physical activity programs in HICs (mostly the

United States) showed significant positive improvements in body weight, cardiometabolic risk factors, physical activity and fitness, and diet quality as well as lower absenteeism and job stress (Conn and others 2009). A systematic review of 17 studies in Europe focusing on promoting a healthy diet in the workplace found limited to moderate evidence of effectiveness for prevention of obesity and obesity-related conditions (Maes and others 2012). Another systematic review of 16 studies, mostly in Europe and North America, found that diet-based worksite interventions of moderate methodological quality led to positive changes in fruits, vegetables, and total fat intake (Mhurchu, Aston, and Jebb 2010). To improve effectiveness, future programs should aim to intervene at multiple levels of the worksite environment and ensure stronger adherence to established quality criteria.

Urban Planning

Evidence from various countries supports the relationship between physically active modes of transport and obesity. An analysis of aggregate cross-sectional health and travel data from the United States, 14 comparison HICs, and 47 large U.S. cities found a significant inverse relationship between active travel and self-reported obesity at all three geographic levels (Pucher and others 2010). A systematic review of 43 incidental physical activity community interventions from high-income economies or regions (Australia; Canada; Europe; Japan; New Zealand; the United Kingdom; the United States; and Hong Kong SAR, China) found that, primarily, active transport (walking, bicycling) interventions and, secondarily, children's play interventions, and to a lesser extent, use of stairs can be effective ways of increasing physical activity (Reynolds and others 2014). Comparisons were control groups that did not receive the intervention or baseline data of participants acting as their own control.

Given the potential for health and environmental benefits, governments should promote and facilitate the use of public transportation and bicycles by providing incentives, such as discounted transportation fares, bicycle-sharing programs, cycling safety classes, and secure bicycle parking. Lower health care premiums for active commuting in countries where health care is not state run would also be beneficial. Using public transportation encourages people to be more active generally, by walking and standing, than if they were using cars. Creating a central policy for urban transportation could be a first step for some countries. Governments should also mandate the construction of sidewalks and safe bicycle lanes and the construction of buildings with features that promote fitness, such as accessible staircases. Urban planning initiatives at the national or regional level should also encourage the development of safe, pedestrian-friendly communities with green spaces and access to public transportation. A systematic review found that physical changes to the built environment can increase urban green space and encourage physical activity (Hunter and others 2015). Careful evaluation of the effectiveness and cost-effectiveness of such policies is needed to support policy strategies.

Popular Weight-Loss Diets

Numerous branded weight-loss programs are broadly available to the general public in many countries, providing structured dietary and lifestyle recommendations via popular books and in-person or online behavioral support. Limited data are available for evaluating the clinical effectiveness of these strategies. However, a recent meta-analysis of trials examining the impact of popular self-administered brand-name diets on body weight compared with no diet found losses in body weight ranging from 4.10 to 6.55 kilograms after 12 months, with no appreciable difference between diets (Johnston and others 2014). Whether such programs are sustainable is not known.

Pharmacological Strategies

Lifestyle interventions for weight loss are often characterized by high rates of recidivism or weight regain, which may be due in part to complex metabolic processes and biological adaptations that defend against subsequent weight loss and promote weight regain. The primary aim of pharmacological treatment for obesity is to suppress the biological drivers of weight gain or dampen the counterregulatory response to weight loss and thereby enable patients to achieve and sustain clinically meaningful reductions in body weight.

Currently, five drugs have been approved by the U.S. Food and Drug Administration for chronic weight management in obese adults: orlistat, lorcaserin, phentermine/topiramate extended release, naltrexone/bupropion extended release (Kakkar and Dahiya 2015), and most recently, liraglutide. Very little data are available regarding the approval, availability, and use of these therapies in LMICs. For countries where these drugs are available, drug safety monitoring systems should be implemented—if not already in existence—to ensure safety of use. A recent report from India documented orlistat abuse in a case of bulimia nervosa and noted that the drug is available over the counter

(Deb, Gupta, and Varshney 2014). Use of anti-obesity medications in conjunction with lifestyle modification can lead to weight loss in the range of 5 percent to 15 percent (Kakkar and Dahiya 2015). One long-term study found that, compared with lifestyle changes alone, orlistat plus lifestyle changes resulted in a greater reduction in the incidence of type 2 diabetes over four years and produced greater weight loss in a clinically representative obese population (Torgerson and others 2004). However, further studies are needed to assess the long-term benefits and cost-effectiveness of these new agents as well as potential pharmacological interactions and adverse effects. Several anti-obesity therapies have been taken off the market because of significant side effects (Kakkar and Dahiya 2015), underscoring the importance of close monitoring and evaluation.

Bariatric Surgery

Management of obesity usually begins in primary care, but surgical approaches for weight loss may be considered when initial measures have failed or the patient's degree of obesity and presence of comorbid conditions are great. The most common types of bariatric surgical procedures include sleeve gastrectomy and gastric bypass along with adjustable gastric banding, which is technically a medical device. Evidence from trials in HICs has shown that these strategies are clinically effective for moderately to severely obese patients compared with nonsurgical interventions (Picot and others 2009). However, further research is needed to provide data on patient quality of life, impact of surgeon experience on outcome, late complications leading to reoperation, duration of comorbid condition remission, and resource use.

The strength of the evidence for these select interventions has been summarized based on data from the Australian Assessing Cost-Effectiveness (ACE) in Obesity and ACE Prevention studies (Gortmaker and others 2011), which assessed the effectiveness and cost-effectiveness of various obesity prevention interventions in Australia (table 7.1). A scale from 1 to 5 was used to rank evidence (with 1 = strongest; 5 = weakest), and the assessment was made by a stakeholders' group. Strategies with the greatest strength of evidence included gastric banding in children and adults, pharmacologic therapy (orlistat), combined diet and exercise, weight-loss diets (low fat, Weight Watchers), and a family-based targeted intervention for obese children. The evidence for unhealthful food and beverage taxes and front-of-package nutrition labeling was considered weak, suggesting a need for additional data.

COST-EFFECTIVENESS FOR SELECT INTERVENTIONS

The gap between available and required resources to tackle the global burden of obesity is very large and expected to continue growing if measures are not taken to abate current trends. Cost-effectiveness analysis is critical to help policy makers with resource allocation and to identify interventions and policies that could be scaled up in countries at different income levels. Policy makers need to weigh the relative benefits of effective interventions reaching a modest number of people against less effective interventions reaching a wider population. However, few obesity prevention interventions or policy strategies have been subjected to rigorous economic evaluation. In this section, we summarize findings from two studies that have evaluated the cost-effectiveness of select obesity prevention interventions using the cost of disability-adjusted life years (DALYs) averted in Australia (Gortmaker and others 2011) and in six LMICs (Brazil, China, India, Mexico, the Russian Federation, and South Africa) as part of a joint Organisation for Economic Co-operation and Development (OECD) and WHO analysis (Cecchini and others 2010).

ACE Obesity Study

In the ACE study, a decision threshold of $A 50,000 (US$49,500) per DALY averted was used to establish whether an intervention was cost-effective, which is in line with empirical evidence on what constitutes acceptable value for money in Australia. Use of standard methods improves the comparability of results, although lower strength of evidence for many interventions limits the generalizability of findings, and costs can vary.

Of the 20 interventions evaluated, 8 were found to improve health and save costs: taxes on unhealthful foods and beverages, front-of-package nutrition labeling, reduction of advertising of unhealthful foods and beverages to children, school-based education programs to reduce television viewing, multifaceted school-based programs including nutrition and physical activity, school-based education programs to reduce the consumption of sugar-sweetened beverages, family-based targeted programs for obese children, and multifaceted school-based targeted programs for overweight and obese children (table 7.1). Gastric banding in adults and adolescents as well as family-based, general practitioner–mediated programs for overweight and obese children were found to be very cost-effective in that they improved health at a cost of less than $A 10,000 per DALY averted, while multifacted school-based programs without a

Table 7.1 Effectiveness and Cost-Effectiveness of Select Obesity Prevention Interventions from the Australian Assessing Cost-Effectiveness (ACE) in Obesity and ACE Prevention Studies

Intervention	Target population	Strength of evidence[a]	Net cost per DALY averted ($A millions)[b]
Taxes on unhealthy foods and beverages	Adults	4	Cost saving
Front-of-package nutritional labeling	Adults	5	Cost saving
Reduction of advertising of junk food and beverages to children	Children (ages 0–14 years)	2	Cost saving
School-based education programs to reduce television viewing	Primary schoolchildren (ages 8–10 years)	3	Cost saving
Multifaceted school-based programs including nutrition and physical activity	Primary schoolchildren (age 6 years)	3	Cost saving
School-based education programs to reduce consumption of sugar-sweetened beverages	Primary schoolchildren (ages 7–11 years)	3	Cost saving
Family-based targeted programs for obese children	Obese children (ages 10–11 years)	1	Cost saving
Multifaceted school-based targeted programs	Overweight or obese primary schoolchildren (ages 7–10 years)	3	Cost saving
Gastric banding: Adolescents	Severely obese adolescents (ages 14–19 years)	1	4,400
Family-based physician-mediated programs	Overweight or moderately obese children (ages 5–9 years)	3	4,700
Gastric banding: Adults	Adults with BMI > 35 kilograms per square meter	1	5,800
Multifaceted school-based programs without a functioning physical activity component	Primary schoolchildren (age 6 years)	3	21,300
Diet and exercise	Adults with BMI > 25 kilograms per square meter	1	28,000
Low-fat diets	Adults with BMI > 25 kilograms per square meter	1	37,000
Active After-School Communities program	Primary schoolchildren (ages 5–11 years)	5	82,000
Weight Watchers	Adults	1	84,000
Lighten Up to a healthier lifestyle weight-loss program	Adults	4	94,000
TravelSmart schools	Primary schoolchildren (ages 10–11 years)	4	117,000
Orlistat	Adults with BMI > 30 kilograms per square meter	1	700,000
Walking School Bus program	Primary schoolchildren (ages 5–7 years)	3	760,000

Source: Gortmaker and others 2011.

Note: BMI = body mass index; DALY = disability-adjusted life year.

a. Strength of evidence is based on criteria adopted in ACE Prevention Study. 1 = sufficient evidence of effectiveness. Effectiveness is shown by sufficient evidence from well-designed research that the effect is unlikely to be due to chance and is unlikely to be a result of bias. 2 = likely to be effective. Effectiveness results are based on sound theoretical rationale and program logic, indirect or parallel evidence for outcomes, or epidemiological modeling of the desired outcome using a mix of evidence types or levels. The effect is unlikely to be due to chance. 3 = limited evidence of effectiveness. Limited effectiveness is demonstrated by limited evidence from studies of varying quality. 4 = may be effective. Effectiveness is similar to evidence of strength 2, but is potentially not significant and bias cannot be excluded as a possible explanation. 5 = inconclusive or inadequate evidence.

b. Net cost per DALY averted = gross costs minus cost offsets divided by number of DALYs saved (costs only for reductions in obesity-related disease and not including unrelated health care costs).

functioning physical activity component, diet and exercise, and low-fat diets were found to improve health at a cost of between $A 10,000 and $A 50,000 per DALY averted. The top three cost-saving interventions—food and beverage tax, nutritional labels, and reduction in advertising to children, all of which are environmental—showed modest effects at the individual level but were highly cost-effective because benefits accrue to the entire population and the cost of implementation is relatively low. However, these interventions vary in their effectiveness and in the likelihood of implementation. In Australia, regulation of advertising is not on the political agenda, which means that reducing advertising to children, one of the most cost-effective interventions, is unlikely. Also, policy makers in Australia considered the evidence for front-of-package nutrition labeling to be insufficient to warrant support, despite plausible outcomes.

Overall, based on assessments made in the ACE study, policy approaches generally showed greater cost-effectiveness than either health promotion or clinical interventions. To prevent obesity, policy makers should consider the strategies found to be cost saving or highly cost-effective. However, the decision about whether to implement a specific obesity prevention strategy in a given country will be based on a combination of factors aside from cost-effectiveness, including the strength and generalizability of the evidence base, feasibility of implementation, impacts on equity, and acceptability to stakeholders. Because the evidence base is constantly evolving, particular emphasis should be given to identifying updated studies in the field. A good example of updated studies pertains to trials examining the effectiveness of low-fat diets on weight loss. Although the ACE study found strong evidence that low-fat diets are effective among overweight adults, recent meta-analyses of trials found negligible effects, suggesting that low-fat diets may not be an effective strategy for weight control (Tobias and others 2015). Other than for this intervention, data from the ACE study are generally consistent with data from other HICs for the same interventions.

OECD and WHO Study

In the OECD and WHO study, seven interventions aimed at tackling rapidly escalating rates of obesity through healthy dietary habits and increased physical activity—school-based health promotion, worksite interventions, mass media campaigns, counseling of individuals at risk in primary care, fiscal measures affecting the price of fruits and vegetables and foods high in fat, regulation of food advertising to children, and food labeling—were evaluated for their cost-effectiveness for preventing related chronic diseases (stroke, ischemic heart disease, and cancer, including lung, colorectal, and female breast cancer) in two time periods—20 years and 50 years—in six LMICs. Additionally, a prevention strategy combining a mass media campaign, fiscal measures, regulation of food advertising, and food labeling was assessed on the basis of the assumption that the effects of the individual interventions, measured by the relative risk of risk factors or chronic diseases, would combine multiplicatively. The analysis was based on a microsimulation model (chronic disease prevention model) that implements a causal web of lifestyle risk factors for selected chronic diseases. Whereas individual-level effectiveness was based mostly on studies from high-income settings, country-specific information was used to establish potential population coverage and to adapt effectiveness to the local distribution of risk factors.

Based on U.S. dollars per DALY averted, relative to a comparator situation of treatment only and no prevention, fiscal measures were consistently cost saving in all LMICs considered and generated the largest (for example, in China) or second largest health effects in both 20 years and 50 years (table 7.2). The health effect of fiscal measures was substantially lower in India than in other countries because Indians consume fewer foods high in fat. Food labeling was also cost saving in many settings, but with smaller health effects than fiscal measures. Regulation of food advertising to children and mass media campaigns had very favorable cost-effectiveness ratios. In 50 years, regulation of food advertising was cost saving in several countries, although its health effect was still very small compared with other interventions. Worksite health promotion initiatives had favorable cost-effectiveness, with quicker health returns than regulation of advertising, although returns were lower in some countries over the entire simulation. Physician counseling of individuals at risk in primary care was one of the most effective interventions, but its health effect was greatest and cost-effectiveness was highest in countries where a larger proportion of the population had regular access to primary care physicians and facilities. School-based interventions consistently had unfavorable cost-effectiveness ratios up to 50 years from their initial implementation. However, the cost-effectiveness of interventions targeting young children tends to improve in a longer timeframe (greater than 50 years), as these interventions realize their full potential in improving health. A multiple-intervention strategy would achieve substantially larger health gains than would individual interventions, often with an even more favorable cost-effectiveness profile. Such a strategy would be cost saving in about half the countries examined.

Taken together, findings from these two studies suggest that the most cost-effective approaches to preventing

Table 7.2 Cost-Effectiveness Ratios of Select Obesity Prevention Interventions after 20 Years and 50 Years in Seven Countries: Organisation for Economic Co-operation (OECD) and WHO Analysis

Strategy and time period	Brazil	China	India	Mexico	Russian Federation	South Africa	United Kingdom
20 years							
School-based interventions	a	704,863	a	a	830,177	a	a
Worksite interventions	8,270	7,785	6,151	37,912	6,187	25,409	45,630
Mass media campaigns	5,074	7,188	15,552	6,858	12,911	23,221	25,897
Fiscal measures	Cost saving	Cost saving	Cost saving	Cost saving	Cost saving	Cost saving	Cost saving
Physician counseling	8,503	9,390	6,155	23,811	5,982	23,841	25,284
Food advertising regulation	Cost saving	556	3,186	11,151	5,718	13,241	25,672
Food labeling	9,962	71	952	3,974	396	7,953	12,577
50 years							
School-based interventions	93,350	35,174	59,665	235,957	26,114	153,233	152,989
Worksite interventions	3,541	3,393	4,491	16,932	2,926	14,561	20,506
Mass media campaigns	1,994	3,177	8,575	2,778	5,822	15,211	13,796
Fiscal measures	Cost saving	Cost saving	Cost saving	Cost saving	Cost saving	Cost saving	Cost saving
Physician counseling	5,156	5,718	5,553	15,108	4,331	16,591	15,731
Food advertising regulation	Cost saving	Cost saving	332	3,415	552	3,352	4,278
Food labeling	Cost saving	Cost saving	776	Cost saving	Cost saving	3,927	5,268
Cost-effectiveness threshold (US$ per DALY)[b]	15,000	5,000	2,500	20,000	15,000	15,000	50,000

Source: Cecchini and others 2010.

Note: WHO = World Health Organization. Cost-effectiveness ratios are expressed in U.S. dollars per disability-adjusted life year (DALY) averted and represent the net cost of gaining one additional year of healthy life, relative to a no-prevention or treatment-only scenario.

a. Cost-effectiveness ratio is higher than US$1 million per DALY averted.

b. For countries other than the United Kingdom, the guideline amount of three times gross domestic product per capita (in 2005 U.S. dollars) is used as a cost-effectiveness threshold. In the United Kingdom, the National Institute for Health and Clinical Excellence uses a threshold of US$50,000 per DALY averted to denote that an intervention is cost-effective.

obesity and downstream chronic disease are price interventions and regulation, such as taxes on unhealthful foods and beverages and subsidies on healthy foods, food labeling, and regulation of advertising of unhealthful foods and beverages. As the OECD and WHO study found, fiscal measures are the only interventions likely to pay for themselves since they can generate larger savings in health expenditures than the costs of delivery. What sets these interventions apart from other more targeted strategies is their greater coverage in the population and relatively low cost of implementation. These strategies could feasibly be added to existing measures for preventing chronic disease, such as demand-reduction strategies for tobacco and alcohol (that is, higher excise taxes, advertising bans, and improved labeling) and salt-reduction strategies (via mass media campaigns or regulation of the salt content in manufactured foods). A strategy of several interventions would generate larger health gains and have a more cost-effective profile than

would individual interventions. School-based interventions can be cost-effective strategies for preventing obesity, but their impact on future chronic disease risk may not be realized until many decades later. Regulation of food advertising to children would be a more effective and efficient strategy for targeting children.

CONCLUSIONS

Obesity is a major contributor to preventable disease and death across the globe and poses a nearly unprecedented challenge to those tasked with addressing it at the public health, health care provider, and individual levels. It is a complex condition resulting from myriad compounding physiological, environmental, behavioral, and sociopolitical factors. Although economic growth and urbanization have reduced food insecurity and improved quality of life for many, they have also provided access to low-cost foods that are low in nutritional value and high in energy and increased the consumption of refined grains, red and processed meats, unhealthful fats, and sugar-sweetened beverages, all of which are associated with weight gain. At the same time, these processes have created environments that promote sedentary lifestyles, reduced physical labor, and increased automated transportation, collectively leading to positive energy balance and weight gain.

Given the scope and complexity of the global increase in obesity, interventions and policies across multiple levels are needed to have a measurable impact on reversing this trend. Such strategies should include coordinated efforts from the international community, governments, food industry, health care providers, schools, urban planners, agriculture and food production and services sectors, media, communities, and individuals.

Based on our summary of epidemiological evidence, various interventions at the population level, including nutritional and agricultural policies, food labeling and advertising, mass media campaigns, school and workplace interventions, and urban planning have the potential to prevent obesity by improving diet, physical activity, or both. Of these approaches, based on limited data from modeling studies in HICs, the most cost-effective include taxes on unhealthful foods and beverages, subsidies on healthy foods, food labeling, and regulation of advertising of unhealthful foods and beverages, particularly to children. These strategies can achieve wide coverage at a relatively low implementation

cost and could feasibly be added to existing measures for preventing chronic diseases (table 7.3). Although the strength of the evidence for these strategies is weak, particularly from LMICs, implementation should not be discouraged given the potential economic gains as well as the potential for beneficial interactions among combinations of strategies.

School and workplace interventions are also cost-effective and may be useful in LMIC communities that are also managing undernutrition since healthy options that provide adequate nutrition can be provided and outcomes can be monitored carefully. Because many LMICs are experiencing nutrition transitions characterized by high intake of refined grains, poor-quality carbohydrate foods that are high in added sugar, and sugar-sweetened beverages, strategies that encourage the intake of high-quality carbohydrate foods, such as whole grains, fruits, and vegetables, should be made a priority, as should ensuring access to safe drinking water, since water is the optimal beverage for hydration. These recommendations would also address nutrient inadequacy.

Regarding interventions to treat obesity, while the evidence is considered strong for the benefits of surgery, pharmacological approaches, and weight-loss diets, the benefits need to be weighed against cost-effectiveness. Feasibility for use in LMICs would also need to be evaluated. Fewer options exist for managing and treating obesity; given the metabolic challenges in losing weight and high costs associated with obesity, prevention should be the goal of governments. Implementing a strategy of

Table 7.3 Recommended Strategies for Obesity Prevention

Strategy	Description	Cost-effectiveness
Taxation of unhealthful foods and beverages and subsidies for healthful foods	Regulation of food consumption and production should be aligned with evidence-based national dietary goals. Taxation, subsidies, and price adjustments can provide incentives for healthy choices and deter unhealthful choices.	✓✓
Food labeling	Nutritional labeling of foods can guide consumers in making healthy and informed dietary choices. Menu labeling in restaurants can positively influence food choices and intake. Awareness campaigns should precede or accompany labeling initiatives.	✓✓
Regulation of food and beverage advertising to children	Regulation of advertising targeted to children should be adopted globally to reduce the adverse effects of marketing unhealthful foods and beverages to children.	✓✓
School and workplace interventions	Nutritional and physical activity education and improved standards of school meal programs, including healthy vending policies, should be part of the global childhood obesity prevention agenda. Workplace environments should facilitate access to healthy food options and promote active living.	✓

Note: ✓✓ = most cost-effective; ✓ = cost-effective. Of the six domains (nutritional and agricultural policies, food labeling, food advertising, school and workplace interventions, mass media, and urban planning) considered in our summary of population-level interventions to improve diet and physical activity for obesity prevention, the most cost-effective approaches were taxes on unhealthful foods and beverages or subsidies on healthy foods, food labeling, and regulation of advertising of unhealthful foods and beverages. These strategies can achieve large coverage at a relatively low implementation cost and could feasibly be added to existing measures for preventing obesity and chronic disease. School and workplace interventions are also cost-effective in the long run and may be particularly useful in communities that are also managing undernutrition since healthy options that provide adequate nutrition can be provided.

several interventions is recommended because multifaceted interventions would garner larger gains than individual approaches.

The majority of evidence related to obesity risk factors, intervention effectiveness, and cost-effectiveness is from studies conducted in HICs, and notable gaps are evident in knowledge from LMICs. Nevertheless, translational approaches should be used to implement evidence-based interventions in these settings rather than waiting for local evidence. Continued surveillance of obesity and national health outcomes is also necessary to monitor and evaluate programs while maintaining awareness among the public and within governments.

NOTES

World Bank Income Classifications as of July 2014 are as follows, based on estimates of gross national income (GNI) per capita for 2013:

- Low-income countries (LICs) = US$1,045 or less
- Middle-income countries (MICs) are subdivided:
  (a) lower-middle-income = US$1,046 to US$4,125
  (b) upper-middle-income (UMICs) = US$4,126 to US$12,745
- High-income countries (HICs) = US$12,746 or more.

1. For some preliminary results of the effects of a tax on sugar-sweetened beverages and energy-dense nonstaple foods in Mexico, see the website of Mexico's National Institute of Public Health (http://www.insp.mx/epppo /blog/preliminares-bebidas-azucaradas.html).

REFERENCES

Afshin, A., R. Micha, M. Webb, S. Capewell, L. Whitsel, and others. 2017. "Diet and Nutrition." In *Disease Control Priorities* (third edition): Volume 5, *Cardiovascular, Respiratory, and Related Disorders*, edited by D. Prabhakaran, S. Anand, T. A. Gaziano, J.-C. Mbanya, Y. Wu, and R. Nugent. Washington, DC: World Bank.

Albuquerque, D., E. Stice, R. Rodriguez-Lopez, L. Manco, and C. Nóbrega. 2015. "Current Review of Genetics of Human Obesity: From Molecular Mechanisms to an Evolutionary Perspective." *Molecular Genetics and Genomics* 290 (4): 1191–221.

Bellamy, L., J. P. Casas, A. D. Hingorani, and D. Williams. 2009. "Type 2 Diabetes Mellitus after Gestational Diabetes: A Systematic Review and Meta-Analysis." *The Lancet* 373 (9677): 1773–79.

Berkey, C. S., H. R. Rockett, and G. A. Colditz. 2008. "Weight Gain in Older Adolescent Females: The Internet, Sleep, Coffee, and Alcohol." *Journal of Pediatrics* 153 (5): 635–39.

Bhardwaj, S., A. Misra, L. Khurana, S. Gulati, P. Shah, and others. 2008. "Childhood Obesity in Asian Indians: A Burgeoning

Cause of Insulin Resistance, Diabetes, and Sub-Clinical Inflammation." *Asia Pacific Journal of Clinical Nutrition* 17 (Suppl 1): 172–75.

Brewis, A. A., S. T. McGarvey, J. Jones, and B. A. Swinburn. 1998. "Perceptions of Body Size in Pacific Islanders." *International Journal of Obesity and Related Metabolic Disorders* 22 (2): 185–89.

Brownson, R. C., T. K. Boehmer, and D. A. Luke. 2005. "Declining Rates of Physical Activity in the United States: What Are the Contributors?" *Annual Review of Public Health* 26 (1): 421–43.

Carnethon, M. R., P. J. De Chavez, M. L. Biggs, C. E. Lewis, V. Guajardo-Barron, and others. 2012. "Association of Weight Status with Mortality in Adults with Incident Diabetes." *JAMA* 308 (6): 581–90.

Cecchini, M., F. Sassi, J. A. Lauer, Y. Y. Lee, V. Guajardo-Barron, and others. 2010. "Tackling of Unhealthy Diets, Physical Inactivity, and Obesity: Health Effects and Cost-Effectiveness." *The Lancet* 376 (9754): 1775–84.

Clark, S. E., C. Hawkes, S. M. Murphy, K. A. Hansen-Kuhn, and D. Wallinga. 2012. "Exporting Obesity: U.S. Farm and Trade Policy and the Transformation of the Mexican Consumer Food Environment." *International Journal of Occupational and Environmental Health* 18 (1): 53–65.

Colchero, M. A., B. M. Popkin, J. A Rivera, and S. W. Ng. 2016. "Beverage Purchases from Stores in Mexico under the Excise Tax on Sugar Sweetened Beverages: Observational Study." *BMJ* 352: h6704.

Conn, V. S., A. R. Hafdahl, P. S. Cooper, L. M. Brown, and S. L. Lusk. 2009. "Meta-Analysis of Workplace Physical Activity Interventions." *American Journal of Preventive Medicine* 37 (4): 330–39.

Danaei, G., E. L. Ding, D. Mozaffarian, B. Taylor, J. Rehm, and others. 2009. "The Preventable Causes of Death in the United States: Comparative Risk Assessment of Dietary, Lifestyle, and Metabolic Risk Factors." *PLoS Medicine* 6 (4): e1000058.

Darmon, N., and A. Drewnowski. 2008. "Does Social Class Predict Diet Quality?" *American Journal of Clinical Nutrition* 87 (5): 1107–17.

Deb, K. S., R. Gupta, and M. Varshney. 2014. "Orlistat Abuse in a Case of Bulimia Nervosa: The Changing Indian Society." *General Hospital Psychiatry* 36 (5): 549. e3–4.

de Onis, M., M. Blossner, and E. Borghi. 2010. "Global Prevalence and Trends of Overweight and Obesity among Preschool Children." *American Journal of Clinical Nutrition* 92 (5): 1257–64.

Ezzati, M., S. Vander Hoorn, C. M. Lawes, R. Leach, W. P. T. James, and others. 2005. "Rethinking the 'Diseases of Affluence' Paradigm: Global Patterns of Nutritional Risks in Relation to Economic Development." *PLoS Medicine* 2 (5): e133.

Farshchi, H. R., M. A. Taylor, and I. A. Macdonald. 2005. "Deleterious Effects of Omitting Breakfast on Insulin Sensitivity and Fasting Lipid Profiles in Healthy Lean Women." *American Journal of Clinical Nutrition* 81 (2): 388–96.

Finucane, M. M., G. A. Stevens, M. J. Cowan, G. Danaei, J. K. Lin, and others. 2011. "National, Regional, and Global

Trends in Body-Mass Index since 1980: Systematic Analysis of Health Examination Surveys and Epidemiological Studies with 960 Country-Years and 9.1 Million Participants." *The Lancet* 377 (9765): 557–67.

Global BMI Mortality Collaboration. 2016. "Body-Mass Index and All-Cause Mortality: Individual-Participant-Data Meta-Analysis of 239 Prospective Studies in Four Continents." *The Lancet*. Epub ahead of print July 13. pii: S0140-6736(16)30175-1.

Gortmaker, S. L., B. A. Swinburn, D. Levy, R. Carter, P. L. Mabry, and others. 2011. "Changing the Future of Obesity: Science, Policy, and Action." *The Lancet* 378 (9793): 838–47.

Gregori, D., S. Ballali, M. G. Vecchio, A. S. Scire, F. Foltran, and others. 2014. "Randomized Controlled Trials Evaluating Effect of Television Advertising on Food Intake in Children: Why Such a Sensitive Topic Is Lacking Top-Level Evidence?" *Ecology of Food and Nutrition* 53 (5): 562–77.

Gross, L. S., L. Li, E. S. Ford, and S. Liu. 2004. "Increased Consumption of Refined Carbohydrates and the Epidemic of Type 2 Diabetes in the United States: An Ecologic Assessment." *American Journal of Clinical Nutrition* 79 (5): 774–79.

Harris, J., P. Kaufman, S. Martinez, and C. Price. 2002. *The U.S. Food Marketing System, 2002.* Agricultural Economic Report 811. Washington, DC: U.S. Department of Agriculture Economic Research Service.

Hawkes, C. 2006. "Uneven Dietary Development: Linking the Policies and Processes of Globalization with the Nutrition Transition, Obesity, and Diet-Related Chronic Diseases." *Global Health* 2 (March): 4.

———. 2007. "Regulating and Litigating in the Public Interest. Regulating Food Marketing to Young People Worldwide: Trends and Policy Drivers." *American Journal of Public Health* 97 (11): 1962–73.

Hu, F. B. 2008. *Obesity Epidemiology.* New York: Oxford University Press.

Hu, E. A., A. Pan, V. S. Malik, and Q. Sun. 2012. "White Rice Consumption and Risk of Type 2 Diabetes: Meta-Analysis and Systematic Review." *British Medical Journal* 344 (March): e1454.

Hunter, R. F., H. Christian, J. Veitch, T. Astell-Burt, J. S. Hipp, and others. 2015. "The Impact of Interventions to Promote Physical Activity in Urban Green Space: A Systematic Review and Recommendations for Future Research." *Social Science and Medicine* 124 (January): 246–56.

Johnston, B. C., S. Kanters, K. Bandayrel, P. Wu, F. Naji, and others. 2014. "Comparison of Weight Loss among Named Diet Programs in Overweight and Obese Adults: A Meta-Analysis." *JAMA* 312 (9): 923–33.

Kakkar, A. K., and N. Dahiya. 2015. "Drug Treatment of Obesity: Current Status and Future Prospects." *European Journal of Internal Medicine* 26 (2): 89–94.

Kearney, J. 2010. "Food Consumption Trends and Drivers." *Philosophical Transactions of the Royal Society of London Series B, Biological Sciences* 365 (1554): 2793–807.

Kelly, T., W. Yang, C. S. Chen, K. Reynolds, and J. He. 2008. "Global Burden of Obesity in 2005 and Projections to 2030." *International Journal of Obesity* 32 (9): 1431–37.

Kjellstrom T., C. Hakansta, and C. Hogstedt. 2007. "Globalisation and Public Health: Overview and a Swedish Perspective." *Scandinavian Journal of Public Health* 70 (December): 2–68.

Kuczmarski, R. J., C. L. Ogden, L. M. Grummer-Strawn, K. M. Flegal, S. S. Guo, and others. 2000. "CDC Growth Charts: United States." *Advance Data* 314: 1–27.

Lakshmi, S., B. Metcalf, C. Joglekar, C. S. Yajnik, C. H. Fall, and others. 2012. "Differences in Body Composition and Metabolic Status between White U.K. and Asian Indian Children (EarlyBird 24 and the Pune Maternal Nutrition Study)." *Pediatric Obesity* 7 (5): 347–54.

Lobstein, T., R. Jackson-Leach, M. L. Moodie, K. D. Hall, S. L. Gortmaker, and others. 2015. "Child and Adolescent Obesity: Part of a Bigger Picture." *The Lancet* 385: 2510–20.

Long, M. W., D. K. Tobias, A. L. Cradock, H. Batchelder, and S. L. Gortmaker. 2015. "Systematic Review and Meta-Analysis of the Impact of Restaurant Menu Calorie Labeling." *American Journal of Public Health* 105 (5): e11–24.

Low, K. G., S. Charanasomboon, C. Brown, G. Hiltunen, K. Long, and others. 2003. "Internalization of the Thin Ideal, Weight, and Body Image Concerns." *Social Behavior and Personality: An International Journal* 31 (1): 81–89.

Maes, L., E. Van Cauwenberghe, W. Van Lippevelde, H. Spittaels, E. De Pauw, and others. 2012. "Effectiveness of Workplace Interventions in Europe Promoting Healthy Eating: A Systematic Review." *European Journal of Public Health* 22 (5): 677–83.

Malik, V. S., W. C. Willett, and F. B. Hu. 2013. "Global Obesity: Trends, Risk Factors, and Policy Implications." *Nature Reviews: Endocrinology* 9 (1): 13–27.

Mattei, J., V. S. Malik, N. M. Wedick, F. B. Hu, D. Spiegelman, and others. 2015. "Reducing the Global Burden of Type 2 Diabetes by Improving the Quality of Staple Foods: The Global Nutrition and Epidemiologic Transition Initiative." *Globalization and Health* 11 (1): 23.

Mhurchu, C. N., L. M. Aston, and S. A. Jebb. 2010. "Effects of Worksite Health Promotion Interventions on Employee Diets: A Systematic Review." *BMC Public Health* 10 (February): 62.

Misra, A., and L. Khurana. 2008. "Obesity and the Metabolic Syndrome in Developing Countries." *Journal of Clinical Endocrinology and Metabolism* 93 (11 Suppl 1): S9–30.

Monteiro, C. A., E. C. Moura, W. L. Conde, and B. M. Popkin. 2004. "Socioeconomic Status and Obesity in Adult Populations of Developing Countries: A Review." *Bulletin of the World Health Organization* 82 (12): 940–46.

Muntner, P., D. Gu, R. P. Wildman, J. Chen, W. Qaan, and others. 2005. "Prevalence of Physical Activity among Chinese Adults: Results from the International Collaborative Study of Cardiovascular Disease in Asia." *American Journal of Public Health* 95 (9): 1631–36.

NCD Risk Factor Collaboration. 2016. "Trends in Adult Body-Mass Index in 200 Countries from 1975 to 2014: A Pooled Analysis of 1,698 Population-Based Measurement Studies with 19.2 Million Participants." *The Lancet* 387 (10026): 1377–96.

Patel, S. R., and F. B. Hu. 2008. "Short Sleep Duration and Weight Gain: A Systematic Review." *Obesity* 16 (3): 643–53.

Picot, J., J. Jones, J. Colquitt, E. Gospodarevskaya, E. Loveman, and others. 2009. "The Clinical Effectiveness and Cost-Effectiveness of Bariatric (Weight Loss) Surgery for Obesity: A Systematic Review and Economic Evaluation." *Health Technology Assessment* 13 (41): 1–190, 215–357, iii–iv.

Popkin, B. M. 2009. *The World Is Fat.* New York: Penguin Group.

Popkin, B. M., L. S. Adair, and S. W. Ng. 2012. "Global Nutrition Transition and the Pandemic of Obesity in Developing Countries." *Nutrition Reviews* 70 (1): 3–21.

Popkin, B. M., W. Conde, N. Hou, and C. Monteiro. 2006. "Is There a Lag Globally in Overweight Trends for Children Compared with Adults?" *Obesity* 14 (10): 1846–53.

Pucher, J., R. Buehler, D. R. Bassett, and A. L. Dannenberg. 2010. "Walking and Cycling to Health: A Comparative Analysis of City, State, and International Data." *American Journal of Public Health* 100 (10): 1986–92.

Qi, Q., A. Y. Chu, J. H. Kang, M. K. Jensen, G. C. Curhan, and others. 2012. "Sugar-Sweetened Beverages and Genetic Risk of Obesity." *New England Journal of Medicine* 367 (15): 138–96.

Reynolds, R., S. McKenzie, S. Allender, K. Brown, and C. Foulkes. 2014. "Systematic Review of Incidental Physical Activity Community Interventions." *Preventive Medicine* 67 (October): 46–64.

Rosenheck, R. 2008. "Fast Food Consumption and Increased Caloric Intake: A Systematic Review of a Trajectory towards Weight Gain and Obesity Risk." *Obesity Reviews* 9 (6): 535–47.

Sallis, J. F., F. Bull, R. Guthold, G. W. Heath, S. Inoue, and others. 2016. "Progress in Physical Activity over the Olympic Quadrennium." Physical Activity Series 2 Executive Committee. *The Lancet.* 388 (10051): 1325–36. doi:10.1016/S0140-6736(16)30581-5. Epub July 28.

Siegel, K., K. M. Narayan, and S. Kinra. 2008. "Finding a Policy Solution to India's Diabetes Epidemic." *Health Affairs* 27 (4): 1077–90.

Sinclair, S. E., M. Cooper, and E. D. Mansfield. 2014. "The Influence of Menu Labeling on Calories Selected or Consumed: A Systematic Review and Meta-Analysis." *Journal of the Academy of Nutrition and Dietetics* 114 (9): 1375–88.e15.

Singh, A. 2005. "Review of Urban Transportation in India." *Journal of Public Transportation* 8 (1): 75–97.

Stuckler, D., M. McKee, S. Ebrahim, and S. Basu. 2012. "Manufacturing Epidemics: The Role of Global Producers in Increased Consumption of Unhealthy Commodities Including Processed Foods, Alcohol, and Tobacco." *PLoS Medicine* 9 (6): e1001235.

Sturm, R., and A. Hattori. 2013. "Morbid Obesity Rates Continue to Rise Rapidly in the United States." *International Journal of Obesity* 37 (6): 889–91.

Tobias, D., M. Chen, J. E. Manson, D. S. Ludwig, W. Willett, and others. 2015. "Effect of Low-Fat Diet Interventions versus Other Diet Interventions on Long-Term Weight Change in Adults: A Systematic Review and Meta-Analysis." *The Lancet Diabetes and Endocrinology* 3 (12): 968–79.

Tobias, D., A. Pan, and F. B. Hu. 2014. "BMI and Mortality among Adults with Incident Type 2 Diabetes." *New England Journal of Medicine* 370 (14): 1363–64.

Torgerson, J. S., J. Hauptman, M. N. Boldrin, and L. Sjöström. 2004. "XENical in the Prevention of Diabetes in Obese Subjects (XENDOS) Study: A Randomized Study of Orlistat as an Adjunct to Lifestyle Changes for the Prevention of Type 2 Diabetes in Obese Patients." *Diabetes Care* 27 (1): 155–61.

UN (United Nations) Department of Economic and Social Affairs. 2009. *World Urbanization Prospects: The 2009 Revision.* New York: United Nations Population Division.

UN Population Fund. 2007. "Unleashing the Potential of Urban Growth." In *State of the World Population 2007*, chapter 1. New York: United Nations Population Fund.

U.S. DHHS (United States Department of Health and Human Services). 2008. *Physical Activity Guidelines for Americans.* Washington, DC: U.S. DHHS. http://health.gov/paguidelines /pdf/paguide.pdf.

Wang, Y., L. Cai, Y. Wu, R. F. Wilson, C. Weston, and others. 2015. "What Childhood Obesity Prevention Programmes Work? A Systematic Review and Meta-Analysis." *Obesity Reviews* 16 (7): 547–65.

Wang, Y., J. Mi, X. Y. Shan, Q. J. Wang, and K.-Y. Ge. 2007. "Is China Facing an Obesity Epidemic and the Consequences? The Trends in Obesity and Chronic Disease in China." *International Journal of Obesity* 31 (1): 177–88.

Whitlock, G., S. Lewington, P. Sherliker, R. Clarke, J. Emberson, and others. 2009. "Body-Mass Index and Cause-Specific Mortality in 900,000 Adults: Collaborative Analyses of 57 Prospective Studies." *The Lancet* 373 (9669): 1083–96.

WHO (World Health Organization). 1995. *Physical Status: The Use and Interpretation of Anthropometry.* Technical Report Series 854. Geneva: WHO.

———. 2000. *Obesity: Preventing and Managing the Global Epidemic. Report of a WHO Consultation.* Geneva: WHO.

———. 2009. *Global Health Risks: Mortality and Burden of Disease Attributable to Selected Major Risks.* Geneva: WHO.

———. 2010. *Set of Recommendations on the Marketing of Foods and Non-Alcoholic Beverages to Children.* Geneva: WHO. http://whqlibdoc.who.int/publications/2010 /9789241500210_eng.pdf?ua=1.

WHO Europe. 2006. *Food and Nutrition Policy for Schools: A Tool for the Development of School Nutrition Programmes in the WHO European Region.* Copenhagen: WHO Europe.

WHO Expert Consultation. 2004. "Appropriate Body-Mass Index for Asian Populations and Its Implications for Policy and Intervention Strategies." *The Lancet* 363 (9403): 157–63.

World Cancer Research Fund International. 2016. *NOURISHING Framework, Restrict Food Marketing.* London: World Cancer Research Fund International. http:// www.wcrf.org/int/policy/nourishing-framework/restrict -food-marketing.

Zhai, F., D. Fu, S. Du, K. Ge, C. Chen, and others. 2002. "What Is China Doing in Policy-Making to Push Back the Negative Aspects of the Nutrition Transition?" *Public Health Nutrition* 5 (1A): 269–73.

Chapter 8

Ischemic Heart Disease: Cost-Effective Acute Management and Secondary Prevention

Sagar B. Dugani, Andrew E. Moran, Robert O. Bonow, and Thomas A. Gaziano

INTRODUCTION

Cardiovascular disease (CVD) is the single most important cause of death worldwide; in 2010, it resulted in 16 million deaths and the loss of 293 million disability-adjusted life years (DALYs) (Lozano and others 2012; Murray and others 2012). CVD involves conditions that affect the vasculature that supplies the heart, brain, and other vital organs (Roth and others 2015). Of all of the causes of CVD, ischemic heart disease (IHD) remains the major contributor to mortality and morbidity. IHD results from delivery of insufficient oxygen to meet the demands of the heart and largely manifests as angina, acute myocardial infarction, and ischemic heart failure.

Over the past two decades, although age-standardized IHD mortality has decreased in most regions, the global burden of IHD has increased by 29 percent to 29 million DALYs, in part because of a larger aging population and overall population growth (Lozano and others 2012; Moran, Forouzanfar, and others 2014a; Murray and others 2012). IHD is projected to be a major cause of death in 2030, along with unipolar depressive disorders and human immunodeficiency virus/acquired immune deficiency syndrome (HIV/AIDS) (Mathers and Loncar 2006).

This chapter reviews the global burden of IHD, with a focus on low- and middle-income countries (LMICs).

We review the cost-effective management of acute IHD and subsequent secondary prevention; primary prevention is discussed in chapter 22 (Jeemon and others 2017). The chapter concludes with a discussion of the challenges that IHD poses to the global community and of solutions that may help reduce attendant mortality and morbidity.

Data Sources

Data for mortality and DALYs come from the Global Burden of Diseases, Injuries, and Risk Factors Study 2010 (GBD 2010), which obtained and analyzed mortality data from 187 countries from 1980 to 2010 (Lozano and others 2012; Murray and Lopez 2013; Murray and others 2012). Although the study made extensive efforts to standardize the mortality data, these estimates should be interpreted cautiously; methodologies for coding deaths vary globally and can result in significant misclassification of the cause of death (Pagidipati and Gaziano 2013). The World Bank has divided the world into seven regions: high-income countries (HICs) and six geographic regions of LMICs. Our information on demographic and social indices is obtained from the World Bank's World Development Indicators; data on gross national income (GNI) per capita are obtained from the Atlas method using 2011 U.S. dollar values.

Corresponding author: Thomas A. Gaziano, Division of Cardiology, Brigham and Women's Hospital, Harvard Medical School, Boston, Massachusetts, United States; tgaziano@partners.org.

MANIFESTATIONS OF ISCHEMIC HEART DISEASE

The most common causes of CVD morbidity and mortality are IHD, stroke (chapter 9, Yan and others 2017), and congestive heart failure (chapter 10, Huffman and others 2017); IHD is a major contributor in most world regions. IHD shares several risk factors with peripheral arterial disease, discussed in chapter 14 (Sampson and others 2017).

Two important manifestations of IHD are angina and acute myocardial infarction. Angina is the characteristic chest pain of IHD that develops when atherosclerosis causes partial occlusion of one or more coronary arteries, leading to insufficient oxygen supply to the heart muscle (ischemia). In chronic stable angina, chest pain follows a predictable exertional pattern with the patient aware of activities that trigger it (Kumar and Cannon 2009a, 2009b; Ohman 2016). Those with chronic stable angina have an annual mortality rate of less than 2 percent. Individuals with chronic stable angina or those who were previously asymptomatic may develop acute chest pain of varying intensity either at rest or with minimal activity. Such events are termed *acute coronary syndrome* (ACS) and include unstable angina, non-ST-elevation myocardial infarction (collectively referred to as NSTE-ACS), and ST-elevation myocardial infarction (STEMI). ACS may be diagnosed by symptoms, characteristic electrocardiogram changes, and elevated serum levels of cardiac biomarkers such as troponin T or I and creatine phosphokinase.

Accordingly, unstable angina is defined as the presence of cardiac symptoms in the absence of elevated cardiac biomarkers; non-ST-elevation myocardial infarction is defined as the presence of cardiac symptoms and elevated cardiac biomarkers in the absence of ST-segment elevations on an electrocardiogram; STEMI is defined as the presence of cardiac symptoms and elevated cardiac biomarkers, along with ST-segment elevations in two or more contiguous leads (Anderson and others 2013; Arbab-Zadeh and others 2012; Crea and Liuzzo 2013; Libby 2013; Thygesen and others 2012). A proportion of acute IHD events, including most sudden cardiac deaths, occurs outside of the clinical and diagnostic setting and cannot be classified into ACS categories.

RISK FACTORS FOR ISCHEMIC HEART DISEASE

Traditional Risk Factors

The development of IHD is associated with several traditional risk factors: hypertension (chapter 22, Jeemon and others 2017), hyperlipidemia (chapter 22, Jeemon and others), type 2 diabetes mellitus (chapter 12, Ali and others), obesity (chapter 7, Malik and Hu 2017), suboptimal diet (chapter 6, Afshin and others 2017), physical activity (chapter 5, Bull and others 2017) and lifestyle, and smoking (chapter 4, Roy and others 2017). The GBD assessed the global burden of these risk factors over 20 years (Lim and others 2012). Health care providers and policy makers are working with government- and nongovernment-based stakeholders to develop interventions to curb the rise in these risk factors that impose significant health and economic burdens. Nontraditional risk factors, such as major depression, socioeconomic deprivation, air pollution, and alcohol abuse, are associated with IHD risk and are described in chapter 16 (Magee and others 2017) and in other chapters in this volume. They are also discussed in *Disease Control Priorities*, third edition, volume 4, *Mental, Neurological, and Substance Use Disorder* (Patel and others 2015).

HIV/AIDS and IHD

With improved management of HIV and AIDS, CVD among those receiving antiretroviral medications is a potential risk (Casper and others, forthcoming). In rural South Africa, the number of CVD-related deaths among men older than age 65 years is increasing; however, for men between ages 50 and 64 years, CVD-related deaths have been halved, likely because of the concomitant rise in HIV/AIDS-related mortality (Tollman and others 2008). HIV-seropositive men have a higher prevalence of dyslipidemia, diabetes, peripheral artery disease, and high baseline lipid levels and lipoprotein(a) (Mauss and others 2008; Palacios and others 2008) attributable to smoking, to antiretroviral medications that cause dyslipidemia, and to HIV/AIDS as an independent risk factor for CVD. These trends suggest that closer monitoring is required in HIV/AIDS patients given that their increased life expectancy from improved treatment makes them more likely to have CVDs seen in non-HIV populations.

GLOBAL BURDEN OF ISCHEMIC HEART DISEASE

Globally, CVD death rates in HICs are declining. However, the high global burden of CVD is driven by deaths among the 85 percent of the world's population that lives in LMICs. The age-adjusted death rate for CVD has decreased by 21 percent, but the number of deaths has increased by 31 percent. The age-adjusted death rate for IHD fell by 19 percent from 131 deaths per 100,000 population to 106 deaths per 100,000 population; however, the total number of deaths increased by 35 percent. The apparent paradox can be explained in large part by overall population growth and aging, as well as by improvements in prevention and case-fatality rates. In both 1990 and 2010, IHD was the single most important cause of death (Lozano and others 2012). Although global trends show a larger IHD burden in LMICs compared with HICs, significant variation in the IHD burden occurs across the six LMIC regions and among countries within a given region or World Bank income category (Moran, Forouzanfar, and others 2014a, 2014b) (map 8.1, figures 8.1 and 8.2).

High-Income Countries

In 2010, CVD was responsible for approximately 36 percent of deaths in HICs; more than 50 percent of these deaths were caused by IHD. The age-standardized loss in DALYs attributed to IHD decreased; France, Japan, and the Republic of Korea reported the lowest DALYs lost among HICs (Moran, Tzong, and others 2014).

East Asia and Pacific

In 1990, IHD was the fourth major cause of death in East Asia and Pacific; in 2010, it was the leading cause.

The mortality trends in 2010 from IHD varied among the subregions in East Asia and Pacific. IHD was the second major cause of death in East Asia, the fourth major cause in South-East Asia, and the fifth major cause in Oceania.

China, which accounts for approximately 70 percent of the region's population, has seen a rapid transition in health in recent decades (Yang and others 2013; Zhang, Lu, and Liu 2008). In 1990, lower respiratory tract infections were the leading cause of death; strokes were the second leading cause of death, accounting for 1.3 million deaths. In 2010, however, stroke-related deaths increased by 35 percent to 1.7 million, making stroke the leading cause of death. IHD, in contrast, was the seventh major cause of death in 1990, accounting for 450,000 deaths; in 2010, it became the second leading cause, claiming approximately 950,000 lives. From 1984 to 1999, the incidence of coronary heart disease (CHD) increased by 2.7 percent annually for men and 1.2 percent annually for women (Zhang, Lu, and Liu 2008).

Map 8.1 Ischemic Heart Disease per 100,000 Population, Both Genders, All Ages, 2010

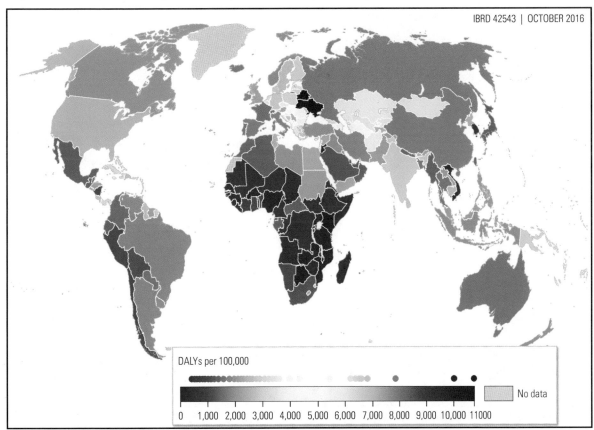

Source: IHME website, http://vizhub.healthdata.org/gbd-compare/.

Note: DALYs = Disability-adjusted life years. Map shows number of DALYs lost per 100,000 population. Each dot in key represents a country and the distribution by each color and number.

Figure 8.1 Global Variation in Mortality from Ischemic Heart Disease in Men, 1990 and 2010

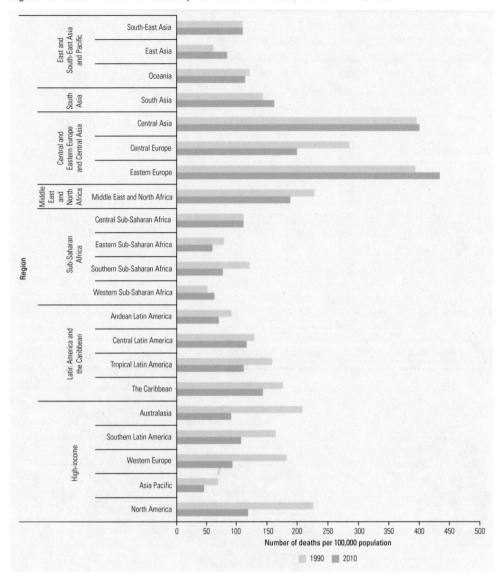

Source: Moran, Forouzanfar, and others 2014b.

Europe and Central Asia

The rate of CVD mortality is highest in Europe and Central Asia: 866 per 100,000 population in Eastern Europe and 604 per 100,000 population in Central Asia. In 2010, CVD accounted for nearly 66 percent of deaths, most of which were due to IHD. The number of CVD-related deaths varies across countries in this region. In Belarus, Bulgaria, the Russian Federation, and Ukraine, CVD rates have reached an alarming 800 per 100,000 for men (Mirzaei and others 2009).

Latin America and the Caribbean

Latin America and the Caribbean has a high CVD burden (Glassman and others 2010). In 2010, IHD was the region's leading cause of DALYs, increasing 36 percent from 1990 (IHME 2013). IHD accounted for 100 deaths per 100,000 population in the Caribbean and for approximately 14 percent of all deaths in Central Latin America. Mortality rates in these regions have increased over the past two decades. It is interesting to note that southern Latin America experienced a decrease in IHD mortality rates

Figure 8.2 Global Variation in Mortality from Ischemic Heart Disease in Women, 1990 and 2010

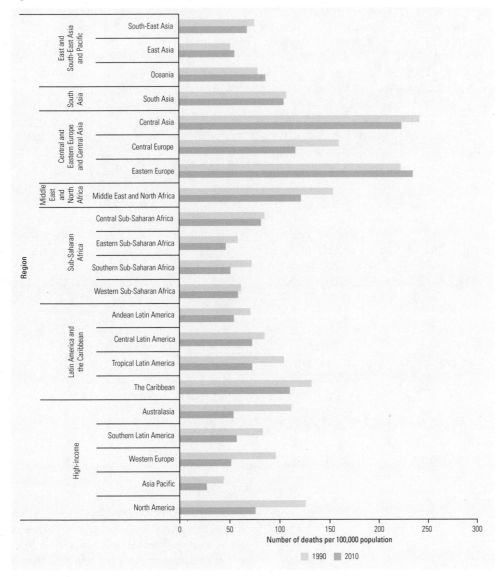

Source: Moran, Forouzanfar, and others 2014b.

from 1990 to 2010. In a nationwide comparative observational study examining five regions in Brazil from 2000 to 2010, 627,786 men and 452,690 women died because of IHD, absolute increases of 19 percent and 17 percent for men and women, respectively (Baena and others 2013).

Middle East and North Africa

In 2010, CVD was responsible for 199 deaths per 100,000 population in the Middle East and North Africa. Of these, IHD claimed 93 deaths per 100,000 population, representing a 15 percent increase in IHD mortality rates

since 1990. In addition to increased mortality, CVD was responsible for 17.2 million DALYs lost, of which 6.8 million were attributed to IHD. A study of the 22 Arab League countries (comprising 5 low-income countries, 11 middle-income countries, and 6 HICs) showed that IHD was responsible for 14.3 percent of deaths in 2010, making it the leading cause of death. Furthermore, IHD was the leading cause of DALYs lost in men (and accounted for 6 percent of DALYs lost) and was the third leading cause of DALYs lost for women (Mokdad and others 2014).

South Asia

CVD accounted for 20 percent of all deaths in South Asia, and IHD was responsible for more than 50 percent of these deaths. In 2010, IHD was responsible for 1.8 million, or 10.6 percent of all deaths. CVD was responsible for 60.5 million DALYs lost in 2010. India, with a population of 1.2 billion, has an extremely high burden of IHD. In 1990, 1.18 million people died because of IHD; in 2010, this number increased to 2.03 million (Gupta and others 2008). A large cross-sectional study showed that CVD causes an estimated 25 percent of deaths in India, and 51 percent of CVD deaths occur in those younger than age 70 years (Reddy and others 2007). In Pakistan, the burden is equally high: approximately 20 percent of adults have IHD (Jafar, Qadri, and Chaturvedi 2008). By 2025, an estimated 3.87 million premature deaths in Pakistan will be due to CVD, cancers, and chronic respiratory diseases in people ages 30–69 years (Jafar and others 2013). These trends threaten significant economic consequences if they are not reversed.

Sub-Saharan Africa

Overall, Africa has a high CVD burden (Gaziano 2008). Of all subregions in Sub-Saharan Africa, southern Africa has the highest number of CVD deaths at 13.0 percent; in western Africa, CVD accounts for 7.5 percent of deaths. Overall across Sub-Saharan Africa, the mortality rates are lower than global averages, with the exception of southern Africa, where the rates have increased from 129 per 100,000 to 136 per 100,000 population.

ECONOMIC BURDEN OF ISCHEMIC HEART DISEASE

The economic burden of IHD is significant and can be measured in at least three ways:

- By financial costs that are incurred in the health care system and described in cost-of-illness studies
- By microeconomic studies that assess the household impact of health events, such as myocardial infarctions
- By macroeconomic analyses that assess worker productivity or loss of economic growth caused by individuals or their caregivers being partially or completely out of work because of illness.

The literature on the first and second measures in LMICs is sparse, and no microeconomic studies focus exclusively on IHD (Huffman and others 2011; Murphy and others 2013; Schieber and others 2007). Many LMICs lack extensive insurance plans, and government-funded programs may be inadequate, forcing individuals

to pay out of pocket for health services in the acute setting and for medications and outpatient follow-up (Kruk, Goldmann, and Galea 2009; Leive and Xu 2008; Xu and others 2003).

Relatively more information is available on the economic burden from a macroeconomic perspective (Gaziano and others 2010). In China, the annual direct costs of CVD are estimated to be more than US$40 billion, or 4 percent of GNI. In South Africa, 25 percent of health care expenditure is devoted to CVD. There are relatively few cost-of-illness studies in other regions, but information on the costs associated with risk factors for IHD is available. Globally, health care costs related to hypertension are an estimated US$370 billion and are expected to rise to US$1 trillion in direct costs and up to US$4 trillion in indirect costs (Gaziano and others 2009). In HICs, 2 percent to 4 percent of health care expenses are devoted to the management of obesity-related illnesses. Although data are not available for all six LMIC regions, estimates from Latin America and the Caribbean indicate that diabetes-related costs are US$10 billion. The cost of long-term management of IHD is equally high. Heart failure, the most common sequela of IHD, costs an estimated US$108 billion annually worldwide (Cook and others 2014; Miller and others 2009; Safraj, Ajay, and Prabhakaran 2013) and is discussed in chapter 10 in this volume (Huffman and others 2017).

INTERVENTIONS

Success in improving CVD mortality rates depends on improved primary and secondary prevention strategies. Accordingly, 25 percent to 50 percent of the reduction in mortality is related to treatments; the remainder is due to changes in risk factors (Ford and Capewell 2011). Improvements in acute care reduce case fatality, but they also increase the size of the chronic IHD population in need of secondary prevention. Strategies to improve primary prevention are described in chapter 22 (Jeemon and others 2017). This chapter discusses individual-level interventions for management of IHD (table 8.1) and population-level interventions for tobacco cessation (table 8.2).

Acute Management

Several factors contribute to the acute management of ACS, starting with the quality of prehospital care available to those experiencing cardiac symptoms. The literature on this topic is sparse, but a survey of emergency medicine leaders in 13 LMICs in Asia, Latin America and the Caribbean, and Sub-Saharan Africa showed that the availability and use of emergency medical transport in LMICs is low, particularly in rural areas,

Table 8.1 Cost-Effectiveness of Interventions for IHD at the Individual Level

	Country or World Bank regions studied	Low-Income Countries		Middle-Income Countries	
		Very cost-effective (up to 1 times GNI per QALY, US$)	Cost-effective (up to 3 times GNI per QALY; that is, up to $3,135, US$)	Very cost-effective (up to 1 times GNI per QALY, US$)	Cost-effective (up to 3 times GNI per QALY; that is, up to $38,238, US$)
Acute management of IHD					
Intervention					
Aspirin + beta-blocker	All non-high-income regions	$11–$22			
Aspirin + beta-blocker + SK	All non-high-income regions	$634–$734			
Aspirin + beta blocker + tPA	All non-high-income regions				$15,860–$18,900
Clopidogrel[a]	China				$17,600
Primary PCI[a]	China				$9,000–$23,000
Coronary artery bypass graft surgery	South Asia, Sub-Saharan Africa, and East Asia and Pacific				$24,000–$33,800 (ICER compared with four medications: aspirin, beta-blocker, statin, and ACE inhibitor)
Secondary prevention of IHD					
Aspirin + beta-blocker + statin + ACE inhibitor	All non-high-income regions	$300–$400			
Aspirin + beta- blocker + statin + ACE inhibitor[a]	China		$3,100	$3,100	
Aspirin + beta- blocker + statin + ACE inhibitor	India			$2,920	
Polypill (aspirin + beta-blocker + statin + ACE inhibitor) to baseline	India			$1,760	
Nicotine-replacement therapy	All non-high-income regions	$55–$761			
Community pharmacist–based smoking cessation program	Thailand	$500 with 0.18 QALY gained (men); $614 with 0.24 QALY gained (women)			
Nicotine-based gum	Seychelles	$599			
Bupropion	Seychelles	$227			
ICD	United States				$17,000
CRT in heart failure	Brazil				$15,700
CRT	Argentina	$34 (ICER compared with medical therapy)			

Note: ACE = angiotensin-converting enzyme; CRT = cardiac resynchronization therapy; GNI = gross national income; ICD = implantable cardioverter defibrillator; ICER = incremental cost-effectiveness ratio; IHD = ischemic heart disease; PCI = percutaneous coronary intervention; QALY = quality-adjusted life year; SK = streptokinase; tPA = tissue plasminogen activator.
a. ICER compared with current treatment.

Table 8.2 Cost-Effectiveness of Interventions for IHD at the Population or Health Systems Level

	Countries or World Bank regions studied	Low-Income Countries		Middle-Income Countries	
		Very cost-effective (up to 1 times GNI per QALY, US$)	Cost-effective (up to 3 times GNI per QALY; that is, up to US$3,135, US$)	Very cost-effective (up to 1 times GNI per QALY, US$)	Cost-effective (up to 3 times GNI per QALY; that is, up to US$38,238)
Secondary prevention of IHD					
Tax increase on tobacco	All non-high-income regions	$3–$42			
Nonprice measure	All non-high-income regions	$54–$674			
Tobacco tax strategy	South Africa	$31			
Tobacco indoor air strategy	South Africa	$410			

Sources: Bitton and Gaziano 2011; Jha and others 2006.
Note: GNI = gross national income; IHD = ischemic heart disease; QALY = quality-adjusted life year.

which is largely attributed to deficiencies in funding and administrative leadership (Nielsen and others 2012). Additional studies are required to understand the availability and barriers to use of formal emergency medical transport systems in these settings. Given the high proportion of patients with ACS who die before coming to the hospital, a modeling study from China estimated that even optimal use of standard hospital-based treatments would have a limited impact on approximately 50 percent of acute IHD mortality (Wang and others 2014).

Where infrastructure exists, the medical management of ACS is well established through clinical trials; it may involve the use of aspirin, beta-blockers, statins, angiotensin receptor blockers (ARBs) or angiotensin-converting enzyme inhibitors (ACE-Is), additional antiplatelet agents, thrombolytics, and anticoagulants.

The availability of and adherence to clinical guidelines vary significantly. A retrospective analysis of studies involving 50,310 STEMI patients from 63 countries showed that the use of aspirin and beta-blockers varies from 75 percent to 95 percent in middle-income countries (Orlandini and others 2006). These findings are consistent with data from the Gulf Registry of Acute Coronary Events (Gulf RACE; 8,176 adults, 6 countries); Acute Coronary Events—A Multinational Survey of Current Management Strategies (ACCESS; 11,731 adults, 19 countries in Africa, Latin America, and the Middle East); and Zyban as an Effective Smoking Cessation Aid (ZESCA; 127 adults, 4 countries) studies that showed that 68 percent to 96 percent of patients received aspirin, beta-blockers, ACE-Is, or statins (ACCESS Investigators 2011; Shimony and others 2014;

Zubaid and others 2009). Several countries have increased the use of evidence-based medications, as seen in the expanded Global Registry of Acute Coronary Events (GRACE2) trial of 31,982 adults in 25 countries (Goodman and others 2009), and in the study of 1,025 patients with ACS managed at a third-level hospital in Lebanon (Abdallah and others 2010). This expansion may be due to effective government-based health care reform, as in Chile (Nazzal and others 2008), or quality improvement measures as in the Brazilian Intervention to Increase Evidence Usage in Acute Coronary Syndromes (BRIDGE-ACS) study of 1,150 patients in Brazil (Berwanger and others 2012).

Despite the availability and use of these medications, certain groups are less likely to receive appropriate therapy. This limited access, which resulted in higher mortality rates, was seen among individuals of lower socioeconomic status in the Treatment and Outcomes of Acute Coronary Syndromes in India (CREATE) prospective registry study (Xavier and others 2008) and among women in a study of six countries in the Middle East and North Africa (El-Menyar and others 2009).

The cost-effectiveness of four incremental strategies for the treatment of ACS has been evaluated:

- Aspirin
- Aspirin + beta-blocker (atenolol)
- Aspirin + beta-blocker (atenolol) + thrombolytic (streptokinase)
- Aspirin + beta-blocker (atenolol) + thrombolytic (tissue plasminogen activator).

The incremental cost per quality-adjusted life year (QALY) gained for aspirin + beta-blocker was less than US$25 for all six LMIC regions; the cost per QALY gained for streptokinase varied from US$630 to US$730; and the incremental cost-effectiveness ratio (ICER) for tissue plasminogen activator was approximately US$16,000 per QALY gained compared with streptokinase. Furthermore, recent Markov modeling of optimal medical management of in-hospital ACS showed that optimal use of aspirin, beta-blockers, ACE-Is, and statins had an ICER of less than US$3,100 (Megiddo and others 2014; Wang and others 2014).

In addition to these medications, management of ACS may require percutaneous coronary intervention (PCI). PCI is a nonsurgical procedure that uses a stent to open occluded coronary arteries. The use of PCI varies by region because thrombolytics, unlike PCI, do not require a dedicated catheterization laboratory onsite with a specialized team. In LMICs, although thrombolytics are more commonly used than PCI, the time to initiation of thrombolytic therapy is longer than in their higher-GNI counterparts: 4.3 hours versus 2.8 hours (Orlandini and others 2006). Delay adversely affects outcomes; the ideal is within 90 minutes and preferably less than six hours from onset of symptoms, because effectiveness declines to near zero at 12 hours from onset of symptoms.

The rates of PCI are higher in the United States than in Eastern Europe (Giugliano and others 2001; Kramer and others 2003). In a study of 13,591 patients enrolled in Ministry of Health hospitals in the National Cardiovascular Disease Database Registry in Malaysia, the use of streptokinase was higher for minorities (Chinese and Indians) than for local Malaysians, who were more likely to get PCI (Lu and Bin Nordin 2013). In India, the overall use of PCI was low, and even lower for those with lower socioeconomic status, reflecting inequity in care even within a country (Xavier and others 2008). In the Thai Registry in Acute Coronary Syndrome (TRACS), the Kerala ACS Registry based in India, and the Gulf RACE study, approximately 40 percent to 80 percent of patients with STEMI received thrombolytic therapy (Mohanan and others 2013; Srimahachota and others 2012; Zubaid and others 2009). Remarkably, in the ACCESS study of 11,731 adults from 19 countries in Africa, Latin America, and the Middle East, approximately 40 percent of adults with confirmed ACS did not receive PCI or thrombolytics, resulting in a higher mortality rate (ACCESS Investigators 2011). In Europe, PCI is emerging as the preferred choice in most countries, with improvements in both time to implant a coronary stent and rates of in-hospital mortality (Kristensen and others 2014; Mandelzweig and others 2006; Schiele and others 2010).

Overall, thrombolysis with streptokinase continues to be a cost-effective strategy in LMICs (Ford and Capewell 2011; Gaziano 2005; Megiddo and others 2014; Sikri and Bardia 2007; Wang and others 2014). From these studies and the GRACE Trial (Fox and others 2003; Goodman and others 2009), it is evident that the use of thrombolytics and PCI varies significantly. In the appropriate ACS setting, PCI can be as cost-effective as medical management (Kuntz and others 1996; Wang and others 2014); however, additional studies are required. In some LMICs, the use and quality of PCI care are improving despite barriers (Ranasinghe and others 2014); in several other countries, including, for example, India, treatment will continue to rely on thrombolytics until PCI-based infrastructure, access to services, and quality of cardiac care improve (Dalal and others 2013). Individuals in several LMICs may live in areas without timely access to PCI facilities; simulation analysis of a hypothetical non-urban population in Canada shows that building a new PCI facility would cost US$7,478 per QALY gained in comparison with ambulance transport (Potter, Weinstein, and Gaziano 2013). Future studies in LMICs are required to estimate costs associated with building new PCI facilities.

In comparison with thrombolytics and PCI, data on the number of coronary artery bypass graft (CABG) operations performed and their outcomes are sparse (Ribeiro and others 2006). The GRACE study based in 14 countries showed that CABG was performed in fewer than 10 percent of patients with ACS (Steg and others 2002). Although CABG is a cost-effective intervention in HICs, its ICER (compared with a combination of aspirin + beta-blocker + ACE-I + statin) may be attractive in middle-income countries (US$24,040–US$72,345 per QALY gained) but may be available only to a smaller proportion of the population (Ford and Capewell 2011; Gaziano 2005).

Regardless of the intervention used, patients may require management in a coronary care unit (CCU) where they can be monitored closely. When appropriately triaged, CCU-level management is cost-effective despite increased staffing and facilities (Kupersmith and others 1995; Weinstein and Stason 1985), but it may not be as widely available in LMICs.

Secondary Prevention

Strategies for the secondary prevention of CVD include population-based and individual-level interventions.

- Population-based interventions are often directed to cessation of tobacco use, reduction in the consumption of dietary salt and trans fatty acids (chapter 6, Afshin and others, increased physical activity (chapter 10, Bull and others 2017), and revision of regional or national government and health policies to improve chronic care services.

- Individual-level interventions are typically seen where access and adherence to essential medications, availability of cardiac resynchronization and defibrillation therapy, and access to and the use of cardiac rehabilitation are all increasing.

Other strategies for the secondary prevention of CVD involve the management of diabetes (chapter 12, Ali and others 2017), obesity (chapter 7, Malik and Hu 2017), and hypertension (chapter 10, Huffman and others 2017).

Smoking

Although tobacco products are a major risk factor for CVD, a significant proportion of the global population continues to smoke (Giovino and others 2012; Jha and Peto 2014; Ng and others 2014). Worldwide, approximately 1.1 billion people smoke; 82 percent of smokers reside in LMICs (Jha and others 2002). Forms of tobacco include bidis, kreteks, hookah pipes, smokeless tobacco, and secondhand smoke, all of which are associated with an increase in CVD (Balbinotto Neto and da Silva 2008; Cronin and others 2012; Gupta, Gupta, and Khedar 2013; Oberg and others 2011; Pell and others 2008; Piano and others 2010). The mortality rate for cigarette smokers is two to three times higher than for similarly aged nonsmokers (Jha and Peto 2014); by 2030, approximately 10 million deaths annually will be attributable to smoking (Jha and Chaloupka 2000). To address the significant mortality and morbidity associated with smoking, the WHO World Health Assembly adopted the Framework Convention on Tobacco Control (FCTC) in 2003, which was the first global tobacco treaty to regulate smoking. Several countries have implemented FCTC measures to curb the use of tobacco and the effects of smoking.

Population-level interventions. The price of tobacco products is a major determinant in smoking uptake and cessation (Jha and Peto 2014). The International Agency for Research on Cancer has shown that a 50 percent increase in inflation-adjusted tobacco prices reduces consumption by 20 percent in LMICs (Jha and Peto 2014). In LMICs, the low specific excise tax is the main reason that cigarettes cost 70 percent less than in HICs (Jha and Peto 2014); it is estimated that a 33 percent price increase worldwide would avert 22 million to 65 million smoking-attributable deaths; 90 percent of these prevented deaths would be in LMICs (Jha and Chaloupka 2000; John 2008;

Kerry and Lee 2007). Some countries, such as Uruguay, have implemented several FCTC measures, for example, banning advertisements, raising taxes, and banning smoking in public places. Over a six-year period, these countries have been able to decrease per-person consumption by 4.3 percent and prevalence of tobacco use by 3.3 percent per year (Abascal and others 2012). Simulation modeling of the effects of tobacco control measures in India shows that increased tobacco taxation and smoke-free laws could potentially avert 25 percent of myocardial infarctions and strokes in that country (Basu and others 2013). Tobacco taxation is the most cost-effective anti-smoking intervention (Ruger and Lazar 2012); however, strong political opposition in many countries remains a major barrier to wider implementation of higher tobacco taxes (Jha and others 2006).

Several other strategies have been implemented to limit the use of tobacco products. One approach is to regulate advertisements and smoking in public spaces. Advertising bans can result in a significant decline in smoking (Blecher 2008; Higashi and others 2011), and legislation-based smoking bans can reduce hospital admissions for cardiac events (Callinan and others 2010). Plain packaging of tobacco products and pictorial warnings can increase smoking cessation, as seen in Australia, Canada, India, and Thailand (Hammond 2010; Wakefield and others 2013). Furthermore, a 15 percent to 30 percent long-term cumulative decline in smoking rates has been seen as a result of effective public health efforts, as has a 6 percent reduction in the demand for tobacco (Jha and Chaloupka 2000; Saffer and Chaloupka 2000; Townsend 1993). In LMICs, mass media campaigns may decrease overall consumption, as was seen in the United States (Bala and others 2013).

Individual-level interventions. Individual-level interventions, including nicotine replacement therapy (NRT) and non-nicotine-based products and behavioral modification, have been implemented (Jha and Chaloupka 2000). A study of 484 smokers in Northern Ireland and London, England, showed that adults randomly assigned to a community-based cessation program had higher abstinence rates at 12 months compared with usual care, 14.3 percent and 2.7 percent, respectively (Maguire, McElnay, and Drummond 2001). Similarly, community-based interventions in Mauritius and South Africa resulted in a 3 percent to 11 percent decrease in smoking (Hodge and others 1996; Rossouw and others 1993; Uusitalo and others 1996). Systematic reviews of studies in HICs and LMICs show that NRT can increase the rate of tobacco-use cessation by 50 percent to 70 percent and is effective in sustaining smoking abstinence (Moore and others 2009; Stead and others 2008).

In addition to NRT, bupropion is a non-nicotine-based medication with similar efficacy to NRT (Hughes and others 2014); however, this medication is not on the WHO's Model List of Essential Medications, and additional studies are required to determine the potential availability of this medication to large populations in LMICs.

Cost-effectiveness. Of the interventions discussed, tobacco taxation is the most cost-effective option to reduce smoking (Gaziano and Pagidipati 2013; Ruger and Lazar 2012), although NRTs are also cost-effective, depending on their price and availability. Jha and others (2006) analyzed the cost-effectiveness of tobacco control using a cohort of smokers in 2000. They calculated that NRT could reduce the number of deaths by 2.9 million to 14.3 million and that a range of nonprice interventions, such as advertising bans, health warnings, and smoke-free laws, could reduce the number of deaths by 5.7 million to 28.6 million. The cost-effectiveness value associated with this reduction is US$3–US$42 per QALY saved for tax increases, not including tax revenue; US$55–US$761 per QALY saved for NRT; and US$54–$674 per QALY saved for other nonprice measures.

Although data on cost-effective interventions in LMICs are limited, a few country-specific studies have been conducted. In South Africa, the tobacco tax and indoor air policies are highly cost-effective, with an ICER of US$31 per DALY averted for the tobacco tax strategy and US$410 per DALY averted for the indoor air strategy (Bitton and Gaziano 2011; Gaziano and Pagidipati 2013). In Thailand, a community pharmacist–based smoking cessation program was cost-effective, resulting in cost savings of US$500 per life-year gained, with an average of 0.18 life-year gained in men, and of US$614 per life-year gained, with an average of 0.24 life-year gained in women (Thavorn and Chaiyakunapruk 2008). In the Seychelles, a cohort study showed that the incremental cost per life-year saved was US$599 for nicotine-based gum and US$227 for bupropion.

These studies show that the effectiveness of a strategy may vary across regions and that additional studies are required to identify cost-effective interventions. The financial investment needed for NRT may be prohibitive on a population scale in some LMICs, but it may be more cost-effective and feasible to treat the smaller, higher-risk population of IHD patients.

Access to Essential Medications for Secondary Prevention

Several evidence-based medication regimens are effective in the secondary prevention of CVD. These include aspirin, beta-blockers, ACEi and ARBs, statins, and more recently, a multidrug combination pill regimen.

Several studies have shown that the use of medications for secondary prevention varies significantly across LMIC regions, despite the inclusion of these agents in the WHO's Model List of Essential Medications (WHO 2013). The WHO study on Prevention of REcurrences of Myocardial Infarction and StrokE (WHO-PREMISE) in 10 LMICs showed that among those with IHD, only 81.2 percent were prescribed aspirin, 48.1 percent a beta-blocker, 39.8 percent an ACE-I, and 29.8 percent a statin (Mendis and others 2005). A survey of nine European countries (EUROASPIRE III study) showed that among patients with IHD, only 71 percent and 78 percent were on a statin and ACEi or ARB, respectively (Kotseva and others 2009). The most recent Prospective Urban and Rural Epidemiological (PURE) study, which enrolled 153,996 adults in 3 HICs and 14 LMICs, showed that only 25.3 percent were on an antiplatelet medication, 17.4 percent on a beta-blocker, 19.5 percent on ACEi or ARBs, and 14.6 percent on a statin (Yusuf and others 2011). The results are less encouraging in India, where a survey of 53 villages observed that 14 percent of those with IHD were on aspirin, 41 percent on blood-pressure-lowering medication, and 5 percent on cholesterol-lowering medication (Joshi and others 2009). Supporting this finding was an observational study of statin use in India, which showed that although the use of statins had increased from 2006 to 2010, only 8 percent of CHD patients were on a statin (Choudhry, Dugani, and others 2014).

Several factors are responsible for the low use of medications, including inadequate availability of and access to affordable medications, low numbers of health care providers, and complicated medication regimens. In many LMICs, the cost of a month's supply of generic secondary prevention medications ranges from 1.5 to 18.4 days' wages of government workers (Mendis and others 2007); the availability of cardiovascular medications, measured by the percentage of facilities in which a medicine is available ranges from 25 percent in the public sector to 60 percent in the private sector (Cameron and others 2011; van Mourik and others 2010). The availability of generic medications had been influenced by the TRIPS (Trade-Related Aspects of Intellectual Property Rights) Agreement of 1995, which obliged World Trade Organization members to protect pharmaceutical patents for 20 years from the date they were filed (Smith, Lee, and Drager 2009). The subsequent Doha Declaration of 2003 granted nations compulsory licenses to domestically manufacture essential medications without permission of patent holders (Beall and Kuhn 2012; Correa 2006; Lybecker and Fowler 2009). Canada was the only country to issue a compulsory license to export generic medications to poorer nations (Lybecker and Fowler 2009), which has helped increase the availability of generic medications in LMICs. More recent studies have shown that from 2001 to 2011, generic medications in the private sectors of 19 LMICs (10 in Latin America and the Caribbean, 8 in the Middle East and North Africa, plus South Africa) represented approximately 70 percent to 80 percent of the market share (Kaplan, Wirtz, and Stephens 2013).

Most patients with CVD require several medications, and a polypill was developed to increase the availability of these medications in LMICs. Polypills have fixed-dose combinations of different cardiac medications; they have the potential to reduce IHD and to become more widely available (Bautista and others 2013; Lonn and others 2010; Wald and Law 2003; Yusuf and others 2009). This development is encouraging, but analysis of studies shows that improved access to pharmaceuticals; improved use of insurance policies; and alignment of incentives for physicians, consumers, and pharmaceutical sellers may be needed to increase the uptake of generic medications (Faden and others 2011; Kaplan and others 2012). Greater availability of trained professionals may help improve patients' access to medications.

Medications are cost-effective in the treatment of myocardial infarction and in the secondary prevention of IHD. Combination therapy consisting of aspirin, ACE-I, a beta-blocker, and a statin is cost-effective in LMICs; combination therapy is associated with a cost of US$350 (range US$300–US$400) per QALY gained, even in the absence of a polypill (Gaziano, Opie, and Weinstein 2006; Gaziano and Pagidipati 2013).

Medication Adherence

Medication adherence refers to whether patients take medications at the required frequency and for the required duration; patients who take the prescribed medications more than 80 percent of the time are considered to be adherent (Ho, Bryson, and Rumsfeld 2009). In addition to having reduced access to affordable medications, approximately 60 percent of people in different regions who are prescribed medications are adherent to the prescribed therapy (Bowry and others 2011; Chowdhury and others 2013). The PURE study observed the lowest medication use in low-income countries, which may be due to several reasons ranging from availability of medications to adherence (Yusuf and others 2011). Medication adherence is associated with a cost reduction of 10.1 percent to 17.8 percent between high- and low- adherence groups (Bitton and others 2013). Adherence is associated with lower mortality rates, as was seen in the international REduction of Atherothrombosis for Continued Health (REACH)

Registry (Kumbhani and others 2013). Overall, medication adherence remains a major challenge, likely further complicated by the complexity of different regimens.

The literature on interventions to improve medication adherence is evolving rapidly. Investigators found that a simple change in prescription length from a 30- to a 60- or 90-day supply could save 1,700–2,500 premature CVD deaths per million patients treated, in addition to up to US$200 per patient over his or her lifetime in reduced costs. In particular, significant savings accrue to patients from reduced time and transportation costs (Gaziano and others 2015). Recent reports of interventions to improve medication adherence suggest that reduced out-of-pocket expenses, better case management, improved patient education with behavioral support, expanded mobile phone messaging—supported by broader practice guidelines as well as regulatory and communication-based policies—may improve medication adherence (de Jongh and others 2012; Laba and others 2013; Tajouri, Driver, and Holmes 2014; Viswanathan and others 2012). In this context, the Post-Myocardial Infarction Free Rx Event and Economic Evaluation (MI FREEE) trial in the United States has shown that elimination of copayments for drugs after a myocardial infarction improved medication adherence to 49.0 percent from 35.9 percent (Choudhry and others 2011), although adherence remained suboptimal. Furthermore, insurance plans that were generous, targeted high-risk patients, offered wellness programs, did not offer disease management programs, and made the benefit available only for medication ordered by mail were associated with significantly higher adherence rates, as much as 4 percentage points to 5 percentage points higher (Choudhry, Fischer, and others 2014). Although these studies are promising, future research will reveal if these models can be successfully replicated in LMICs.

The polypill is a promising intervention for improving adherence. A randomized clinical trial of 2,004 participants in India and Europe showed that use of a polypill containing aspirin, a statin, and two blood-pressure-lowering agents was associated with improved medication adherence compared with usual care, at 86 percent and 65 percent, respectively, resulting in concurrent reduction in systolic blood pressure (by 2.6 millimeters of mercury, a measure of pressure) and LDL cholesterol (4.2 milligrams per deciliter) (Thom and others 2013). Several other secondary prevention trials are underway, including the Indian Polycap-K Trial, the Kanyini Guidelines Adherence with the Polypill Study of indigenous and nonindigenous people in Australia, and the Trial in Secondary Prevention in Spain and Latin American countries (Lonn and others 2010; Sanz and Fuster 2009). These and other studies will provide information on the effectiveness of polypills for the secondary prevention of CVD and may support the suggestion that polypills be included in the WHO's Model List of Essential Medications (Huffman and Yusuf 2014).

Cardiac Rehabilitation

Cardiac rehabilitation programs are professionally supervised programs that provide education and counseling on diet, lifestyle, and physical fitness to patients recovering from myocardial infarctions, PCI, and cardiac surgery, with the goal of reducing the likelihood of future cardiac events. Data on the effectiveness of rehabilitation programs come from studies largely conducted in HICs. Two systematic analyses show that exercise-based rehabilitation programs can reduce hospital readmission rates (Davies and others 2010; Heran and others 2011). A randomized study showed that patients who received cardiac rehabilitation had shorter lengths of hospital stay and reduced cardiac risk factors (Zwisler and others 2008). Recent studies have shown that cardiac rehabilitation programs are offered in LMICs, particularly in Latin America and the Caribbean and in India, and show positive outcomes. Despite these findings, there is a general dearth of rehabilitation programs (Boriani and others 2014; Grace and others 2013; Madan and others 2014; Shanmugasegaram and others 2014) and studies on their cost-effectiveness in different countries, prompting the International Charter on Cardiovascular Prevention and Rehabilitation to call for increased implementation and expansion of programs worldwide (Grace and others 2013).

Cardiac Resynchronization Therapy and Implantable Cardioverter Defibrillators

Cardiac resynchronization therapy (CRT) seeks to improve symptoms in patients with symptomatic heart failure due to systolic dysfunction and a delay between repolarization of the left and right ventricles of the heart. CRT synchronizes the timing of right- and left-ventricular depolarization, and improves contractility and backflow of the blood through leaky mitral valves (known as *mitral regurgitation*) (Strickberger and others 2005). Implantable cardioverter defibrillators (ICDs) are devices to rectify life-threatening abnormal heart rhythms, namely, ventricular tachycardia and ventricular fibrillation. ICDs constantly monitor heart rate and rhythm and deliver electrical pulses to restore normal heart rhythm.

Some of the earliest articles on CRT in the United States showed that ICDs are cost-effective and cost approximately US$17,000 per life-year saved in selected patients (Kuppermann and others 1990). Markov analysis of heart failure patients in Argentina showed that management with optimal medical therapy and CRT is cost-effective compared with optimal medical therapy alone. In the analysis, the ICER was I$38 (international dollars) per year of life gained and US$34 per QALY gained (Poggio and others 2012). In Brazil, Markov analysis of heart failure patients showed that management with ICD is cost-effective (Bertoldi and others 2013; Ribeiro and others 2010) where the ICER of CRT over medical therapy was US$15,723; however, upgrading to CRT in combination with ICD was associated with an ICER of US$84,345, which is well above the WHO willingness-to-pay threshold of Brazil's GDP per capita of US$31,689 (Bertoldi and others 2013). Similar cost-effectiveness was seen in Markov modeling of a European cohort of patients with reduced systolic function; placement of an ICD was associated with an ICER of US$50,161 per QALY gained, suggesting that this is a cost-effective intervention (Smith and others 2013). Additional studies are required to assess whether these interventions are cost-effective in LMICs.

CONCLUSIONS

Several cost-effective interventions are available for acute and chronic management of ACS and for long-term management of IHD risk factors. Most of the data on cost-effectiveness come from studies in HICs; however, emerging literature is directed toward estimating cost-effectiveness at regional and country levels in LMICs (Gaziano and Pagidipati 2013; Huffman and others 2013; Myers and Mendis 2014; Suhrcke, Boluarte, and Niessen 2012).

Acute Care

In acute settings, the medical management of ACS is cost-effective; emerging literature shows that PCI may also be cost-effective, but facilities providing this type of care may not be available in all regions. Furthermore, when appropriately triaged, intensive monitoring with CCU-level care is cost-effective; however, such monitoring requires significant infrastructure and qualified health professionals and is not widely available. Comparative effectiveness and cost-effectiveness information needs to be developed to guide the implementation of ACS care components so that they are widely accessible and equitably distributed.

Long-Term Management

Once patients have been managed in acute settings, subsequent mortality and morbidity can be lowered through a combination of reducing risk factors, increasing access and adherence to medications, and using the placement of CRT and ICDs in areas where advanced care and sub-specialists are available. Smoking is a major risk factor for IHD, and several cost-effective interventions have been identified, including increased tobacco taxes, use of NRT and non-nicotine-based medications, and policies to restrict smoking in public spaces; the combination of these interventions could help reduce IHD-related mortality and morbidity. Combination therapy of aspirin, beta-blockers, ACE-Is, and statins is cost-effective in the chronic management of IHD. However, IHD patients in LMICs have inadequate access to affordable medications and show low adherence to medications even when they can afford them. Interventions are being developed to support patients by increasing medication availability and encouraging adherence.

Finally, when used in the appropriate patients, CRT and ICDs can be cost-effective; however, these interventions are not widely available. The implementation of cost-effective interventions may depend on country- or region-specific factors, and additional studies on interventions and their cost-effectiveness are urgently required to tackle the significant mortality and morbidity associated with IHD.

NOTE

World Bank Income Classifications as of July 2014 are as follows, based on estimates of gross national income (GNI) per capita for 2013:

- Low-income countries (LICs) = US$1,045 or less
- Middle-income countries (MICs) are subdivided:
  (a) lower-middle-income = US$1,046 to US$4,125
  (b) upper-middle-income (UMICs) = US$4,126 to US$12,745
- High-income countries (HICs) = US$12,746 or more.

REFERENCES

Abascal, W., E. Esteves, B. Goja, F. González Mora, A. Lorenzo, and others. 2012. "Tobacco Control Campaign in Uruguay: A Population-Based Trend Analysis." *The Lancet* 380 (9853): 1575–82. doi:10.1016/S0140-6736(12)60826-5.

Abdallah, M., W. Karrowni, W. Shamseddeen, S. Itani, L. Kobeissi, and others. 2010. "Acute Coronary Syndromes: Clinical Characteristics, Management, and Outcomes at the American University of Beirut Medical Center, 2002–2005." *Clinical Cardiology* 33 (1): E6–13. doi:10.1002/clc.20636.

ACCESS Investigators. 2011. "Management of Acute Coronary Syndromes in Developing Countries: Acute Coronary Events—A Multinational Survey of Current Management Strategies." *American Heart Journal* 162 (5): 852–59.e22. doi:10.1016/j.ahj.2011.07.029.

Afshin, A., R. Micha, M. Webb, S. Capewell, L. Whitsel, and others. 2017. "Effectiveness of Dietary Policies to Reduce Noncommunicable Diseases." In *Disease Control Priorities* (third edition): Volume 5, *Cardiovascular, Respiratory, and Related Disorders,* edited by D. Prabhakaran, S. Anand, T. A. Gaziano, J-C. Mbanya, Y. Wu, and R. Nugent. Washington, DC: World Bank.

Ali, M. K., K. R. Siegel, E. Chandrasekar, N. Tandon, P. A. Montoya, and others. 2017. "Diabetes: An Update on the Pandemic and Potential Solutions." In *Disease Control Priorities* (third edition): Volume 5, *Cardiovascular, Respiratory, and Related Disorders,* edited by D. Prabhakaran, S. Anand, T. A. Gaziano, J.-C. Mbanya, Y. Wu, and R. Nugent. Washington, DC: World Bank.

Anderson, J. L., C. D. Adams, E. M. Antman, C. R. Bridges, R. M. Califf, and others. 2013. "2012 ACCF/AHA Focused Update Incorporated into the ACCF/AHA 2007 Guidelines for the Management of Patients with Unstable Angina/Non-ST-Elevation Myocardial Infarction: A Report of the American College of Cardiology Foundation/American Heart Association Task Force on Practice Guidelines." *Journal of the American College of Cardiology* 61 (23): e179–347. doi:10.1016/j.jacc.2013.01.014.

Arbab-Zadeh, A., M. Nakano, R. Virmani, and V. Fuster. 2012. "Acute Coronary Events." *Circulation* 125 (9): 1147–56. doi:10.1161/CIRCULATIONAHA.111.047431.

Baena, C. P., R. Chowdhury, N. A. Schio, A. E. Sabbag, L. C. Guarita-Souza, and others. 2013. "Ischaemic Heart Disease Deaths in Brazil: Current Trends, Regional Disparities and Future Projections." *Heart* 99 (18): 1359–64. doi:10.1136/heartjnl-2013-303617.

Bala, M. M., L. Strzeszynski, R. Topor-Madry, and K. Cahill. 2013. "Mass Media Interventions for Smoking Cessation in Adults." *Cochrane Database of Systematic Reviews* 6: CD004704. doi:10.1002/14651858.CD004704.pub3.

Balbinotto Neto, G., and E. N. da Silva. 2008. "The Costs of Cardiovascular Disease in Brazil: A Brief Economic Comment." *Arquivos Brasileiros de Cardiologia* 91 (4): 198–99.

Basu, S., S. Glantz, A. Bitton, and C. Millett. 2013. "The Effect of Tobacco Control Measures during a Period of Rising Cardiovascular Disease Risk in India: A Mathematical Model of Myocardial Infarction and Stroke." *PLoS Medicine* 10 (7): e1001480. doi:10.1371/journal.pmed.1001480.

Bautista, L. E., L. M. Vera-Cala, D. Ferrante, V. M. Herrera, J. J. Miranda, and others. 2013. "A 'Polypill' Aimed at Preventing Cardiovascular Disease Could Prove Highly Cost-Effective for Use in Latin America." *Health Affairs* 32 (1): 155–64. doi:10.1377/hlthaff.2011.0948.

Beall, R., and R. Kuhn. 2012. "Trends in Compulsory Licensing of Pharmaceuticals since the Doha Declaration: A Database Analysis." *PLoS Medicine* 9 (1): e1001154. doi:10.1371/journal.pmed.1001154.

Bertoldi, E. G., L. E. Rohde, L. I. Zimerman, M. Pimentel, and C. A. Polanczyk. 2013. "Cost-Effectiveness of Cardiac Resynchronization Therapy in Patients with Heart Failure: The Perspective of a Middle-Income Country's Public Health System." *International Journal of Cardiology* 163 (3): 309–15. doi:10.1016/j.ijcard.2011.06.046.

Berwanger, O., H. P. Guimarães, L. N. Laranjeira, A. B. Cavalcanti, A. A. Kodama, and others. 2012. "Effect of a Multifaceted

Intervention on Use of Evidence-Based Therapies in Patients with Acute Coronary Syndromes in Brazil: The BRIDGE-ACS Randomized Trial." *Journal of the American Medical Association* 307 (19): 2041–49. doi:10.1001/jama .2012.413.

Bitton, A., N. K. Choudhry, O. S. Matlin, K. Swanton, and W. H. Shrank. 2013. "The Impact of Medication Adherence on Coronary Artery Disease Costs and Outcomes: A Systematic Review." *American Journal of Medicine* 126 (4): 357.e7–357. e27. doi:10.1016/j.amjmed.2012.09.004.

Bitton, A., and T. A. Gaziano. 2011. "The Cost-Effectiveness of Selective Tobacco Control Policies in South Africa." *Journal of General Internal Medicine* 26 (Suppl): S353–54.

Blecher, E. 2008. "The Impact of Tobacco Advertising Bans on Consumption in Developing Countries." *Journal of Health Economics* 27 (4): 930–42. doi:10.1016/j.jhealeco.2008.02.010.

Boriani, G., P. Cimaglia, M. Biffi, C. Martignani, M. Ziacchi, and others. 2014. "Cost-Effectiveness of Implantable Cardioverter-Defibrillator in Today's World." *Indian Heart Journal* 66 (Suppl 1): S101–4. doi:10.1016/j.ihj.2013.12.034.

Bowry, A. D. K., W. H. Shrank, J. L. Lee, M. Stedman, and N. K. Choudhry. 2011. "A Systematic Review of Adherence to Cardiovascular Medications in Resource-Limited Settings." *Journal of General Internal Medicine* 26 (12): 1479–91. doi:10.1007/s11606-011-1825-3.

Bull, F., S. Goenka, V. Lambert, and M. Pratt. 2017. "Physical Activity for the Prevention of Cardiometabolic Disease." In *Disease Control Priorities* (third edition): Volume 5, *Cardiovascular, Respiratory, and Related Disorders*, edited by D. Prabhakaran, S. Anand, T. A. Gaziano, J-C. Mbanya, Y. Wu, and R. Nugent. Washington, DC: World Bank.

Callinan, J. E., A. Clarke, K. Doherty, and C. Kelleher. 2010. "Legislative Smoking Bans for Reducing Secondhand Smoke Exposure, Smoking Prevalence and Tobacco Consumption." *Cochrane Database of Systematic Reviews* 4: CD005992. doi:10.1002/14651858.CD005992.pub2.

Cameron, A., I. Roubos, M. Ewen, A. K. Mantel-Teeuwisse, H. G. M. Leufkens, and others. 2011. "Differences in the Availability of Medicines for Chronic and Acute Conditions in the Public and Private Sectors of Developing Countries." *Bulletin of the World Health Organization* 89 (6): 412–21. doi:10.2471/BLT.10.084327.

Casper, C., H. Crane, M. Menon, and D. Money. 2017. "HIV/ AIDS Comorbidities: Cancer, Noncommunicable Diseases, and the Impact of HIV/AIDS and other STIs on Reproductive Health." In *Disease Control Priorities* (third edition): Volume 6, *Major Infectious Diseases*, edited by K. C. Holmes, S. Bertozzi, B. Bloom, and P. Jha. Washington, DC: World Bank.

Choudhry, N. K., J. Avorn, R. J. Glynn, E. M. Antman, S. Schneeweiss, and others. 2011. "Full Coverage for Preventive Medications after Myocardial Infarction." *New England Journal of Medicine* 365 (22): 2088–97. doi:10.1056 /NEJMsa1107913.

Choudhry, N. K., S. Dugani, W. H. Shrank, J. M. Polinski, C. E. Stark, and others. 2014. "Despite Increased Use and Sales of Statins in India, per Capita Prescription Rates Remain Far Below High-Income Countries." *Health Affairs* 33 (2): 273–82. doi:10.1377/hlthaff.2013.0388.

Choudhry, N. K., M. A. Fischer, B. F. Smith, G. Brill, C. Girdish, and others. 2014. "Five Features of Value-Based Insurance Design Plans Were Associated with Higher Rates of Medication Adherence." *Health Affairs* 33 (3): 493–501. doi: 10.1377/hlthaff.2013.0060.

Chowdhury, R., H. Khan, E. Heydon, A. Shroufi, S. Fahimi, and others. 2013. "Adherence to Cardiovascular Therapy: A Meta-Analysis of Prevalence and Clinical Consequences." *European Heart Journal* 34 (38): 2940–48. doi:10.1093 /eurheartj/eht295.

Cook, C., G. Cole, P. Asaria, R. Jabbour, and D. P. Francis. 2014. "The Annual Global Economic Burden of Heart Failure." *International Journal of Cardiology* 171 (3): 368–76. doi:10.1016/j.ijcard.2013.12.028.

Correa, C. M. 2006. "Implications of Bilateral Free Trade Agreements on Access to Medicines." *Bulletin of the World Health Organization* 84 (5): 399–404. doi:S0042 -96862006000500021.

Crea, F., and G. Liuzzo. 2013. "Pathogenesis of Acute Coronary Syndromes." *Journal of the American College of Cardiology* 61 (1): 1–11. doi:10.1016/j.jacc.2012.07.064.

Cronin, E. M., P. M. Kearney, P. P. Kearney, P. Sullivan, and I. J. Perry. 2012. "Impact of a National Smoking Ban on Hospital Admission for Acute Coronary Syndromes: A Longitudinal Study." *Clinical Cardiology* 35 (4): 205–9. doi:10.1002/clc.21014.

Dalal, J., P. K. Sahoo, R. K. Singh, A. Dhall, R. Kapoor, and others. 2013. "Role of Thrombolysis in Reperfusion Therapy for Management of AMI: Indian Scenario." *Indian Heart Journal* 65 (5): 566–85. doi:10.1016/j.ihj.2013.08.032.

Davies, E. J., T. Moxham, K. Rees, S. Singh, A. J. Coats, and others. 2010. "Exercise Based Rehabilitation for Heart Failure." *Cochrane Database of Systematic Reviews* (4): CD003331. doi:10.1002/14651858.CD003331.pub3.

de Jongh, T., I. Gurol-Urganci, V. Vodopivec-Jamsek, J. Car, and R. Atun. 2012. "Mobile Phone Messaging for Facilitating Self-Management of Long-Term Illnesses." *Cochrane Database of Systematic Reviews* 12: CD007459. doi:10.1002/14651858 .CD007459.pub2.

El-Menyar, A., M. Zubaid, W. Rashed, W. Almahmeed, J. Al-Lawati, and others. 2009. "Comparison of Men and Women with Acute Coronary Syndrome in Six Middle Eastern Countries." *American Journal of Cardiology* 104 (8): 1018–22. doi:10.1016/j.amjcard.2009.06.003.

Faden, L., C. Vialle-Valentin, D. Ross-Degnan, and A. Wagner. 2011. "The Role of Health Insurance in the Cost-Effective Use of Medicines." Working Paper 2, Review Series on Pharmaceutical Pricing Policies and Interventions, World Health Organization/Health Action International Project on Medicine Prices and Availability, Geneva.

Ford, E. S., and S. Capewell. 2011. "Proportion of the Decline in Cardiovascular Mortality Disease Due to Prevention versus Treatment: Public Health versus Clinical Care." *Annual Review of Public Health* 32: 5–22. doi:10.1146 /annurev-publhealth-031210-101211.

Fox, K. A. A., S. G. Goodman, F. A. Anderson, C. B. Granger, M. Moscucci, and others. 2003. "From Guidelines to Clinical Practice: The Impact of Hospital and Geographical

Characteristics on Temporal Trends in the Management of Acute Coronary Syndromes: The Global Registry of Acute Coronary Events (GRACE)." *European Heart Journal* 24 (15): 1414–24.

Gaziano, T. A. 2005. "Cardiovascular Disease in the Developing World and Its Cost-Effective Management." *Circulation* 112 (23): 3547–53. doi:10.1161/CIRCULATIONAHA.105 .591792.

———. 2008. "Economic Burden and the Cost-Effectiveness of Treatment of Cardiovascular Diseases in Africa." *Heart* 94 (2): 140–44. doi:10.1136/hrt.2007.128785.

Gaziano, T. A., A. Bitton, S. Anand, S. Abrahams-Gessel, and A. Murphy. 2010. "Growing Epidemic of Coronary Heart Disease in Low- and Middle-Income Countries." *Current Problems in Cardiology* 35 (2): 72–115. doi:10.1016/j .cpcardiol.2009.10.002.

Gaziano, T. A., A. Bitton, S. Anand, M. C. Weinstein, and International Society of Hypertension. 2009. "The Global Cost of Nonoptimal Blood Pressure." *Journal of Hypertension* 27: 1472–77.

Gaziano, T. A., S. Cho, S. Sy, A. Pandya, N. S. Levitt, and others. 2015. "Increasing Prescription Length Could Cut Cardiovascular Disease Burden and Produce Savings in South Africa." *Health Affairs* 34: 1578–85.

Gaziano, T. A., L. H. Opie, and M. C. Weinstein. 2006. "Cardiovascular Disease Prevention with a Multidrug Regimen in the Developing World: A Cost-Effectiveness Analysis." *The Lancet* 368 (9536): 679–86. doi:10.1016 /S0140-6736(06)69252-0.

Gaziano, T. A., and N. Pagidipati. 2013. "Scaling Up Chronic Disease Prevention Interventions in Lower- and Middle-Income Countries." *Annual Review of Public Health* 34: 317–35. doi:10.1146/annurev-publhealth-031912-114402.

Giovino, G. A., S. A. Mirza, J. M. Samet, P. C. Gupta, M. J. Jarvis, and others. 2012. "Tobacco Use in 3 Billion Individuals from 16 Countries: An Analysis of Nationally Representative Cross-Sectional Household Surveys." *The Lancet* 380 (9842): 668–79. doi:10.1016/S0140-6736(12)61085-X.

Giugliano, R. P., J. Llevadot, R. G. Wilcox, E. P. Gurfinkel, C. H. McCabe, and others. 2001. "Geographic Variation in Patient and Hospital Characteristics, Management, and Clinical Outcomes in ST-Elevation Myocardial Infarction Treated with Fibrinolysis: Results from InTIME-II." *European Heart Journal* 22 (18): 1702–15. doi:10.1053/euhj.2001.2583.

Glassman, A., T. A. Gaziano, C. P. Bouillon Buendia, and F. C. Guanais de Aguiar. 2010. "Confronting the Chronic Disease Burden in Latin America and the Caribbean." *Health Affairs* 29 (12): 2142–48. doi:10.1377/hlthaff.2010.1038.

Goodman, S. G., W. Huang, A. T. Yan, A. Budaj, B. M. Kennelly, and others. 2009. "The Expanded Global Registry of Acute Coronary Events: Baseline Characteristics, Management Practices, and Hospital Outcomes of Patients with Acute Coronary Syndromes." *American Heart Journal* 158 (2): 193–201.e1–5. doi:10.1016/j.ahj.2009.06.003.

Grace, S. L., D. R. Warburton, J. A. Stone, B. K. Sanderson, N. Oldridge, and others. 2013. "International Charter on Cardiovascular Prevention and Rehabilitation: A Call for Action." *Journal of Cardiopulmonary Rehabilitation and Prevention* 33 (2): 128–31. doi:10.1097/HCR .0b013e318284ec82.

Gupta, R., N. Gupta, and R. S. Khedar. 2013. "Smokeless Tobacco and Cardiovascular Disease in Low and Middle Income Countries." *Indian Heart Journal* 65 (4): 369–77. doi:10.1016/j.ihj.2013.06.005.

Gupta, R., P. Joshi, V. Mohan, K. S. Reddy, and S. Yusuf. 2008. "Epidemiology and Causation of Coronary Heart Disease and Stroke in India." *Heart* 94 (1): 16–26. doi:10.1136 /hrt.2007.132951.

Hammond, D. 2010. "'Plain Packaging' Regulations for Tobacco Products: The Impact of Standardizing the Color and Design of Cigarette Packs." *Salud Pública de México* 52 (Suppl 2): S226–32.

Heran, B. S., J. M. Chen, S. Ebrahim, T. Moxham, N. Oldridge, and others. 2011. "Exercise-Based Cardiac Rehabilitation for Coronary Heart Disease." *Cochrane Database of Systematic Reviews* 7: CD001800. doi:10.1002/14651858 .CD001800.pub2.

Higashi, H., K. D. Truong, J. J. Barendregt, P. K. Nguyen, M. L. Vuong, and others. 2011. "Cost Effectiveness of Tobacco Control Policies in Vietnam: The Case of Population-Level Interventions." *Applied Health Economics and Health Policy* 9 (3): 183–96. doi:10.2165/11539640-000000000-00000.

Ho, P. M., C. L. Bryson, and J. S. Rumsfeld. 2009. "Medication Adherence: Its Importance in Cardiovascular Outcomes." *Circulation* 119 (23): 3028–35. doi:10.1161/CIRCULATIONAHA .108.768986.

Hodge, A. M., G. K. Dowse, H. Gareeboo, J. Tuomilehto, K. G. Alberti, and P. Z. Zimmet. 1996. "Incidence, Increasing Prevalence, and Predictors of Change in Obesity and Fat Distribution over 5 Years in the Rapidly Developing Population of Mauritius." *International Journal of Obesity and Related Metabolic Disorders* 20 (2): 137–46.

Huffman, M. D., A. Baldridge, G. S. Bloomfield, L. D. Colantonio, P. Prabhakaran, and others. 2013. "Global Cardiovascular Research Output, Citations, and Collaborations: A Time-Trend, Bibliometric Analysis (1999–2008)." *PLoS One* 8 (12): e83440. doi:10.1371/journal.pone.0083440.

Huffman, M. D., K. D. Rao, A. Pichon-Riviere, D. Zhao, S. Harikrishnan, and others. 2011. "A Cross-Sectional Study of the Microeconomic Impact of Cardiovascular Disease Hospitalization in Four Low- and Middle-Income Countries." *PLoS One* 6 (6): e20821. doi:10.1371/journal.pone.0020821.

Huffman, M. D., G. A. Roth, K. Sliwa, C. W. Yancy, and D. Prabhakaran. 2017. "Heart Failure." In *Disease Control Priorities* (third edition): Volume 5, *Cardiovascular, Respiratory, and Related Disorders,* edited by D. Prabhakaran, S. Anand, T. A. Gaziano, J.-C. Mbanya, Y. Wu, and R. Nugent. Washington, DC: World Bank.

Huffman, M. D., and S. Yusuf. 2014. "Polypills: Essential Medicines for Cardiovascular Disease Secondary Prevention?" *Journal of the American College of Cardiology* 63 (14): 1368–70. doi:10.1016/j.jacc.2013.08.1665.

Hughes, J. R., L. F. Stead, J. Hartmann-Boyce, K. Cahill, and T. Lancaster. 2014. "Antidepressants for Smoking Cessation." *Cochrane Database of Systematic Reviews* 1: CD000031. doi:10.1002/14651858.CD000031.pub4.

IHME (Institute for Health Metrics and Evaluation). 2013. *The Global Burden of Disease: Generating Evidence, Guiding Policy—Latin America and Caribbean Regional Edition.* Seattle, WA: IHME.

Jafar, T. H., B. A. Haaland, A. Rahman, J. A. Razzak, M. Bilger, and others. 2013. "Non-Communicable Diseases and Injuries in Pakistan: Strategic Priorities." *The Lancet* 381 (9885): 2281–90. doi:10.1016/S0140-6736(13)60646-7.

Jafar, T. H., Z. Qadri, and N. Chaturvedi. 2008. "Coronary Artery Disease Epidemic in Pakistan: More Electrocardiographic Evidence of Ischaemia in Women Than in Men." *Heart* 94 (4): 408–13. doi:10.1136/hrt.2007.120774.

Jha, P., and F. J. Chaloupka. 2000. "The Economics of Tobacco Control." *BMJ* 321 (7257): 358–61.

Jha, P., J. Moore, V. Gajalakshmi, P. C. Gupta, and others. 2006. "Tobacco Addiction." In *Disease Control Priorities in Developing Countries* (second edition), edited by D. T. Jamison, J. Breman, A. R. Measham, G. Alleyne, M. Claeson, D. B. Evans, P. Jha, A. Mills, and P. Musgrove. Washington, DC: World Bank and Oxford University Press.

Jha, P., and R. Peto. 2014. "Global Effects of Smoking, of Quitting, and of Taxing Tobacco." *New England Journal of Medicine* 370 (1): 60–68. doi:10.1056/NEJMra1308383.

Jha, P., M. K. Ranson, S. N. Nguyen, and D. Yach. 2002. "Estimates of Global and Regional Smoking Prevalence in 1995, by Age and Sex." *American Journal of Public Health* 92 (6): 1002–6.

Jeemon, P., R. Gupta, C. Onen, A. Adler, T. A. Gaziano, and others. 2017. "Management of Hypertension and Dyslipidemia for Primary Prevention of Cardiovascular Disease." In *Disease Control Priorities* (third edition): Volume 5, *Cardiovascular, Respiratory, and Related Conditions*, edited by D. Prabhakaran, S. Anand, T. A. Gaziano, J-C. Mbanya, Y. Wu, and R. Nugent. Washington, DC: World Bank.

John, R. M. 2008. "Price Elasticity Estimates for Tobacco Products in India." *Health Policy and Planning* 23 (3): 200–09. doi:10.1093/heapol/czn007.

Joshi, R., C. K. Chow, P. K. Raju, R. Raju, K. S. Reddy, and others. 2009. "Fatal and Nonfatal Cardiovascular Disease and the Use of Therapies for Secondary Prevention in a Rural Region of India." *Circulation* 119 (14): 1950–55. doi:10.1161/CIRCULATIONAHA.108.819201.

Kaplan, W. A., L. S. Ritz, M. Vitello, and V. J. Wirtz. 2012. "Policies to Promote Use of Generic Medicines in Low and Middle Income Countries: A Review of Published Literature, 2000–2010." *Health Policy* 106 (3): 211–24. doi:10.1016/j.healthpol.2012.04.015.

Kaplan, W. A., V. J. Wirtz, and P. Stephens. 2013. "The Market Dynamics of Generic Medicines in the Private Sector of 19 Low and Middle Income Countries between 2001 and 2011: A Descriptive Time Series Analysis." *PLoS One* 8 (9): e74399. doi:10.1371/journal.pone.0074399.

Kerry, V. B., and K. Lee. 2007. "TRIPS, the Doha Declaration and Paragraph 6 Decision: What Are the Remaining Steps for Protecting Access to Medicines?" *Globalization and Health* 3: 3. doi:10.1186/1744-8603-3-3.

Kotseva, K., D. Wood, G. De Backer, D. De Bacquer, K. Pyörälä, and others. 2009. "EUROASPIRE III: A Survey on the Lifestyle, Risk Factors and Use of Cardioprotective Drug Therapies in Coronary Patients from 22 European Countries." *European Journal of Cardiovascular Prevention and Rehabilitation* 16 (2): 121–37. doi:10.1097/HJR.0b013e3283294b1d.

Kramer, J. M., L. K. Newby, W. C. Chang, R. J. Simes, F. Van de Werf, and others. 2003. "International Variation in the Use of Evidence-Based Medicines for Acute Coronary Syndromes." *European Heart Journal* 24 (23): 2133–41.

Kristensen, S. D., K. G. Laut, J. Fajadet, Z. Kaifoszova, P. Kala, and others. 2014. "Reperfusion Therapy for ST Elevation Acute Myocardial Infarction 2010/2011: Current Status in 37 ESC Countries." *European Heart Journal* 35 (29): 1957–70. doi:10.1093/eurheartj/eht529.

Kruk, M. E., E. Goldmann, and S. Galea. 2009. "Borrowing and Selling to Pay for Health Care in Low- and Middle-Income Countries." *Health Affairs* 28 (4): 1056–66. doi:10.1377/hlthaff.28.4.1056.

Kumar, A., and C. P. Cannon. 2009a. "Acute Coronary Syndromes: Diagnosis and Management, Part I." *Mayo Clinic Proceedings* 84 (10): 917–38. doi:10.1016/S0025-6196(11)60509-0.

———. 2009b. "Acute Coronary Syndromes: Diagnosis and Management, Part II." *Mayo Clinic Proceedings* 84 (11): 1021–36. doi:10.1016/S0025-6196(11)60674-5.

Kumbhani, D. J., G. C. Fonarow, C. P. Cannon, A. F. Hernandez, E. D. Peterson, and others. 2013. "Predictors of Adherence to Performance Measures in Patients with Acute Myocardial Infarction." *American Journal of Medicine* 126 (1): 74.e1–9. doi:10.1016/j.amjmed.2012.02.025.

Kuntz, K. M., J. Tsevat, L. Goldman, and M. C. Weinstein. 1996. "Cost-Effectiveness of Routine Coronary Angiography after Acute Myocardial Infarction." *Circulation* 94 (5): 957–65.

Kupersmith, J., M. Holmes-Rovner, A. Hogan, D. Rovner, and J. Gardine. 1995. "Cost-Effectiveness Analysis in Heart Disease, Part III: Ischemia, Congestive Heart Failure, and Arrhythmias." *Progress in Cardiovascular Diseases* 37 (5): 307–46.

Kuppermann, M., B. R. Luce, B. McGovern, P. J. Podrid, J. T. Bigger, and others. 1990. "An Analysis of the Cost Effectiveness of the Implantable Defibrillator." *Circulation* 81 (1): 91–100.

Laba, T.-L., J. Bleasel, J.-A. Brien, A. Cass, K. Howard, and others. 2013. "Strategies to Improve Adherence to Medications for Cardiovascular Diseases in Socioeconomically Disadvantaged Populations: A Systematic Review." *International Journal of Cardiology* 167 (6): 2430–40. doi:10.1016/j.ijcard.2013.01.049.

Leive, A., and K. Xu. 2008. "Coping with Out-of-Pocket Health Payments: Empirical Evidence from 15 African Countries." *Bulletin of the World Health Organization* 86 (11): 849–56. http://www.pubmedcentral.nih.gov/articlerender.fcgi?artid=2649544&tool=pmcentrez&rendertype=abstract.

Libby, P. 2013. "Mechanisms of Acute Coronary Syndromes and Their Implications for Therapy." *New England Journal of Medicine* 368 (21): 2004–13. doi:10.1056/NEJMra1216063.

Lim, S. S., T. Vos, A. D. Flaxman, G. Danaei, K. Shibuya, and others. 2012. "A Comparative Risk Assessment of Burden of Disease and Injury Attributable to 67 Risk Factors and Risk Factor Clusters in 21 Regions, 1990–2010: A Systematic Analysis for the Global Burden of Disease Study 2010."

The Lancet 380 (9859): 2224–60. doi:10.1016/S0140-6736(12)61766-8.

Lonn, E., J. Bosch, K. K. Teo, P. Pais, D. Xavier, and others. 2010. "The Polypill in the Prevention of Cardiovascular Diseases: Key Concepts, Current Status, Challenges, and Future Directions." *Circulation* 122 (20): 2078–88. doi:10.1161/CIRCULATIONAHA.109.873232.

Lozano, R., M. Naghavi, K. Foreman, S. Lim, K. Shibuya, and others. 2012. "Global and Regional Mortality from 235 Causes of Death for 20 Age Groups in 1990 and 2010: A Systematic Analysis for the Global Burden of Disease Study 2010." *The Lancet* 380 (9859): 2095–128. doi:10.1016/S0140-6736(12)61728-0.

Lu, H. T., and R. Bin Nordin. 2013. "Ethnic Differences in the Occurrence of Acute Coronary Syndrome: Results of the Malaysian National Cardiovascular Disease (NCVD) Database Registry (March 2006–February 2010)." *BMC Cardiovascular Disorders* 13 (97). doi:10.1186/1471-2261-13-97.

Lybecker, K. M., and E. Fowler. 2009. "Compulsory Licensing in Canada and Thailand: Comparing Regimes to Ensure Legitimate Use of the WTO Rules." *Journal of Law, Medicine and Ethics* 37 (2): 222–39. doi:10.1111/j.1748-720X.2009.00367.x.

Madan, K., A. S. Babu, A. Contractor, J. P. S. Sawhney, D. Prabhakaran, and others. 2014. "Cardiac Rehabilitation in India." *Progress in Cardiovascular Diseases* 56 (5): 543–50. doi:10.1016/j.pcad.2013.11.001.

Magee, M., M. Ali, D. Prabhakaran, V. S. Ajay, and K. M. Venkat Narayan. 2017. "Integrated Public Health and Health Service Delivery for Noncommunicable Diseases and Comorbid Infectious Diseases and Mental Health." In *Disease Control Priorities* (third edition): Volume 5, *Cardiovascular, Respiratory, and Related Conditions*, edited by D. Prabhakaran, S. Anand, T. A. Gaziano, J-C. Mbanya, Y. Wu, and R. Nugent. Washington, DC: World Bank.

Maguire, T. A., J. C. McElnay, and A. Drummond. 2001. "A Randomized Controlled Trial of a Smoking Cessation Intervention Based in Community Pharmacies." *Addiction* 96 (2): 325–31. doi:10.1080/09652140020021062.

Malik, V. S., and F. B. Hu. 2017. "Obesity Prevention." In *Disease Control Priorities* (third edition): Volume 5, *Cardiovascular, Respiratory, and Related Disorders*, edited by D. Prabhakaran, S. Anand, T. A. Gaziano, J.-C. Mbanya, Y. Wu, and R. Nugent. Washington, DC: World Bank.

Mandelzweig, L., A. Battler, V. Boyko, H. Bueno, N. Danchin, and others. 2006. "The Second Euro Heart Survey on Acute Coronary Syndromes: Characteristics, Treatment, and Outcome of Patients with ACS in Europe and the Mediterranean Basin in 2004." *European Heart Journal* 27 (19): 2285–93. doi:10.1093/eurheartj/ehl196.

Mathers, C. D., and D. Loncar. 2006. "Projections of Global Mortality and Burden of Disease from 2002 to 2030." *PLoS Medicine* 3 (11): e442. doi:10.1371/journal.pmed.0030442.

Mauss, S., F. Berger, G. Schmutz, J. Henke, and W. O. Richter. 2008. "Lipoprotein(a) in Patients Initiating Antiretroviral Therapy." *HIV Medicine* 9 (6): 415–20. doi:10.1111/j.1468-1293.2008.00574.x.

Megiddo, I., S. Chatterjee, A. Nandi, and R. Laxminarayan. 2014. "Cost-Effectiveness of Treatment and Secondary Prevention of Acute Myocardial Infarction in India: A Modeling Study." *Global Heart* 9 (4): 391–98.e3. doi:10.1016/j.gheart.2014.07.002.

Mendis, S., D. Abegunde, S. Yusuf, S. Ebrahim, G. Shaper, and others. 2005. "WHO Study on Prevention of REcurrences of Myocardial Infarction and StrokE (WHO-PREMISE)." *Bulletin of the World Health Organization* 83 (11): 820–29. doi:/S0042-96862005001100011.

Mendis, S., K. Fukino, A. Cameron, R. Laing, A. Filipe, and others. 2007. "The Availability and Affordability of Selected Essential Medicines for Chronic Diseases in Six Low- and Middle-Income Countries." *Bulletin of the World Health Organization* 85 (4): 279–88.

Miller, G., S. Randolph, E. Forkner, B. Smith, and A. D. Galbreath. 2009. "Long-Term Cost-Effectiveness of Disease Management in Systolic Heart Failure." *Medical Decision Making* 29 (3): 325–33. doi:10.1177/0272989X08327494.

Mirzaei, M., A. S. Truswell, R. Taylor, and S. R. Leeder. 2009. "Coronary Heart Disease Epidemics: Not All the Same." *Heart* 95 (9): 740–46. doi:10.1136/hrt.2008.154856.

Mohanan, P. P., R. Mathew, S. Harikrishnan, M. N. Krishnan, G. Zachariah, and others. 2013. "Presentation, Management, and Outcomes of 25,748 Acute Coronary Syndrome Admissions in Kerala, India: Results from the Kerala ACS Registry." *European Heart Journal* 34 (2): 121–29. doi:10.1093/eurheartj/ehs219.

Mokdad, A. H., S. Jaber, M. I. A. Aziz, F. AlBuhairan, A. AlGhaithi, and others. 2014. "The State of Health in the Arab World, 1990–2010: An Analysis of the Burden of Diseases, Injuries, and Risk Factors." *The Lancet* 383 (9914): 309–20. doi:10.1016/S0140-6736(13)62189-3.

Moore, D., P. Aveyard, M. Connock, D. Wang, A. Fry-Smith, and others. 2009. "Effectiveness and Safety of Nicotine Replacement Therapy Assisted Reduction to Stop Smoking: Systematic Review and Meta-Analysis." *BMJ* 338: b1024.

Moran, A. E., M. H. Forouzanfar, G. A. Roth, G. A. Mensah, M. Ezzati, and others. 2014a. "The Global Burden of Ischemic Heart Disease in 1990 and 2010: The Global Burden of Disease 2010 Study." *Circulation* 129 (14): 1493–501. doi:10.1161/CIRCULATIONAHA.113.004046.

Moran, A. E., M. H. Forouzanfar, G. A. Roth, G. A. Mensah, M. Ezzati, and others. 2014b. "Temporal Trends in Ischemic Heart Disease Mortality in 21 World Regions, 1980 to 2010: The Global Burden of Disease 2010 Study." *Circulation* 129 (14): 1483–92. doi:10.1161/CIRCULATIONAHA.113.004042.

Moran, A. E., K. Y. Tzong, M. H. Forouzanfar, G. A. Rothy, G. A. Mensah, and others. 2014. "Variations in Ischemic Heart Disease Burden by Age, Country, and Income: The Global Burden of Diseases, Injuries, and Risk Factors 2010 Study." *Global Heart* 9 (1): 91–99. doi:10.1016/j.gheart.2013.12.007.

Murphy, A., A. Mahal, E. Richardson, and A. E. Moran. 2013. "The Economic Burden of Chronic Disease Care Faced by Households in Ukraine: A Cross-Sectional Matching Study of Angina Patients." *International Journal for Equity in Health* 12: 38. doi:10.1186/1475-9276-12-38.

Murray, C. J. L., and A. D. Lopez. 2013. "Measuring the Global Burden of Disease." *New England Journal of Medicine* 369 (5): 448–57. doi:10.1056/NEJMra1201534.

Murray, C. J. L., T. Vos, R. Lozano, M. Naghavi, A. D. Flaxman, and others. 2012. "Disability-Adjusted Life Years (DALYs) for 291 Diseases and Injuries in 21 Regions, 1990–2010: A Systematic Analysis for the Global Burden of Disease Study 2010." *The Lancet* 380 (9859): 2197–223. doi:10.1016/S0140-6736(12)61689-4.

Myers, L., and S. Mendis. 2014. "Cardiovascular Disease Research Output in WHO Priority Areas between 2002 and 2011." *Journal of Epidemiology and Global Health* 4 (1): 23–28. doi:10.1016/j.jegh.2013.09.007.

Nazzal, N. C., T. P. Campos, H. R. Corbalán, Z. F. Lanas, J. Bartolucci, and others. 2008. "The Impact of Chilean Health Reform on the Management and Mortality of ST Elevation Myocardial Infarction (STEMI) in Chilean Hospitals." *Revista Médica de Chile* 136 (10): 1231–39. doi:/S0034-98872008001000001.

Ng, M., M. K. Freeman, T. D. Fleming, M. Robinson, L. Dwyer-Lindgren, and others. 2014. "Smoking Prevalence and Cigarette Consumption in 187 Countries, 1980–2012." *Journal of the American Medical Association* 311 (2): 183–92. doi:10.1001/jama.2013.284692.

Nielsen, K., C. N. Mock, M. Joshipura, A. M. Rubiano, A. Zakariah, and others. 2012. "Assessment of the Status of Prehospital Care in 13 Low- and Middle-Income Countries." *Prehospital Emergency Care* 16 (3): 381–89. doi:10.3109/10903127.2012.664245.

Oberg, M., M. S. Jaakkola, A. Woodward, A. Peruga, and A. Prüss-Ustün. 2011. "Worldwide Burden of Disease from Exposure to Second-Hand Smoke: A Retrospective Analysis of Data from 192 Countries." *The Lancet* 377 (9760): 139–46. doi:10.1016/S0140-6736(10)61388-8.

Ohman, E. M. 2016. "Chronic Stable Angina." *New England Journal of Medicine* 374: 1167–76.

Orlandini, A., R. Díaz, D. Wojdyla, K. Pieper, F. Van de Werf, and others. 2006. "Outcomes of Patients in Clinical Trials with ST-Segment Elevation Myocardial Infarction among Countries with Different Gross National Incomes." *European Heart Journal* 27 (5): 527–33. doi:10.1093/eurheartj/ehi701.

Pagidipati, N. J., and T. A. Gaziano. 2013. "Estimating Deaths from Cardiovascular Disease: A Review of Global Methodologies of Mortality Measurement." *Circulation* 127 (6): 749–56. doi:10.1161/CIRCULATIONAHA.112.128413.

Palacios, R., I. Alonso, A. Hidalgo, I. Aguilar, M. A. Sánchez, and others. 2008. "Peripheral Arterial Disease in HIV Patients Older Than 50 Years of Age." *AIDS Research and Human Retroviruses* 24 (8): 1043–46. doi:10.1089/aid.2008.0001.

Patel, V., D. Chisholm, T. Dua, R. Laxminarayan, and M. E. Medina-Mora, eds. 2015. *Disease Control Priorities* (third edition): Volume 4, *Mental, Neurological, and Substance Use Disorders*. Washington, DC: World Bank.

Pell, J. P., S. Haw, S. Cobbe, D. E. Newby, A. C. H. Pell, and others. 2008. "Smoke-Free Legislation and Hospitalizations for Acute Coronary Syndrome." *New England Journal of Medicine* 359 (5): 482–91. doi:10.1056/NEJMsa0706740.

Piano, M. R., N. L. Benowitz, G. A. Fitzgerald, S. Corbridge, J. Heath, and others. 2010. "Impact of Smokeless Tobacco Products on Cardiovascular Disease: Implications for Policy, Prevention, and Treatment; A Policy Statement from the American Heart Association." *Circulation* 122 (15): 1520–44. doi:10.1161/CIR.0b013e3181f432c3.

Poggio, R., F. Augustovsky, J. Caporale, V. Irazola, and S. Miriuka. 2012. "Cost-Effectiveness of Cardiac Resynchronization Therapy: Perspective from Argentina." *International Journal of Technology Assessment in Health Care* 28 (4): 429–35. doi:10.1017/S0266462312000505.

Potter, B., M. Weinstein, and T. A. Gaziano. 2013. "Effect of the Rate of Rescue PCI after Thrombolysis on the Cost-Effectiveness of Acute STEMI Management Strategies in Non-Urban Communities." Poster presented at the 35th Annual Meeting of the Society for Medical Decision Making, Baltimore, MD, October 22.

Ranasinghe, I., Y. Rong, X. Du, Y. Wang, R. Gao, and others. 2014. "System Barriers to the Evidence-Based Care of Acute Coronary Syndrome Patients in China: Qualitative Analysis." *Circulation* 7 (2): 209–16. doi:10.1161/CIRCOUTCOMES.113.000527.

Reddy, K. S., D. Prabhakaran, P. Jeemon, K. R. Thankappan, P. Joshi, and others. 2007. "Educational Status and Cardiovascular Risk Profile in Indians." *Proceedings of the National Academy of Sciences of the United States of America* 104 (41): 16263–68. doi:10.1073/pnas.0700933104.

Ribeiro, A. L. P., S. P. L. Gagliardi, J. L. S. Nogueira, L. M. Silveira, E. A. Colosimo, and others. 2006. "Mortality Related to Cardiac Surgery in Brazil, 2000–2003." *Journal of Thoracic and Cardiovascular Surgery* 131 (4): 907–79. doi:10.1016/j.jtcvs.2005.11.022.

Ribeiro, R. A., S. F. Stella, S. A. Camey, L. I. Zimerman, M. Pimentel, and others. 2010. "Cost-Effectiveness of Implantable Cardioverter-Defibrillators in Brazil: Primary Prevention Analysis in the Public Sector." *Value in Health* 13 (2): 160–68. doi:10.1111/j.1524-4733.2009.00608.x.

Rossouw, J. E., P. L. Jooste, D. O. Chalton, E. R. Jordaan, M. L. Langenhoven, and others. 1993. "Community-Based Intervention: The Coronary Risk Factor Study (CORIS)." *International Journal of Epidemiology* 22 (3): 428–38.

Roth, G. A., G. Nguyen, M. H. Forouzanfar, A. H. Mokdad, M. Naghavi, and others. 2015. "Estimates of Global and Regional Premature Cardiovascular Mortality in 2025." *Circulation* 132: 1270–82.

Roy, A., I. Rawal, S. Jabbour, and D. Prabhakaran. 2017. "Tobacco and Cardiovascular Disease: A Summary of Evidence." In *Disease Control Priorities* (third edition): Volume 5, *Cardiovascular, Respiratory, and Related Disorders*, edited by D. Prabhakaran, S. Anand, T. A. Gaziano, J-C. Mbanya, Y. Wu, and R. Nugent. Washington, DC: World Bank.

Ruger, J. P., and C. M. Lazar. 2012. "Economic Evaluation of Pharmaco- and Behavioral Therapies for Smoking Cessation: A Critical and Systematic Review of Empirical Research." *Annual Review of Public Health* 33: 279–305. doi:10.1146/annurev-publhealth-031811-124553.

Saffer, H., and F. Chaloupka. 2000. "The Effect of Tobacco Advertising Bans on Tobacco Consumption." *Journal of Health Economics* 19 (6): 1117–37.

Safraj, S., V. S. Ajay, and D. Prabhakaran. 2013. "Heart Failure: Meeting the Challenges of Surveillance and Knowledge Translation in Resource-Poor Settings." *Current Cardiology Reviews* 9 (2): 99–101.

Sampson, U. K. A., F. G. R. Fowkes, N. G. Naidoo, and M. H. Criqui. 2017. "Peripheral Artery Disease." In *Disease Control Priorities* (third edition): Volume 5, *Cardiovascular, Respiratory, and Related Disorders*, edited by D. Prabhakaran, S. Anand, T. A. Gaziano, J-C. Mbanya, Y. Wu, and R. Nugent. Washington, DC: World Bank.

Sanz, G., and V. Fuster. 2009. "Fixed-Dose Combination Therapy and Secondary Cardiovascular Prevention: Rationale, Selection of Drugs and Target Population." *Nature Clinical Practice Cardiovascular Medicine* 6 (2): 101–10. doi:10.1038/ncpcardio1419.

Schieber, G. J., P. Gottret, L. K. Fleisher, and A. A. Leive. 2007. "Financing Global Health: Mission Unaccomplished." *Health Affairs* 26 (4): 921–34. doi:10.1377/hlthaff.26.4.921.

Schiele, F., M. Hochadel, M. Tubaro, N. Meneveau, W. Wojakowski, and others. 2010. "Reperfusion Strategy in Europe: Temporal Trends in Performance Measures for Reperfusion Therapy in ST-Elevation Myocardial Infarction." *European Heart Journal* 31 (21): 2614–24. doi:10.1093/eurheartj/ehq305.

Shanmugasegaram, S., C. Perez-Terzic, X. Jiang, and S. L. Grace. 2014. "Cardiac Rehabilitation Services in Low- and Middle-Income Countries: A Scoping Review." *Journal of Cardiovascular Nursing* 29 (5): 454–63. doi:10.1097/JCN.0b013e31829c1414.

Shimony, A., S. M. Grandi, L. Pilote, L. Joseph, J. O'Loughlin, and others. 2014. "Utilization of Evidence-Based Therapy for Acute Coronary Syndrome in High-Income and Low/Middle-Income Countries." *American Journal of Cardiology* 113 (5): 793–97. doi:10.1016/j.amjcard.2013.11.024.

Sikri, N., and A. Bardia. 2007. "A History of Streptokinase Use in Acute Myocardial Infarction." *Texas Heart Institute Journal* 34 (3): 318–27.

Smith, R. D., K. Lee, and N. Drager. 2009. "Trade and Health: An Agenda for Action." *The Lancet* 373 (9665): 768–73. doi:10.1016/S0140-6736(08)61780-8.

Smith, T., L. Jordaens, D. A. M. J. Theuns, P. F. van Dessel, A. A. Wilde, and others. 2013. "The Cost-Effectiveness of Primary Prophylactic Implantable Defibrillator Therapy in Patients with Ischaemic or Non-Ischaemic Heart Disease: A European Analysis." *European Heart Journal* 34 (3): 211–19. doi:10.1093/eurheartj/ehs090.

Srimahachota, S., S. Boonyaratavej, R. Kanjanavanit, P. Sritara, R. Krittayaphong, and others. 2012. "Thai Registry in Acute Coronary Syndrome (TRACS): An Extension of Thai Acute Coronary Syndrome Registry (TACS) Group: Lower In-Hospital but Still High Mortality at One-Year." *Journal of the Medical Association of Thailand* 95 (4): 508–18.

Stead, L. F., R. Perera, C. Bullen, D. Mant, and T. Lancaster. 2008. "Nicotine Replacement Therapy for Smoking Cessation." *Cochrane Database of Systematic Reviews* (1): CD000146. doi:10.1002/14651858.CD000146.pub3.

Steg, P. G., R. J. Goldberg, J. M. Gore, K. A. A. Fox, K. A. Eagle, and others. 2002. "Baseline Characteristics, Management Practices, and In-Hospital Outcomes of Patients Hospitalized with Acute Coronary Syndromes in the Global Registry of Acute Coronary Events (GRACE)." *American Journal of Cardiology* 90 (4): 358–63.

Strickberger, S. A., J. Conti, E. G. Daoud, E. Havranek, M. R. Mehra, and others. 2005. "Patient Selection for Cardiac Resynchronization Therapy: From the Council on Clinical Cardiology Subcommittee on Electrocardiography and Arrhythmias and the Quality of Care and Outcomes Research Interdisciplinary Working Group, in Collaboration with the Heart Rhythm Society." *Circulation* 111 (16): 2146–50. doi:10.1161/01.CIR.0000161276.09685.4A.

Suhrcke, M., T. A. Boluarte, and L. Niessen. 2012. "A Systematic Review of Economic Evaluations of Interventions to Tackle Cardiovascular Disease in Low- and Middle-Income Countries." *BMC Public Health* 12: 2–13. doi:10.1186/1471-2458-12-2.

Tajouri, T. H., S. L. Driver, and D. R. Holmes. 2014. "'Take as Directed'—Strategies to Improve Adherence to Cardiac Medication." *Nature Reviews Cardiology* 11 (5): 304–7. doi:10.1038/nrcardio.2013.208.

Thavorn, K., and N. Chaiyakunapruk. 2008. "A Cost-Effectiveness Analysis of a Community Pharmacist–Based Smoking Cessation Programme in Thailand." *Tobacco Control* 17 (3): 177–82. doi:10.1136/tc.2007.022368.

Thom, S., N. Poulter, J. Field, A. Patel, D. Prabhakaran, and others. 2013. "Effects of a Fixed-Dose Combination Strategy on Adherence and Risk Factors in Patients with or at High Risk of CVD: The UMPIRE Randomized Clinical Trial." *Journal of the American Medical Association* 310 (9): 918–29. doi:10.1001/jama.2013.277064.

Thygesen, K., J. S. Alpert, A. S. Jaffe, M. L. Simoons, B. R. Chaitman, and others. 2012. "Third Universal Definition of Myocardial Infarction." *Journal of the American College of Cardiology* 60 (16): 1581–98. doi:10.1016/j.jacc.2012.08.001.

Tollman, S. M., K. Kahn, B. Sartorius, M. A. Collinson, S. J. Clark, and others. 2008. "Implications of Mortality Transition for Primary Health Care in Rural South Africa: A Population-Based Surveillance Study." *The Lancet* 372 (9642): 893–901. doi:10.1016/S0140-6736(08)61399-9.

Townsend, J. 1993. "Policies to Halve Smoking Deaths." *Addiction* 88 (1): 37–46.

Uusitalo, U., E. J. Feskens, J. Tuomilehto, G. Dowse, U. Haw, and others. 1996. "Fall in Total Cholesterol Concentration over Five Years in Association with Changes in Fatty Acid Composition of Cooking Oil in Mauritius: Cross Sectional Survey." *BMJ* 313 (7064): 1044–46.

van Mourik, M. S. M., A. Cameron, M. Ewen, and R. O. Laing. 2010. "Availability, Price and Affordability of Cardiovascular Medicines: A Comparison across 36 Countries Using WHO/HAI Data." *BMC Cardiovascular Disorders* 10: 25. doi:10.1186/1471-2261-10-25.

Viswanathan, M., C. E. Golin, C. D. Jones, M. Ashok, S. J. Blalock, and others. 2012. "Interventions to Improve Adherence to

Self-Administered Medications for Chronic Diseases in the United States: A Systematic Review." *Annals of Internal Medicine* 157 (11): 785–95. doi:10.7326/0003-4819-157-11-201212040-00538.

Wakefield, M. A., L. Hayes, S. Durkin, and R. Borland. 2013. "Introduction Effects of the Australian Plain Packaging Policy on Adult Smokers: A Cross-Sectional Study." *BMJ Open* 3 (7). doi:10.1136/bmjopen-2013-003175.

Wald, N. J., and M. R. Law. 2003. "A Strategy to Reduce Cardiovascular Disease by More Than 80%." *BMJ* 326 (7404): 1419. doi:10.1136/bmj.326.7404.1419.

Wang, M., A. E. Moran, J. Lu, P. G. Coxson, P. A. Heidenreich, and others. 2014. "Cost-Effectiveness of Optimal Use of Acute Myocardial Infarction Treatments and Impact on Coronary Heart Disease Mortality in China." *Circulation: Cardiovascular Quality and Outcomes* 7 (1): 78–85. doi:10.1161/CIRCOUTCOMES.113.000674.

Weinstein, M. C., and W. B. Stason. 1985. "Cost-Effectiveness of Interventions to Prevent or Treat Coronary Heart Disease." *Annual Review of Public Health* 6: 41–63. doi:10.1146/annurev.pu.06.050185.000353.

WHO (World Health Organization). 2013. "WHO Model List of Essential Medicines." Geneva, WHO. http://www.who.int/iris/bitstream/10665/93142/1/EML_18_eng.pdf?ua=1.

Xavier, D., P. Pais, P. J. Devereaux, C. Xie, D. Prabhakaran, and others. 2008. "Treatment and Outcomes of Acute Coronary Syndromes in India (CREATE): A Prospective Analysis of Registry Data." *The Lancet* 371 (9622): 1435–42. doi:10.1016/S0140-6736(08)60623-6.

Xu, K., D. B. Evans, K. Kawabata, R. Zeramdini, J. Klavus, and others. 2003. "Household Catastrophic Health Expenditure: A Multicountry Analysis." *The Lancet* 362 (9378): 111–17. doi:10.1016/S0140-6736(03)13861-5.

Yan, L. L., C. Li, J. Chen, R. Luo, J. Bettger, and others. 2017. "Stroke." In *Disease Control Priorities* (third edition): Volume 5, *Cardiovascular, Respiratory, and Related Disorders*, edited by D. Prabhakaran, S. Anand, T. A. Gaziano, J-C. Mbanya, Y. Wu, and R. Nugent. Washington, DC: World Bank.

Yang, G., Y. Wang, Y. Zeng, G. F. Gao, X. Liang, and others. 2013. "Rapid Health Transition in China, 1990–2010: Findings from the Global Burden of Disease Study 2010." *The Lancet* 381 (9882): 1987–2015. doi:10.1016/S0140-6736(13)61097-1.

Yusuf, S., S. Islam, C. K. Chow, S. Rangarajan, G. Dagenais, and others. 2011. "Use of Secondary Prevention Drugs for Cardiovascular Disease in the Community in High-Income, Middle-Income, and Low-Income Countries (the PURE Study): A Prospective Epidemiological Survey." *The Lancet* 378 (9798): 1231–43. doi:10.1016/S0140-6736(11)61215-4.

Yusuf, S., P. Pais, R. Afzal, D. Xavier, K. Teo, and others. 2009. "Effects of a Polypill (Polycap) on Risk Factors in Middle-Aged Individuals without Cardiovascular Disease (TIPS): A Phase II, Double-Blind, Randomised Trial." *The Lancet* 373 (9672): 1341–51. doi:10.1016/S0140-6736(09)60611-5.

Zhang, X.-H., Z. L. Lu, and L. Liu. 2008. "Coronary Heart Disease in China." *Heart* 94 (9): 1126–31. doi:10.1136/hrt.2007.132423.

Zubaid, M., W. A. Rashed, W. Almahmeed, J. Al-Lawati, K. Sulaiman, and others. 2009. "Management and Outcomes of Middle Eastern Patients Admitted with Acute Coronary Syndromes in the Gulf Registry of Acute Coronary Events (Gulf RACE)." *Acta Cardiologica* 64 (4): 439–46.

Zwisler, A.-D. O., A. M. B. Soja, S. Rasmussen, M. Frederiksen, S. Abedini, and others. 2008. "Hospital-Based Comprehensive Cardiac Rehabilitation versus Usual Care among Patients with Congestive Heart Failure, Ischemic Heart Disease, or High Risk of Ischemic Heart Disease: 12-Month Results of a Randomized Clinical Trial." *American Heart Journal* 155 (6): 1106–13. doi:10.1016/j.ahj.2007.12.033.

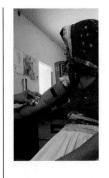

Chapter **9**

Stroke

Lijing L. Yan, Chaoyun Li, Jie Chen, Rong Luo, Janet Bettger,
Yishan Zhu, Valery Feigin, Martin O'Donnell,
J. Jaime Miranda, Dong Zhao, and Yangfeng Wu

INTRODUCTION

According to the World Health Organization's Global Health Estimates, stroke was the second-leading cause of death and the third-leading cause of disability-adjusted life years (DALYs) lost globally in 2012. In certain low- and middle-income countries (LMICs), such as China, the disease burden of stroke increased significantly over the past two decades, accounting for the most years of life lost in 2010. This chapter—the first on stroke in the history of the *Disease Control Priorities* publications—presents evidence on the disease burden of stroke, describing the epidemiology, disability, and socioeconomic burdens, then discusses modifiable and other risk factors for stroke. The chapter describes primary prevention, treatment, and management of stroke during the acute phase as well as secondary prevention and rehabilitation, with a focus on cost-effective strategies in LMICs, where such evidence exists. The chapter concludes with recommendations for policy makers and future research directions.

There are two main types of stroke—ischemic, including transient ischemic attack, and hemorrhagic, including intracerebral and subarachnoid. The term *stroke* refers to all subtypes. The two main subtypes are distinguished from one another when appropriate because the etiology and management of these subtypes can be very different. Within the hemorrhagic subtype, we focus mainly on intracerebral hemorrhage, given that subarachnoid hemorrhage occurs spontaneously, usually from a ruptured cerebral aneurysm, or results from a head injury.

DISEASE BURDEN

Existing Evidence

In 2010, there were 16.9 million cases of incident stroke; an additional 33 million stroke survivors were alive worldwide, more than half of them in LMICs (Feigin and others 2014). A systematic review of 12 population-based studies from 10 LMICs and 44 studies from 18 high-income countries (HICs) found significant disparities in stroke incidence trends between HICs and LMICs. Over the past four decades, stroke incidence decreased 42 percent in HICs but increased more than 100 percent in LMICs. From 2000 to 2008, estimated stroke incidence rates in LMICs surpassed those in HICs by approximately 20 percent (Feigin and others 2009).

Stroke mortality was highest in Central, Southeast, and East Asia; Central and Eastern Europe; and central Sub-Saharan Africa; it was lowest in HICs, Latin America, western Sub-Saharan Africa, and South Asia (map 9.1) (Feigin and others 2014). However, estimated mortality may be unreliable because few LMICs have the necessary funding and resources either to establish surveillance networks or to register data on stroke mortality.

Corresponding author: Yangfeng Wu, The George Institute for Global Health at Peking University Health Science Center; Department of Epidemiology and Biostatistics, Peking University School of Public Health, Beijing, China; ywu@georgeinstitute.org.cn.

Map 9.1 Age-Standardized Stroke Mortality per 100,000 Population, 2010

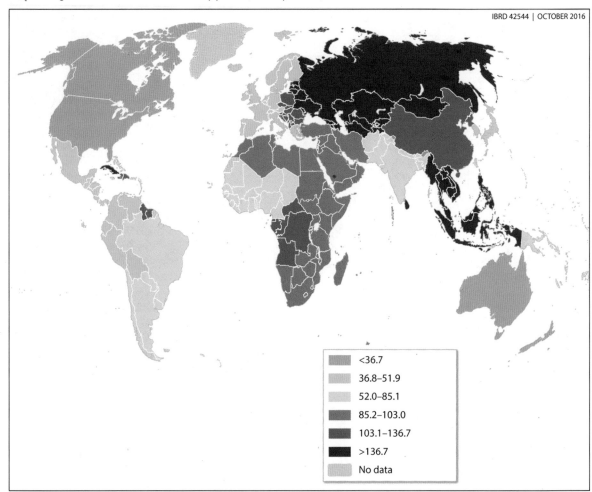

IBRD 42544 | OCTOBER 2016

	<36.7
	36.8–51.9
	52.0–85.1
	85.2–103.0
	103.1–136.7
	>136.7
	No data

Source: Feigin and others 2014.

Projections indicate that stroke incidence, mortality, and DALYs will continue to rise in LMICs and that by 2030 there will be almost 12 million stroke deaths, 70 million stroke survivors, and more than 200 million DALYs lost globally each year. The heavy and increasing global burden of stroke reflects a pressing need for well-designed and comparable surveillance systems to track current trends and for prevention, treatment, and management programs to curb and treat strokes worldwide, especially in LMICs.

Impact on Disability

Disability often persists for a long time, sometimes permanently, after a stroke. According to an international survey of 11 sites in seven LMICs, stroke is the fourth-largest contributor to disability among people older than age 65 years (Sousa and others 2009).

Yet the impact of stroke on disability could be underestimated because the impact of limb paralysis or weakness is not accounted for and the extent of cognitive impairment is not always fully assessed.

SOCIAL AND ECONOMIC BURDEN

Stroke results in substantial social and economic burdens around the world. The burden on caregivers is increasingly recognized as a significant health problem. Caregiving has been linked to higher rates of depression, anxiety, cardiovascular disease (CVD), general ill health, and mortality.

The economic burden of stroke is also significant. An international comparison of cost studies showed that national health systems spent, on average, 0.27 percent of gross domestic product on stroke and that stroke care accounted for about 3 percent of total health care expenditures (Evers and others 2004). In the United States in 2008, the total direct and indirect costs of stroke were estimated to be US$65.5 billion (Rosamond and others 2008). In the 27 European Union countries, the total annual costs of stroke were estimated to be US$35.8 billion: US$24.6 billion (68.5 percent) for direct and US$11.3 billion (31.5 percent) for indirect costs (Allender, Scarborough, and Peto 2008). In China, the average cost for a stroke admission in 2004 was twice the annual income of rural residents, and the cost of stroke care for government-funded hospitals increased 117 percent annually between 2003 and 2007. The current literature provides no comprehensive analysis of the economic burden of stroke in LMICs, but it is reasonable to assume that it will continue to rise if current trends in stroke incidence and mortality persist and if prevention and control efforts are not intensified.

RISK FACTORS

Increased stroke incidence is associated with aging and urbanization and propelled by the increasing prevalence of key modifiable risk factors, especially in LMICs.

Modifiable Risk Factors

The INTERSTROKE Study, a large international case-control study of risk factors for incidence of stroke in 22 countries, including LMICs, found evidence of 10 significant modifiable risk factors, including history of hypertension, current smoking, diabetes mellitus, waist-to-hip ratio, diet risk score, physical inactivity, alcohol intake, psychosocial stress and depression, cardiac causes, and ratio of apolipoproteins B to A1 (O'Donnell and others 2010). All 10 risk factors were significant predictors of ischemic stroke; hypertension, smoking, waist-to-hip ratio, diet, and alcohol intake were significant predictors of hemorrhagic stroke. Table 9.1 summarizes evidence-based estimates of relative risks, odds ratios, and hazard ratios associated with risk factors for stroke.

High Blood Pressure

High blood pressure is the leading risk factor for stroke, accounting for an estimated 52 percent of all stroke deaths (O'Donnell and others 2010). Lower blood pressure is associated not only with a lower risk of stroke, but also with a lower risk of reoccurrence among stroke survivors.

Table 9.1 Relative Risks, Odds Ratios, or Hazard Ratios of Risk Factors for Stroke

Risk factor	Reference	Type of study	Results
High blood pressure	Di Legge and others 2012	Review	A close, progressive, and approximately linear relationship exists between blood pressure levels and primary incidence of stroke.
	Prospective Studies Collaboration 1995	Review	A fivefold difference in stroke risk exists between the highest blood pressure categories (usual diastolic blood pressure of 102 mmHg) and the lowest ones (usual diastolic blood pressure of 75 mmHg).
	Lewington and others 2002	Meta-analysis	At ages 40–69 years, each difference of 20 mmHg in usual systolic blood pressure is associated with a more than twofold difference in the stroke death rate.
	Asia Pacific Cohort Studies Collaboration 1998	Cohort studies	Each 5 mmHg lower increment of usual diastolic blood pressure is associated with lower risk of both nonhemorrhagic (odds ratio of 0.61; 95% CI, 0.57–0.66) and hemorrhagic stroke (odds ratio of 0.54; 95% CI, 0.50–0.58).
Tobacco use	Thun and others 2013	Cohort studies	In contemporary cohorts, male and female current smokers have similar relative risks for death from stroke (1.92 for men and 2.10 for women).
	Jha and others 2013	Cohort study	Adjusted hazard ratios for death from stroke among current smokers compared with persons who never smoked is 3.2 (99% CI, 2.2–4.7) for women and 1.7 (99% CI, 1.0–2.8) for men.
	Shah and Cole 2010	Review	Current smokers have at least a two- to fourfold higher risk of stroke than lifelong nonsmokers or individuals who have not smoked for more than 10 years.

table continues next page

Table 9.1 Relative Risks, Odds Ratios, or Hazard Ratios of Risk Factors for Stroke (continued)

Risk factor	Reference	Type of study	Results
Diabetes mellitus	Luitse and others 2012	Review	People with diabetes have more than double the risk of ischemic stroke relative to individuals without diabetes.
	Banerjee and others 2012	Cohort study	Compared with nondiabetic participants, those with diabetes for 0–5 years (adjusted hazard ratio of 1.7), 5–10 years (1.8), and more than 10 years (3.2) are at increased risk of ischemic stroke.
Diet and nutrition	Sharma and others 2013	Cohort study	High consumption of fruits and vegetables is associated with lower risk of stroke; adherence to the U.S. Department of Agriculture dietary recommendations for vegetable intake among women is associated with a reduced risk of fatal stroke, although this result is not statistically significant (relative risk of 0.84; 95% CI, 0.68–1.04).
	He and others 1999	Cohort study	Among overweight persons, a 100 mmol higher sodium intake is associated with a 32% increase (relative risk of 1.32; 95% CI, 1.07–1.64) in stroke incidence and 89% increase (relative risk of 1.89; 95% CI, 1.31–2.74) in stroke mortality.
	Nagata and others 2004	Cohort study	Associations between sodium intake and death from ischemic stroke are significantly positive (hazard ratio of 3.22; 95% CI, 1.22–8.53).
Overweight and obesity	Yan and others 2006	Cohort study	Overweight and obesity increases the risk of stroke not only through its impacts on other risk factors but also independently.
Physical activity	Lee, Folsom, and Blair 2003	Meta-analysis	Highly active individuals have a 27% lower risk of stroke incidence or mortality (relative risk of 0.73; 95% CI, 0.67–0.79) than less-active individuals, with moderately active individuals compared with inactive persons (relative risks were 0.83 [95% CI, 0.76–0.89] for cohort, 0.52 [95% CI, 0.40–0.69] for case control, and 0.80 [95% CI, 0.74–0.86] for the two combined).
Age	Manolio and others 1996	Cohort study	Risk of stroke approximately doubles for each successive decade of life after age 65.
Gender	Reeves and others 2008	Review	Women have more stroke events because of their longer life expectancy and older age at the time of stroke onset; stroke-related outcomes, including disability and quality of life, are poorer in women than in men.
	Appelros, Stegmayr, and Terent 2009	Systematic review	Stroke is more common among men, but women become more severely ill; incidence and prevalence rates of men are 33% and 41% higher, respectively, than those of women; stroke is more severe in women, with a case fatality at one month of 24.7% compared with 19.7% for men.
Atrial fibrillation	Wolf, Abbott, and Kannel 1991	Cohort study (Framingham Study)	In persons with coronary heart disease or cardiac failure, atrial fibrillation doubles the stroke risk in men and trebles the risk in women; in older patients ages 80–89 years, the attributable risk of stroke from atrial fibrillation is 23.5%.

Note: CI = confidence interval; mmHG = millimeters of mercury, a measure of pressure; mmol = millimoles.

Tobacco Use

Smoking is an independent and important risk factor for both ischemic and hemorrhagic stroke in all regions, with a stronger association with incident ischemic stroke. Smokers have stroke risk two times higher than non-smokers. Cigarette smoking accounts for 12 percent to 14 percent of all stroke deaths. In addition to smoking, exposure to environmental tobacco smoke—secondhand or passive smoking—is also a substantial risk factor for stroke.

Diabetes Mellitus

Diabetes is a well-recognized independent risk factor for stroke and also a strong predictor of worse long-term outcomes of stroke. Diabetes increases the risk of ischemic stroke more than hemorrhagic stroke, resulting in a higher ratio of ischemic to hemorrhagic stroke in people with diabetes compared with the general population. The duration of diabetes is also an important factor contributing to the risk of stroke. In addition, a prediabetic state is associated with increased stroke risk.

Diet and Nutrition

Adequate consumption of fruits and vegetables—at least five servings a day—is associated with lower risk of stroke, a relationship consistent across ethnic groups. Minerals such as sodium and potassium also affect the risk of stroke. Excess sodium intake is considered the greatest factor leading to high blood pressure. Despite ongoing controversies regarding whether low salt intake (less than 3 grams per day) is a health risk (O'Donnell and others 2014) and the lack of direct trial data on sodium and hard outcomes (for example, mortality or morbidity), studies have shown that higher levels of sodium intake are associated with a higher risk of stroke, and higher levels of potassium intake are associated with a lower risk of stroke (He and others 1999; Nagata and others 2004). Other dietary factors, such as moderation of alcohol intake and vegetarian diets, may affect the risk of stroke, but the evidence is insufficient to make specific recommendations.

Overweight and Obesity

Overweight and obesity are risk factors for many chronic conditions, including stroke. Higher body mass index, a common measure of overweight and obesity, has been shown to increase the risk of stroke independently as well as through its impact on other risk factors such as blood pressure and lipids (Yan and others 2006).

Physical Activity

Physical inactivity is associated with numerous adverse health effects, including stroke. A large and generally consistent body of evidence from prospective observational studies indicates that routine physical activity can prevent stroke (Lee, Folsom, and Blair 2003). The benefits can be obtained from a variety of activities, including leisure time physical activity, occupational activity, and walking. Overall, the relationship between activity and stroke is not influenced by gender or age.

OTHER RISK FACTORS

In addition to modifiable risk factors, factors such as age, gender, and race or ethnicity are related to hereditary or natural processes and cannot be modified. The cumulative effects of aging on the cardiovascular system and the progressive nature of stroke risk factors over a prolonged period substantially increase the risks of both ischemic and hemorrhagic stroke. Men and women have significantly different risks for the incidence, mortality, severity, and recovery from stroke. Worldwide, stroke is more common in men than in women, but the difference tends to decrease with age. Some systematic reviews have reported that stroke-related outcomes, including disability and quality of life, are consistently poorer in women than in men and that case fatality at one month is higher among women (Appelros, Stegmayr, and Terent 2009).

Atrial fibrillation is the most common cardiac rhythm abnormality among adults and accounts for 20 percent of all ischemic strokes. One of the complications of atrial fibrillation is the development of thromboembolism leading to stroke. A pooled analysis of atrial fibrillation studies suggests that paroxysmal atrial fibrillation carries risk of stroke similar to the risk from sustained atrial fibrillation (Laupacis and others 1994).

Many studies have investigated novel factors for stroke, including hyperhomocysteinemia, obstructive sleep apnea, air pollution, psychosocial factors such as depression and stress, and genetic factors. These factors are not discussed further in this chapter because of lack of conclusive evidence.

PREVENTION AND TREATMENT OF STROKE

Stroke prevention and control involve surveillance, screening, diagnosis, primary and secondary prevention, management in the acute phase, and poststroke rehabilitation. Innovative system-based solutions beyond these approaches, such as task-shifting and task-sharing, are needed to achieve better prevention and control. These solutions are discussed in detail in chapters 16 and 17 of this volume (Magee and others 2017; Joshi and others 2017).

Surveillance, Screening, and Diagnosis

Surveillance

Few LMICs have the necessary funding and resources either to establish surveillance networks or to register data for detecting health trends in the population. The World Health Organization recommends a stepwise stroke surveillance approach (STEPS Stroke) for collecting data and monitoring trends. STEPS Stroke recommends collecting three types of data: information on stroke patients admitted to heath facilities (step 1), number of fatal stroke events in the community (step 2), and estimated number of nonfatal stroke events in the community (step 3). A study synthesizing STEPS Stroke surveillance in nine sites in India, the Islamic Republic of Iran, Mozambique, Nigeria, and the Russian Federation showed that STEPS Stroke surveillance is possible and feasible in low-resource settings (Truelsen and others 2007).

Screening

Screening for stroke risk factors provides an excellent opportunity to identify and educate persons at high risk.

It usually includes surveys of demographic and lifestyle information; blood pressure measurement; carotid bruit detection; cholesterol measurement; blood glucose tests; and education on warning signs or symptoms, such as transient ischemic attack, and heart-related symptoms, such as atrial fibrillation.

Similar to surveillance initiatives, a stepwise approach is suggested for screening. At a most basic level, screening for risk factors may include collection of information on demographics and lifestyle, such as diet, physical activity, and smoking or alcohol use. A second tier of screening might include data obtained from physical examination, including height, weight, girth, and blood pressure measurements. A final tier might include laboratory measures, such as blood glucose and cholesterol levels. In resource-poor settings, where clinical tests may be inaccessible and unaffordable, patient history and physical examinations are more cost-effective than laboratory measures (Olson and Roth 2007).

Congleton, Small, and Freeman (2013) report that in eastern North Carolina, where previous stroke mortality had been 12 percent higher than in the rest of the state, stroke prevalence and mortality declined after approximately 4,900 community outreach risk factor screenings were conducted between 2007 and 2011. The cost-effectiveness of national stroke screening has not been analyzed comprehensively in LMICs, but it is reasonable to assume that targeted or opportunistic screening would decrease the stroke burden in LMICs. China launched the Stroke Screening, Prevention, and Treatment Project in 2009 to establish a nationwide stroke screening network consisting of nearly 140 stroke screening centers in selected hospitals, aiming to standardize evidence-based stroke care throughout China and explore the need to establish an electronic national stroke registry. However, many LMICs have no stroke screening projects, which is likely attributable to limited resources and lack of awareness of the benefits of screening.

Diagnosis

The American Heart Association and the American Stroke Association introduced best-practice guidelines for stroke diagnosis that include patient history, physical examination, neurological examination and use of stroke scales, and diagnostic tests. Neurological examinations should be performed if patient history and physical examination are suggestive of a stroke, and the National Institutes of Health Stroke Scale or other standardized stroke scales can assist in estimating the severity of stroke. Brain imaging can distinguish ischemic stroke from intracranial hemorrhage and identify the subtype of stroke and often its cause; vascular imaging may identify the site and cause of arterial obstruction and also identify patients at high risk of stroke recurrence. Computed tomography (CT) scanning, magnetic resonance imaging, Doppler ultrasound, CT angiography, and magnetic resonance angiography are widely used in HICs to determine the subtypes and causes of stroke.

The most widely used strategy for stroke diagnosis is immediate CT scanning. However, the expense of CT equipment for health care facilities and the cost of individual use of CT scanning for patients are still high for low-resource countries and areas. Moreover, CT scanning is not sensitive for old hemorrhage, a condition that requires the use of other technologies such as magnetic resonance imaging and digital subtraction angiography, which may not be available in resource-poor countries. The need to develop and distribute accessible, inexpensive, and reliable diagnostic equipment and technologies continues to present a growing challenge to LMICs.

Primary Prevention

The main primary preventive approaches for stroke are the promotion and maintenance of a healthy lifestyle and blood pressure control. A healthy lifestyle includes not smoking (and stopping smoking for smokers); not engaging in binge drinking; being physically active; and eating a healthy diet characterized by adequate intake of fruits and vegetables, reduced intake of dietary trans fat, and reduced intake of sodium. Prevention strategies for CVD may target persons at high risk or whole populations. Although clinical guidelines recommend targeting persons at high risk as the primary strategy, most CVD events occur in individuals who are at low to moderate absolute risk of CVD; therefore, prevention strategies based on the high-risk approach might have a limited impact on reducing stroke risk in populations. Which strategy is more cost-effective remains debatable, and a more sensible approach may be a combination of the two.

Tobacco Control

Tobacco control is ranked as the most important of five priority interventions for preventing noncommunicable diseases (Beaglehole and others 2011). According to a microsimulation model based on Indian data, smoke-free legislation and tobacco taxation in combination could avert 25 percent of myocardial infarction and stroke if the effects of the interventions were additive (Basu and others 2013). These approaches are likely to be more effective than brief cessation advice provided by health care providers, mass media campaigns, and advertising bans. Cessation advice is considered the least-effective strategy at the population level.

High Blood Pressure Prevention and Control

Reducing blood pressure has been demonstrated to reduce the risk of stroke effectively. In a meta-analysis of 11 clinical trials on reducing blood pressure and stroke among Asian populations, a 10 millimeters of mercury (mmHg) reduction in systolic blood pressure was associated with a 30 percent reduction in risk of stroke, regardless of the antihypertensive agent used (renin-angiotensin blockers, calcium-channel blockers, or diuretics) (Yano and others 2013). Another meta-analysis involving 19 trials indicated that a 7 mmHg and 5 mmHg reduction in systolic and diastolic blood pressure, respectively, reduced the relative risk of stroke by 22 percent (Xie and others 2015).

All clinical guidelines and expert consensus statements on prevention of stroke place great emphasis on preventing and controlling high blood pressure. Both a health care provider–centered high-risk approach as well as population-based measures for preventing hypertension in the general population are needed. Many LMICs, such as Brazil, China, Mexico, and Thailand, have initiated nationwide programs for preventing and managing high blood pressure through a combination of public health, clinical, and health system approaches. Both monitoring and evaluation of the long-term cost-effectiveness of these programs are necessary, as are developing and refining evidence-based, feasible, sustainable, and specific measures to guide their implementation.

Sodium Reduction

A particularly cost-effective strategy for reducing blood pressure is to reduce sodium intake. Achievement of actual and sustained reduction in sodium intake remains a challenge for both researchers and policy makers because of the well-established difficulty of changing lifelong dietary habits. More emphasis is needed on programs that discourage younger generations from establishing high-sodium dietary patterns earlier in life.

The use of low-sodium high-potassium salt substitutes, a safe product commercially available for many years, remains useful for circumventing the need to change dietary habits. In HICs, more than 70 percent of sodium intake comes from processed prepackaged food; persons in HICs probably would not benefit from the use of salt substitutes as much as persons in LMICs, where the majority of sodium intake comes from salt added during cooking. A meta-analysis of six clinical trials found that salt substitutes reduce systolic blood pressure by an average of 4.9 mmHg and diastolic blood pressure by 1.5 mmHg in adults, compared with salt (Peng and others 2014). These trials on salt substitutes—to be substantiated in the future by larger trials on hard outcomes, such as a trial of 21,000 patients currently under way in rural China—suggest that a policy of subsidizing and promoting salt substitutes may be useful for reducing sodium intake, blood pressure, and stroke incidence in LMICs.

Pharmaceutical Treatments

In addition to lifestyle modifications, another mainstay strategy for primary prevention of stroke is the use of pharmaceutical means to address hypertension, dyslipidemia (high cholesterol), and atrial fibrillation. The most compelling evidence—from multiple randomized clinical trials or meta-analyses—recommends treating hypertensive patients primarily with thiazide-type diuretics, as well as angiotensin-converting enzyme inhibitors, angiotensin II receptor blockers, beta blockers, calcium channel blockers, or a combination, with the aim of achieving blood pressure goals set in the eighth report of the Joint National Committee on Prevention, Detection, Evaluation, and Treatment of High Blood Pressure (James and others 2014). In patients with coronary heart disease or diabetes, the recommended treatment is a 3-hydroxy-3-methyl-glutaryl coenzyme-A reductase inhibitor (statin) medication, with the aim of reaching low-density lipoprotein–cholesterol goals set in the National Cholesterol Education Program guidelines (Expert Panel on Detection, Evaluation, and Treatment of High Blood Cholesterol in Adults 2001). In contrast, intensive glucose therapy in patients with type 2 diabetes did not significantly reduce the incidence of stroke or other macrovascular events, according to the ACCORD or ADVANCE trials (ADVANCE Collaborative Group and others 2008).

The awareness, treatment, and control rates of hypertension and statin use in LMICs are universally lower than in HICs. To close the gap between guidelines and practice, LMICs need to find innovative and effective strategies for overcoming many health system and socioeconomic barriers, such as the prevalence of curative, acute care–oriented systems with limited resources and capacity, to improve identification of those at risk and to develop more comprehensive medication formularies on public and private health and pharmacy insurance plans.

Polypill Use

Polypill was originally proposed in the early 2000s and is estimated to have reduced ischemic heart disease events and stroke by more than 70 percent each as, respectively, either a secondary prevention drug among persons with vascular disease (Yusuf 2002) or as a primary prevention measure (Wald and Law 2003). The concept of a fixed-dose combination drug has been controversial since its inception and sparked many debates and several clinical trials intended to test the efficacy of polypill in similar but slightly different formulations. Trials (TIPS, UMPIRE, and IMPACT) conducted in India, New Zealand, and three European countries (Ireland, the Netherlands, and the United Kingdom) focused on improving risk factors (Mohan 2009; Selak and others 2011; Thom and others 2013). Their results showed smaller-than-theorized improvements in blood pressure and lipid levels, but the relative and absolute benefits of polypill on clinical outcomes are likely to be larger in high-risk than in low-risk subgroups. However, the differences are not statistically significant.

Although these initial results are not as promising as expected, controversies regarding polypill are likely to continue given its multifaceted appeal for overcoming the problems of polypharmacy, low cost, and large anticipated effects. At the same time, unresolved issues with polypill include the need to define its optimal components and to evaluate the pharmacodynamics and pharmacokinetics of a multiple-component formulation. Ongoing and future trials and hard outcomes are needed to establish safety and effectiveness. The cost-effectiveness of such a strategy in LMICs also needs to be established. Meanwhile, a balanced view regarding its role in the primary prevention of stroke is warranted. Polypill use should not lead to reduced emphasis on healthy lifestyle measures because these are the mainstays of stroke prevention.

Atrial Fibrillation Control

Prevention is one of the best protections against stroke caused by recurrent atrial fibrillation. Antiplatelet compounds such as aspirin are indicated for atrial fibrillation patients with a low to moderate risk of thrombosis and can reduce the risk of stroke from atrial fibrillation by 20 percent to 25 percent. Anticoagulation using vitamin K antagonists (most commonly warfarin in the United States and some other countries and acenocoumarol and phenprocoumon in Europe) has been the treatment of choice for preventing embolic events in patients with atrial fibrillation and a moderate to high risk of thrombosis, reducing the risk of stroke by up to 62 percent (Finsterer and Stollberger 2008). However, warfarin has significant limitations, including bleeding, need for continued follow-up blood tests, and drug-drug interactions. Although newer anticoagulants such as rivaroxaban and dabigatran have been developed, they potentially cause significant bleeding.

Because of their limitations, effective use of warfarin or other anticoagulants has faced many barriers,

especially in LMICs. In health resource–limited settings such as China, new oral anticoagulants were not found to be cost-effective because of their high price. The left atrial appendage is the site of thrombus formation in the majority of strokes associated with atrial fibrillation. Closure or exclusion of the left atrial appendage has emerged as an alternative therapeutic approach to medical therapy, but its safety and effectiveness are yet to be fully established.

Community-Based Education

Community education encompasses all approaches that are concerned with screening, awareness raising, health education on risk factors, ways to reduce disease risks, and other health-promotion activities conducted in communities. A systematic review of peer-reviewed articles published between 1999 and 2006 on the topic of public education for stroke prevention included 32 studies on educational programs. Seven educational programs were judged successful using the evaluation criteria. They included two large-scale programs and five narrowly targeted programs (Wilson and others 2007). A community-based intervention trial was conducted in two communities (one intervention, one control) in three cities in China. Regular health education and health-promotion activities were conducted between 1991 and 2000 in the intervention communities, but no special action was taken in the control communities. Over the 10 years of the intervention, incident risk of strokes decreased by 11.4 percent, 13.2 percent, and 7.2 percent, respectively, in the three intervention communities compared with controls (Wang and Shuaib 2007).

Digital Health Strategies

Digital health is a promising field that involves the use of new information and communication technologies to improve health care management for both providers and patients. So far, no clear consensus has emerged regarding its terminology or definition. Other terminology includes e-Health, telemedicine, and mHealth. In this chapter, digital health is used to encompass all related terms.

Digital health is often associated with improved clinical decision making and increased efficiency for health care providers. For example, electronic health records, which are replacing traditional paper-based health records, integrate and organize patient health information so that every health provider involved in a patient's care can have the same accurate and up-to-date information.

The growing global burden of stroke requires innovative, effective, and widely available strategies for stroke prevention. Mobile technologies, such as the recently introduced Stroke Riskometer application (app), offer an opportunity to address these issues (Feigin and Norrving 2014; Parmar and others 2015). Digital health makes it possible to individualize interventions for physical activity and dietary behavior change. Some digital health apps have already been developed to address stroke prevention, based on the Framingham Heart Study stroke prediction algorithm; these apps have been enhanced by data on major risk factors for stroke. Users can identify their personal risk factors, their absolute risk of stroke, and their relative risk compared with persons of the same age and gender; knowledge of one's relative risk may be more motivating for behavior change than knowledge of absolute risk. Digital health programs in LMICs have the potential to expand access to prevention and treatment services by using ubiquitous and low-cost communication infrastructure. However, more research on the effectiveness of digital health and best strategies for implementation is needed to harness its potential for stroke prevention and control.

Cost-Effectiveness

Few cost-effectiveness studies compare multiple prevention strategies in LMICs. A review of nine studies that evaluated 14 comparative strategies for CVD (both heart disease and stroke) in Argentina concluded that salt reduction in breads, antihypertensive treatment, mass educational campaigns, and polypill strategies could be considered cost-effective. However, the authors cautioned that the economic evidence available to guide CVD resource allocation in Argentina seems to be limited (Colantonio, Marti, and Rubinstein 2010).

Treatment during the Acute Stage

Ischemic Stroke

The evidence regarding treatment in the acute stage of stroke is limited and based on a few small randomized trials, extrapolation of results from larger trials, and two well-conducted nonrandomized studies (Rothwell, Algra, and Amarenco 2011). A combination of preventive treatments (antiplatelet agents, antihypertensive treatment and statins, and anticoagulation and carotid endarterectomy, as appropriate) started quickly in specialist units appears to be effective.

Carotid endarterectomy has been shown in randomized trials to be highly effective when done within two weeks after a nondisabling stroke, although there is uncertainty about the safety of the intervention in the first 48 hours. Additionally, two trials with a total of 40,000 randomized patients showed that oral aspirin within 48 hours of onset of major ischemic stroke reduced 14-day morbidity and mortality, mostly by reducing the risk of a

recurrent stroke. However, intensive lowering of blood pressure during the acute phase of ischemic stroke was not found to reduce the risk of recurrent stroke or death.

Intravenous tissue plasminogen activator (tPA), administered within 4.5 hours of symptom onset, is the only therapeutic agent approved for achieving arterial recanalization in acute ischemic stroke. Current major guidelines recommend the use of a standard dose (0.9 milligram per kilogram of body weight; maximum of 90 milligrams) of tPA. However, the recommended dosage of tPA in Asian populations varies, partly influenced by the treatment costs of this expensive medicine and the perceived racial differences in treatment response. In Japan, the only approved dosage of tPA is 0.6 milligram per kilogram of body weight; one of the reasons for using such a low dosage is treatment response. Consensus regarding the optimal dosage of tPA is wanting, and ongoing trials should begin to demonstrate whether low-dose tPA could be effective and for which populations. Based on reported use, tPA for acute ischemic stroke is available to some patients in approximately one-third of countries globally.

Hemorrhagic Stroke

Results of data from 404 hemorrhagic stroke patients showed that early (within six hours of onset) intensive blood pressure–lowering treatment (target systolic blood pressure of 140 mmHg) attenuated hematoma growth for 72 hours. There were no appreciable effects on perihematomal edema (Anderson and others 2010). A larger trial based on 2,794 hemorrhagic stroke patients did not find that intensive lowering of blood pressure within one hour reduced the primary outcome of death or severe disability. Additional analyses indicated improved functional outcomes with intensive lowering of blood pressure (Anderson and others 2010).

Stroke Units

Organized inpatient stroke unit care is provided by multidisciplinary teams that exclusively manage stroke patients in a dedicated ward, with a mobile team, or within a generic disability service (a mixed rehabilitation ward). Stroke units have long been shown to be an effective care-delivery model that improves clinical outcomes for stroke patients. The Stroke Unit Trialists' Collaboration published a series of Cochrane reviews on stroke units. This systematic review of randomized trials in 1997 indicated that stroke patients who were managed in an organized setting (stroke unit) were less likely to die, remain physically dependent, or require long-term institutional care, compared with patients managed in a conventional care setting (Stroke Unit Trialists' Collaboration 1997). Further analyses showed that organized inpatient stroke unit care probably benefited a wide range of stroke patients in a variety of ways—for example, reducing death from secondary complications and reducing the need for institutional care through a reduction in disability. The review, published in 2002 and updated in 2007 and in 2013 (Stroke Unit Trialists' Collaboration 2002, 2007, 2013), concluded that stroke patients who received organized inpatient care in a stroke unit were more likely to be alive, independent, and living at home one year after the stroke. The benefits were most apparent in units based in discrete wards. No systematic increase in the length of inpatient stay was observed. Evidence of care in stroke units is limited in LMICs, where establishing such units is a challenge in itself, possibly due to lack of specialists, capacity, and other system-level barriers. More translational studies are needed to assess whether and how stroke units can be implemented in resource-limited settings.

Secondary Prevention

Secondary prevention of stroke is of particular importance because of the high risk of recurrent stroke, which occurs in approximately a third of stroke survivors in five years. Evidence-based guidelines for secondary prevention stress the benefits of a healthy lifestyle, including a healthy diet, appropriate physical activity, and no smoking, similar to the guidelines described for primary prevention.

Blood Pressure Control

Control of high blood pressure remains the most important strategy for secondary prevention of stroke. Existing evidence shows that lowering blood pressure with lifestyle changes and antihypertensive medicines protects against stroke recurrence. No comprehensive data are available on how well blood pressure treatment has been achieved among stroke patients in LMICs; however, it is intuitively logical that the situation is worse in LMICs than in HICs, because of the higher prevalence of stroke, more limited access to high-quality health care, and lower affordability of medicine, especially in rural areas.

Antiplatelet and Lipid-Lowering Therapies

Antiplatelet and lipid-lowering therapies are effective treatments for secondary prevention of ischemic stroke. Major clinical guidelines for secondary prevention of stroke recommend aspirin as the mainline antiplatelet therapy and statins as lipid-lowering therapy. However, uptake has been low for aspirin and even lower for statins, especially in LMICs. A study of 4,782 ischemic stroke inpatients in urban China in 2006 showed that use of antiplatelet therapy and lipid-lowering therapy declined substantially after discharge, from 81 percent and 31 percent, respectively, in hospital to 66 percent and 17 percent, respectively, a year later. Unlike the controversy surrounding use of polypill for primary prevention, polypill for secondary prevention has special appeal in LMICs because of its relative ease of use, effectiveness, and low cost. How to overcome barriers in its production, distribution, and sustained use by patients is a key issue that needs to be addressed to reap its population-wide benefits.

Homocysteine-Lowering Therapy

Elevated circulating homocysteine level has been postulated as a risk factor for CVD. However, an updated Cochrane review published in 2013 that included 12 trials (4 new trials since the last review in 2009) found no support for homocysteine-lowering therapy in the form of vitamin B6, B9, or B12 supplements, either alone or in combination, for preventing cardiovascular events (Martí-Carvajal and others 2013). The review included 47,429 participants either with or without CVD, suggesting that the finding of lack of effectiveness may apply to both primary and secondary intervention to prevent myocardial infarction and stroke. New trials are underway in China to evaluate the combined effect of folic acid and B vitamins for secondary prevention of stroke.

Surgery for Carotid Stenosis

Surgical interventions for symptomatic or asymptomatic carotid stenosis may be one option for certain patients. The less-invasive carotid artery stenting was not inferior to traditional carotid endarterectomy. However, the cost is much higher for stenting than for endarterectomy. More evidence is needed to determine whether and under what circumstances surgical interventions for carotid stenosis are useful.

Self-Management and Family Support

Community-based self-management intervention—a promising strategy for addressing chronic conditions across the world—emphasizes patient responsibility and action in concert with community health care providers. Self-management in stroke involves conscious efforts by patients themselves to deal with stroke-induced impairments, threat of stroke recurrence, and challenges of long-term recovery. Patients require a combination of information, support, and education about behavior change, tailored to the beliefs, attitudes, and cognitions of those who have had a stroke, their social circles, and health care providers. Three key dimensions affect stroke self-management equally: individual capacity, support for self-management, and self-management environment.

Each component has the potential to facilitate or hinder successful self-management.

Self-management interventions have been demonstrated to reduce the risk of stroke recurrence and to have a positive impact on the use of health care resources, which is of great significance for resource-scarce settings. However, the benefits of self-management are inconclusive. The latest systematic review reported that only six of nine randomized controlled studies and three of six nonrandomized trials found that benefits were associated with poststroke self-management (Lennon, McKenna, and Jones 2013). None of the trials was conducted in LMICs, further limiting conclusions for resource-poor settings.

Between 25 percent and 74 percent of stroke survivors require help with daily living activities from informal caregivers, often family members. Results from the London Stroke Carers Training Course (LSCTC), which is a systematic, structured, training program delivered in a stroke unit for caregivers, showed a reduction in caregiver burden, anxiety, and depression and an improvement in psychological outcomes for patients, when compared with usual care. However, the Training Programme for Caregivers of Inpatients after Stroke, a large-scale, robust trial, showed no significant differences between the LSCTC and usual care on any of the assessed outcomes. Currently, the RECOVER (clinicaltrials.gov registration number NCT02247921) and ATTEND (trial registration number ACTRN12613000078752) trials are being implemented in China and India to determine whether stroke recovery care at home given by a trained family member is an effective, affordable strategy for persons who have suffered a disabling stroke. The results of these two trials will provide strong evidence on the effects of caregiver training programs in LMICs.

Rehabilitation

Although stroke is experienced as an acute event, stroke survivors live with long-term consequences and often manage their resulting limitations and health status as a chronic condition. As the population of elderly stroke survivors increases, and the number of survivors with disability and chronic care needs grows, rehabilitation care and therapy will play an increasingly important role. Stroke rehabilitation can be provided in inpatient, home, and community-based programs and may include physical, occupational, speech, and recreational therapies. The availability of and access to rehabilitation services and care for patients making the transition from acute care hospitalization varies dramatically around the globe, especially in LMICs. Factors contributing to the limited availability and accessibility of rehabilitation services include poor physician knowledge of the role of rehabilitation; lack of a rehabilitation component in the standard of care; long interval from stroke onset to admission to rehabilitation; infrequent, unskilled, and short-lived provision of rehabilitation care; and inadequate public insurance or financial support for rehabilitation care. This section discusses both care delivery and discipline-specific rehabilitation interventions. Table 9.2 summarizes various models of care delivery currently in practice.

Table 9.2 Models of Care Delivery for Stroke Rehabilitation

Model of care delivery	Description	General evidence	LMIC relevance and evidence	Evidence gap
Stroke unit	Provided in hospitals by nurses, doctors, and therapists specializing in care for stroke patients	Improved likelihood of survival, return home, and independence after a stroke (Stroke Unit Trialists' Collaboration 1997)	None	The extent to which organized stroke unit care is or can be provided globally
Multidisciplinary inpatient rehabilitation services	Therapy and treatment provided primarily to address mobility, self-care, cognition, communication, and mental health before patients return home	Functional improvements from admission to discharge negatively associated with number of days from stroke onset to admission to rehabilitation (Gökkaya and others 2006)	In Thailand, stroke survivors improved in activities of daily living, psychological status, and quality of life (Kuptniratsaikul and others 2009); in China, neurologic function significantly improved (Research Group of the Standardized Tertiary Rehabilitation Program in Cerebral Diseases' Patients 2006).	The effectiveness of task-shifting and cross-training of health care providers to provide rehabilitation therapies

table continues next page

Table 9.2 Models of Care Delivery for Stroke Rehabilitation (continued)

Model of care delivery	Description	General evidence	LMIC relevance and evidence	Evidence gap
Early supported discharge	Supports patients who return home from the hospital earlier than usual with continued care and rehabilitation from teams of therapists, nurses, and doctors in the home	Long-term dependence, admission to institutional care, and length of hospital stay could be reduced with a structured and coordinated model of early supported discharge, especially for stroke patients with mild to moderate disability (Fearon and Langhorne 2012)	Results from pilot studies, including RECOVER and ATTEND trials in China and India, are to be reported.	Implementation and evaluation needed in LMICs
Home- and community-based rehabilitation	Therapy and treatment provided for community-dwelling stroke survivors in or outside the home	Improved and maintained independence in activities of daily living in the year following a stroke (Outpatient Service Trialists 2003)	In the Islamic Republic of Iran, treatment group had better basic and instrumental activities-of-daily-living performance than controls (Sahebalzamani, Aliloo, and Shakibi 2009).	Understanding needed of therapeutic benefit or harm of rehabilitation provided to stroke survivors living at home a year or longer after the stroke
Telerehabilitation	Information technologies used for communications between patients and caregivers in remote locations	No sufficient evidence to draw conclusions on the effectiveness of telerehabilitation on mobility, health-related quality of life, or participant satisfaction with the intervention (Laver and others 2013)	May be especially relevant for LMICs where expertise or resources do not reach the country's borders.	Globally, further assessment needed of feasibility and effectiveness

Note: LMICs = low- and middle-income countries.

Physical, Occupational, or Movement Therapy

Several interventions to improve physical function in the upper or lower limbs and activities of daily living have been studied in LMICs. Studies examining physical therapy in LMICs showed that patient outcomes improved significantly over time, including as measured by the Barthel index, Mini-Mental State Examination, and Stroke Rehabilitation Assessment of Movement. The research to date demonstrates interest in examining the efficacy and effectiveness of physical rehabilitation and medicine; however, studies are often hampered by low quality and significant limitations.

Speech Therapy or Cognitive Rehabilitation

No individual studies were identified for "rehabilitation of speech and language disorders," and systematic reviews have not identified any studies from LMICs that meet inclusion criteria for specific questions related to speech and language or cognition. Given that an estimated 67 percent of stroke patients experience cognitive challenges, such as decreased attention and poor recall, this gap in the evidence requires attention from researchers.

Cost-Effectiveness

Cost-effectiveness studies of rehabilitation services in LMICs are also lacking. Investigators from Thailand reported that the cost of the acute phase of care was higher than that of the subacute phase, with differences by disability level (Khiaocharoen, Pannarunothai, and Zungsontiporn 2012). Compared with conventional hospital care, home-based rehabilitation for ischemic stroke patients resulted in a greater number of patients avoiding disability at a lower cost. Despite large gaps in stroke rehabilitation research, studies have increasingly included rehabilitation outcomes or evaluations of rehabilitation and therapy services. There is also tremendous opportunity in stroke rehabilitation research, and the intersection of disciplines and policy agendas provides the ideal platform for continued growth and success.

CONCLUSIONS AND RECOMMENDATIONS

Over the past two decades, the incidence, prevalence, and mortality rates of stroke declined in most HICs, but rose in LMICs. The absolute number of people annually affected by stroke, living with stroke, and dying from stroke is increasing worldwide. Globally, stroke was the second-leading cause of death and the third-leading cause of DALYs lost in 2010. Major modifiable risk factors for stroke include high blood pressure, tobacco use, diet (high salt intake, in particular), physical inactivity, overweight and obesity, diabetes, and atrial fibrillation.

For stroke prevention and control, evidence shows the following:

- Surveillance to obtain current epidemiological data, screening for risk factors, and accurate diagnoses are important for preventing and controlling stroke. LMICs face challenges in all three activities because of lack of resources, awareness, and technical capacity. Screening is most successful in high-risk groups; its value to risk reduction in the general population is debatable. The development and distribution of accessible (mobile), inexpensive, and reliable diagnostic equipment and technologies is clearly a pressing need in LMICs. Maintaining a healthy lifestyle, such as no tobacco use, a healthy diet, physical activity, and weight control, are important strategies for both primary and secondary prevention of stroke.
- Population-based strategies, such as a tobacco tax, universal sodium reduction, and subsidies for healthy dietary choices such as fruits and vegetables, appear to be cost-effective options for LMICs. These strategies do not rely on screening for high-risk individuals, shift the distribution of risk factors in the population downward, and substantially reduce disease risk. However, no trial evidence or rigorous cost-effectiveness analyses are yet available to support these claims.
- Recent trials of intensive blood pressure control in the acute stage of hemorrhagic stroke found improvements in functional outcomes and health-related quality of life, although the impact on severe disability and death was not significant (Anderson and others 2013). Nevertheless, controlling high blood pressure is critically important for preventing and controlling stroke in general.
- Besides lifestyle modification and blood pressure control, additional primary prevention strategies for stroke include community-based education programs and prevention and management of atrial fibrillation through maintenance of a healthy lifestyle and use of pharmaceuticals, such as anticoagulants.
- Digital health technology, such as tablet-based risk-assessment tools, mobile phone apps for physicians, and text messaging interventions, is a new approach to stroke prevention and control. Many studies on digital health, including some in LMICs,

are ongoing; these studies are expected to provide best evidence on how to use these technological tools for prevention and control of noncommunicable diseases.

- In addition to specific surgical procedures and medications for stroke, organized inpatient stroke care units have repeatedly been found to provide higher-quality care that leads to better patient outcomes.
- Evidence to support the use of the polypill for secondary prevention of stroke (as well as other CVDs) is emerging, although its use for primary prevention remains controversial.
- Patients with chronic conditions like stroke may require lifelong pharmaceutical treatment, lifestyle maintenance and self-management skills, and caregiver and family support skills to achieve optimal health outcomes. Evidence in LMICs is lacking, but it is anticipated that LMICs will face special challenges in this regard because the health literacy and self-efficacy of patients are typically lower.
- Rehabilitation improves physical, speech, and cognitive functioning of patients disabled by stroke. It is not clear which mode of delivery is best for LMICs, but home- or community-based services and telerehabilitation may hold particular promise.
- System-based solutions need to address health system barriers to efficiency and lack of capacity and human resources to prevent and control stroke, as well as address other public health problems. Such solutions are needed to underpin any specific approach. For example, the shifting and sharing of tasks among specialists and community health care workers have received considerable attention as system-based solutions.

Evidence on the cost-effectiveness of specific strategies in LMICs is limited. Nevertheless, prompt attention to and action on what is known—the importance of controlling tobacco use, reducing sodium intake, controlling blood pressure, and promoting a healthy diet and physical activity—will contribute to curbing the rising epidemic of stroke in the coming years.

NOTE

World Bank Income Classifications as of July 2014 are as follows, based on estimates of gross national income (GNI) per capita for 2013:

- Low-income countries (LICs) = US$1,045 or less
- Middle-income countries (MICs) are subdivided:
  (a) lower-middle-income = US$1,046 to US$4,125
  (b) upper-middle-income (UMICs) = US$4,126 to US$12,745
- High-income countries (HICs) = US$12,746 or more.

REFERENCES

ADVANCE Collaborative Group, A. Patel, S. MacMahon, J. Chalmers, B. Neal, and others. 2008. "Intensive Blood Glucose Control and Vascular Outcomes in Patients with Type 2 Diabetes." *New England Journal of Medicine* 358 (24): 2560–72.

Allender, S., P. Scarborough, and V. Peto. 2008. "European Cardiovascular Disease Statistics 2008." European Heart Network, Brussels.

Anderson, C. S., E. Heeley, Y. Huang, J. Wang, C. Stapf, and others. 2013. "Rapid Blood-Pressure Lowering in Patients with Acute Intracerebral Hemorrhage." *New England Journal of Medicine* 368 (25): 2355–65.

Anderson, C. S., Y. Huang, H. Arima, E. Heeley, C. Skulina, and others. 2010. "Effects of Early Intensive Blood Pressure–Lowering Treatment on the Growth of Hematoma and Perihematomal Edema in Acute Intracerebral Hemorrhage: The Intensive Blood Pressure Reduction in Acute Cerebral Haemorrhage Trial (INTERACT)." *Stroke* 41 (2): 307–12.

Appelros, P., B. Stegmayr, and A. Terent. 2009. "Sex Differences in Stroke Epidemiology: A Systematic Review." *Stroke* 40 (4): 1082–90.

Asia Pacific Cohort Studies Collaboration. 1998. "Blood Pressure, Cholesterol, and Stroke in Eastern Asia. Eastern Stroke and Coronary Heart Disease Collaborative Research Group." *The Lancet* 352 (9143): 1801–7.

Banerjee, C., Y. P. Moon, M. C. Paik, T. Rundek, C. Mora-McLaughlin, and others. 2012. "Duration of Diabetes and Risk of Ischemic Stroke: The Northern Manhattan Study." *Stroke* 43 (5): 1212–17.

Basu, S., S. Glantz, A. Bitton, and C. Millett. 2013. "The Effect of Tobacco Control Measures during a Period of Rising Cardiovascular Disease Risk in India: A Mathematical Model of Myocardial Infarction and Stroke." *PLoS Medicine* 10 (7): e1001480.

Beaglehole, R., R. Bonita, R. Horton, C. Adams, G. Alleyne, and others. 2011. "Priority Actions for the Non-Communicable Disease Crisis." *The Lancet* 377 (9775): 1438–47.

Colantonio, L. D., S. G. Marti, and A. L. Rubinstein. 2010. "Economic Evaluations on Cardiovascular Preventive Interventions in Argentina." *Expert Review of Pharmacoeconomics and Outcomes Research* 10 (4): 465–73.

Congleton, T. M., C. W. Small, and S. D. Freeman. 2013. "Stroke Risk Factors Screening and Education: A Regional Strategy to Address Stroke Prevalence and Mortality in Eastern North Carolina." *Stroke* 44 (2 Meeting Abstracts): AWP345.

Di Legge, S., G. Koch, M. Diomedi, P. Stanzione, and F. Sallustio. 2012. "Stroke Prevention: Managing Modifiable Risk Factors." *Stroke Research and Treatment* 2012: 391538.

Evers, S. M., J. N. Struijs, A. J. Ament, M. L. van Genugten, J. H. Jager, and others. 2004. "International Comparison of Stroke Cost Studies." *Stroke* 35 (5): 1209–15.

Expert Panel on Detection, Evaluation, and Treatment of High Blood Cholesterol in Adults. 2001. "Executive Summary of the Third Report of the National Cholesterol Education Program (NCEP) Expert Panel on Detection, Evaluation, and Treatment of High Blood Cholesterol in Adults (Adult Treatment Panel III)." *Journal of the American Medical Association* 285 (19): 2486–97.

Fearon, P., and P. Langhorne. 2012. "Early Supported Discharge Trialists: Services for Reducing Duration of Hospital Care for Acute Stroke Patients." *Cochrane Database of Systematic Reviews* 9: CD000443.

Feigin, V. L., M. H. Forouzanfar, R. Krishnamurthi, G. A. Mensah, and M. Connor. 2014. "Global and Regional Burden of Stroke during 1990–2010: Findings from the Global Burden of Disease Study 2010." *The Lancet* 383 (9913): 245–54.

Feigin, V. L., C. M. Lawes, D. A. Bennett, S. L. Barker-Collo, and V. Parag. 2009. "Worldwide Stroke Incidence and Early Case Fatality Reported in 56 Population-Based Studies: A Systematic Review." *The Lancet Neurology* 8 (4): 355–69.

Feigin, V. L., and B. Norrving. 2014. "A New Paradigm for Primary Prevention Strategy in People with Elevated Risk of Stroke." *International Journal of Stroke* 9 (5): 624–26.

Finsterer, J., and C. Stollberger. 2008. "Strategies for Primary and Secondary Stroke Prevention in Atrial Fibrillation." *Netherlands Journal of Medicine* 66 (8): 327–33.

Gökkaya, N., M. Aras, D. Cardenas, and A. Kaya. 2006. "Stroke Rehabilitation Outcome: The Turkish Experience." *International Journal of Rehabilitation Research* 29 (2): 105–11.

He, J., L. G. Ogden, S. Vupputuri, L. A. Bazzano, C. Loria, and others. 1999. "Dietary Sodium Intake and Subsequent Risk of Cardiovascular Disease in Overweight Adults." *Journal of the American Medical Association* 282 (21): 2027–34.

James, P. A., S. Oparil, B. L. Carter, W. C. Cushman, C. Dennison-Himmelfarb, and others. 2014. "2014 Evidence-Based Guideline for the Management of High Blood Pressure in Adults: Report from the Panel Members Appointed to the Eighth Joint National Committee (JNC 8)." *Journal of the American Medical Association* 311 (5): 507–20.

Jha, P., C. Ramasundarahettige, V. Landsman, B. Rostron, M. Thun, and others. 2013. "21st-Century Hazards of Smoking and Benefits of Cessation in the United States." *New England Journal of Medicine* 368 (4): 341–50.

Joshi, R., A. P. Kengne, F. Hersch, M. B. Weber, H. McGuire, and A. Patel. 2017. "Innovations in Community-Based Health Care for Cardiometabolic and Respiratory Diseases." In *Disease Control Priorities* (third edition): Volume 5, *Cardiovascular, Respiratory, and Related Disorders*, edited by D. Prabhakaran, S. Anand, T. A. Gaziano, J.-C. Mbanya, Y. Wu, and R. Nugent. Washington, DC: World Bank.

Khiaocharoen, O., S. Pannarunothai, and C. Zungsontiporn. 2012. "Cost of Acute and Sub-Acute Care for Stroke Patients." *Journal of the Medical Association of Thailand* 95 (10): 1266–77.

Kuptniratsaikul, V., A. Kovindha, P. Dajpratham, and K. Piravej. 2009. "Main Outcomes of Stroke Rehabilitation: A Multi-Centre Study in Thailand." *Journal of Rehabilitation Medicine* 41 (1): 54–58.

Laupacis, A., G. Boysen, S. Connolly, M. Ezekowitz, R. Hart, and others. 1994. "Risk-Factors for Stroke and Efficacy of Antithrombotic Therapy in Atrial-Fibrillation: Analysis of Pooled Data from 5 Randomized Controlled Trials." *Archives of Internal Medicine* 154 (13): 1449–57.

Laver, K. E., D. Schoene, M. Crotty, S. George, N. A. Lannin, and others. 2013. "Telerehabilitation Services for Stroke." *Cochrane Database of Systematic Reviews* 12: CD010255.

Lee, C. D., A. R. Folsom, and S. N. Blair. 2003. "Physical Activity and Stroke Risk: A Meta-Analysis." *Stroke* 34 (10): 2475–81.

Lennon, S., S. McKenna, and F. Jones. 2013. "Self-Management Programmes for People Post Stroke: A Systematic Review." *Clinical Rehabilitation* 27 (10): 867–78.

Lewington, S., R. Clarke, N. Qizilbash, R. Peto, R. Collins, and others. 2002. "Age-Specific Relevance of Usual Blood Pressure to Vascular Mortality: A Meta-Analysis of Individual Data for One Million Adults in 61 Prospective Studies." *The Lancet* 360 (9349): 1903–13.

Luitse, M. J., G. J. Biessels, G. E. Rutten, and L. J. Kappelle. 2012. "Diabetes, Hyperglycaemia, and Acute Ischaemic Stroke." *The Lancet Neurology* 11 (3): 261–71.

Magee, M., M. Ali, D. Prabhakaran, V. S. Ajay, and K. M. Venkat Narayan. 2017. "Integrated Public Health and Health Service Delivery for Noncommunicable Diseases and Comorbid Infectious Diseases and Mental Health." In *Disease Control Priorities* (third edition): Volume 5, *Cardiovascular, Respiratory, and Related Disorders*, edited by D. Prabhakaran, S. Anand, T. A. Gaziano, J.-C. Mbanya, Y. Wu, and R. Nugent. Washington, DC: World Bank.

Manolio, T. A., R. A. Kronmal, G. L. Burke, D. H. O'Leary, and T. R. Price. 1996. "Short-Term Predictors of Incident Stroke in Older Adults: The Cardiovascular Health Study." *Stroke* 27 (9): 1479–86.

Martí-Carvajal, A. J., I. Solà, D. Lathyris, D.-E. Karakitsiou, and D. Simancas-Racines. 2013. "Homocysteine-Lowering Interventions for Preventing Cardiovascular Events." *Cochrane Database of Systematic Reviews* 4: CD006612.

Mohan, V. 2009. "Effects of a Polypill (Polycap) on Risk Factors in Middle-Aged Individuals without Cardiovascular Disease (TIPS): A Phase II, Double-Blind, Randomised Trial." *The Lancet* 373 (9672): 1341–51.

Nagata, C., N. Takatsuka, N. Shimizu, and H. Shimizu. 2004. "Sodium Intake and Risk of Death from Stroke in Japanese Men and Women." *Stroke* 35 (7): 1543–47.

O'Donnell, M., A. Mente, S. Rangarajan, M. J. McQueen, X. Wang, and others. 2014. "Urinary Sodium and Potassium Excretion, Mortality, and Cardiovascular Events." *New England Journal of Medicine* 371 (7): 612–23.

O'Donnell, M. J., D. Xavier, L. Liu, H. Zhang, S. L. Chin, and others. 2010. "Risk Factors for Ischaemic and Intracerebral Haemorrhagic Stroke in 22 Countries (The INTERSTROKE Study): A Case-Control Study." *The Lancet* 376 (9735): 112–23.

Olson, D. P., and K. E. Roth. 2007. "Diagnostic Tools and the Hands-on Physical Examination." *Virtual Mentor* 9 (2): 113–18.

Outpatient Service Trialists. 2003. "Therapy-Based Rehabilitation Services for Stroke Patients at Home." *Cochrane Database of Systematic Reviews* 1: CD002925.

Parmar, P., R. Krishnamurthi, M. A. Ikram, A. Hofman, S. S. Mirza, and others. 2015. "The Stroke Riskometer (TM) App: Validation of a Data Collection Tool and Stroke Risk Predictor." *International Journal of Stroke* 10 (2): 231–44.

Peng, Y. G., W. Li, X. X. Wen, Y. Li, J. H. Hu, and others. 2014. "Effects of Salt Substitutes on Blood Pressure: A Meta-Analysis of Randomized Controlled Trials." *American Journal of Clinical Nutrition* 100 (6): 1448–54.

Prospective Studies Collaboration. 1995. "Cholesterol, Diastolic Blood Pressure, and Stroke: 13,000 Strokes in 450,000 People in 45 Prospective Cohorts; Prospective Studies Collaboration." *The Lancet* 346 (8991–8992): 1647–53.

Reeves, M. J., C. D. Bushnell, G. Howard, J. W. Gargano, P. W. Duncan, and others. 2008. "Sex Differences in Stroke: Epidemiology, Clinical Presentation, Medical Care, and Outcomes." *The Lancet Neurology* 7 (10): 915–26.

Research Group of the Standardized Tertiary Rehabilitation Program in Cerebral Diseases' Patients. 2006. "Effects Study of Standardized Tertiary Rehabilitation on Promoting of the Neurological Functions in Stroke Patients with Hemiplegia." *Zhonghua yi xue za zhi* 86 (37): 2621.

Rosamond, W., K. Flegal, K. Furie, A. Go, K. Greenlund, and others. 2008. "Heart Disease and Stroke Statistics—2008 Update: A Report from the American Heart Association Statistics Committee and Stroke Statistics Subcommittee." *Circulation* 117 (4): e25–146.

Rothwell, P. M., A. Algra, and P. Amarenco. 2011. "Medical Treatment in Acute and Long-Term Secondary Prevention after Transient Ischaemic Attack and Ischaemic Stroke." *The Lancet* 377 (9778): 1681–92.

Sahebalzamani, M., L. Aliloo, and A. Shakibi. 2009. "The Efficacy of Self-Care Education on Rehabilitation of Stroke Patients." *Saudi Medical Journal* 30 (4): 550–54.

Selak, V., C. R. Elley, S. Crengle, M. Harwood, R. Doughty, and others. 2011. "IMProving Adherence using Combination Therapy (IMPACT): Design and Protocol of a Randomised Controlled Trial in Primary Care." *Contemporary Clinical Trials* 32 (6): 909–15.

Shah, R. S., and J. W. Cole. 2010. "Smoking and Stroke: The More You Smoke the More You Stroke." *Expert Review of Cardiovascular Therapy* 8 (7): 917–32.

Sharma, S., M. Pakserescht, K. Cruickshank, D. M. Green, and L. N. Kolonel. 2013. "Adherence to the USDA Dietary Recommendations for Fruit and Vegetable Intake and Risk of Fatal Stroke among Ethnic Groups: A Prospective Cohort Study." *BMC Neurology* 13: 120.

Sousa, R. M., C. P. Ferri, D. Acosta, E. Albanese, M. Guerra, and others. 2009. "Contribution of Chronic Diseases to Disability in Elderly People in Countries with Low and Middle Incomes: A 10/66 Dementia Research Group Population-Based Survey." *The Lancet* 374 (9704): 1821–30.

Stroke Unit Trialists' Collaboration. 1997. "Collaborative Systematic Review of the Randomised Trials of Organised Inpatient (Stroke Unit) Care after Stroke. Stroke Unit Trialists' Collaboration." *BMJ* 314 (7088): 1151–59.

———. 2002. "Organised Inpatient (Stroke Unit) Care for Stroke." *Cochrane Database of Systematic Reviews* (1): CD000197.

———. 2007. "Organised Inpatient (Stroke Unit) Care for Stroke." *Cochrane Database of Systematic Reviews* (4): CD000197.

———. 2013. "Organised Inpatient (Stroke Unit) Care for Stroke." *Cochrane Database of Systematic Reviews* (9): CD000197.

Thom, S., N. Poulter, J. Field, A. Patel, D. Prabhakaran, and others. 2013. "Effects of a Fixed-Dose Combination Strategy on Adherence and Risk Factors in Patients with or at High Risk of CVD: The UMPIRE Randomized Clinical Trial." *Journal of the American Medical Association* 310 (9): 918–29.

Thun, M. J., B. D. Carter, D. Feskanich, N. D. Freedman, R. Prentice, and others. 2013. "50-Year Trends in Smoking-Related Mortality in the United States." *New England Journal of Medicine* 368 (4): 351–64.

Truelsen, T., P. U. Heuschmann, R. Bonita, G. Arjundas, P. Dalal, and others. 2007. "Standard Method for Developing Stroke Registers in Low-Income and Middle-Income Countries: Experiences from a Feasibility Study of a Stepwise Approach to Stroke Surveillance (STEPS Stroke)." *The Lancet Neurology* 6 (2): 134–39.

Wald, N. J., and M. R. Law. 2003. "A Strategy to Reduce Cardiovascular Disease by More Than 80%." *BMJ* 326 (7404): 1419.

Wang, C. X., and A. Shuaib. 2007. "Neuroprotective Effects of Free Radical Scavengers in Stroke." *Drugs and Aging* 24 (7): 537–46.

Wilson, D. L., R. J. Beyth, P. Linn, and P. Berger. 2007. "Systematic Review of Public Education and Policy for Stroke Prevention." *Current Drug Targets* 8 (7): 874–79.

Wolf, P. A., R. D. Abbott, and W. B. Kannel. 1991. "Atrial Fibrillation as an Independent Risk Factor for Stroke: The Framingham Study." *Stroke* 22 (8): 983–88.

Xie, X., E. Atkins, J. Lv, A. Bennett, B. Neal, and others. 2015. "Effects of Intensive Blood Pressure Lowering on Cardiovascular and Renal Outcomes: Updated Systematic Review and Meta-Analysis." *The Lancet* 387 (10017): 435–43. doi:10.1016/S0140-6736(15)00805-3.

Yan, L. L., M. L. Daviglus, K. Liu, J. Stamler, R. Wang, and others. 2006. "Midlife Body Mass Index and Hospitalization and Mortality in Older Age." *Journal of the American Medical Association* 295 (2): 190–98.

Yano, Y., A. Briasoulis, G. L. Bakris, S. Hoshide, J.-G. Wang, and others. 2013. "Effects of Antihypertensive Treatment in Asian Populations: A Meta-Analysis of Prospective Randomized Controlled Studies (CARdiovascular protectioN Group in Asia: CARNA)." *Journal of the American Society of Hypertension* 8 (2): 103–16.

Yusuf, S. 2002. "Two Decades of Progress in Preventing Vascular Disease." *The Lancet* 360 (9326): 2–3.

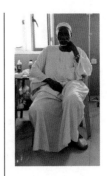

Chapter **10**

Heart Failure

Mark D. Huffman, Greg A. Roth, Karen Sliwa, Clyde W. Yancy, and Dorairaj Prabhakaran

INTRODUCTION

This chapter presents data on the efficacy, effectiveness, and cost-effectiveness of priority heart failure–related interventions. Heart failure is a clinical syndrome in which the heart is unable to meet the metabolic demands of the body because of functional limitations in ventricular filling (diastole), ejection (systole), or both (Yancy and others 2013). Heart failure is a heterogeneous, progressive, chronic disease with protean symptoms, including fatigue; breathlessness at rest or with exertion; and fluid retention in the lungs, abdomen, or extremities. The stages and functional classes of heart failure are detailed in box 10.1.

Causes of Heart Failure

Often, heart failure is an end-stage manifestation of other forms of heart disease, such as ischemic heart disease, usually the result of reduced or obstructed blood flow to the heart; hypertensive heart disease, associated with cardiac damage resulting from high blood pressure; or valvular heart disease, characterized by damage to one or more of the four cardiac valves. There are marked differences according to geographic region (Callender and others 2014; Sliwa and Stewart 2014).

Other causes include the following:

- Primary heart muscle abnormalities known as cardiomyopathies, for example, dilated, familial, peripartum, and infiltrative cardiomyopathies

- Heart muscle toxins, for example, alcohol or cocaine use, as well as cancer therapies
- Specific or severe inflammation, for example, myocarditis, AIDS (acquired immune deficiency syndrome), and Chagas disease.

Diagnosis

Heart failure is diagnosed through a careful history and physical examination, but additional diagnostics—including B-type natriuretic peptide and echocardiography—are frequently performed (McMurray and others 2012; Yancy and others 2013). Five-year mortality rates continue to be estimated at 50 percent in high-income countries (HICs) (Loehr and others 2008), reflecting the severity of a heart failure diagnosis. Long-term outcome data are not available for individuals living in low- and middle-income countries (LMICs) but are assumed to be similarly high, if not higher. Hospitalization for acute heart failure symptoms that typically require intravenous diuretic therapy is a particularly high-risk event, with one-year mortality estimates of 30 percent among older adults in the United States; this rate has not changed substantially between 1998 and 2008 (Chen and others 2011).

BURDEN OF DISEASE

Global Burden

Global estimates of the disease burden of heart failure are difficult to capture, in part because heart failure may be considered both a mode of death (for example, heart

Corresponding author: Mark D. Huffman, MD, MPH, Northwestern University Feinberg School of Medicine, Chicago, Illinois, United States, m-huffman@northwestern.edu.

Stages and Functional Classes of Heart Failure

The American Heart Association and the American College of Cardiology have developed a system to classify heart failure into one of four stages. This classification scheme describes the inviolate progression of clinical manifestations of heart failure based on risk for subsequent fatal and nonfatal events, including hospitalization due to acute heart failure.

- Stage A applies to individuals with heart failure risk factors.
- Stage B applies to individuals with cardiac structural abnormalities without symptoms.
- Stage C applies to individuals with current or previous heart failure symptoms.
- Stage D applies to individuals with end-stage heart failure.

This classification scheme is complemented by the New York Heart Association functional classification scheme, which is widely used by clinicians for risk stratification and treatment decision making. The New York Heart Association functional classification is restricted to patients with stages B, C, or D heart failure:

- Class I applies to individuals with no functional limitations.
- Class II applies to individuals with slight functional limitations.
- Class III applies to individuals with marked functional limitations.
- Class IV applies to individuals with severe limitations upon undertaking any activity or while at rest.

Source: Yancy and others 2013.

failure in a patient with end-stage ischemic heart disease, valvular heart disease, or hypertensive heart disease) and an underlying disease process that causes death or disability (for example, cardiomyopathy or primary heart muscle disorder) (Stevens, King, and Shibuya 2010). Mortality data are generally limited to deaths attributable to underlying disease processes.

According to the World Health Organization (WHO), an estimated 482,000 individuals (0.8 percent of total deaths) died as the result of cardiomyopathy, myocarditis, or endocarditis in 2015 (WHO 2015a) (table 10.1). The majority of these deaths occurred among men compared with women (58 percent versus 42 percent), and among individuals living in LMICs compared with individuals living in HICs (88 percent versus 12 percent). Because of population growth and aging, the estimated number of deaths is projected to reach 576,000 by 2030, which would be 0.8 percent of total deaths. This estimate does not reflect the burden and costs of heart failure caused by other, more common causes, including ischemic heart disease, hypertensive heart disease, and valvular heart disease.

Hypertensive heart disease is categorized separately and caused an estimated 1,137,000 deaths (2.0 percent of total deaths) in 2015 (table 10.1). The majority of these deaths occurred among women compared with men (57 percent versus 43 percent), and among individuals living in LMICs compared with individuals living

in HICs (80 percent versus 20 percent). Because of population growth and aging, this estimate is projected to reach 1.5 million by 2030, which would be 2.1 percent of total deaths.

The Global Burden of Disease Study Investigators estimated that 61.7 million individuals had symptomatic heart failure from any cause in 2013, which is a substantial increase from 31.4 million estimated in 1990 (table 10.2) (GBD Study 2013 Collaborators 2015). The investigators used all available hospital-based data, a literature review, and a DisMod state transition model to create this estimate in total and for individual causes.

Regional Burden of Disease

A systematic review of the same Global Burden of Disease Study methodology describes the geographic variation in major risk factors (figure 10.1) (Khatibzadeh and others 2012). Although the presence of multiple risk factors was common, hypertension was reported as a risk factor in 17 percent of cases, with a higher age- and gender-adjusted prevalence in Eastern and Central Europe (35 percent, 95 percent confidence interval [CI] 33–37 percent) and Sub-Saharan Africa (33 percent, 95 percent CI 30–36 percent). Ischemic heart disease was reported as a risk factor in 52 percent of patients with heart failure in HICs but only 5 percent of patients with

Table 10.1 Population and Mortality Estimates (2015) and Projections (2030) for Cardiomyopathy, Myocarditis, Endocarditis, and Hypertensive Heart Disease

	2015			2030		
	Population	Deaths attributable to cardiomyopathy, myocarditis, or endocarditis	Deaths attributable to hypertensive heart disease	Population	Deaths attributable to cardiomyopathy, myocarditis, or endocarditis	Deaths attributable to hypertensive heart disease
Global men	3,655,810,000	278,055	488,881	4,170,366,000	327,081	625,483
Global women	3,592,760,000	203,664	648,049	4,113,006,000	248,470	831,823
Global total	*7,248,570,000*	*481,720*	*1,136,930*	*8,283,372,000*	*575,551*	*1,457,306*
High-income men	555,410,000	50,239	84,763	591,660,000	56,048	100,911
High-income women	563,034,000	38,565	137,564	595,773,000	41,888	150,650
High-income total	*1,118,444,000*	*88,804*	*222,327*	*1,187,434,000*	*97,936*	*251,561*
LMI-AFR men	472,224,000	36,361	25,818	657,536,000	58,455	41,185
LMI-AFR women	628,815,000	30,527	69,171	653,881,000	48,459	119,186
LMI-AFR total	*943,520,000*	*66,888*	*94,989*	*1,311,417,000*	*106,914*	*160,372*
LMI-AMR men	303,611,000	21,803	55,680	341,868,000	26,098	75,542
LMI-AMR women	311,305,000	16,548	67,153	352,013,000	20,358	88,349
LMI-AMR total	*614,917,000*	*38,351*	*122,834*	*693,881,000*	*46,456*	*163,892*
LMI-SEAR men	979,685,000	74,042	127,215	1,119,437,000	91,416	177,272
LMI-SEAR women	941,076,000	44,754	139,359	1,085,709,000	59,256	198,416
LMI-SEAR total	*1,920,761,000*	*118,796*	*266,574*	*2,205,146,000*	*150,672*	*375,687*
LMI-EUR men	196,322,000	44,314	37,641	200,123,000	34,826	37,175
LMI-EUR women	214,911,000	27,805	51,344	218,087,000	24,257	50,072
LMI-EUR total	*411,234,000*	*72,119*	*88,985*	*418,210,000*	*59,083*	*87,247*
LMI-EMR men	304,165,000	21,136	34,596	381,747,000	29,556	51,076
LMI-EMR women	298,489,000	18,251	42,108	376,438,000	27,095	67,407
LMI-EMR total	*602,655,000*	*39,387*	*76,703*	*758,185,000*	*56,651*	*118,483*
LMI-WPR men	844,393,000	30,160	123,168	877,995,000	30,682	142,321
LMI-WPR women	792,647,000	27,214	141,350	831,104,000	27,157	157,743
LMI-WPR total	*1,637,040,000*	*57,375*	*264,518*	*1,709,099,000*	*57,839*	*300,064*

Source: WHO 2015a.
Note: AFR = Africa; AMR = the Americas; EMR = Eastern Mediterranean Region; EUR = Europe; LMI = low- and middle-income; SEAR = South-East Asia Region; WPR = Western Pacific Region.

Table 10.2 Prevalence and Causes of Symptomatic Heart Failure in 1990 and 2013 Based on Estimates Derived from the Global Burden of Disease Study

	Prevalence (%), 1990	Prevalence (%), 2013
Ischemic heart disease	10,298,900 (32.8)	20,372,600 (33.0)
Hypertensive heart disease	5,128,400 (16.3)	10,906,900 (17.7)
Other cardiovascular disease	4,117,600 (13.1)	95,421,000 (15.5)
Cardiomyopathy and myocarditis	4,077,600 (13.0)	7,629,900 (12.4)
Chronic obstructive pulmonary disease	3,036,500 (9.7)	5,846,400 (9.5)

table continues next page

Table 10.2 Prevalence and Causes of Symptomatic Heart Failure in 1990 and 2013 Based on Estimates Derived from the Global Burden of Disease Study **(continued)**

	Prevalence (%), 1990	Prevalence (%), 2013
Rheumatic heart disease	2,837,800 (9.0)	4,274,000 (6.9)
Endocrine, metabolic, blood, and immune disorders	338,200 (1.1)	852,400 (1.4)
Congenital heart anomalies	495,900 (1.6)	621,700 (1.0)
Iron-deficiency anemia	373,200 (1.2)	446,600 (0.7)
Chagas disease	280,100 (0.9)	383,900 (0.6)
Endocarditis	136,200 (0.4)	250,200 (0.4)
Other hemoglobinopathies and hemolytic anemias	93,000 (0.3)	216,600 (0.4)
Thalassemias	96,400 (0.3)	117,800 (0.2)
Interstitial lung disease and pulmonary sarcoidosis	51,300 (0.2)	102,100 (0.2)
Other pneumoconiosis	16,200 (0.1)	37,700 (0.1)
Glucose-6-phosphate dehydrogenase deficiency	8,100 (<0.1)	20,400 (<01)
Silicosis	10,800 (<0.1)	16,200 (<0.1)
Coal workers' pneumoconiosis	5,800 (<0.1)	9,000 (<0.1)
Iodine deficiency	4,300 (<0.1)	6,900 (<0.1)
Asbestosis	2,400 (<0.1)	4,100 (<0.1)
Total	31,408,500	61,657,600

Source: GBD 2015.

Figure 10.1 Age- and Gender-Adjusted Proportional Contribution of Six Heart Failure Risk Factors

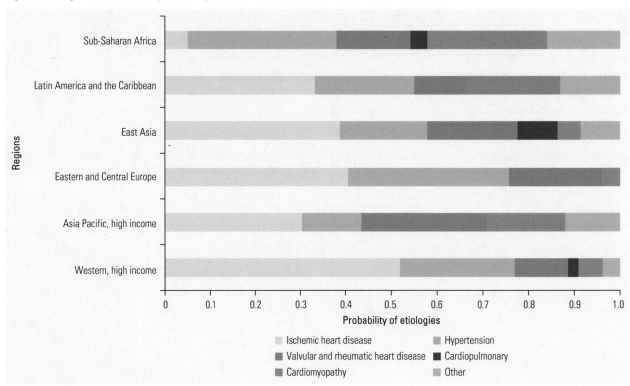

Source: Khatibzadeh and others 2012.
Note: Regions of the world are according to the Global Burden of Disease 2005 classifications.

heart failure in Sub-Saharan Africa. The diversity of causes and the relative weights across regions suggest that optimal prevention and treatment strategies may vary substantially.

HEART FAILURE INTERVENTIONS

Methods

To evaluate potential individual, health system, and health policy interventions to reduce the burden and costs of heart failure, we performed a systematic review of interventions by searching MEDLINE through September 15, 2013, with the assistance of an information specialist. Our search strategy was based on Khatibzadeh and others (2012). We restricted our search to the English language and to those studies published after 1980. Our initial search produced 12,747 results. Restricting the search to *systematic* reviews by filtering with the term systematic produced 396 results. One author reviewed titles and abstracts from these results and selected full-text reports based on perceived relevance, quality, and scalability. We did not include strategies targeting distal heart failure risk factors, such as the prevention and control of ischemic heart disease or rheumatic heart disease or their risk factors (stage A heart failure), because these topics are covered in other chapters of this volume. (See chapters 8 and 11 in this volume [Dugani and others 2017; Watkins and others 2017]).

The MEDLINE search was complemented by another search in August 2014 on http://www .healthsystemsevidence.org, using the term *heart failure*. This search produced 49 systematic reviews of effects of interventions (1997–2003) and 44 economic evaluations (2003–14), all of which were reviewed by one author. Two studies were reported in both categories (N = 91). Individual reports were included on the basis of their publication date (more recent publications were selected over reports from earlier years if the topics were similar) and quality (reports with higher ratings using the A Measurement Tool to Assess Systematic Reviews [AMSTAR] instrument, a reliable and valid tool for assessing systematic review quality [Shea and others 2009], were selected over reports with lower AMSTAR ratings if the topics were similar). The systematic reviews of effects of interventions fell into the broad domains of telemonitoring and self-monitoring, disease management programs, and clinic-based arrangements. Among the economic analyses, only one report came from an upper-middle-income country (China). No results from low- or lower middle-income countries were retrieved.

Recommended Pharmacologic Interventions

Pharmacotherapy for heart failure has demonstrated benefits for individuals with heart failure with reduced left-ventricular ejection fraction (ejection fraction < 40 percent). Individuals with heart failure with preserved ejection fraction (ejection fraction ≥ 40 percent) may derive symptomatic benefit from diuretics for management of intravascular volume, but other agents have largely failed to improve clinical outcomes in these patients. This threshold for ejection fraction was initially based on the concept that heart failure could be attributable only to a low ejection fraction, or low pumping function of the heart. Later research demonstrated the high prevalence of heart failure attributable to poor filling of the heart (Redfield and others 2003). Each of the drug classes outlined in subsequent sections is included in the most recent version of the WHO's Model List of Essential Medicines, reflecting the expectation of the general availability of these drugs, even in LMICs (WHO 2015b).

Diuretics

Diuretics work by promoting water loss through the kidneys, thereby increasing urine output and decreasing intravascular volume. Common side effects include electrolyte disturbances and abnormalities in renal function, particularly at higher doses. Diuretics have become a mainstay in the treatment of heart failure. Diuretics have substantial effects in key areas:

- Reducing mortality (odds ratio [OR] 0.24, 95 percent CI 0.07–0.83; three trials, 202 participants)
- Reducing hospital admissions for worsening heart failure (OR 0.07, 95 percent CI 0.01–0.52; two trials, 169 participants)
- Increasing exercise capacity (weighted mean difference 0.72 units, 95 percent CI 0.40–1.04; four trials, 91 participants) in patients with chronic heart failure symptoms.

However, trials have been generally few, small, and of short duration (4–24 weeks) (Faris and others 2012). Diuretics are widely available and relatively inexpensive.

Beta Blockers

Beta blockers work by reducing the effects of neurohormonal stress that develops from heart failure with reduced ejection fraction, helping the heart strengthen over time. Beta blockers have become an integral part of chronic pharmacotherapy for patients with heart failure who have reduced ejection fraction. Data from 22 randomized controlled trials that included 10,480 participants demonstrated a reduction in all-cause mortality with beta blockers compared with placebo (458 deaths out of 5,657 participants [8 percent] versus 635 deaths in 4,951 participants [13 percent]; OR 0.63, 95 percent CI 0.55–0.72). Similar reductions have been demonstrated for heart failure–related hospitalizations (11 percent versus 17 percent; OR 0.63, 95 percent CI 0.56–0.71) (Shibata, Flather, and Wang 2001). Some beta blockers appear to be more effective than others in head-to-head trials (Poole-Wilson and others 2003). However, a network meta-analysis suggests that the effects of atenolol, bisoprolol, bucindolol, carvedilol, metoprolol, and nebivolol may be similar in their effects on mortality and ejection fraction (Chatterjee and others 2013).

In patients with Chagas cardiomyopathy, only two trials evaluated the effects of beta blockers in 69 participants; both trials had a high risk of bias. There was no evidence that beta blockers lowered all-cause mortality compared with placebo (two deaths among 34 participants [5.9 percent] versus three deaths among 35 participants [5.9 percent]; relative risk [RR] 0.69, 95 percent CI 0.12–3.88, heterogeneity measured by $I^2 = 0$ percent) (Hidalgo and others 2012). These trials did not report the effects on cardiovascular disease mortality or nonfatal events and should not be considered conclusive.

Angiotensin-Converting Enzyme Inhibitors and Angiotensin Receptor Blockers

Angiotensin-converting enzyme inhibitors (ACEi) also work by reducing the effects of neurohormonal stress that develop from heart failure with reduced ejection fraction and help the heart to strengthen over time. ACEi are another integral part of the chronic pharmacotherapy regimen for patients with heart failure who have reduced ejection fraction. Among patients with heart failure with reduced ejection fraction, data from 32 trials randomizing 7,205 participants demonstrated a reduction in all-cause mortality (15.5 percent versus 21.9 percent; OR 0.77, 95 percent CI 0.67–0.88). ACEi have demonstrated a similar effect on the risk of heart failure–related hospitalizations (OR 0.65, 95 percent CI 0.57–0.74), compared with placebo (Garg and Yusuf 1995).

Even among individuals with left-ventricular systolic dysfunction or reduced ejection fraction without symptoms of heart failure (stage B heart failure), ACE inhibitors have been demonstrated to reduce the incidence of heart failure among 4,228 participants randomized to ACEi compared with control (20.7 percent versus 30.2 percent) (SOLVD Investigators 1992).

For patients who cannot tolerate ACEi because of side effects—including allergic reactions such as angioedema, elevated serum potassium levels, or abnormal renal function—angiotensin receptor blockers (ARBs) are frequently recommended, although similar side effects can occur (Yancy and others 2013). Among patients with heart failure, data from nine trials randomizing 4,643 participants demonstrated a reduction in all-cause mortality with ARBs (RR 0.87, 95 percent CI 0.76–1.00) (Heran and others 2012). Among patients with heart failure who have reduced ejection fraction, candesartan has been shown to reduce the risk of heart failure–related hospitalization (RR 0.71, 95 percent CI 0.61–0.82). However, candesartan increased the risk of hospitalization for other causes (RR 1.12, 95 percent CI 1.00–1.25) (Heran and others 2012).

Combination therapy with ACEi and ARBs is not recommended because it is associated with increased risk of hyperkalemia, hypotension, and renal failure, without reducing all-cause mortality (Makani and others 2013). Some evidence indicates that this combination may reduce heart failure–related hospitalizations (RR 0.83, 95 percent CI 0.71–0.97) (Shibata, Tsuyuki, and Wiebe 2008).

Mineralocorticoid Receptor Antagonists

A systematic review and meta-analysis of 19 trials demonstrated a 20 percent reduction in all-cause death from mineralocorticoid receptor antagonists in patients with left-ventricular systolic dysfunction (RR 0.80, 95 percent CI 0.74–0.87) compared with placebo (Ezekowitz and McAlister 2009). Although these drugs have potent effects, are widely available, inexpensive, and cost effective (Glick and others 2002; Zhang and others 2010), they require echocardiography for demonstrating a reduced ejection fraction and monitoring of serum electrolytes and serum creatinine because of increased risks for hyperkalemia and acute kidney injury. Similar monitoring is typically recommended for ACEi and ARBs. Side effects also include gynecomastia. Early detection of these laboratory abnormalities, usually through blood testing one week after initiation of treatment, helps minimize clinical adverse events, including arrhythmia and renal failure. However, the need for laboratory monitoring may limit the scalability of these drugs.

Other Potential Pharmacological Interventions

Digoxin

Digoxin works by blocking ion channel pumps to improve the heart's function. Digoxin does not have an effect on mortality in individuals with heart failure (OR 0.98, 95 percent CI 0.89–1.09; eight studies, 7,755 participants). However, evidence suggests that digoxin reduces heart failure–related hospitalization rates (OR 0.68, 95 percent CI 0.61–0.75; four studies, 7,262 participants) (Hood and others 2014). These trials were largely performed before widespread neurohormonal blockade with beta blockers and ACE inhibitors in patients with left-ventricular systolic dysfunction. The independent effect of digoxin in patients treated with beta blockers and ACEi is uncertain.

Digoxin is widely available and relatively inexpensive, but the high frequency of adverse effects severely limits its widespread use. Digoxin is largely reserved for rate control of atrial fibrillation when other agents are ineffective or contraindicated (for example, calcium channel blockers in patients with left-ventricular systolic dysfunction). Investigators have become interested in its potential for treatment of acute heart failure (Gheorghiade and Braunwald 2009), but large-scale trials of this strategy have yet to be performed.

Anticoagulants

Anticoagulants work by thinning the blood and preventing the development of clots. They are commonly used for individuals with abnormal heart rhythms for stroke prevention but have been considered in patients with heart failure with reduced ejection. Only two small randomized trials (N = 324 participants) with substantial heterogeneity (I^2 = 82 percent) have reported results on the potential effects of anticoagulation in patients with heart failure in normal sinus rhythm. Compared with placebo, there is no convincing evidence that anticoagulation reduces all-cause mortality (RR 0.66, 95 percent CI 0.36–1.18) or cardiovascular disease mortality in patients with heart failure (RR 0.98, 95 percent CI 0.58–1.65) (Lip, Wrigley, and Pisters 2012). However, anticoagulation is associated with a substantial increase in major bleeding (RR 5.98, 95 percent CI 1.71–20.93). Accordingly, it is not recommended for the prevention of thromboembolic events in patients with heart failure. It is unlikely that further trials evaluating anticoagulation in patients with heart failure in sinus rhythm will be performed. Similarly, routine aspirin use is not recommended in patients with heart failure because of the lack of efficacy in preventing thromboembolic events, unless the patients have a comorbid condition for which aspirin is recommended, for example, ischemic heart disease (Yancy and others 2013).

Inotropes

Inotropes work by increasing the heart's pumping function or rate, by reducing the pressure inside the heart so it can pump more easily, or by increasing blood pressure when it is low. For patients who are hospitalized with severe left-ventricular systolic dysfunction and low blood pressure attributable to low cardiac output, short-term

use of intravenous inotropes can be considered to preserve end-organ function (Yancy and others 2013). However, trials have not demonstrated improvements in fatal or nonfatal events with inotropes (Cuffe 2002; Schaink 2012). Outside of these conditions, inotropes can be harmful.

Recommended Nonpharmacologic Interventions

Noninvasive Positive Pressure Ventilation

Compared with standard medical care, noninvasive positive pressure ventilation has been associated with lower rates of in-hospital mortality (RR 0.66, 95 percent CI 0.48–0.89) and endotracheal intubation (RR 0.52, 95 percent CI 0.36–0.75) in patients hospitalized for heart failure based on data from 32 trials enrolling 2,916 participants (Vital, Ladeira, and Atallah 2013). Noninvasive positive pressure ventilation was also associated with fewer adverse events, including respiratory failure and coma, compared with usual care. This intervention requires specialized personnel (respiratory therapist) and equipment, but it is less invasive than endotracheal intubation and more scalable as an adjunct to medical therapy for hospital-based management of acute heart failure. The availability of noninvasive positive pressure ventilation equipment and personnel in LMICs is uncertain. However, data on stable, outpatient heart failure patients with reduced ejection fraction (less than 45 percent) and predominantly central sleep apnea have not demonstrated benefits from this intervention (Cowie 2015).

Exercise-Based Rehabilitation

Exercise-based rehabilitation for patients with heart failure has been studied in 25 trials enrolling 1,871 participants. There is no evidence of overall reduction in all-cause mortality (RR 0.93, 95 percent CI 0.67–1.27). In trials with more than one year of follow-up (six trials, 2,845 participants), the effect size was modestly increased (RR 0.88, 95 percent CI 0.75–1.01) (Taylor and others 2014). Exercise training reduced hospitalization in 12 trials that included 1,036 participants (RR 0.61, 95 percent CI 0.46–0.80). Exercise training also improved the health-related quality of life in 13 trials that included 1,270 participants (weighted mean difference in Minnesota Living with Heart Failure −5.8 points, 95 percent CI −9.2 to −2.4) (Taylor and others 2014). An incremental cost-effectiveness ratio of US$1,773 (1998 U.S. dollars) per life year gained was reported in one trial with 15.5 years of follow-up among 99 participants. The HF-ACTION trial of 2,331 participants with heart failure in the United States demonstrated lower expenditures from high-cost inpatient procedures for individuals randomized to the exercise group (US$4,300 in 2008); however, these savings were offset by increased costs related to participants' time, travel, and parking (Reed and others 2010).

Devices

Implantable cardioverter defibrillators continuously detect heart rhythm and have the capacity to charge and shock when potentially fatal heart rhythm abnormalities are detected. Compared with usual care, implantable cardioverter defibrillators are associated with a 31 percent (95 percent CI 21–40 percent) lower risk of all-cause mortality in patients with heart failure with reduced ejection fraction ≤ 35 percent (10 studies enrolling 8,606 participants) (Uhlig and others 2013). Although adverse events such as device or lead infection occur in fewer than 5 percent of patients, approximately 20 percent of patients who receive an implantable cardioverter defibrillator will receive at least one inappropriate shock, meaning that the device will deliver an electrical shock to the patient at a time when it is not needed.

Patients with heart failure with reduced ejection fraction and evidence of ventricular dyssynchrony (when the electrical conduction systems of the right and left ventricles depolarize at least 120 milliseconds apart from one another) benefit from cardiac resynchronization therapy, which uses a pacemaker lead in both the left and right ventricles to synchronize ventricular depolarization and thereby contraction. Rivero-Ayerza and others (2006) evaluated five trials of 2,371 patients and found that, compared with the control, cardiac resynchronization was associated with a reduction in all-cause mortality (17 percent versus 21 percent; OR 0.71, 95 percent CI 0.57–0.88) and heart failure–associated mortality (7 percent versus 10 percent; OR 0.62, 95 percent CI 0.45–0.84). However, data on the availability of device-based therapies in LMICs are limited.

Advanced Heart Failure Therapies

Advanced heart failure therapies for patients with end-stage heart failure, such as ventricular reconstruction, implantable ventricular assist devices, or heart transplantation, have very limited availability in most LMICs and are beyond the scope of this chapter.

HEALTH SERVICE ARRANGEMENTS

Takeda and others (2012) evaluated three types of health service arrangements for patients with heart failure across 25 trials of nearly 6,000 patients:

- Case management with telephone and home visit support from specialty nurses (17 studies)

- Clinic-based interventions, including vertical, specialized heart failure clinics (six studies)
- Multidisciplinary care by a team of physicians, nurses, dieticians, and pharmacists (two studies).

Case Management Interventions

Case management interventions were associated with a reduction in all-cause mortality reduction at 12 months (OR 0.66, 95 percent CI 0.47–0.91) but not at six months. Case management was associated with a reduction in heart failure readmission rates at both six months (OR 0.64, 95 percent CI 0.46–0.88) and 12 months (OR 0.47, 95 percent CI 0.30–0.76). There was no evidence that vertical-type heart failure clinic-based interventions improved mortality or heart failure readmissions. Multidisciplinary interventions to bridge the gap between hospital admission and discharge home care were associated with reductions in heart failure readmission rates (OR 0.46, 95 percent CI 0.46–0.69). A systematic review demonstrated that weekly, but not monthly, heart failure clinics were associated with reductions in unplanned hospitalizations (RR 0.42, 95 percent CI 0.27–0.65; three studies); these reports were from HICs (Thomas and others 2013).

Inglis and others (2011) performed a systematic review of the potential effects of telemonitoring (11 studies, 2,710 participants) and structured telephone support (16 studies, 5,613 participants). Telemonitoring was associated with a reduction in all-cause mortality (RR 0.66, 95 percent CI 0.54–0.81) and heart failure–related hospitalizations (RR 0.79, 95 percent CI 0.67–0.94). Costs related to hospital admissions or health care were lower in individuals randomized to telemonitoring compared with usual care (range 14–86 percent). Structured telephone support demonstrated a less robust effect on mortality but similar effect on hospitalization. Both strategies appear to increase evidence-based prescribing as the mechanism of effect.

Quality Improvement through Care Pathways

Heart failure quality-improvement programs are typically multifaceted strategies to improve evidence-based medication prescribing. One such strategy includes care pathways, or algorithms. A systematic review of seven randomized and quasi-randomized trials in HICs that included 3,690 participants with heart failure demonstrated a 55 percent reduction in in-hospital mortality (RR 0.45, 95 percent CI 0.21–0.94) and a 19 percent reduction in readmission (RR 0.81, 95 percent

CI 0.66–0.99) with the use of care pathways. The weighted mean length of hospital stay was reduced by 1.9 days (95 percent CI 1.3–2.4), but costs were similar (Kul and others 2012). There are no reports of similar randomized or quasi-randomized trials in LMICs, but data in box 10.2 demonstrate the current state of the science.

Box 10.3 provides a recent, specific example of presentation, management, and outcomes among individuals hospitalized for heart failure in India, a middle-income country.

Box 10.2

Systematic Review of Heart Failure Presentation, Management, and Outcomes in Low- and Middle-Income Countries

Callender and others (2014) described data on heart failure presentation, management, and outcomes among low- and middle-income countries (LMICs) from 1995 to 2014, including 42 studies of acute (hospitalized) heart failure (25 LMICs; N = 232,500 patients) and 11 studies of chronic heart failure (14 LMICs; N = 5,358 patients). Mean ejection fraction was 38 percent (range 27–57 percent) and 48 percent (range 29–55 percent) among acute and chronic heart failure patients, respectively. Ischemic heart disease was the most common cause of heart failure in all regions except Sub-Saharan Africa and the Americas, where hypertension was the most common cause. Mean length of hospital stay was 10 days (range 3–23 days), and mean in-hospital mortality was 8 percent (95 percent CI 6–10 percent). Diuretics were prescribed in

69 percent of patients (range 60–78 percent); ACE inhibitors were prescribed in 57 percent of patients (range 49–64 percent); beta blockers were prescribed in 34 percent of patients (range 28–41 percent); and mineralocorticoid receptor antagonists were prescribed in 32 percent (range 25–39 percent).

For context, in the EuroHeart Failure II Survey (Nieminen and others 2006) of acute heart failure patients admitted to hospitals across 30 European countries, discharge medication rates for patients with heart failure with reduced ejection fraction were generally higher (ACE inhibitors 71 percent; beta blockers 61 percent; mineralocorticoid receptor antagonists 48 percent) than the rates reported by Callender and others (2014). However, those rates may have changed over the ensuing decade.

Box 10.3

Case Study: Trivandrum Heart Failure Registry

Harikrishnan and others (2015) described the in-hospital and short-term outcomes among 1,205 consecutive admissions from 13 urban and 5 rural hospitals in Trivandrum, India, with a primary diagnosis of heart failure from January to December 2013. Ischemic heart disease was the underlying etiology of 72 percent of admissions, and heart failure with preserved ejection fraction (> 45 percent) constituted 26 percent of the sample. The median length of hospital stay was 6 days (interquartile range = 4–9 days), and in-hospital mortality rate was 8.5 percent (95 percent CI

6.9–10.0 percent). The all-cause mortality rate at 90 days was 2.43 deaths per 1,000 person-days (95 percent CI 2.11–2.78). Older age, lower education, poor ejection fraction, higher serum creatinine, New York Heart Association functional class IV, and not receiving guideline-based medical treatment were associated with higher risk of 90-day mortality.

These data demonstrate opportunities for improving in-hospital heart failure care in a low- and middle-income country setting.

Integration and Prioritization

The interventions discussed can be viewed through the lens of the WHO's building blocks for health systems framework (http://www.who.int/healthinfo/systems/monitoring/en/) to help guide their integration and prioritization (box 10.4, table 10.3). Because of the morbid nature of heart failure, early diagnosis and medical therapy are crucial to altering the natural history, particularly in patients with reduced ejection fraction in whom the majority of the interventions have been shown to be more effective compared with individuals with preserved ejection fraction.

Box 10.4

Health System Capacity Needs for Integrating and Prioritizing Interventions for Patients with Heart Failure, According to the World Health Organization's Building Blocks for Health Systems Framework

Service delivery
- Clinic and hospital facilities are required for initial diagnosis and treatment of patients with heart failure.
- Self-management supported by telemonitoring, ideally with multidisciplinary teams, improves outcomes, primarily through prescription of evidence-based drugs.
- Quality improvement programs that use care pathways have substantial potential to improve in-hospital quality of care and outcomes.

Health workforce
- Key staff members include physicians and nurses, particularly those with training in echocardiography. Ancillary staff members, including dieticians, psychologists, and pharmacists, can improve general self-care and self-management in a team-based care model.

Health information systems
- Information systems need to identify heart failure as an underlying disease process and mode of death for estimating disease burden.
- Ejection fraction, typically derived from echocardiography, is essential for matching drug therapy with underlying disease process.

Access to essential medicines and technologies
- Several medications have independently demonstrated improvements in survival among patients with heart failure with reduced ejection fraction, highlighting how important pharmacologic therapy is for such patients. Strategies to improve adherence to medication regimens, including fixed-dose combination therapies, are important to optimize their use and effectiveness.
- Echocardiography, which can be performed by both doctors and nurses, is an essential technology for diagnosis of heart failure.
- Noninvasive positive pressure ventilation is a relatively low-cost and effective, yet underutilized, option for preventing death and the need for intubation among patients with acute (stage C or D) heart failure.

Financing
- Strategies to reduce the financial burden of access to clinicians, echocardiography, and essential medicines, with an emphasis on reducing point-of-service costs, will likely lead to improved process and outcome measures.

Leadership and governance
- Patients with heart failure are cared for by primary care physicians and specialists, where available, and their teams in both inpatient and outpatient settings. Leadership and governance structures of health systems will need to rely upon these groups to execute any proposed health service changes.

Table 10.3 Priority Interventions for Patients with Heart Failure

Intervention	Effect on mortality (range)	Effect on heart failure hospitalization (range)	Study
Pharmacologic			
Diuretics	OR = 0.27 (0.07–0.83)	OR = 0.07 (0.01–0.52)	Faris and others 2012
Beta blockers*	OR = 0.63 (0.55–0.72)	OR = 0.63 (0.56–0.71)	Shibata, Flather, and Wang 2001
ACE inhibitors*	OR = 0.77 (0.67–0.88)	OR = 0.65 (0.57–0.74)	Garg and Yufus 1995
Mineralocorticoid receptor antagonists*	RR = 0.80 (0.74–0.87)	RR = 0.77 (0.68–0.87)	Ezekowitz and McAlister 2009
Nonpharmacologic			
Noninvasive positive pressure ventilation	RR = 0.66 (0.48–0.89)	Not applicable	Vital, Ladeira, and Atallah 2013
Implantable cardioverter defibrillator*	RR = 0.69 (0.60–0.89)		Uhlig and others 2013
Cardiac resynchronization therapy*	RR = 0.71 (0.57–0.88)		Rivero-Ayerza and others 2006
Health system arrangements			
Multidisciplinary team management		OR = 0.40 (0.30–0.76)	Thomas and others 2013
Telemonitoring	RR = 0.66 (0.54–0.81)	RR = 0.79 (0.67–0.94)	Inglis and others 2010
Care pathways	RR = 0.45 (0.21–0.94)	RR = 0.81 (0.66–0.99)	Kul and others 2012

Note: ACE = angiotensin-converting enzyme; OR = odds ratio; RR = relative risk.
*Denotes interventions wherein benefits are limited to patients with heart failure with reduced ejection fraction.

COST-EFFECTIVENESS AND EXTENDED COST-EFFECTIVENESS OF POTENTIAL INTERVENTIONS

Screening for Suspected Heart Failure

Kwan and others (2013) developed a nurse-led, echocardiographic screening method for heart failure diagnosis and treatment in rural Rwanda for patients suspected of having heart failure. Nurses were provided with diagnostic criteria to categorize patients as either having cardiomyopathy, hypertensive heart disease, mitral stenosis, other valvular abnormalities, or isolated right heart failure. Beyond volume management for all patients, the investigators provided a general therapeutic plan based on the underlying heart failure etiology and

estimated the annual cost to be US$315 in 2010 U.S. dollars per patient (table 10.4).

Treatment for Heart Failure

Diuretics

The mainstay for heart failure includes diuretics in patients with heart failure with either reduced or preserved ejection fraction. While diuretics have been shown to be cost-effective for managing hypertension in HICs (Tran and others 2007) and LMICs (Alefan and others 2009), they have not been evaluated in a cost-effectiveness analysis for heart failure. However, given that patients with heart failure have much higher risk and costs associated with the condition, and that the

Table 10.4 Annual Costs of Heart Failure Diagnostics and Treatment in Rwanda

Program costs	Annual cost per patient (2010 US$)
Typical medical regimen	40
• Furosemide 40 mg twice daily	
• Lisinopril 20 mg daily	
• Carvedilol 25 mg twice daily	
Laboratory testing and imaging (including point-of-care chemistries and echocardiography)	59
Transport subsidy ($3 per visit, 12 visits)	36
Community health worker ($30 per month divided among five patients)	72
Advanced NCD clinician salary ($10,000/year)	33
Marginal cost of hospitalization (five days/year at $15 per day)	75
Total	*315*

Source: Kwan and others 2013.
Note: mg = milligram; NCD = noncommunicable disease.

relative risk reduction for heart failure is similar to that for those with hypertension, it is safe to infer their overall cost-effectiveness. All other agents for heart failure have then been compared with a baseline of diuretic therapy.

ACE Inhibitors

ACE inhibitors are an integral part of the treatment of patients with heart failure, both reducing costly admissions and prolonging life (table 10.5). Cost-effectiveness studies dating back to the 1990s have shown ACE inhibitors to be either highly cost-effective or cost saving in HICs (Butler and Fletcher 1996; Paul and others 1994; Tsevat and others 1995). Further work in LMICs has confirmed the use of ACE inhibitors as cost saving when added to diuretics in all six LMIC regions (Gaziano 2005) or extremely cost-effective (US$50 per disability-adjusted life year [DALY] averted) when access to hospitals was limited.

Beta Blockers

Beta blockers are equally integral for the management of patients with heart failure with reduced ejection fraction. In HICs, similar cost-effectiveness results for carvedilol were seen in the late 1990s (Delea and others 1999) and for metoprolol in the early 2000s (Levy and others 2001) of less than US$30,000 per quality-adjusted life year (QALY) to as low as US$4,000 per QALY.

However, these studies used costs of up to US$500–US$1,000 per year. When analyses were repeated using generic pricing in all six LMIC regions, the incremental cost-effectiveness ratios were extremely favorable, ranging from US$124 to US$219 per DALY averted in all regions (Gaziano 2005).

Mineralocorticoid Agents

Mineralocorticoid agents have a favorable health profile in patients with reduced systolic function heart failure, reducing both all-cause mortality and hospitalizations. Although eplerenone has proven to be cost-effective in HICs (McKenna and others 2010; Weintraub and others 2005), it has not been evaluated for cost-effectiveness in LMICs. One limitation to its use is an additional requirement for blood monitoring of renal function and electrolytes.

Devices

Devices such as the implantable cardioverter defibrillator for those with advanced heart failure have been cost-effective in HICs. When implantable cardioverter defibrillators were compared with best medical therapy for those with heart failure in Brazil, the cost was US$50,000 per QALY for those with advanced heart failure (Ribeiro and others 2010). When implantable cardioverter defibrillators for those with heart failure were evaluated, the incremental cost-effectiveness ratio dropped to US$32,000 per QALY (Bertoldi and others 2013). When implantable cardiac resynchronization therapy (CRT) was compared with medical therapy in Brazil in those with advanced heart failure, CRT was even more cost-effective, at US$17,700 per QALY in 2012 U.S. dollars. When implantable cardioverter defibrillator and CRT capabilities were combined in the same device for those with heart failure, the incremental cost-effectiveness ratio was nearly US$33,000 per QALY. Similar values for CRT of US$34,000 per QALY were observed in Argentina (Poggio and others 2012).

CONCLUSIONS

Heart failure is a progressive, highly morbid condition that can result from underlying cardiovascular diseases, such as ischemic heart disease or hypertensive heart disease, or from underlying heart muscle abnormalities, such as cardiomyopathies. The predominant underlying causes of heart failure vary substantially by region. Several inexpensive therapies can improve the natural history of heart failure, particularly in the presence of left-ventricular systolic dysfunction. While the

Table 10.5 Incremental Cost-Effectiveness Ratios for Heart Failure Treatment, Compared with No Treatment, by Region
US$/DALY averted

Region	Medical therapy for AMI compared with baseline of no treatment				Medical therapy and CABG for IHD compared with baseline of no treatment, hospital access				Medical therapy and CABG for IHD compared with baseline of no treatment, limited hospital access			ACEi and BBs for CHF compared with baseline of diuretics, hospital access		ACEi and BBs for CHF compared with baseline of diuretics, limited hospital access	
	ASA	ASA, BB	ASA, BB, SK	ASA, BB, TPA	ASA, BB	ASA, BB, ACEi	ASA, BB, ACEi, Statin	CABG	ASA, BB	ASA, BB, ACEi	ASA, BB, Statin	ACEi	ACEi, MET	ACEi	ACEi, MET
East Asia and the Pacific	13	15	672	15,867	Cost saving	781	1,914	33,846	461	942	2,220	Cost saving	189	27	274
Europe and Central Asia	19	21	722	15,878	Cost saving	866	2,026	47,942	530	1,097	2,470	Cost saving	144	30	275
Latin America and the Caribbean	20	22	734	15,887	Cost saving	821	1,942	62,426	545	1,111	2,497	Cost saving	124	31	275
Middle East and North Africa	17	20	715	15,893	Cost saving	672	1,686	72,345	527	996	2,305	Cost saving	128	29	275
South Asia	9	11	638	15,860	Cost saving	715	1,819	24,040	386	828	2,034	Cost saving	219	25	273
Sub-Saharan Africa	9	11	634	15,862	Cost saving	660	1,720	26,813	389	783	1,955	Cost saving	218	25	273

Source: Gaziano and others 2006.

Note: ACEi = angiotensin-converting enzyme inhibitors; AMI = acute myocardial infarction; ASA = aspirin; BB = beta blocker; CABG = coronary artery bypass graft surgery; CHF = congestive heart failure; DALY = disability-adjusted life year; IHD = ischemic heart disease; MET = metoprolol; SK = streptokinase; TPA = tissue plasminogen activator. The intervention in the first column of each set of strategies is compared with the baseline of no treatment; each successive intervention for each set of strategies is compared with the intervention immediately to its left.

prevention of heart failure is ideal, we propose a resource-stratified approach to integrate and adopt interventions, including coprimary strategies to diagnose patients early in the disease course and to improve initiation and adherence to medication regimens.

Effective Strategies

Nurse-based screening with echocardiography and biomarker testing for diagnosis of heart failure appears promising, but human resource availability and economic costs are likely to be variable.

Diuretics are inexpensive, effective therapies that should be available for all patients with heart failure. Diuretics should be complemented by medical therapy using beta blockers, ACE inhibitors, and mineralocorticoid receptor antagonists in patients with heart failure with reduced ejection fraction.

Noninvasive positive pressure ventilation is an effective, yet likely underutilized, therapy for patients with acute respiratory distress secondary to heart failure, particularly in middle-income countries. Effectiveness and cost-effectiveness of cardioverter defibrillators require further study.

Beta blockers, ACE inhibitors, and mineralocorticoid receptor antagonists generally should be favored over digoxin for treatment of heart failure because of their superior mid- and long-term effectiveness compared with digoxin, and because of the narrow therapeutic index and high adverse event rate associated with digoxin.

Strategies to Avoid

Inotropic agents are frequently used in patients hospitalized with heart failure and cardiogenic shock, yet they have failed to demonstrate benefits.

Routine oral anticoagulation in patients with severe left-ventricular systolic dysfunction has not been demonstrated to improve outcomes. Anticoagulation should be reserved for patients with evidence of ventricular thrombi.

Future Directions

Policies related to the prevention, treatment, and control of cardiovascular risk factors and cardiovascular disease may favorably influence age-adjusted heart failure incidence and prevalence. Whether these policies lead to overall reductions in heart failure and heart failure–related costs, particularly in the presence of aging populations, remains uncertain.

Heart failure screening is generally restricted to patients presenting with symptoms. However, the influence of health system arrangements for screening and ultimately diagnosing patients with heart failure, including the availability of advanced diagnostic services such as biomarker testing and echocardiography at various health system levels, warrants further study to understand where best to place available diagnostics. Facilities or systems that can link patients from diagnostics to treatment will likely be effective for longitudinal care.

Long-term heart failure treatment is based on the provision and use of essential medications that need to be available, accessible, and affordable. Long-term adherence to complex medication regimens remains difficult for most patients, and strategies that use nonphysician health workers, that lower out-of-pocket spending, or that lower the number of pills used each day (such as fixed-dose combinations) appear to improve adherence (Nieuwlaat and others 2014). Updated local and regional health policy and cost-effectiveness models may be useful methods for evaluating the effect of health system arrangements for acute and chronic treatment on outcomes and costs.

NOTE

World Bank Income Classifications as of July 2014 are as follows, based on estimates of gross national income (GNI) per capita for 2013:

- Low-income countries (LICs) = US$1,045 or less
- Middle-income countries (MICs) are subdivided:
  (a) lower-middle-income = US$1,046 to US$4,125
  (b) upper-middle-income (UMICs) = US$4,126 to US$12,745
- High-income countries (HICs) = US$12,746 or more.

REFERENCES

Alefan, Q., M. I. M. Ibrahim, T. A. Razak, and A. Ayub. 2009. "Cost-Effectiveness of Antihypertensive Treatment in Malaysia." *Malaysian Journal of Pharmaceutical Sciences* 7 (2): 137–52.

Bertoldi, E. G., L. E. Rohde, L. I. Zimerman, M. Pimentel, and C. A. Polanczyk. 2013. "Cost-Effectiveness of Cardiac Resynchronization Therapy in Patients with Heart Failure: The Perspective of a Middle-Income Country's Public Health System." *International Journal of Cardiology* 163 (3): 309–15. ISSN 0167–5273.

Butler, J. R., and P. J. Fletcher. 1996. "A Cost-Effectiveness Analysis of Enalapril Maleate in the Management of Congestive Heart Failure in Australia." *Australian and New Zealand Journal of Medicine* 26 (1): 89–95.

Callender, T., M. Woodward, G. Roth, F. Farzadfar, J.-C. Lemarie, and others. 2014. "Heart Failure Care in Low- and Middle-Income Countries: A Systematic Review and Meta-Analysis." *PLoS Medicine* 11 (8): e1001699. doi:10.1371/journal.pmed .1001699.

Chatterjee, S., G. Biondi-Zoccai, A. Abbate, F. D'Ascenzo, D. Castagno, and others. 2013. "Benefits of Beta Blockers in Patients with Heart Failure and Reduced Ejection Fraction: Network Meta-Analysis." *BMJ* 346 (1): f55–55. doi:10.1136 /bmj.f55.

Chen, J., S.-L. T. Normand, Y. Wang, and H. M. Krumholz. 2011. "National and Regional Trends in Heart Failure Hospitalization and Mortality Rates for Medicare Beneficiaries, 1998–2008." *Journal of the American Medical Association* 306 (15): 1669–78. doi:10.1001/jama.2011.1474.

Cowie, M. R., H. Woehrle, K. Wegscheider, C. Angermann, M. P. d'Ortho, and others. 2015. "Adaptive Servo-Ventilation for Central Sleep Apnea in Systolic Heart Failure." *New England Journal of Medicine* 373(12): 1095-105. doi:10.1056 /NEJMoa1506459. Epub September 1. PubMed PMID: 26323938; PubMed Central PMCID: PMC4779593.

Cuffe, M. S. 2002. "Short-Term Intravenous Milrinone for Acute Exacerbation of Chronic Heart Failure." *Journal of the American Medical Association* 287 (12): 1541–47. doi:10.1001/jama.287.12.1541.

Delea, T. E., M. Vera-Llonch, R. E. Richner, M. B. Fowler, and G. Oster. 1999. "Cost Effectiveness of Carvedilol for Heart Failure." *American Journal of Cardiology* 83 (6): 890–96.

Dugani, S. B., A. E. Moran, R. O. Bonow, and T. A. Gaziano. 2017. "Ischemic Heart Disease: Cost-Effective Management and Secondary Prevention." In *Disease Control Priorities* (third edition): Volume 5 *Cardiovascular, Respiratory, and Related Disorders,* edited by D. Prabhakaran, S. Anand, T. A. Gaziano, J.-C. Mbanya, R. Nugent, and Y. Wu. Washington, DC: World Bank.

Ezekowitz, J. A., and F. A. McAlister. 2009. "Aldosterone Blockade and Left Ventricular Dysfunction: A Systematic Review of Randomized Clinical Trials." *European Heart Journal* 30 (4): 469–77.

Faris, R. F., M. Flather, H. Purcell, P. A. Poole-Wilson, and A. J. S. Coats. 2012. "Diuretics for Heart Failure." *Cochrane Database of Systematic Reviews* 2: CD003838. doi:10.1002 /14651858.CD003838.pub3.

Garg, R., and S. Yusuf. 1995. "Overview of Randomized Trials of Angiotensin-Converting Enzyme Inhibitors on Mortality and Morbidity in Patients with Heart Failure. Collaborative Group on ACE Inhibitor Trials." *Journal of the American Medical Association* 273 (18): 1450–56. doi:10.1001/jama.273.18.1450.

Gaziano, T. A. 2005. "Cardiovascular Disease in the Developing World and Its Cost-Effective Management." *Circulation* 112 (23): 3547–553.

Gaziano, T. A., K. S. Reddy, F. Paccaud, S. Horton, and V. Chaturvedi. 2006. "Cardiovascular Disease." In *Disease Control Priorities in Developing Countries* (second edition), edited by D. T. Jamison, J. Breman, A. R. Meashamm, G. Alleyne, M. Claeson, D. Evans, P. Jha, A. Mills, and

P. Musgrove. Washington, DC: Oxford University Press and World Bank.

GBD (Global Burden of Disease Study 2013 Collaborators). 2015. "Global, Regional, and National Incidence, Prevalence, and Years Lived with Disability for 301 Acute and Chronic Diseases and Injuries in 188 Countries, 1990–2013: A Systematic Analysis for the Global Burden of Disease Study 2013." *The Lancet* 386 (9995): 743–800. doi:10.1016 /S0140-6736(15)60692-4).

Gheorghiade, M., and E. Braunwald. 2009. "Reconsidering the Role for Digoxin in the Management of Acute Heart Failure Syndromes." *Journal of the American Medical Association* 302 (19): 2146–47.

Glick, H. A., S. M. Orzol, J. F. Tooley, W. J. Remme, S. Sasayama, and others. 2002. "Economic Evaluation of the Randomized Aldactone Evaluation Study (RALES): Treatment of Patients with Severe Heart Failure." *Cardiovascular Drugs and Therapy* 16 (1): 53–59.

Harikrishnan, S., G. Sanjay, T. Anees, S. Viswanathan, G. Vijayaraghavan, and others. 2015. "Clinical Presentation, Management, In-Hospital and 90-Day Outcomes of Heart Failure Patients in Trivandrum, Kerala, India: The Trivandrum Heart Failure Registry." *European Journal of Heart Failure* 17 (8): 794–800. doi:10.1002/ejhf.283.

Heran, B. S., V. M. Musini, K. Bassett, R. S. Taylor, and J. M. Wright. 2012. "Angiotensin Receptor Blockers for Heart Failure." *Cochrane Database of Systematic Reviews (Online)* 4 (4): CD003040. doi:10.1002/14651858. CD003040.pub2.

Hidalgo, R., A. J. Martí-Carvajal, J. S. W. Kwong, D. Simancas-Racines, and S. Nicola. 2012. "Pharmacological Interventions for Treating Heart Failure in Patients with Chagas Cardiomyopathy." *Cochrane Database of Systematic Reviews* 11 (11). doi:10.1002/14651858.CD009077.pub2.

Hood, W. B., Jr, A. L. Dans, G. H. Guyatt, R. Jaeschke, and J. J. McMurray. 2014. "Digitalis for Treatment of Heart Failure in Patients in Sinus Rhythm." *Cochrane Database of Systematic Reviews* 4: CD002901. doi:10.1002/14651858 .CD002901.pub3.

Inglis, S. C., R. A. Clark, F. A. McAlister, J. Ball, C. Lewinter, and others. 2010. "Structured Telephone Support or Telemonitoring Programmes for Patients with Chronic Heart Failure." *Cochrane Database of Systematic Reviews (Online)* 8. doi:10.1002/14651858.CD007228.pub2.

Inglis, S. C., R. A. Clark, F. A. McAlister, S. Stewart, and J. G. F. Cleland. 2011. "Which Components of Heart Failure Programmes Are Effective? A Systematic Review and Meta-Analysis of the Outcomes of Structured Telephone Support or Telemonitoring as the Primary Component of Chronic Heart Failure Management in 8323 Patients: Abridged Cochrane Review." *European Journal of Heart Failure* 13 (9): 1028–40. doi:10.1093/eurjhf/hfr039.

Khatibzadeh, S., F. Farzadfar, J. Oliver, M. Ezzati, and A. Moran. 2012. "Worldwide Risk Factors for Heart Failure: A Systematic Review and Pooled Analysis." *International Journal of Cardiology* 168 (2): 1186–94. doi:10.1016/j .ijcard.2012.11.065.

Kul, S., A. Barbieri, E. Milan, I. Montag, K. Vanhaecht, and others. 2012. "Effects of Care Pathways on the In-Hospital Treatment of Heart Failure: A Systematic Review." *BMC Cardiovascular Disorders* 12: 81. doi:10.1186/1471-2261-12-81.

Kwan, G. F., A. K. Bukhman, A. C. Miller, G. Ngoga, J. Mucumbitsi, and others. 2013. "A Simplified Echocardiographic Strategy for Heart Failure Diagnosis and Management within an Integrated Noncommunicable Disease Clinic at District Hospital Level for Sub-Saharan Africa." *Journal of the American College of Cardiology: Heart Failure* 1 (3): 230–36. doi:10.1016/j.jchf.2013.03.006.

Levy, A. R., A. H. Briggs, C. Demers, and B. J. O'Brien. 2001. "Cost-Effectiveness of Beta-Blocker Therapy with Metoprolol or with Carvedilol for Treatment of Heart Failure in Canada." *American Heart Journal* 142 (3): 537–43.

Lip, G. Y., B. J. Wrigley, and R. Pisters. 2012. "Anticoagulation versus Placebo for Heart Failure in Sinus Rhythm." *Cochrane Database of Systematic Reviews* 6: CD003336. doi:10.1002/14651858.CD003336.pub2.

Loehr, L. R., W. D. Rosamond, P. P. Chang, A. R. Folsom, and L. E. Chambless. 2008. "Heart Failure Incidence and Survival (from the Atherosclerosis Risk in Communities Study)." *American Journal of Cardiology* 101 (7): 1016–22. doi:10.1016/j.amjcard.2007.11.061.

Makani, H., S. Bangalore, K. A. Desouza, A. Shah, and F. H. Messerli. 2013. "Efficacy and Safety of Dual Blockade of the Renin-Angiotensin System: Meta-Analysis of Randomised Trials." *BMJ* 346: f360.

McKenna, C., J. Burch, S. Suekarran, S. Walker, A. Bakhai, and others. 2010. "A Systematic Review and Economic Evaluation of the Clinical Effectiveness and Cost-Effectiveness of Aldosterone Antagonists for Postmyocardial Infarction Heart Failure." *Health Technology Assessment* 14 (24): 1–162.

McMurray, J. J. V., S. Adamopoulos, S. D. Anker, A. Auricchio, M. Böhm, and others. 2012. "ESC Guidelines for the Diagnosis and Treatment of Acute and Chronic Heart Failure 2012: The Task Force for the Diagnosis and Treatment of Acute and Chronic Heart Failure 2012 of the European Society of Cardiology: Developed in Collaboration with the Heart Failure Association (HFA) of the ESC." *European Heart Journal* 33 (14): 1787–847. doi:10.1093/eurheartj/ehs104.

Nieminen, M. S., D. Brutsaert, K. Dickstein, H. Drexler, F. Follath, and others. 2006. "EuroHeart Failure Survey II (EHFS II): A Survey on Hospitalized Acute Heart Failure Patients: Description of Population." *European Heart Journal* 27 (22): 2725–36.

Nieuwlaat, R., N. Wilczynski, T. Navarro, N. Hobson, R. Jeffery, and others. 2014. "Interventions for Enhancing Medication Adherence." *Cochrane Database of Systematic Reviews* 11: CD000011. doi:10.1002/14651858.CD000011.pub4.

Paul, S. D., K. M. Kuntz, K. A. Eagle, and M. C. Weinstein. 1994. "Costs and Effectiveness of Angiotensin Converting Enzyme Inhibition in Patients with Congestive Heart Failure." *Archives of Internal Medicine* 154: 1143–49.

Poggio, R., F. Augustovsky, J. Caporale, V. Irazola, and S. Miriuka. 2012. "Cost-Effectiveness of Cardiac Resynchronization Therapy: Perspective from Argentina." *International Journal of Technology Assessment in Health Care* 28 (4): 429–35.

Poole-Wilson, P. A., K. Swedberg, J. G. F. Cleland, A. Di Lenarda, P. Hanrath, and others. 2003. "Comparison of Carvedilol and Metoprolol on Clinical Outcomes in Patients with Chronic Heart Failure in the Carvedilol or Metoprolol European Trial (COMET): Randomised Controlled Trial." *The Lancet* 362 (9377): 7–13.

Redfield, M. M., S. J. Jacobsen, J. C. Burnett Jr., D. W. Mahoney, K. R. Bailey, and others. 2003. "Burden of Systolic and Diastolic Ventricular Dysfunction in the Community: Appreciating the Scope of the Heart Failure Epidemic." *Journal of the American Medical Association* 289 (2): 194–202.

Reed, S. D., D. J. Whellan, Y. Li, J. Y. Friedman, S. J. Ellis, and others. 2010. "Economic Evaluation of the HF-ACTION (Heart Failure: A Controlled Trial Investigating Outcomes of Exercise Training) Randomized Controlled Trial: An Exercise Training Study of Patients with Chronic Heart Failure." *Circulation: Cardiovascular Quality and Outcomes* 3 (4): 374–81. doi:10.1161/CIRCOUTCOMES.109.907287.

Ribeiro, R. A., S. F. Stella, S. A. Camey, L. I. Zimerman, M. Pimentel, and others. 2010. "Cost-Effectiveness of Implantable Cardioverter-Defibrillators in Brazil: Primary Prevention Analysis in the Public Sector." *Value in Health* 13 (2): 160–68.

Rivero-Ayerza, M., D. A. M. J. Theuns, H. M. Garcia-Garcia, E. Boersma, M. Simoons, and others. 2006. "Effects of Cardiac Resynchronization Therapy on Overall Mortality and Mode of Death: A Meta-Analysis of Randomized Controlled Trials." *European Heart Journal* 27 (22): 2682–88. doi:10.1093/eurheartj/ehl203.

Shea, B. J., C. Hamel, G. A. Wells, L. M. Bouter, E. Kristjansson, and others. 2009. "AMSTAR Is a Reliable and Valid Measurement Tool to Assess the Methodological Quality of Systematic Reviews." *Journal of Clinical Epidemiology* 62(10): 1013-20. PMID: 19230606.

Schaink, A. 2012. *Inotropic and Vasoactive Agents for In-Hospital Heart Failure Management: A Rapid Review*. Toronto: Health Quality Ontario.

Shibata, M. C., M. D. Flather, and D. Wang. 2001. "Systematic Review of the Impact of Beta Blockers on Mortality and Hospital Admissions in Heart Failure." *European Journal of Heart Failure* 3 (3): 351–57.

Shibata, M. C., R. T. Tsuyuki, and N. Wiebe. 2008. "The Effects of Angiotensin-Receptor Blockers on Mortality and Morbidity in Heart Failure: A Systematic Review." *International Journal of Clinical Practice* 62 (9): 1397–402. doi:10.1111/j.1742-1241.2008.01806.x.

SOLVD Investigators. 1992. "Effect of Enalapril on Mortality and the Development of Heart Failure in Asymptomatic Patients with Reduced Left Ventricular Ejection Fractions: The SOLVD Investigators." *New England Journal of Medicine* 327 (10): 685–91. doi:10.1056/NEJM199209033271003.

Sliwa, K., and S. Stewart. 2014. "Heart Failure in the Developing World." In *Heart Failure: A Companion to Braunwald's Heart Disease*, edited by D. L. Mann, 410–20. Philadelphia: Elsevier.

Stevens, G. A., G. King, and K. Shibuya. 2010. "Deaths from Heart Failure: Using Coarsened Exact Matching to Correct Cause-of-Death Statistics." *Population Health Metrics* 8: 6. doi:10.1186/1478-7954-8-6.

Takeda, A., S. J. C. Taylor, R. S. Taylor, F. Khan, H. Krum, and others. 2012. "Clinical Service Organisation for Heart Failure." *Cochrane Database of Systematic Reviews* 9 (9): CD002752. doi:10.1002/14651858.CD002752.pub3.

Taylor, R. S., V. A. Sagar, E. J. Davies, S. Briscoe, A. J. S. Coats, and others. 2014. "Exercise-Based Rehabilitation for Heart Failure." *Cochrane Database of Systematic Reviews* 4 (4): CD003331. doi:10.1002/14651858.CD003331.pub4.

Thomas, R., A. Huntley, M. Mann, D. Huws, S. Paranjothy, and others. 2013. "Specialist Clinics for Reducing Emergency Admissions in Patients with Heart Failure: A Systematic Review and Meta-Analysis of Randomised Controlled Trials." *Heart* 99 (4): 233–39.

Tran, K., C. Ho, H. Z. Noorani, K. Cimon, A. Hodgson, and others. 2007. *Thiazide Diuretics as First-Line Treatment for Hypertension: Meta-Analysis and Economic Evaluation.* Technology Report Number 95. Ottawa, Ontario: Canadian Agency for Drugs and Technologies in Health.

Tsevat, J., D. Duke, L. Goldman, M. A. Pfeffer, G. A. Lamas, and others. 1995. "Cost-Effectiveness of Captopril Therapy after Myocardial Infarction." *Journal of the American College of Cardiology* 26 (4): 914–19.

Uhlig, K., E. M. Balk, A. Earley, R. Persson, A. C. Garlitski, and others. 2013. *Assessment on Implantable Defibrillators and the Evidence for Primary Prevention of Sudden Cardiac Death.* Technology Assessment Project ID: CRDT0511. Rockville, MD: Agency for Healthcare Research and Quality. http:// www.cms.gov/medicare/coverage/determinationprocess /downloads/id91TA.pdf.

Vital, F. M. R., M. T. Ladeira, and Á. N. Atallah. 2013. "Non-Invasive Positive Pressure Ventilation (CPAP or Bilevel NPPV) for Cardiogenic Pulmonary Oedema." *Cochrane Database of Systematic Reviews* 5: CD005351. doi:10.1002/14651858.CD005351.pub3.

Watkins, D., B. Hasan, B. Mayosi, G. Buhkman, J. A. Marin-Neto, and others. 2017. "Structural Heart Disease." In *Disease Control Priorities* (third edition): Volume 5 *Cardiovascular, Respiratory, and Related Disorders,* edited by D. Prabhakaran, S. Anand, T. A. Gaziano, J.-C. Mbanya, Y. Wu, and R. Nugent. Washington, DC: World Bank.

Weintraub, W. S., Z. Zhang, E. M. Mahoney, P. Kolm, J. A. Spertus, and others. 2005. "Cost-Effectiveness of Eplerenone Compared with Placebo in Patients with Myocardial Infarction Complicated by Left Ventricular Dysfunction and Heart Failure." *Circulation* 111 (9): 1106–13.

WHO (World Health Organization). 2015a. "Global Health Estimates." WHO, Geneva. http://www.who.int/healthinfo /global_burden_disease/en.

———. 2015b. "WHO Model List of Essential Medicines." 19th List. WHO, Geneva. http://www.who.int/medicines /publications/essentialmedicines/EML_2015_FINAL _amended_NOV2015.pdf?ua=1.

Yancy, C. W., M. Jessup, B. Bozkurt, J. Butler, D. E. Casey Jr., and others. 2013. "2013 ACCF/AHA Guideline for the Management of Heart Failure: A Report of the American College of Cardiology Foundation/ American Heart Association Task Force on Practice Guidelines." *Circulation* 128 (16): E240–327. doi:10.1161/ CIR.0b013e31829e8776.

Zhang, Z., E. M. Mahoney, P. Kolm, J. Spertus, J. Caro, and others. 2010. "Cost Effectiveness of Eplerenone in Patients with Heart Failure after Acute Myocardial Infarction Who Were Taking Both ACE Inhibitors and Beta-Blockers: Subanalysis of the EPHESUS." *American Journal of Cardiovascular Drugs* 10 (1): 55–63. doi:10.2165/11319940 -000000000-00000.

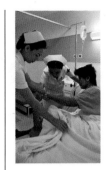

Chapter **11**

Structural Heart Diseases

David A. Watkins, Babar Hasan, Bongani Mayosi,
Gene Bukhman, J. Antonio Marin-Neto, Anis Rassi Jr.,
Anis Rassi, and R. Krishna Kumar

INTRODUCTION

Structural heart diseases constitute a large proportion of the burden of cardiovascular disease in low- and middle-income countries (LMICs). Some conditions, such as rheumatic heart disease (RHD) and Chagas disease (CD), are associated with poverty and are preventable. Congenital heart disease (CHD), in contrast, is prevalent in all regions, but treatment is more readily available in higher-income countries. All structural heart diseases have a progressive course in the absence of prevention or surgical treatment.

This chapter summarizes the key clinical and public health issues around three key groups of structural heart disease: major congenital heart defects, RHD, and CD. Although advanced surgical care for these conditions is a rapidly evolving topic, this chapter emphasizes the importance of primary prevention and early detection, which are the missing links in many programs. These activities have particular relevance in resource-constrained settings, where access to advanced surgical and interventional care is not feasible.

CONGENITAL HEART DISEASE

The Condition

Incidence and Natural History

CHD is the most common single congenital anomaly. The overall incidence of CHD is approximately 8–10 per 1,000 live births; 5–6 per 1,000 require specialized

interventions, and approximately 50 percent of these are patients during the neonatal or early infancy period of critical CHD (Hoffman and Kaplan 2002). Systematic efforts have been made to determine the burden of CHD in selected LMICs (Saxena and others 2015). Vaidyanathan and others (2011) reported 425 babies (7.75 percent) with CHD of the 5,487 consecutive newborns screened at a community hospital in Kerala, India. Of these, 17 (0.31 percent) had major CHD that was likely to require correction through heart surgery or catheter procedure; the rest had minor lesions, most of which normalized without intervention by age six weeks (Vaidyanathan and others 2011). The incidence among live births in China was similar to that in high-income countries (HICs)—8.2 per 1,000 live births—although a much higher incidence was seen among stillbirths, 168.8 per 1,000 (Yang and others 2009).

Most forms of CHD in HICs are also encountered in LMICs, but the outcomes vary in LMICs depending on the availability of facilities and expertise (Kumar 2003; Kumar and Shrivastava 2008). Table 11.1 summarizes the natural history and modified natural history, following surgery or catheter intervention, of common forms of CHD.

Global Burden and Geography

The World Health Organization (WHO) estimates that 230,000 deaths or 20.3 million disability-adjusted life-years (DALYs) from CHD occurred globally in 2000 and 234,000 deaths or 19.8 million DALYs occurred in 2012, corresponding to 0.4 percent of total deaths and

Corresponding author: David A. Watkins, Department of Medicine, University of Washington, Seattle, WA, United States; davidaw@uw.edu.

Table 11.1 Broad Categories of Congenital Heart Disease, Classified According to Natural History

Broad category	Implications for survival and treatment	Examples[a]
Critical CHD	Incompatible with survival without specific intervention in newborn period or early infancy	Transposition of the great arteries, obstructed TAPVC, duct-dependent pulmonary or systemic circulation
Major CHD	Intervention is required, often in early infancy, for optimal long-term outcome	TOF, DORV, large VSD and PDA, complete atrioventricular canal, truncus arteriosus, aorto-pulmonary window, single ventricle physiology, unobstructed TAPVC, ALCAPA, severe outflow tract obstructions
CHD that typically manifests at an older age	Diagnosis seldom made in early childhood; intervention required to prevent long-term sequelae in adulthood	Moderate or large ASD, some forms of coarctation, some patients with Ebstein's anomaly, relatively less severe forms of aortic and pulmonary valve stenosis, congenitally corrected transposition of the great arteries with intact ventricular septum
Minor CHD	Long-term, symptom-free survival can be expected without any specific intervention in most cases	Small left-to-right shunts (ASD, VSD, PDA), bicommissural aortic valve

Note: ALCAPA = anomalous coronary artery from pulmonary artery; ASD = atrial septal defect; CHD = congenital heart disease; DORV = double outlet right ventricle; PDA = patent ductus arteriosus; TAPVC = total anomalous pulmonary venous communication; TOF = tetralogy of Fallot; VSD = ventricular septal defect.

a. These examples are not a comprehensive list of conditions; many conditions are not listed. Numerous combinations are possible.

0.7 percent of DALYs in each year. The impact of the congenital anomalies varies by geographic region. They account for 510 DALYs per 100,000 population in the Middle East and North Africa, but only 260 DALYs per 100,000 population in East Asia and Pacific (WHO 2015).

Risk Factors

Genetic predisposition, in conjunction with environmental factors, appears to explain the occurrence of CHD. The recurrence risk in siblings of an affected individual is 1 percent to 6 percent when neither parent is affected (Burn and others 1998; Calcagni and others 2007); if more than one sibling is affected, this risk can increase to 10 percent (Nora and Nora 1988). Obstructive left-heart lesions generally have a higher risk of recurrence, compared with other forms of CHD (Lewin and others 2004); an estimated 20 percent of the first-degree relatives of patients with obstructive left-heart lesions may have undiagnosed CHD, such as bicuspid aortic valve (Kerstjens-Frederikse and others 2011). CHD has also been been associated with environmental factors such as folate deficiency, maternal diabetes, and use of specific medications or alcohol during pregnancy (Blue and others 2012). Table 11.2 summarizes the risk factors.

Trends

CHD is unlikely to be perceived as a pediatric health priority in regions with high infant mortality, defined as greater than 20 per 1,000 live births. However, as infant mortality from communicable diseases continues to decline in most regions, CHD is likely to emerge as a

significant health problem among infants and newborns in regions witnessing rapid and substantial human and economic development (Boutayeb 2006). Furthermore, the number of children born with CHD in LMICs is several times that in HICs because of population size, and birth rates are higher in most LMICs because of the higher numbers of women of reproductive age and higher fertility rates compared to HICs (UN 2014).

Interventions, Platforms, and Policies

Relatively modest benefits can be achieved by antenatal prevention efforts, but most of the postnatal interventions for CHD, whether screening or treatment, imply some availability of advanced, specialized surgical care.

CHD Prevention

Only 20 percent of cases have an identifiable cause; multifactorial inheritance has been proposed for cases of unknown etiology (Blue and others 2012). Genetic counseling and better family planning measures can help prevent CHD, especially if multiple family members are affected and a specific, inheritable, genetic disorder is identified. Consanguinity is a challenging problem and can be approached through educational programs targeted to the regions and communities where it is more frequently prevalent (Stoll and others 1999). Folate deficiency, use of certain medications during pregnancy, maternal diabetes, and phenylketonuria are also modifiable risk factors. Despite the limited

Table 11.2 Etiology of CHD: Prenatal Exposure to Acquired Factors

Risk factors	Associations with CHD
Diabetes and obesity	Various forms of CHD are linked with maternal gestational and pregestational diabetes or obesity, including transposition of the great arteries, ASD, VSD, hypoplastic left heart syndrome, cardiomyopathy, and PDA.
Phenylketonuria	Phenylketonuria is associated with a more than sixfold increase in the risk of CHD, specifically VSD, TOF, PDA, and single ventricle.
Febrile illnesses in the first trimester	Any febrile illness during the first trimester of pregnancy may result in a twofold increase in the risk of CHD.
Rubella	Specific cardiac manifestations of rubella embryopathy include PDA, pulmonary valve abnormalities, peripheral pulmonary stenosis, and VSD.
Epilepsy	The association may be a result of the risk of CHD from anticonvulsant medications.
Lupus (apart from typical symptoms of SLE, it may be useful to ask for history of previous abortions)	Maternal SLE is associated with risk of complete heart block in the offspring.
Vitamin deficiency	Multivitamin supplements, including folic acid derivatives, have been shown to protect against occurrence of CHD; multivitamins may reduce the risk of CHD associated with febrile illnesses in the first trimester.
Alcohol consumption	Muscular VSD
Maternal use of folate	Decreased risk of conotruncal anomalies
Prenatal exposure to medications in the first trimester, including anticonvulsants, NSAIDs, trimethoprim-sulphonamide, thalidomide, and vitamin A cogenors	Ebstein's anomaly, VSD, and ASD

Source: Blue and others 2012.
Note: ASD = atrial septal defect; CHD = congenital heart disease; NSAIDs = nonsteroidal anti-inflammatory drugs; PDA = patent ductus arteriosus; SLE = systemic lupus erythematosus; TOF = tetralogy of Fallot; VSD = ventricular septal defect.

and inconclusive evidence, several general recommendations can be made for women during early pregnancy (Blue and others 2012):

- Daily folic acid and vitamin B12 supplementation in the preconception and periconception period
- Completion of rubella vaccination before pregnancy
- Optimal management of metabolic disorders, such as diabetes and phenylketonuria, before and during pregnancy
- Avoidance of medication associated with CHD before and during pregnancy, if possible.

CHD Screening

Prenatal diagnosis and postnatal screening protocols have helped in the early detection of CHD, especially those cases with critical duct-dependent lesions in HICs. In most LMICs, however, timely diagnosis of CHD is uncommon, and late presentation is the norm. Critical CHD may first manifest with hypoxemia, hypotension, or both and is frequently misdiagnosed as neonatal sepsis or pneumonia (Saxena 2005). Many pediatricians and primary care providers in LMICs do not regularly consider CHD to be a significant cause of neonatal and early infant morbidity and mortality, and intense targeted education and awareness are needed.

The relatively low overall prevalence of CHD and low positive predictive value of screening tests should be considered when evaluating whether to implement a screening program (Zühlke and Vaidyanathan 2013). Screening can be accomplished prenatally using fetal echocardiogram or in newborns using physical exam and pulse oximetry.

Prenatal Screening. Fetal echocardiography is often used to screen for CHD after 14–16 weeks gestation and is best suited for relatively severe forms of CHD. The test is time consuming, and accuracy is considerably influenced by operator expertise and quality of equipment (Sharland 2010), which are low in many LMICs. Nuchal translucency seen on first trimester antenatal ultrasound (appearing as a collection of fluid under the skin behind the fetal neck) may be an alternative screening test (Hyett and others 1999), but its sensitivity is low and its utility is probably limited (Makrydimas, Sotiriadis, and Ioannidis 2003). The treatment options in the event of a positive screening test are also limited. Termination of pregnancy may be an option in countries where it is legally permissible and screening is initiated before 20–24 weeks of gestation. Screening beyond the 20–24 week limit implies the capacity to refer patients to deliver at a center with a comprehensive pediatric heart program. Early referral for delivery overcomes the logistical challenges of transporting a newborn with CHD. Improved postnatal outcomes in prenatally diagnosed cases of CHD have not been consistently demonstrated (Sharland 2010).

Neonatal Screening. The identification of critical CHD soon after birth could substantially reduce mortality, but babies with critical CHD are not always immediately symptomatic. Early postnatal pulse oximetry has a higher sensitivity and specificity than clinical examination for detecting CHD (Vaidyanathan and others 2011). A meta-analysis of screening studies from HICs demonstrated that pulse oximetry was 76.5 percent sensitive and 99.9 percent specific for CHD (Thangaratinam and others 2012); however, the positive predictive value of screening in LMICs is poorly understood. Studies of pulse oximetry screening in resource-limited settings have yielded disappointing results (Saxena and others 2015; Vaidyanathan and others 2011).

Although physical examination has low sensitivity and specificity, one study demonstrated several findings that could identify patients with CHD (Vaidyanathan and others 2011). In these cases, follow-up examination is required at six weeks of life because certain defects—such as large ventricular septal defect and patent ductus arteriosus—can only be detected at that time. To date, routine physical examination screening programs in LMICs have not been evaluated.

Finally, while routine screening echocardiograms for all newborns is impractical, the use of echocardiography has value in cases where pulse oximetry or clinical examination suggests a higher than usual probability of CHD. Unfortunately, the barriers to widespread availability of echocardiography include high equipment costs and limited operator expertise (Kumar and Shrivastava 2008).

Screening of Infants and Toddlers. Screening modalities have not been systematically evaluated in this age group. Perhaps the best opportunity for screening for CHD is during routine immunization. A combination of clinical examination and pulse oximetry can be considered in this age group. It may be necessary to develop a simple clinical protocol and then validate it (Directorate General of Health Services 2006).

Screening of School Children. Cardiac auscultation is likely to be the most practical strategy for screening school children given that the utility of pulse oximetry in this group is very limited. CHD screening can potentially be integrated with screening for RHD, undernutrition, obesity, and hypertension (Thakur and others 1997). Children who are underweight and those with limited physical capacity need to be reevaluated, and the capacity to refer for confirmatory echocardiography is required for suspected cases.

CHD Care and Treatment: Curative and Palliative

Management of CHD requires the building of surgical programs (figure 11.1) and skill sets that take decades to develop. Comprehensive pediatric heart care with facilities to treat even the most complicated lesions, however, is realistic only in selected centers in LMICs, usually limited to large cities (Kumar and Shrivastava 2008). Most LMICs have varying degrees of resources for treatment. These limitations apply to treatment of cases identified by screening, so consideration needs to be given to treatment availability before initiation of a new screening program. Furthermore, identification of a large number of CHD cases by screening will put additional pressure on specialized centers in LMICs to expand care.

Depending on the type of defect, surgical procedures are designed to either restore normal anatomy or physiology (or both) or palliate by improving physiology. The latter is more realistic for severe defects that lead to single ventricle physiology. The majority of CHDs require open-heart cardiac surgery, although increasing numbers of patients are being managed using catheter-based procedures. The cost of surgical interventions increases incrementally as CHD becomes more complex, and outcomes are often less than ideal. Many CHDs require multiple operations, often into adolescence or adulthood. In most cases, surgical intervention requires lifelong medical supervision to monitor for potential complications (Zühlke, Mirabel, and Marijon 2013).

Several new pediatric heart programs have been established in LMICs, such as in China, India, and Vietnam, and increasing numbers of heart operations and catheter interventions are being performed. Still, few comprehensive pediatric heart centers with the capability for infant and newborn heart surgery exist in LMICs; many of these centers, especially in India, are in the private sector and financially out of the reach of average families (Kumar and Shrivastava 2008; Saxena 2005). Existing centers are clustered in selected cities and regions with relatively better human development indices, and many children in Asia, Africa, and South America have no access to pediatric heart care (Zühlke, Mirabel, and Marijon 2013).

Figure 11.1 Organization of Resources Needed to Provide Surgical Care for Structural Heart Diseases

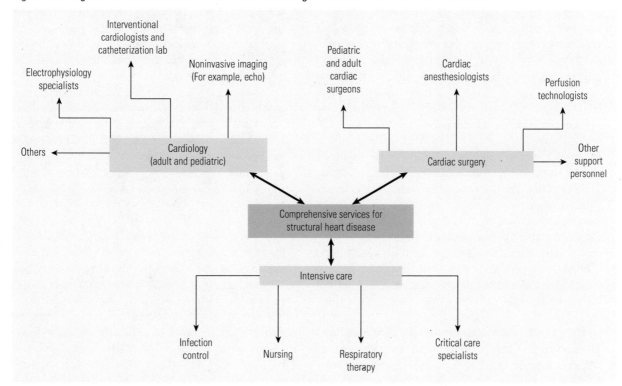

Source: Kumar and Shrivastava 2008.

Early initiation of treatment for children with CHD is widely recommended, but it is unrealistic in many LMICs, where treatment strategies and thresholds are significantly restricted. Palliation as the final path or as a bridge to complete repair at an older age may be the only realistic option in centers with limited resources (Kumar and Tynan 2005; Pinto and Dalvi 2004). Surgery may be offered as an alternative to the less invasive option of catheter closure of heart defects because of the cost of imported hardware (Kumar and Tynan 2005; Vida and others 2006).

Summary of Costs and Cost-Effectiveness of CHD Interventions

Cost of CHD Care

By means of semistructured interviews, Raj and others (2015) explored the direct and indirect expenses, sources of financing, and perceived financial stress of surgery for CHD on 464 Indian families whose children underwent surgery. They found that the surgery imposed a substantial economic burden on the health care infrastructure and affected families. The mean hospital expenses for the admission and surgery (including indirect costs to the family) accounted for an average of 0.93 (interquartile range 0.52–1.49) times the annual family income of patients (Raj and others 2015). Selected centers in LMICs have developed low-cost alternatives to expand the capacity to treat patients. These approaches include reuse of hardware (Kumar and Tynan 2005), development of novel devices and surgical prosthetics (Bhuvaneshwar and others 1996), and alternatives to the cardiopulmonary bypass circuit (Kreutzer and others 2005; Rasheed and others 2014).

Cost-Effectiveness of CHD Screening

Most cost-effectiveness analyses of CHD screening have been conducted in HICs and the results do not appear to be cost-effective using acceptability thresholds in LMICs. Modeling studies based in the United Kingdom and the United States have demonstrated that screening would generate more false than true positives and would only avert a handful of deaths annually, with incremental cost-effectiveness ratios (ICERs) exceeding US$40,000 per life year gained (Peterson and others 2013; Roberts and others 2012). Universal newborn oximetry screening is recommended in many HICs (Thangaratinam and others 2012); however, cost-effectiveness data from

LMICs are sparse, and published HIC ICERs would not be "acceptable" in LMICs. Furthermore, given the poor sensitivity and positive predictive value of the test in resource-limited environments (Vaidyanathan and others 2011), it is unclear that universal pulse oximetry screening can be recommended in LMICs.

CHD Programs in Low- and Middle-Income Countries
A Guatemalan experience demonstrates how a successful CHD program can be developed in a low-resource setting (Larrazabal and others 2007). The key aspect of the program was the creation of a self-sustaining endowment fund to support the cost of care, since 95 percent of patients required subsidized care. Monetary donations were collected through the Friends of Aldo Castenada Foundation. Individuals invested in stocks and company shares, and the interest returns on these investments were placed back into the endowment fund. The goal was to let the interest money accumulate. This fund was then used to share the cost of care with government-subsidized insurance and patient copays.

Bakshi and others (2007) reported that accumulative experience led to satisfactory neonatal CHD surgical outcomes in a center in southern India. Postoperative mortality decreased from 21.4 percent to 4.3 percent, although the prevalence of postoperative infections remained high. Similarly, the experience of the Amrita Institute of Medical Sciences in Kochi, India, has demonstrated that developing a pediatric heart center in a low-resource setting is feasible and can provide high-quality surgical care (Reddy and others 2015).

CHD Conclusions and Recommendations
Congenital heart disease contributes significantly to morbidity and mortality among children in LMICs. CHD is likely to surface as a pediatric health priority in many regions in the near future because of declining mortality from infectious diseases. Unfortunately, routine screening for CHD before or shortly after birth may not be realistic in many countries, and access to surgical care is limited, even for existing cases. Despite the limited and inconclusive evidence, a few general recommendations can be made:

- *Address modifiable risk factors for CHD whenever possible.* Several of these risk factors are routinely addressed by high-quality prenatal care—for example, folate supplementation, education about teratogens, and management of maternal weight and gestational diabetes—and investment in prenatal care can be a first step to addressing CHD in the absence of treatment options.

- *All countries can begin to consider building capacity for the treatment of CHD.* It may not be possible to meet the ideal requirement of one center per 5 million population (Davis and others 1996), but a limited number of regional centers could develop expertise in advanced CHD care and training. These centers do need to include investments in nonsurgical physician expertise, such as cardiovascular imaging and anesthesia, as well as nonphysician expertise, such as critical care nursing. Governments could subsidize such centers to serve as a source of local data on disease burden, educate local pediatricians to recognize CHD, and develop innovative and low-cost therapies and management protocols.

- *The decision to initiate universal screening for CHD is context and resource dependent.* The lack of an effective screening tool makes CHD screening difficult, and no cost-effectiveness studies have assessed CHD screening in LMICs. However, targeted efforts to improve awareness of early diagnosis and management among pediatricians are likely to improve detection in symptomatic infants and newborns. Cost-effectiveness studies of CHD screening could be considered in settings where surgical capacity exists.

- *Careful case selection needs to be part of any scale-up of surgical care for CHD.* The specific treatment strategy could be individualized, depending on resources, disease characteristics, comorbidities, and local medical expertise. Given the extraordinary clinical variety of CHDs, this task is likely to be daunting. Nevertheless, conditions such as ventricular septal defects, which can be corrected through a single operation, could receive higher priority; multistage palliative operations, such as those for hypoplastic left heart syndrome, could receive lower priority. No therapy may be the only realistic option in settings with significant resource limitations. Although philanthropy or charity can provide substantial help in providing care to families who cannot afford such therapies, donor exhaustion makes such sources unreliable. Endowments-based charity accounts, which are self-sustaining, may be more beneficial.

- *Consideration should be given to financing of CHD diagnosis and treatment.* In LMICs, cardiovascular care, including CHD surgery, is infrequently covered by public finance or other subsidized insurance systems; the inclusion of CHD care may allow a larger proportion of affected children to benefit from definitive treatment. However, in countries with very constrained budgets, public finance may not be financially sustainable and could detract from more pressing priorities for universal coverage.

RHEUMATIC HEART DISEASE

The Condition

Pathogenesis and Natural History

RHD, a chronic inflammatory disease of the heart valves, is the result of untreated group A streptococcal throat infection (pharyngitis). The streptococcus produces an abnormal immune response in susceptible individuals, typically between the ages of 5 and 15 years. This immune response manifests as acute rheumatic fever (ARF), and severe and recurrent episodes of rheumatic fever (RF) increase the likelihood of heart valve damage (Marijon and others 2012). RHD remains the most common cause of acquired heart disease in children and young adults in LMICs (Carapetis and others 2005).

RHD classically presents as progressive shortness of breath between the ages of 20 years and 50 years. It is slightly more common in women than men; in many women, its first manifestation is during pregnancy as the physiologic stress on the heart increases (Sliwa and others 2010). The clinical period is preceded by a long latent and asymptomatic period, however—perhaps as long as 10 years—especially for well-tolerated patterns of valve disease (Marijon and others 2012). This latent period poses significant barriers to clinical screening and preventive treatment, because individuals are often otherwise healthy. Many patients first present for care in advanced heart failure or with other complications, such as heart valve bacterial infection (endocarditis) or stroke due to atrial fibrillation (Sliwa and others 2010).

Global Burden and Geography of RHD

RHD is the most common cause of valvular heart disease in LMICs. There were an estimated 372,000 deaths or 14.3 million DALYs from RHD globally in 2000 and 337,000 deaths or 12.0 million DALYs in 2012 (WHO 2015). Most contemporary reports on RHD have come from South Asia, the Pacific Islands, and Sub-Saharan Africa; many indigenous communities in Asia and Pacific show a high prevalence of ARF and RHD risk factors (Carapetis and others 2005; Omurzakova and others 2009). The burden of RHD as measured by prevalence is an active topic in the literature (Zühlke and Steer 2013). Studies using echocardiography-based methods of measuring prevalence in schoolchildren have demonstrated a 10-fold higher prevalence of valvular abnormalities, compared with prevalence reported using clinical diagnostic methods (Marijon and others 2007). Little is known about the natural history of these asymptomatic cases compared with the smaller number of symptomatic cases that have traditionally been reported (Zühlke and Mayosi 2013).

Risk Factors

The most important risk factor for ARF seems to be proximity to other individuals with streptococcal pharyngitis—a situation seen in overcrowded areas with inadequate sanitation, such as among the urban poor (Robertson and Mayosi 2008). Other risk factors that correlate with poverty include undernutrition, low maternal educational level, and unemployment (Longo-Mbenza and others 1998). In HICs, the incidence of ARF began to decline before the discovery of penicillin, and this observation has prompted the hypothesis that economic development and sanitation are as important as antibiotic treatment in eradicating RHD (Gordis 1985). Genetic factors also may increase the risk of ARF (Engel and others 2011), which helps account for the empirical observation that, at most, 3 percent to 5 percent of individuals with untreated streptococcal pharyngitis will develop ARF, and even fewer will progress to RHD (Michaud, Rammohan, and Narula 1999).

Trends

The burden of RHD in both deaths and DALYs appears to be declining, but newer methods of measuring prevalence may lead to revisions of these estimates. Nevertheless, the decrease in burden is consistent with overall trends in economic development and global health gains during the past two decades. The distribution of these health gains remains unclear, particularly among the poorest and most remote populations. For example, in 2005, mortality from RHD in rural Ethiopia was 12.5 percent per year (Gunther, Asmera, and Parry 2006). Finally, declining mortality rates imply an increasing prevalence and an increasing case load on health systems in LMICs.

Interventions, Platforms, and Policies

RHD Interventions

Primary Prevention. Table 11.3 summarizes the key points of intervention in the natural history of ARF and RHD, covering primary and secondary prevention, surgical treatment, and *primordial prevention*, the latter referring to measures that reduce the incidence of streptococcal transmission in the general population. Research on primary prevention conducted in the 1950s among American military recruits demonstrated that penicillin treatment of streptococcal pharyngitis could reduce the risk of ARF by about 80 percent (Robertson, Volmink, and Mayosi 2005). Although most of the effectiveness data on primary prevention are older and of lower quality, penicillin is widely regarded as the mainstay of prevention and remains in all major clinical guidelines (Marijon and others 2012).

Table 11.3 Major Categories of Interventions for the Prevention and Control of RHD

Intervention	Rationale	Estimated efficacy or effectiveness	Comments
Vaccination against group A streptococcus	Prevent streptococcal sore throat infection	100 percent (theoretical) efficacy at preventing strep throat and ARF or RHD	No vaccine has yet been developed to cover all major serotypes affecting LMICs.
Primary prevention of ARF with benzathine penicillin G	Prevent development of first episode of ARF	80 percent relative risk reduction	Most trials conducted in 1950s and 1960s in young American males.
Secondary prevention of ARF and RHD with benzathine penicillin G	Prevent recurrent episodes of ARF and recurrent and progressive heart valve damage	55 percent relative risk reduction (penicillin vs. control); 87 percent to 98 percent relative risk reduction (injectable versus oral penicillin)	Trials are generally of poor quality and heterogeneous methodology, making results difficult to extrapolate.
Surgical and percutaneous management of established RHD	Palliate cases of advanced RHD with heart failure	Variable effectiveness: Depends on severity of disease, number of heart valves involved, and surgical technique	No controlled trials comparing surgical treatment to no therapy or to medical therapy. Percutaneous treatment of mitral stenosis can be very effective in well-selected cases but generally requires surgical capacity as a backup.

Note: ARF = acute rheumatic fever; LMICs = low- and middle-income countries; RF = rheumatic fever; RHD = rheumatic heart disease.

Secondary Prevention. Early studies of individuals with a documented history of ARF demonstrated that regular secondary preventive therapy with penicillin—especially injectable benzathine penicillin—could reduce the risk of recurrent ARF and, by inference, RHD (Manyemba and Mayosi 2002). The rationale for secondary prevention is that it eliminates streptococcal colonization and thereby persistent subclinical inflammation and progressive valve damage (Majeed and others 1986). Sufficient evidence indicates that secondary prevention programs produce low rates of ARF recurrence in patients receiving continuous secondary prophylaxis. However, the quality of controlled studies is suboptimal, and it has been difficult to quantify the relationship between ARF recurrences averted and reductions in incident RHD (Manyemba and Mayosi 2002). Despite these evidence gaps, there is strong consensus globally that secondary prevention is effective and that further trials on its effectiveness would not be ethical.

Limitations of the Evidence for Prevention. From the policy standpoint, interpreting and applying the literature on primary and secondary prevention poses several challenges.

- The studies are all of poor quality and are more than 20 years old; nearly all were conducted in HICs. These trials used older formulations of penicillin that are no longer in widespread use, limiting the usefulness of these data in contemporary economic models.

- There is no evidence that primary or secondary prevention reduces RHD mortality, and no such trials are likely to be performed in children for ethical reasons.
- No studies have been conducted for secondary prevention in adults with ARF and RHD, who constitute the majority of cases today.
- An exclusive primary prevention strategy could miss a substantial proportion of cases because 50 percent to 75 percent of ARF cases may have no history of symptomatic pharyngitis.
- Adherence to a regimen of three- or four-weekly penicillin injections for secondary prevention is often difficult to achieve in practice (Gunther, Asmera, and Parry 2006; WHO 1992).
- Despite aggressive prevention efforts, many patients with established RHD require surgical intervention when valve dysfunction becomes severe and symptomatic (Zühlke and others 2015).

Cardiac Surgery. For individuals with established RHD, surgical and percutaneous techniques are available to repair, replace, or palliate damaged valves. The mitral valve is most commonly affected by RHD and is the most frequent target of surgical and catheter-based interventions; the aortic and tricuspid valves are also susceptible. In general, patients with more than one valve involved have a poorer prognosis, even with adequate access to surgery (Marijon and others 2012).

For patients with isolated mitral stenosis (narrowed mitral valve) and favorable valve characteristics, catheter-based dilation (percutaneous balloon valvulotomy) has become the treatment standard—at least in settings with access to state-of-the-art equipment and interventional cardiologists. However, percutaneous procedures should be performed in centers with cardiothoracic surgical expertise in case of complications (figure 11.1). An alternative to percutaneous valvulotomy is closed mitral valvulotomy, which can be performed by a general or cardiothoracic surgeon in a center with fewer resources.

For many LMICs, however, the scale-up of open-heart surgical services may be the most important option for patients with advanced RHD. Given the prevalence of unfavorable mitral stenosis, mitral incompetence (which cannot currently be treated by catheter-based methods), and multivalvular disease, most patients with RHD are not eligible for minimally invasive techniques and eventually require surgical valve replacement. Valve replacement is palliative rather than curative; most patients require lifelong anticoagulation and are exposed to high complication rates (Marijon and others 2012).

Primordial Prevention. A final intervention for RHD, although theoretical at present, is a vaccine against group A streptococcus—primordial prevention. Vaccine research and development has been ongoing for years, with promising results in select populations from phase II clinical trials (Bisno and others 2005). Unfortunately, the global distribution of streptococcal serotypes is very different from those investigated in clinical trials (Steer and others 2009); an array of serotypes—more than could feasibly have been included in any previously developed multivalent vaccine—have been implicated in ARF. Efforts are underway to ensure the development of a vaccine that will be effective in LMICs (Dale and others 2013).

RHD Delivery Platforms

The potential delivery platforms for RHD-related interventions can be classified as follows:

- Community-based efforts to educate children, parents, and educators about sore throat, ARF, and RHD
- Provision of primary and secondary prophylaxis in outpatient settings, primarily in primary care settings
- Third-level care at specialized or referral facilities that offer cardiology and cardiac surgery services.

Community-Based Primary and Secondary Prevention. Successful ARF and RHD programs have implemented a comprehensive approach that integrates community-based education and awareness with the scale-up of sore throat treatment to increase primary prevention and case finding of patients with ARF and RHD to build disease registers and increase secondary prevention. The WHO recommends a comprehensive approach to RHD control modeled after these types of programs (WHO 2004).

Unfortunately, as of 2012, ARF and RHD prevention had not been included in standard guidelines and protocols for child health, such as the Integrated Management of Childhood Illness program. This omission is partly because most child health programs focus on those under age five years, and streptococcal sore throat and ARF are uncommon in this group. Accordingly, although the RHD community has produced many resources for managing sore throat and developing secondary prevention programs (Wyber 2013), these resources have yet to be integrated with other child and adolescent health interventions. Partners in Health has developed an integrated model for noncommunicable diseases that includes RHD, factoring in such issues as registration, supply chain management, and adherence support at both first- and second-level hospitals (Partners in Health 2011). However, this model has not yet been applied in a broad range of settings.

Secondary Prevention Using Echocardiography. Following the publication of echocardiography screening studies (Marijon and others 2007), many research groups attempted to develop active case finding programs to increase secondary prevention using echocardiography in community and school settings.[1] This approach was adopted by the Stop RHD A.S.A.P. Programme at the University of Cape Town (Robertson, Volmink, and Mayosi 2006) and by similar programs in the South Pacific (Lawrence and others 2013). Controversy remains about the long-term impact and cost-effectiveness of these programs because the natural history of cases detected by echocardiogram—and the effectiveness of secondary prophylaxis in this group—is unknown (Zühlke and Mayosi 2013).

Surgical Care Platforms. Although some countries have the capacity for specialized surgical and catheter-based interventions, at least in urban centers, the ratio of the population to the number of centers is grossly inequitable; only a handful of centers exist in all of Sub-Saharan Africa other than South Africa (Zühlke, Mirabel, and Marijon 2013). Three models of initiatives have helped ameliorate this situation:

- Some well-selected cases are transferred for surgery on a philanthropic basis to Europe and the United States; a variant of this model is for visiting surgeons to set up temporary services in-country in conjunction with charitable organizations.[2]

- Using South-South collaboration, patients are referred to high-volume regional or continental centers, such as in India or Sudan.[3] Unfortunately, many countries have national referral boards that finance out-of-country transfers on an extremely limited basis, and these referrals are likely to be somewhat biased against the rural poor who are less likely to receive a diagnosis or to benefit from advocacy efforts.
- Lower-income countries start to build surgical platforms in their own countries (Binagwaho and others 2013), although this model can be resource intensive and may detract from other health priorities.

ARF and RHD Public Policies for Prevention and Control

The WHO's comprehensive set of guidelines on RF and RHD for LMICs (WHO 2004) recommended a package of several types of activities within an integrated RHD program (table 11.4). The evidence for these public health initiatives largely came from Latin America and the Caribbean during the 1970s and 1980s, when ARF was essentially eradicated and the prevalence of severe RHD was dramatically reduced (Bach and others 1996; Nordet and others 2008). Although the decline in ARF and RHD in most regions has tracked closely with social and economic development, the role of primordial measures—policies dealing with risk factors such as overcrowding, sanitation and hygiene, and poor nutrition—is unclear, yet is likely to be significant (Gordis 1985).

There have been recent efforts to develop policies for ARF and RHD prevention and control in Africa. A technical consultation initiated by the African Union in 2015 produced a set of seven key actions for ARF and RHD (Watkins, Zühlke, and others 2016). In addition to the elements recommended by the WHO (2004) report, this consultation stressed the need to ensure adequate supplies of high-quality penicillin, which has recently experienced poor availability globally. It also highlighted the many points of integration with reproductive and maternal health services and with other noncommunicable diseases. These recommendations have since been adopted in a resolution signed by all African heads of state, and implementation plans are currently being developed in collaboration with the WHO.

Table 11.4 Components of an Integrated Program on ARF and RHD Prevention and Control

Component activity	Elements	Comments
Planning phase	Establishment of a national advisory committee; assessment of disease burden; stepwise implementation, monitoring, and evaluation	Program should be multisectoral, engaging stakeholders in ministries of health and education, and streamlined into existing infrastructure.
Primary prevention	Training of health care providers to accurately detect and treat streptococcal pharyngitis; ensuring adequate supply of and affordability of penicillin	Most effective when the importance of primary prevention is integrated into a public education program.
Secondary prevention	Establishment of national, regional, and local disease registers; active case finding, surveillance, and follow-up of existing cases	Particular focus should be given to cases at risk of poor adherence to regular prophylaxis.
Provider training	Training health care workers on primary and secondary prevention as appropriate, as well as management of anaphylactic reactions to penicillin	Engagement of public health nurses is essential in areas with physician shortages.
Health education	Regular educational activities to be carried out in schools and using local and nationwide print and electronic media programs	Messaging should summarize importance of primary and secondary prevention, promote health-seeking behavior for sore throat, and encourage efforts to limit spread of infection.
Epidemiologic surveillance	Regular audits of disease registers and conduct of prevalence studies (resources permitting), including microbiological surveillance	Reports should note seasonal frequency, distribution of cases, and streptococcal serotypes implicated.
Community engagement	Major stakeholders include health and educational administrators, school teachers and school health services, and families of patients.	Active screening of school children for RHD may be indicated in high-prevalence settings.

Source: Adapted from WHO 2004.
Note: ARF = acute rheumatic fever; RHD = rheumatic heart disease.

Summary of Costs and Cost-Effectiveness of RHD Interventions

Economic Burden of RHD

Appropriate management of RHD involves access to primary as well as specialized care, and long-term use of medications; for many individuals, it also involves one or more major surgeries. RHD results in both direct and indirect losses in productivity due to chronic disability. Only one study of the economic impact of RHD in an LMIC was identified. This study, in Brazil, demonstrated high rates of health care utilization, school and work absenteeism, and direct medical costs of approximately US$151,300 per 100 patients annually (Terreri and others 2001).

Cost of RHD Interventions

Published estimates of RHD intervention costs to the health system are scarce. One study reported primary, secondary, and tertiary prevention costs to Pondicherry Union Territory, India (population 974,345), as totaling approximately US$6.2 million, US$5.0 million, and US$8.8 million, respectively (Soudarssanane and others 2007). Irlam and others (2013) gathered primary cost data as part of a clinical cost-effectiveness analysis of primary prevention strategies in South Africa. Watkins and others (2015) reanalyzed data from Cuba and found that a combined primary and secondary prevention program cost approximately US$0.07 per year per at-risk child ages 5–14 years. Finally, it should be noted that although the prevalence of RHD is thought to be highest in low-income countries, the direct cost of RHD to the health system is probably higher in middle-income countries, where tertiary cardiology and cardiac surgery services are available and are being widely provided for persons with RHD.

Cost-Effectiveness of Primary RHD Prevention

In low-prevalence settings with inexpensive throat culture media, the most cost-effective strategy for ARF prevention is to screen with a rapid antigen test and send positive screens for throat culture, withholding treatment unless throat cultures are positive (Shulman and others 2012). In contrast, Irlam and others (2013) evaluated a clinical decision rule developed for low-resource settings. They compared treat-all and treat-none strategies to five algorithms that combined decision-rule cutoffs, with or without culture. In their high-prevalence setting (15.3 percent streptococcal pharyngitis), the most cost-effective strategy was to treat individuals with a decision-rule score of two or higher, without microbiologic confirmation. The ICER for this approach was US$145 per quality-adjusted life year, and it dominated

all other strategies up to a willingness-to-pay threshold of US$60,000. These results have yet to be replicated in other countries.

Cost-Effectiveness of Secondary RHD Prevention

The evidence for the cost-effectiveness of secondary prevention is based primarily on the results of a multicountry study conducted by the WHO in the late 1970s to scale up secondary prevention. Over 5,500 patient-years were observed in the study. The cost of secondary prevention resources was much lower than the averted cost of hospitalizations for recurrent ARF, making the program cost saving by definition (Strasser and others 1981).

Some studies have attempted to model the cost-effectiveness of echocardiography to identify RHD cases and scale-up of secondary prevention, compared with other primary and secondary prevention strategies (Manji and others 2013). However, these studies rely on natural history assumptions that have not been borne out by long-term follow-up of echocardiography screening studies (Zühlke and Mayosi 2013).

Comparative Cost-Effectiveness of RHD Interventions

Several studies provide insights into the tradeoffs between various prevention and treatment strategies.

- Watkins and others (2015) demonstrated that a comprehensive approach to ARF and RHD control in Cuba—including both primary and secondary prevention at the community level—was cost saving. However, much of the savings were from cardiac surgery costs averted, and these savings may not be relevant to a country without these high health system costs.
- Soudarssanane and others (2007) compared primary and secondary prevention and surgery as isolated interventions, measuring benefits as gains in labor productivity and monetary value of deaths averted in a benefit-cost framework. They cited benefit-cost ratios of 1.56 for primary prevention, 1.07 for secondary prevention, and 0.12 for surgery and argued that primary prevention was the most cost-effective of the three approaches.
- A similar approach, with a narrower cost-effectiveness framework, was used as part of the first Disease Control Priorities project (Michaud, Rammohan, and Narula 1999). The study compared the cost-effectiveness of a theoretical vaccine to primary, secondary, and tertiary strategies in low- versus high-endemicity settings. Secondary prevention dominated primary prevention and surgery, while a theoretical vaccine was probably cost-effective compared with secondary prevention. This study extrapolated cost data from the early 1990s and,

compared with more recent work, used fairly crude assumptions in the model (Irlam and others 2013).
- Watkins, Lubinga, and others (forthcoming) updated this analysis using contemporary data on disease epidemiology and costs as well as a lifetime horizon model. They found that, in a hypothetical African country, scale-up of primary prevention would be cost saving and secondary prevention would be very cost-effective, with ICERs less than per capita gross domestic product of LMICs in Sub-Saharan Africa. Scale-up of surgery by referral to international sites (for example, in India) could be cost-effective in some contexts, but building an in-country surgical center would probably not be cost-effective and would have a large budgetary impact.

However, building cardiac surgery capacity in low-resource settings might yield economies of scope and scale and educational output with regard to training surgeons and cardiologists; these are benefits that cannot be included in a narrow cost-effectiveness analysis around RHD. Accordingly, decisions about building cardiac surgery should ideally use a benefit-cost analysis approach that accounts for the added benefits outside of the domain of RHD.

RHD Conclusions and Recommendations

RHD remains one of the most important cardiovascular conditions globally. Public policies to address ARF and RHD need to balance the lower costs and higher benefits of preventing future cases of RHD with the ethical obligation to consider advanced medical and surgical treatment of existing cases. Policy decisions are context specific and often made in an environment of high uncertainty.

We make the following general recommendations for countries seeking to increase their capacity to address the challenges of ARF and RHD:

- *All countries in endemic regions could implement steps to measure and monitor the burden of ARF and RHD.* Vital statistics, disease notification systems, and disease registers can be important sources of data for tracking ARF and RHD at a local level, and notification and registries can support primary and secondary prevention efforts.
- *Primary prevention could be a high priority and could be integrated into existing child and adolescent health interventions.* The successful control of ARF and RHD in several Latin American countries was predicated on combining primary and secondary prevention within existing care delivery programs. Such programs are likely to be synergistic when combined with secondary prevention (Watkins and others 2015).

- *The foundation of secondary prevention could be passive case finding through disease registries.* Active case finding through echocardiography-based screening has not yet been demonstrated to improve clinical outcomes; it should only be considered in the context of a well-functioning disease registry with adequate rates of adherence.
- *All countries in endemic regions could assess capacity for scaling up surgical care.* Some countries may find that establishing a surgical center is cost-effective and can strengthen health services for other diseases. Others may continue to rely on philanthropic care. A third model, particularly for very poor nations in Sub-Saharan Africa, would be to strengthen referral pathways to regional centers of excellence and provide greater financial protection for patients and families in need. In all of these cases, given the impact of surgery on premature child and young adult mortality, provision of surgery will likely lead to a positive return on investment.

CHAGAS HEART DISEASE

The Condition

Pathogenesis and Natural History

CD is caused by infection with the protozoan parasite *Trypanosoma cruzi* (*T. cruzi*), and runs through acute and chronic phases. Diagnosis in the acute phase is rare since most patients are asymptomatic or experience a nonspecific flu-like episode. After the acute phase, a latent or indeterminate form of the disease occurs in which patients also remain asymptomatic. When the determinate forms appear late in the natural history of the infection, chronic Chagas cardiomyopathy (CCC) is the most common and ominous form of the disease (Rassi, Rassi, and Marin-Neto 2010).

Organ damage during the acute phase is associated with high-grade parasitemia, intense tissue parasitism, and the immuno-inflammatory response to the parasite, mainly in the heart, gastrointestinal tract, and central nervous system. Although several mechanisms may contribute to the pathogenesis of CCC, the consensus is that parasite persistence and the parasite-driven immune response are key factors (Marin-Neto and others 2007) along with neurogenic depopulation caused by the parasite, which may trigger malignant arrhythmia and sudden death (Marin-Neto and others 1992).

Although patients with the indeterminate form of CD—including those with any abnormality on highly sensitive blood tests—have a good prognosis, epidemiological studies in endemic areas have shown that, in 1 percent to 3 percent each year, the disease evolves from the indeterminate to the determinate forms (Sabino and others 2013). Accordingly, even patients with the indeterminate form require yearly follow-up (Rassi, Rassi, and Marin-Neto 2010). Major risk factors for mortality in patients with CCC are clinical heart failure, cardiomegaly, left ventricular systolic dysfunction, and nonsustained ventricular tachycardia (Rassi, Rassi, and Marin-Neto 2009; Rassi, Rassi, and Rassi 2007). A risk score for predicting mortality in patients with CCC has been developed (Rassi and others 2006) and validated (Rocha and Ribeiro 2006).

Global Burden and Geography

CD accounted for 9,000 deaths and 571,000 DALYs in 2000 and 8,000 deaths and 528,000 DALYs in 2012 (WHO 2015). Despite a substantial reduction in the number of individuals infected with *T. cruzi* worldwide—from between 16 million and 18 million in the 1990s to between 8 million and 10 million in the mid-2000s—CD still represents the third-largest tropical disease burden, after malaria and schistosomiasis. Most infections occur through vector-borne transmission by Triatominae insects; transmission can also occur through blood transfusion, from mother to infant, by ingestion of food or liquid contaminated with *T. cruzi*, and rarely by organ transplantation and accidents among laboratory personnel who work with live parasites (Rassi, Rassi, and Marin-Neto 2010).

Formerly, the disease was confined to socially underdeveloped rural areas in almost all Latin American and the Caribbean countries. However, because of the migration from endemic countries, CD has become a potential public health problem in nonendemic regions, including Australia, Europe, Japan, and the United States (Schmunis 2007). Transmission risk in HICs occurs mostly through the nonvector mechanisms; these are becoming increasingly important even in endemic regions where recent vector transmission programs have been successful.

Interventions, Platforms, and Policies

CD requires interventions at multiple levels. Vector control and prevention of transmission from nonvectorial mechanisms are the two essential strategies aimed at primary prevention. Reduction of domiciliary vector infestation by spraying of insecticides, improvement in housing conditions, and education of individuals at risk are the key measures. Most national vector control programs in Latin America and the Caribbean have been initiated centrally and have involved three successive stages:

- Rapid and aggressive mass insecticide spraying
- Respraying of houses with residual infestation
- Subsequent community surveillance.

The classic example is the Brazilian experience during the 1970s and 1980s, which resulted in near eradication of the vector by the mid-2000s (Moncayo and Silveira 2009). These measures, coupled with serological screening of blood donors, have markedly reduced transmission of the parasite in many endemic countries (Rassi, Rassi, and Marin-Neto 2010). Additionally, trypanocide treatment before pregnancy has been demonstrated to prevent congenital transmission in affected women treated before they become pregnant (Fabbro and others 2014).

Secondary prevention includes screening and finding cases of *T. cruzi* infection at an early asymptomatic stage of the disease to offer specific therapy. The mainstay of secondary prevention is treating patients with the indeterminate form of the disease with a trypanocidal agent such as benznidazole or nifurtimox. The backbone of secondary prevention lies in the attempt to eradicate *T. cruzi*, to prevent chronic organ damage in the infected host, and to interrupt the epidemiological chain (Rassi, Rassi, and Marin-Neto 2010). However, a clinical trial of benznidazole for CCC demonstrated reductions in parasitemia but no reduction in the progression of cardiac disease over five years (Morillo and others 2015). Advanced medical or surgical prevention strategies aim to reduce morbidity and mortality related to congestive heart failure (see chapter 10 of this volume, Huffman and others 2017), valvular disease, and cardiac arrhythmias (Sosa-Estani, Colantonio, and Segura 2012).

Summary of Costs and Cost-Effectiveness of Interventions

Economic Burden of CD

A recent Markov simulation model estimated the global and regional health and economic burden of CD from the societal perspective to be US$7.2 billion per year and US$188.8 billion for the lifetimes of the whole population of individuals infected (Lee and others 2013). More than 10 percent of these costs were accrued in nonendemic countries. Most of the economic costs arose from lost productivity caused directly by early cardiovascular mortality (Lee and others 2013). Another study addressed the cost of treating patients with CCC who were admitted with decompensated heart failure as compared with other etiologies of acute heart failure. They found that treating CCC was more expensive and mortality was higher in this population at follow-up (Abuhab and others 2013). Finally, a Colombian study estimated that the average lifetime cost of a patient with CCC was US$14,501 (Castillo-Riquelme and others 2008).

Cost-Effectiveness of Interventions for CD

Economic evaluations of CD interventions have focused predominantly on vector control efforts, such as insecticide spraying programs. The economic impact of the Brazilian program was also assessed using both cost-effectiveness and benefit-cost strategies. The program cost US$57 per DALY averted or saved US$25 for every dollar spent on prevention, making it economically very attractive (Moncayo and Silveira 2009).

In Colombia, one study used subnational survey data to assess the incremental cost-effectiveness of spraying versus doing nothing, demonstrating that geographical variation (for example, in higher- versus lower-endemicity regions) had a large effect on the ICER and that resources should be allocated accordingly (Castillo-Riquelme and others 2008). Investigators from Argentina retrospectively assessed the cost-effectiveness of shifting from a vertical (centralized) vector control approach to a community-based, horizontal approach (including a mixed approach incorporating both elements). They found that a mixed approach—a vertical attack phase followed by horizontal surveillance phase led by communities and primary health care centers—would be more cost-effective than either fully horizontal or vertical approaches (Vazquez-Prokopec and others 2009).

Finally, one study of a hypothetical CD vaccine demonstrated that, under a wide variety of assumptions about coverage, effectiveness, and cost, such a vaccine would be very cost-effective and even cost saving (Lee and others 2010). Unfortunately, very little has been written about the cost-effectiveness of secondary or tertiary prevention strategies, which are likely to be relatively more important in the face of decreasing incidence.

CD Conclusions and Recommendations

CD remains an important cause of cardiovascular morbidity and mortality in countries in Latin America and the Caribbean. However, the rapid rollout of effective vector control efforts has led to a dramatic reduction in the incidence of CD and could lead to reductions in CCC in the long term.

We make the following recommendations to endemic countries:

- *Insecticide spraying programs are very cost-effective.* Policy makers in regions where *T. cruzi* is still endemic could embrace a mixed vertical and horizontal approach to vector control. The experiences of Argentina and Brazil can serve as models for other countries.

- *More research is needed on the cost-effectiveness of secondary and tertiary prevention before specific recommendations can be made.* Little is known about the cost-effectiveness of screening individuals and blood bank supplies for evidence of *T. cruzi* or treating CCC with advanced cardiac technologies, such as pacemakers. Prevention of congenital CD may be a high priority area from an equity standpoint. Future research could examine the tradeoffs between ongoing prevention efforts and treatment of existing cases.

CONCLUSIONS

Structural heart diseases are unique because they predominantly affect younger populations and thus contribute substantially to the years of life lost from cardiovascular disease in LMICs. Preventive measures exist for all three conditions, and they are most effective for RHD and CD. Interest is growing in screening programs for structural heart diseases, yet the role of screening is limited in settings where access to advanced medical and surgical care is not available. Most individuals with advanced structural heart disease require surgery, which poses particular challenges in limited-resource settings and provides additional rationale for scaling up cost-effective primary prevention efforts. Our discussion of these three conditions provides decision makers with a framework for public policy that takes into consideration the resources available in various settings. Our recommendations for prevention and management will need to be contextualized to individual settings and integrated into broader cardiovascular disease control policy frameworks.

NOTES

World Bank Income Classifications as of July 2014 are as follows, based on estimates of gross national income (GNI) per capita for 2013:

- Low-income countries (LICs) = US$1,045 or less
- Middle-income countries (MICs) are subdivided:
  (a) lower-middle-income = US$1,046 to US$4,125
  (b) upper-middle-income (UMICs) = US$4,126 to US$12,745
- High-income countries (HICs) = US$12,746 or more.

1. See the World Heart Federation's website at http://www.world-heart-federation.org/what-we-do/applied-research/rheumatic-heart-disease-demonstration-projects/.
2. See the Chain of Hope at http://www.chainofhope.org/.
3. For example, see the Salaam Centre for Cardiac Surgery at http://salamcentre.emergency.it.

REFERENCES

Abuhab, A., E. Trindade, G. B. Aulicino, S. Fujii, E. A. Bocchi, and others. 2013. "Chagas' Cardiomyopathy: The Economic Burden of an Expensive and Neglected Disease." *International Journal of Cardiology* 168 (3): 2375–80.

Bach, J. F., S. Chalons, E. Forier, G. Elana, J. Jouanelle, and others. 1996. "10-Year Educational Programme Aimed at Rheumatic Fever in Two French Caribbean Islands." *The Lancet* 347 (9002): 644–48.

Bakshi, K. D., B. Vaidyanathan, K. R. Sundaram, S. J. Roth, K. Shivaprakasha, and others. 2007. "Determinants of Early Outcome after Neonatal Cardiac Surgery in a Developing Country." *Journal of Thoracic and Cardiovascular Surgery* 134 (3): 765–71.

Bhuvaneshwar, G. S., C. V. Muraleedharan, G. A. Vijayan, R. S. Kumar, and M. S. Valiathan. 1996. "Development of the Chitra Tilting Disc Heart Valve Prosthesis." *Journal of Heart Valve Disease* 5 (4): 448–58.

Binagwaho, A., E. Rusingiza, J. Mucumbitsi, C. M. Wagner, and J. D. Swain. 2013. "Uniting to Address Pediatric Heart Disease in Africa: Advocacy from Rwanda." *South African Heart Journal* 10 (2): 440–64.

Bisno, A. L., F. A. Rubin, P. P. Cleary, J. B. Dale, for the National Institute of Allergies and Infectious Diseases. 2005. "Prospects for a Group A Streptococcal Vaccine: Rationale, Feasibility, and Obstacles: Report of a National Institute of Allergy and Infectious Diseases Workshop." *Clinical Infectious Diseases* 41 (8): 1150–56.

Blue, G. M., E. P. Kirk, G. F. Sholler, R. P. Harvey, and D. S. Winlaw. 2012. "Congenital Heart Disease: Current Knowledge about Causes and Inheritance." *Medical Journal of Australia* 197 (3): 155–59.

Boutayeb, A. 2006. "The Double Burden of Communicable and Non-Communicable Diseases in Developing Countries." *Transactions of the Royal Society of Tropical Medicine and Hygiene* 100 (3): 191–99.

Burn, J., P. Brennan, J. Little, S. Holloway, R. Coffey, and others. 1998. "Recurrence Risks in Offspring of Adults with Major Heart Defects: Results from First Cohort of British Collaborative Study." *The Lancet* 351 (9099): 311–16.

Calcagni, G., M. C. Digilio, A. Sarkozy, B. Dallapiccola, and B. Marino. 2007. "Familial Recurrence of Congenital Heart Disease: An Overview and Review of the Literature." *European Journal of Pediatrics* 166 (2): 111–16.

Carapetis, J. R., A. C. Steer, E. K. Mulholland, and M. Weber. 2005. "The Global Burden of Group A Streptococcal Diseases." *The Lancet Infectious Diseases* 5 (11): 685–94.

Castillo-Riquelme, M., F. Guhl, B. Turriago, N. Pinto, F. Rosas, and others. 2008. "The Costs of Preventing and Treating Chagas Disease in Colombia." *PLoS Neglected Tropical Diseases* 2 (11): e336.

Dale, J. B., V. A. Fischetti, J. R. Carapetis, A. C. Steer, S. Sow, and others. 2013. "Group A Streptococcal Vaccines: Paving a Path for Accelerated Development." *Vaccine* 31 (Suppl 2): B216–22.

Davis, J. T., H. D. Allen, J. D. Powers, and D. M. Cohen. 1996. "Population Requirements for Capitation Planning in Pediatric Cardiac Surgery." *Archives of Pediatrics and Adolescent Medicine* 150 (3): 257–59.

Directorate General of Health Services. 2006. *Indian Public Health Standards for Primary Health Centers, Guidelines 2006*. New Delhi: Directorate General of Health Services, Government of India. http://www.iapsmgc.org/userfiles /4IPHS_for_PHC.pdf.

Engel, M. E., R. Stander, J. Vogel, A. A. Adeyemo, and B. M. Mayosi. 2011. "Genetic Susceptibility to Acute Rheumatic Fever: A Systematic Review and Meta-Analysis of Twin Studies." *PLoS One* 6 (9): e25326.

Fabbro, D. L., E. Danesi, V. Olivera, M. O. Codebo, S. Denner, and others. 2014. "Trypanocide Treatment of Women Infected with *Trypanosoma cruzi* and its Effect on Preventing Congenital Chagas." *PLoS Neglected Tropical Diseases* 8 (11): e3312.

Gordis, L. 1985. "The Virtual Disappearance of Rheumatic Fever in the United States: Lessons in the Rise and Fall of Disease. T. Duckett Jones Memorial Lecture." *Circulation* 72 (6): 1155–62.

Gunther, G., J. Asmera, and E. Parry. 2006. "Death from Rheumatic Heart Disease in Rural Ethiopia." *The Lancet* 367 (9508): 391.

Hoffman, J. I., and S. Kaplan. 2002. "The Incidence of Congenital Heart Disease." *Journal of the American College of Cardiology* 39 (12): 1890–900.

Huffman, M. D., G. A. Roth, K. Sliwa, C. W. Yancy, and D. Prabhakaran. 2017. "Heart Failure." In *Disease Control Priorities* (third edition): Volume 5, *Cardiovascular, Respiratory, and Related Diseases*, edited by D. Prabhakaran, S. Anand, T. A. Gaziano, J.-C. Mbanya, Y. Wu, and R. Nugent. Washington, DC: World Bank.

Hyett, J., M. Perdu, G. Sharland, R. Snijders, and K. H. Nicolaides. 1999. "Using Fetal Nuchal Translucency to Screen for Major Congenital Cardiac Defects at 10–14 Weeks of Gestation: Population Based Cohort Study." *British Medical Journal* 318 (7176): 81–85.

Irlam, J., B. M. Mayosi, M. Engel, and T. A. Gaziano. 2013. "Primary Prevention of Acute Rheumatic Fever and Rheumatic Heart Disease with Penicillin in South African Children with Pharyngitis: A Cost-Effectiveness Analysis." *Circulation: Cardiovascular Quality and Outcomes* 6 (3): 343–51.

Kerstjens-Frederikse, W. S., G. J. Du Marchie Sarvaas, J. S. Ruiter, P. C. Van Den Akker, A. M. Temmerman, and others. 2011. "Left Ventricular Outflow Tract Obstruction: Should Cardiac Screening Be Offered to First-Degree Relatives?" *Heart* 97 (15): 1228–32.

Kreutzer, C., G. Zapico, J. L. Simon, A. J. Schlichter, and G. O. Kreutzer. 2005. "A Simplified and Economic Technique for Immediate Postcardiotomy Pediatric Extracorporeal Membrane Oxygenation." *ASAIO Journal* 51 (5): 659–62.

Kumar, R. K. 2003. "Congenital Heart Disease Management in the Developing World (Letter)." *Pediatric Cardiology* 24 (311): 13.

Kumar, R. K. and S. Shrivastava. 2008. "Paediatric Heart Care in India." *Heart* 94 (8): 984–90.

Kumar, R. K., and M. J. Tynan. 2005. "Catheter Interventions for Congenital Heart Disease in Third World Countries." *Pediatric Cardiology* 26 (3): 241–49.

Larrazabal, L. A., K. J. Jenkins, K. Gauvreau, V. L. Vida, O. J. Benavidez, and others. 2007. "Improvement in Congenital Heart Surgery in a Developing Country: The Guatemalan Experience." *Circulation* 116 (17): 1882–87.

Lawrence, J. G., J. R. Carapetis, K. Griffiths, K. Edwards, and J. R. Condon. 2013. "Acute Rheumatic Fever and Rheumatic Heart Disease: Incidence and Progression in the Northern Territory of Australia, 1997 to 2010." *Circulation* 128 (5): 492–501.

Lee, B. Y., K. M. Bacon, M. E. Bottazzi, and P. J. Hotez. 2013. "Global Economic Burden of Chagas Disease: A Computational Simulation Model." *The Lancet Infectious Diseases* 13 (4): 342–84.

Lee, B. Y., K. M. Bacon, D. L. Connor, A. M. Willig, and R. R. Bailey. 2010. "The Potential Economic Value of a *Trypanosoma cruzi* (Chagas Disease) Vaccine in Latin America." *PLoS Neglected Tropical Diseases* 4 (12): e916.

Lewin, M. B., K. L. McBride, R. Pignatelli, S. Fernbach, A. Combes, and others. 2004. "Echocardiographic Evaluation of Asymptomatic Parental and Sibling Cardiovascular Anomalies Associated with Congenital Left Ventricular Outflow Tract Lesions." *Pediatrics* 114 (3): 691–96.

Longo-Mbenza, B., M. Bayekula, R. Ngiyulu, V. E. Kintoki, N. F. Bikangi, and others. 1998. "Survey of Rheumatic Heart Disease in School Children of Kinshasa Town." *International Journal of Cardiology* 63 (3): 287–94.

Majeed, H. A., A. M. Yousof, F. A. Khuffash, A. R. Yusuf, S. Farwana, and others. 1986. "The Natural History of Acute Rheumatic Fever in Kuwait: A Prospective Six Year Follow-Up Report." *Journal of Chronic Diseases* 39 (5): 361–69.

Makrydimas, G., A. Sotiriadis, and J. P. Ioannidis. 2003. "Screening Performance of First-Trimester Nuchal Translucency for Major Cardiac Defects: A Meta-Analysis." *American Journal of Obstetrics and Gynecology* 189 (5): 1330–35.

Manji, R. A., J. Witt, P. S. Tappia, Y. Jung, A. H. Menkis, and others. 2013. "Cost-Effectiveness Analysis of Rheumatic Heart Disease Prevention Strategies." *Expert Review of Pharmacoeconomics and Outcomes Research* 13 (6): 715–24.

Manyemba, J., and B. M. Mayosi. 2002. "Penicillin for Secondary Prevention of Rheumatic Fever." *Cochrane Database of Systematic Reviews* 3: CD002227.

Marijon, E., M. Mirabel, D. S. Celermajer, and X. Jouven. 2012. "Rheumatic Heart Disease." *The Lancet* 379 (9819): 953–64.

Marijon, E., P. Ou, D. S. Celermajer, B. Ferreira, A. O. Mocumbi, and others. 2007. "Prevalence of Rheumatic Heart Disease Detected by Echocardiographic Screening." *New England Journal of Medicine* 357 (5): 470–76.

Marin-Neto, J. A., E. Cunha-Neto, B. C. Maciel, and M. V. Simoes. 2007. "Pathogenesis of Chronic Chagas Heart Disease." *Circulation* 115 (9): 1109–23.

Marin-Neto, J. A., P. Marzullo, C. Marcassa, L. Gallo Júnior, B. C. Maciel, and others. 1992. "Myocardial Perfusion Abnormalities in Chronic Chagas' Disease as Detected by Thallium-201 Scintigraphy." *American Journal of Cardiology* 69 (8): 780–84.

Michaud, C., R. Rammohan, and J. Narula. 1999. "Cost-Effectiveness Analysis of Intervention Strategies for Reduction of the Burden of Rheumatic Heart Disease." In *Rheumatic Fever*, edited by J. Narula, R. Virmani, K. S, Reddy, and R. Tandon, 485–97. Washington, DC: American Registry of Pathology.

Moncayo, A., and A. C. Silveira. 2009. "Current Epidemiological Trends for Chagas Disease in Latin America and Future Challenges in Epidemiology, Surveillance and Health Policy." *Memorias do Instituto Oswaldo Cruz* 104 (Suppl 1): 17–30.

Morillo, C. A., J. A. Marin-Neto, A. Avezum, S. Sosa-Estani, A. Rassi Jr., and others. 2015. "Randomized Trial of Benznidazole for Chronic Chagas' Cardiomyopathy." *New England Journal of Medicine* 373 (14): 1295–306.

Nora, J. J., and A. H. Nora. 1988. "Update on Counseling the Family with a First-Degree Relative with a Congenital Heart Defect." *American Journal of Medical Genetics* 29 (1): 137–42.

Nordet, P., R. Lopez, A. Duenas, and L. Sarmiento. 2008. "Prevention and Control of Rheumatic Fever and Rheumatic Heart Disease: The Cuban Experience (1986–1996–2002)." *Cardiovascular Journal of Africa* 19 (3): 135–40.

Omurzakova, N. A., Y. Yamano, G. M. Saatova, M. I. Mirzakhanova, S. M. Shukurova, and others. 2009. "High Incidence of Rheumatic Fever and Rheumatic Heart Disease in the Republics of Central Asia." *International Journal of Rheumatic Diseases* 12 (2): 79–83.

Partners in Health. 2011. "The Partners in Health Guide to Chronic Care Integration for Endemic Non-Communicable Diseases, Rwanda Edition." In *Cardiac, Renal, Diabetes, Pulmonary, and Palliative Care*, edited by G. Bukhman and A. Kidder. Boston, MA: Partners in Health.

Peterson, C., S. D. Grosse, M. E. Oster, R. S. Olney, and C. H. Cassell. 2013. "Cost-Effectiveness of Routine Screening for Critical Congenital Heart Disease in US Newborns." *Pediatrics* 132 (3): e595–603.

Pinto, R. I., and B. Dalvi. 2004. "Transcatheter Guidewire Perforation of the Pulmonary Valve as a Palliative Procedure in Pulmonary Atresia with Intact Interventricular Septum." *Indian Heart Journal* 56 (6): 661–63.

Raj, M., M. Paul, A. Sudhakar, A. A. Varghese, A. C. Haridas, and others. 2015. "Micro-Economic Impact of Congenital Heart Surgery: Results of a Prospective Study from a Limited-Resource Setting." *PLoS One* 10 (6): e0131348.

Rasheed, R., O. Hidayat, M. Amanullah, and B. S. Hasan. 2014. "Conversion of Cardiac Bypass into an Extracorporeal Membrane Oxygenation Circuit: A Case from Pakistan." *Journal of the Pakistan Medical Association* 64 (5): 589–92.

Rassi, A. Jr., A. Rassi, W. C. Little, S. S. Xavier, S. G. Rassi, and others. 2006. "Development and Validation of a Risk Score for Predicting Death in Chagas' Heart Disease." *New England Journal of Medicine* 355 (8): 799–808.

Rassi, A. Jr., A. Rassi, and J. A. Marin-Neto. 2009. "Chagas Heart Disease: Pathophysiologic Mechanisms, Prognostic Factors and Risk Stratification." *Memorias do Instituto Oswaldo Cruz* 104 (Suppl 1): 152–58.

———. 2010. "Chagas Disease." *The Lancet* 375 (9723): 1388–402.

Rassi, A. Jr., A. Rassi, and S. G. Rassi. 2007. "Predictors of Mortality in Chronic Chagas Disease: A Systematic Review of Observational Studies." *Circulation* 115 (9): 1101–08.

Reddy, S. N., M. Kappanayil, R. Balachandran, A. Sudhakar, G. S. Sunil, and others. 2015. "Preoperative Determinants of Outcomes of Infant Heart Surgery in a Limited-Resource Setting." *Seminars in Thoracic and Cardiovascular Surgery* 27: 331–38.

Roberts, T. E., P. M. Barton, P. E. Auguste, L. J. Middleton, A. T. Furmston, and others. 2012. "Pulse Oximetry as a Screening Test for Congenital Heart Defects in Newborn Infants: A Cost-Effectiveness Analysis." *Archives of Disease in Childhood* 97 (3): 221–26.

Robertson, K. A., and B. M. Mayosi. 2008. "Rheumatic Heart Disease: Social and Economic Dimensions." *South African Medical Journal* 98 (10): 780–81.

Robertson, K. A., J. A. Volmink, and B. M. Mayosi. 2005. "Antibiotics for the Primary Prevention of Acute Rheumatic Fever: A Meta-Analysis." *BMC Cardiovascular Disorders* 5 (1): 11.

———. 2006. "Towards a Uniform Plan for the Control of Rheumatic Fever and Rheumatic Heart Disease in Africa— The Awareness Surveillance Advocacy Prevention (A.S.A.P.) Programme." *South African Medical Journal/Suid-Afrikaanse tydskrif vir geneeskunde* 96 (3 Pt 2): 241.

Rocha, M. O., and A. L. Ribeiro. 2006. "A Risk Score for Predicting Death in Chagas' Heart Disease." *New England Journal of Medicine* 355 (23): 2488–89; author reply 90–91.

Sabino, E. C., A. L. Ribeiro, V. M. Salemi, C. Di Lorenzo Oliveira, A. P. Antunes, and others. 2013. "Ten-Year Incidence of Chagas Cardiomyopathy among Asymptomatic *Trypanosoma cruzi*-Seropositive Former Blood Donors." *Circulation* 127 (10): 1105–15.

Saxena, A. 2005. "Congenital Heart Disease in India: A Status Report." *Indian Journal of Pediatrics* 72 (7): 595–98.

Saxena, A., A. Mehta, S. Ramakrishnan, M. Sharma, S. Salhan, and others. 2015. "Pulse Oximetry as a Screening Tool for Detecting Major Congenital Heart Defects in Indian Newborns." *Archives of Disease in Childhood Fetal and Neonatal Edition* 100 (5): F416–21.

Schmunis, G. A. 2007. "Epidemiology of Chagas Disease in Non-Endemic Countries: The Role of International Migration." *Memorias do Instituto Oswaldo Cruz* 102 (Suppl 1): 75–85.

Sharland, G. 2010. "Fetal Cardiac Screening: Why Bother?" *Archives of Disease in Childhood Fetal and Neonatal Edition* 95 (1): F64–68.

Shulman, S. T., A. L. Bisno, H. W. Clegg, M. A. Gerber, E. L. Kaplan, and others. 2012. "Clinical Practice Guideline for the Diagnosis and Management of Group A Streptococcal Pharyngitis: 2012 Update by the Infectious Diseases Society of America." *Clinical Infectious Diseases: An Official Publication of the Infectious Diseases Society of America* 55 (10): 1279–82.

Sliwa, K., M. Carrington, B. M. Mayosi, E. Zigiriadis, R. Mvungi, and S. Stewart. 2010. "Incidence and Characteristics of Newly Diagnosed Rheumatic Heart Disease in Urban African Adults: Insights from the Heart of Soweto Study." *European Heart Journal* 31 (6): 719–27.

Sosa-Estani, S., L. Colantonio, and E. L. Segura. 2012. "Therapy of Chagas Disease: Implications for Levels of Prevention." *Journal of Tropical Medicine* 2012: 292138.

Soudarssanane, M. B., M. Karthigeyan, T. Mahalakshmy, A. Sahai, S. Srinivasan, and others. 2007. "Rheumatic Fever and Rheumatic Heart Disease: Primary Prevention Is the Cost Effective Option." *Indian Journal of Pediatrics* 74 (6): 567–70.

Steer, A. C., I. Law, L. Matatolu, B. W. Beall, and J. R. Carapetis. 2009. "Global emm Type Distribution of Group A Streptococci: Systematic Review and Implications for Vaccine Development." *The Lancet Infectious Diseases* 9 (10): 611–16.

Stoll, C., Y. Alembik, M. P. Roth, and B. Dott. 1999. "Parental Consanguinity as a Cause for Increased Incidence of Births Defects in a Study of 238,942 Consecutive Births." *Annales de Genetique* 42 (3): 133–39.

Strasser, T., N. Dondog, A. E. Kholy, R. Gharagozloo, V. V. Kalbian, and others. 1981. "The Community Control of Rheumatic Fever and Rheumatic Heart Disease: Report of a WHO International Cooperative Project." *Bulletin of the World Health Organization* 59 (2): 285–94.

Terreri, M. T., M. B. Ferraz, J. Goldenberg, C. Len, and M. O. E. Hilario. 2001. "Resource Utilization and Cost of Rheumatic Fever." *Journal of Rheumatology* 28 (6): 1394–97.

Thakur, J. S., P. C. Negi, S. K. Ahluwalia, and R. Sharma. 1997. "Integrated Community-Based Screening for Cardiovascular Diseases of Childhood." *World Health Forum* 18 (1): 24–27.

Thangaratinam, S., K. Brown, J. Zamora, K. S. Khan, and A. K. Ewer. 2012. "Pulse Oximetry Screening for Critical Congenital Heart Defects in Asymptomatic Newborn Babies: A Systematic Review and Meta-Analysis." *The Lancet* 379 (9835): 2459–64.

UN (United Nations). 2014. *World Population Prospects: The 2012 Revision*. New York: UN.

Vaidyanathan, B., G. Sathish, S. T. Mohanan, K. R. Sundaram, K. K. Warrier, and others. 2011. "Clinical Screening for Congenital Heart Disease at Birth: A Prospective Study in a Community Hospital in Kerala." *Indian Pediatrics* 48 (1): 25–30.

Vazquez-Prokopec, G. M., C. Spillmann, M. Zaidenberg, U. Kitron, and R. E. Gurtler. 2009. "Cost-Effectiveness of Chagas Disease Vector Control Strategies in Northwestern Argentina." *PLoS Neglected Tropical Diseases* 3 (1): e363.

Vida, V. L., J. Barnoya, M. O'Connell, J. Leon-Wyss, L. A. Larrazabal, and others. 2006. "Surgical Versus Percutaneous Occlusion of Ostium Secundum Atrial Septal Defects: Results and Cost-Effective Considerations in a Low-Income Country." *Journal of the American College of Cardiology* 47 (2): 326–31.

Watkins, D. A., S. J. Lubinga, B. M. Mayosi, and J. B. Babigumira. Forthcoming. "A Cost-Effectiveness Tool to Guide the Prioritization of Interventions for Rheumatic Fever and Rheumatic Heart Disease Control in African Nations." *PLoS Neglected Tropical Diseases*.

Watkins, D. A., M. Mvundura, P. Nordet, and B. M. Mayosi. 2015. "A Cost-Effectiveness Analysis of a Program to Control Rheumatic Fever and Rheumatic Heart Disease in Pinar del Rio, Cuba." *PLoS One* 10 (3): e0121363.

Watkins, D. A., L. J. Zühlke, M. Engel, R. Daniels, V. Francis, and others. 2016. "Seven Key Actions to Eradicate Rheumatic Heart Disease in Africa: The Addis Ababa Communiqué." *Cardiovascular Journal of Africa* 27: 1–5.

WHO (World Health Organization). 1992. "WHO Programme for the Prevention of Rheumatic Fever/Rheumatic Heart Disease in Developing Countries: Report from Phase I (1986–90)." *Bulletin of the World Health Organization* 70 (2): 213–18.

———. 2004. *Rheumatic Fever and Rheumatic Heart Disease.* Technical Report Series 923. Geneva: WHO.

———. 2015. *Global Health Estimates.* Geneva: WHO. http://www.who.int/healthinfo/global_burden_disease/en/.

Wyber, R. 2013. "A Conceptual Framework for Comprehensive Rheumatic Heart Disease Control Programs." *Global Heart* 8 (3): 241–46.

Yang, X. Y., X. F. Li, X. D. Lu, and Y. L. Liu. 2009. "Incidence of Congenital Heart Disease in Beijing, China." *Chinese Medical Journal* 122 (10): 1128–32.

Zühlke, L. J., M. E. Engel, G. Karthikeyan, S. Rangarajan, P. Mackie, and others. 2015. "Characteristics, Complications, and Gaps in Evidence-Based Interventions in Rheumatic Heart Disease: The Global Rheumatic Heart Disease Registry (the REMEDY Study)." *European Heart Journal* 36: 1115–22a.

Zühlke, L. J., and B. M. Mayosi. 2013. "Echocardiographic Screening for Subclinical Rheumatic Heart Disease Remains a Research Tool Pending Studies of Impact on Prognosis." *Current Cardiology Reports* 15 (3): 343.

Zühlke, L. J., M. Mirabel, and E. Marijon. 2013. "Congenital Heart Disease and Rheumatic Heart Disease in Africa: Recent Advances and Current Priorities." *Heart* 99 (21): 1554–61.

Zühlke, L. J., and A. C. Steer. 2013. "Estimates of the Global Burden of Rheumatic Heart Disease." *Global Heart* 8 (3): 189–95.

Zühlke, L. J., and B. Vaidyanathan. 2013. "Is It Time for Developing Countries to Adopt Neonatal Pulse Oximetry Screening for Critical Congenital Heart Disease?" *SA Heart* 10: 454–61.

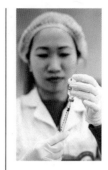

Chapter **12**

Diabetes: An Update on the Pandemic and Potential Solutions

Mohammed K. Ali, Karen R. Siegel, Eeshwar Chandrasekar,
Nikhil Tandon, Pablo Aschner Montoya, Jean-Claude Mbanya,
Juliana Chan, Ping Zhang, and K. M. Venkat Narayan

INTRODUCTION

Diabetes mellitus is a chronic metabolic disease with deadly, disabling, and costly consequences for individuals, families, communities, and countries. Although they are phenotypically distinct, diabetes subtypes (type 1, type 2, gestational, and other forms) are all defined by elevated blood glucose levels. Approximately 95 percent of diabetes cases worldwide are type 2 diabetes (previously known as *adult-onset* or *non-insulin-dependent* diabetes), which is the focus of this chapter. Type 1 diabetes (previously known as *insulin-dependent* diabetes) most commonly begins in childhood and adolescence. Gestational diabetes refers to elevated blood glucose levels during pregnancy among women without previous diabetes and is associated with fetal, birthing, and early childhood complications as well as higher risk of the mother developing postgestation diabetes.

The growth of diabetes and its impacts have accelerated worldwide since the end of the twentieth century (NCD-RisC 2016), likely correlated with expansion of diabetes risk factors, especially population aging and obesity. Diabetes is a multifactorial condition. Because genetic, epigenetic, lifestyle, economic, and psychosocial factors all contribute to the development of diabetes (McCarthy 2010; Stumvoll, Goldstein, and van Haeften 2005), preventing and managing the condition require action at policy, program, clinical practice, and individual levels (Hill and others 2013).

Reliable and meaningful estimates of burdens, risk factors, and effectiveness and cost-effectiveness of interventions as well as evaluations of existing policies, are limited; data are especially scarce in low- and middle-income countries (LMICs). This chapter focuses on what can and should be done to address diabetes. We present the available data regarding global burdens and trends in diabetes; review available evidence and assess the effectiveness and cost-effectiveness of interventions to prevent, detect, and control diabetes; and report summary expert opinions regarding the priority and feasibility of implementing these interventions. Assimilating evidence from countries at different income levels, we provide global perspectives on the diabetes pandemic, recommend priority interventions, and identify remaining data gaps.

GLOBAL BURDEN

Distribution and Prevalence

An estimated 415 million people—8.8 percent of the world's adult population—have diabetes (IDF 2015), and 75 percent of people with diabetes live in LMICs. Worldwide, specific populations and geographies

Corresponding author: Mohammed K. Ali, Hubert Department of Global Health, Rollins School of Public Health, Emory University, Atlanta, Georgia, United States; mkali@emory.edu.

experience very high prevalence of diabetes, notably the Western Pacific (for example, the Federated States of Micronesia) and Indian Ocean islands (for example, Mauritius), the Middle East (for example, Kuwait), North Africa (for example, the Arab Republic of Egypt), Native Americans, and urban South Asia (Ali, Bhaskarapillai, and others 2016; IDF 2015; Knowler and others 1978; Zabetian and others 2013). In addition, the world's most populous countries, such as China (Yang and others 2010), India (Anjana and others 2011), and the United States (CDC 2016), have very high absolute numbers of people with diabetes: 92.4 million, 65.1 million, and 29 million, respectively.

Worldwide, an estimated 46.5 percent of people with blood glucose levels in the diabetes range are undiagnosed (IDF 2015). It is estimated that, on average, one-quarter of people with diabetes in HICs are undiagnosed; in LMICs, in contrast, two-thirds to three-quarters are undiagnosed.

Globally, an equally high number of people are at high risk for developing diabetes because they have higher-than-normal fasting (impaired fasting glucose [IFG]) or postprandial (impaired glucose tolerance [IGT]) blood glucose levels, or both, or high glycated hemoglobin levels. Having any of these high-risk conditions is called prediabetes and puts individuals at 5–12 times higher annual risk of developing diabetes than the general population (Gerstein and others 2007). Although IFG and IGT may be phenotypically different and represent different pathophysiologies, accurate global estimates regarding the distribution of these subtypes of prediabetes are not available because the blood tests required to diagnose prediabetes are relatively expensive and logistically inconvenient to administer. Furthermore, standardizing and verifying whether individuals are fasting can be challenging. Estimates from the International Diabetes Federation (IDF) do not include individuals with isolated IFG (iIFG) or fully capture those with combined IFG-IGT; the IDF estimates that 318 million people (6.7 percent of the adult population) worldwide have some form of IGT (IDF 2015). This lack of data has major implications for understanding the natural history of different types of diabetes and implementing appropriate interventions.

Complications

Diabetes is associated with acute and chronic complications. Acutely, people with diabetes can experience fluctuations in blood glucose levels that require medical attention. Because people with type 1 diabetes require insulin treatment, acute complications occur more commonly in that population and can be fatal if untreated.

Long-standing and poorly controlled diabetes—both types 1 and 2—is associated with increased risks of neurological, renal, ophthalmic, cardiovascular, cognitive, and psychiatric illnesses, and even cancers and infections. Despite our understanding of how diabetes progresses and increases the risk of complications, the understanding of the global distribution of diabetes complications is limited. In most LMICs, testing instruments (for example, retinal cameras) and technical capacity to operate and interpret the tests are too costly or scarce.

Diabetes leads to loss of sensory and motor function as well as poor circulation of the hands and feet, increasing the risks of infection, poor wound healing, and eventual amputation. Diabetes is a leading cause of chronic kidney disease (CKD) and end-stage renal disease (ESRD), requiring dialysis or transplantation. Retinopathy, cataracts, and glaucoma related to diabetes are very common and lead to visual disturbance and blindness. Coronary heart disease, heart failure, and stroke are two to four times more common among persons with diabetes than among similar persons without diabetes. Persons with diabetes often have comorbid depression and a higher risk of developing dementia. The coexistence of depression and diabetes markedly increases the risk of mortality as well as loss of productivity in persons who are gainfully employed; the increasingly early onset of diabetes and depression is a major concern in this context. There is also growing appreciation of a link between diabetes and cancers, particularly because people with diabetes are living longer and are less likely to die from cardiovascular disease (CVD) or CKD (Gregg, Cheng, and others 2012; Gregg and others 2014; Gregg, Sattar, and Ali 2016). In addition, diabetes and cancers share some risk factors such as older age; tobacco use; and oxidant rich, low-fiber diets (Giovannucci and others 2010).

Diabetes and infections increasingly occur together. This is particularly relevant for LMICs, which face a substantial residual burden of infectious diseases. It is not clear whether people with diabetes have more infections, but the coexistence of diabetes and tuberculosis and group B streptococci (Dooley and Chaisson 2009; Magee, Blumberg, and Narayan 2011) is of policy importance because of the added health system burden when these interactions occur. In particular, the coexistence of tuberculosis and diabetes may be associated with poorer recovery and higher risk of tuberculosis relapse, resistance, and death, although the data are inconclusive, as discussed in greater detail in chapter 16 of this volume (Magee and others 2016). Diabetes reportedly occurs increasingly among people infected with human immunodeficiency virus (HIV); this metabolic dysfunction may be related to the HIV infection itself, higher life expectancy with HIV treatments, the treatments themselves, or some combination of these factors (Ali, Magee, and others 2014). The long-term implications of these interactions are actively evolving.

Whether acute, chronic, or infectious, complications increase the use and cost of health care, decrease productivity and quality of life, and increase the risk of mortality for people with diabetes. Though type 1 diabetes is not a focus of this chapter, it is important to note that the disease occurs earlier in life than type 2 diabetes; therefore, if it is poorly controlled, people with type 1 diabetes have more years lived with disability and are at risk for more years of life lost. This is an important policy consideration.

Mortality

Worldwide, life expectancy has been rising. Even mortality rates attributable to other leading noncommunicable diseases, such as CVD, stroke, some cancers, and chronic respiratory disease, have been declining (Ali and others 2015). However, both the age-standardized mortality rate and absolute number of deaths from diabetes have been rising.

Some regional variation is evident in deaths attributable to diabetes, as shown in table 12.1. North Africa and the Middle East, Latin America and the Caribbean, and the Western Pacific regions have the highest proportions of and increases in deaths attributable to diabetes (IDF 2015). South Asia has the highest absolute number, with almost 25 percent of all diabetes deaths globally.

However, the magnitude of deaths attributable to diabetes is probably underestimated because death certifications and mortality approximations list only one cause of death. At least half of all deaths in people with diabetes are related to CVD (Geiss, Herman, and Smith 1995; IDF 2015; Moss, Klein, and Klein 1991), and CKD contributes significantly to deaths among people with diabetes (Levitt 2008; Zimmet 2009); however, these deaths are assigned to CVD or CKD, not diabetes. The World Health Organization (WHO) estimates that deaths attributable to diabetes amounted to 2.8 percent of all deaths globally in 2010, not including deaths attributable to CVD and CKD (32.0 percent and 1.5 percent, respectively). However, diabetes contributes to at least 21 percent of coronary heart disease and 13 percent of stroke mortality worldwide (Danaei and others 2006). Incorporating these aspects, the IDF estimates that diabetes is responsible for 5 million adult deaths annually, or 8.4 percent of all deaths globally (IDF 2015; Roglic and others 2005).

Morbidity and Disability

In addition to shortening life expectancy by 7–15 years (Franco and others 2007; Morgan, Currie, and Peters 2000), diabetes is associated with considerable morbidity and disability. Disability-adjusted life years (DALYs) reflect the combined burdens of disability and premature mortality associated with different diseases. Earlier age of onset of diabetes increases the duration of exposure to diabetes, the associated disability (Bardenheier and others 2016), and the risk

Table 12.1 Percentage of All Deaths and DALYs Lost Attributable to Diabetes, Globally and by Region

	WHO Estimates[a]		IDF Estimates	
Region	DALYs lost	Deaths	Region	Deaths
Global	2.1	2.9	Global	8.4
Latin America	3.4	5.9	South and Central America	~12.0
Eastern and South-East Asia	3.2	3.9	South-East Asia	~14.0
South Asia	1.6	2.6	Western Pacific	~16.0
Middle East and North Africa	3.1	4.1	Middle East and North Africa	~13.0
Sub-Saharan Africa	0.8	1.8	Africa	~8.5
Eastern and Central Europe	2.3	1.1	Europe	~10.5
High-income countries	2.8	2.7	North America	~13.5

Sources: IDF 2013; WHO 2014.
Note: DALYs = disability-adjusted life years; IDF = International Diabetes Federation; WHO = World Health Organization. Estimates are approximations where IDF- and WHO-defined regions are different.
a. Does not include deaths or DALYs lost attributable to chronic kidney disease or cardiovascular diseases attributable to diabetes.

of an early death. Globally, diabetes accounted for 2.1 percent of DALYs lost from all diseases in 2010, with Latin America experiencing the highest (3.4 percent) and Sub-Saharan Africa experiencing the lowest (0.8 percent) DALYs from diabetes.

Diabetes-related disability can be temporary or permanent and can have physical (Lavigne and others 2003; Tunceli and others 2007), psychological (Degmecic and others 2014; McKellar, Humphreys, and Piette 2004; Nicolucci and others 2013; Piette, Richardson, and Valenstein 2004), and social impacts on functioning (Lavigne and others 2003). With regard to physical manifestations, diabetic neuropathy and foot disease accounted for more than half of all diabetes-related years lived with disability, while amputation, vision loss, and CKD attributable to diabetes accounted for 5 percent each (Vos and others 2012). Even in the absence of physical complications or disability, self-care of diabetes itself requires structure and diligence: persons requiring insulin have to monitor their glucose meticulously and time their dietary intake; may experience episodes of hypoglycemia or hyperglycemia; and are advised to undertake routine preventive medical visits, such as annual eye exams (Brod and others 2014; Fu and others 2009; Nicolucci and others 2013). Some studies report that 20 percent of persons with diabetes and their families experience some form of social stigma and discrimination (Kovacs Burns and others 2013; Nicolucci and others 2013), although these incidents are context-dependent. Adults with diabetes experience more depression, anxiety, and cognitive dysfunction than their nondiabetic counterparts. These psychosocial issues negatively affect their social integration, quality of relationships (Aalto, Uutela, and Kangas 1996; Hempler, Ekholm, and Willaing 2013), and self management, creating a vicious cycle.

Economic Burdens

Diabetes is associated with high and long-standing direct medical and nonmedical costs for patients and their caregivers. Worldwide, an estimated 12 percent of all annual direct medical expenditures (an estimated US$673 billion), including outpatient consultations, diagnostic testing, medications, emergency visits, and inpatient procedures and care, are for diabetes (IDF 2015).

Diabetes is also associated with substantial indirect costs (lost productivity attributable to absenteeism, suboptimal work performance, and premature deaths) as well as intangible costs (related to psychosocial harm). Both of these costs are difficult to quantify empirically.

CONSIDERATIONS IN LMICS

Worldwide, the patterns of morbidity and mortality associated with diabetes vary because of differences in populations (differences in maternal and childhood nutrition, exposure to infectious diseases, and level of awareness and health literacy), behavior (likelihood of seeking health care), health financing (health care coverage through public payer or insurance schemes), physical access to care, health facility resources and infrastructure (ability to support high-quality and effective lifestyle interventions and self-management), provider clinical practices, mechanisms for monitoring and delivering quality care, and policies to support diabetes prevention and management. In LMICs, it is especially hard to quantify these factors given the general lack of robust population-based longitudinal data. However, significant and lofty barriers in LMICs clearly have to be overcome to manage diabetes more effectively.

Most LMICs face two significant challenges: (1) lack of coverage of routine tests and inability of patients to pay for them, leading to a high proportion of undiagnosed cases; and (2) limited access to routine care and medications such as insulin that can be life-saving, as well as a general lack of human and infrastructural resources (refrigeration for insulin, for example), leading to poor health outcomes (Beran and Yudkin 2006; Beran, Yudkin, and de Courten 2005; Sobngwi and others 2012). The issue of affordable access to insulin is especially acute for type 1 diabetes because this lifelong medicine is essential for keeping these patients alive.

There are very few, if any, data from LMICs regarding coverage or access to health services and treatments. A WHO study in four LMIC regions showed generally low availability of insulin in both the public and private health sectors, and the cost of a one-month supply of insulin was equivalent to several days of a person's wages (Mendis and others 2007). A 47-country survey conducted by IDF Europe (n.d.) is also illustrative of major disparities in availability, accessibility, and affordability of medications to control diabetes across country-income groups. The data reflect varying levels of annual spending per capita on diabetes (from less than US$100 in the Kyrgyz Republic to US$9,000 in Switzerland) and public financing of diabetes care (from 22 percent in Georgia to 85 percent in the Netherlands). Financial or geographic barriers to accessing medications and preventive services result in suboptimal care (Beran and Yudkin 2006; Beran, Yudkin, and de Courten 2005; Zhang and others 2012) and delayed presentation, giving rise to disabling and expensive-to-treat complications.

EFFECTIVENESS OF INTERVENTIONS

In the past half century, well-conducted studies from across the world have created a strong base of evidence about interventions that can help prevent diabetes among high-risk individuals (Gillies and others 2007; Knowler and others 2002; Tuomilehto and others 2001). In addition, robust data from trials and epidemiological studies—conducted largely in high-income settings—have shown that proactively and intensively managing diabetes lowers the risk of cardiovascular, kidney, eye, and limb diseases and of death (Holman and others 2008; Nathan and others 2005). Interventions to address diabetes, their efficacy, the level of evidence to support these interventions, and the few studies of this nature from LMICs are cataloged in annex 12A.

Fewer data are available from LMICs themselves to aid decision makers in these contexts. Ongoing studies are evaluating the implementation of diabetes prevention in South Africa (Pengpid, Peltzer, and Skaal 2014) and Brazil (Pimentel and others 2010); other studies are piloting novel approaches to preventing diabetes (Hegde and others 2013; McDermott 2012; McDermott and others 2014), but data are as yet unavailable or the sample sizes are too small to support generalizations. However, as annex 12A shows, the estimated effects in LMICs are comparable to those in HICs. The major considerations regarding the use of HIC data for LMIC settings are possible differences in the patterns of disease and comorbidities, as well as possible differences in accessibility, availability, affordability, and implementation capacity in lower-resource settings (Basu and others 2015).

Screening for Prediabetes and Diabetes

Diabetes meets many of the criteria for screening (Wilson and Jungner 1968), with (1) reliable tests to identify elevated glucose, (2) a precursor phase (prediabetes), and (3) interventions to delay onset and manage the disease (DCCT Research Group 1993; UKPDS Group 1998b). However, screening for diabetes and prediabetes continues to be a fiercely debated topic (Echouffo-Tcheugui and others 2011; Engelgau and Gregg 2012; Engelgau, Narayan, and Herman 2000). Lack of consensus surrounds two issues: the long-term benefits of screening for hard outcomes like CVD or mortality (Norris and others 2008; Rahman and others 2012) and the possible harm it could cause, such as increased anxiety or discrimination (Paddison and others 2011; Park and others 2008); and the cost-effectiveness of screening.

Not understanding the condition or knowing that one is affected causes two types of difficulties. First, high blood glucose can progressively damage tissues and lead to complications; according to studies in both the United States and India, up to 30 percent of people with newly diagnosed diabetes already were experiencing retinopathy, nephropathy, and CVD at the time of diagnosis (Casagrande, Cowie, and Fradkin 2013; Unnikrishnan and others 2007). Second, not knowing or understanding one's condition precludes adopting healthful behaviors or seeking care, both of which are needed to manage diabetes.

For these reasons, early detection is thought to confer opportunities to intervene earlier, slow disease progression, address comorbidities like hypertension that commonly coexist with prediabetes and diabetes, and possibly even lower the growing costs of managing diabetes and its complications. Furthermore, studies have shown that screening has minimal psychological impacts (Eborall, Davies, and others 2007; Eborall, Griffin, and others 2007; Echouffo-Tcheugui and others 2011) and causes no significant harm, especially if testing is targeted to high-risk individuals (those with established diabetes risk factors like age over 40 years, minority ethnicity, family history of diabetes, obesity, physical inactivity, other cardiometabolic risk factors like dyslipidemia, or history of gestational diabetes) rather than universal (Selph and others 2015).

The cost-effectiveness of screening depends on both the yield in the population offered testing and the cost-effectiveness of the intervention (Glumer and others 2006; Waugh and others 2007). Given that interventions to prevent diabetes among persons with prediabetes is so cost-effective (DPP Research Group 2012), screening for both prediabetes and diabetes is more cost-effective than screening for diabetes alone (Echouffo-Tcheugui and others 2011; Gillies and others 2008; Hoerger and others 2004; Khunti and others 2012). Ultimately, clinical guidelines play a role in whether and how clinicians offer testing for different conditions, and guidelines will depend on yield, availability of tools for testing, and resources and interventions to address the condition in the given locality. This last issue should not be taken lightly—there are few or no data for many countries around the world regarding the adequacy and readiness of health systems to cope with increased numbers of people with prediabetes and diabetes needing intervention if a widespread screening policy or program were adopted.

Preventing Diabetes

Large randomized controlled trials (RCTs) in China (Pan and others 1997), Finland (Tuomilehto and others 2001), India (Ramachandran and others 2006), Japan (Kosaka, Noda, and Kuzuya 2005), and the United States

(Knowler and others 2002) have shown that, among individuals with established IGT, structured approaches to modifying behavior (exercising more, consuming fewer high-energy calories, increasing fiber intake, and modest weight loss) lowered the incidence of diabetes by approximately 30 percent to 60 percent compared with simple advice regarding diet and exercise. These structured interventions included regular counseling or coaching sessions delivered by health (or allied health) professionals and weight monitoring, as well as extended support in some cases. The applicability of evidence from trials in people with IGT to those with iIFG—the most prevalent form of prediabetes in many parts of the world—remains open for investigation.

These lifestyle interventions are also associated with long-term benefits, including greater likelihood of regression to normal blood glucose levels (Perreault and others 2009), sustained reductions in diabetes incidence, better cardiometabolic control, and fewer long-term eye complications and cardiovascular deaths (Gong and others 2011; Li and others 2014).

Data also show that pharmaceutical agents to lower glucose, lose weight, or both (for example, biguanides) in people with prediabetes can lower diabetes incidence (Gillies and others 2007).

Managing Diabetes

To manage diabetes and prevent diabetes-related complications, large RCTs—again, largely from HICs—have assessed the benefits of lifestyle interventions; surgical procedures; and pharmaceutical approaches to lowering blood glucose, blood pressure, and lipid levels; as well as avoiding tobacco.

A trial to assess whether intensive lifestyle interventions could lower CVD found no effect at 9.6 years of follow-up (Look AHEAD Research Group 2006, 2013). However, intensive lifestyle modification and weight loss have been associated with a four to six times higher (partial or complete) remission from diabetes (7 percent to 12 percent for intervention vs. 2 percent for control arm participants) (Gregg, Chen, and others 2012); less need for medication and health care (Redmon and others 2010); less loss of mobility (Rejeski and others 2012); less new sleep apnea and higher remission from obstructive sleep apnea (Foy and others 2011); 34 percent lower incidence of depression (Wing 2010); 31 percent lower incidence of ESKD (Otto and others 2007); 14 percent lower incidence of retinopathy (O'Riordan 2013); delayed bone loss (Lipkin and others 2014); and improved patient-reported quality of life, particularly physical function (Look AHEAD Research Group 2014). Given the high

personal and monetary costs of these morbidities, lifestyle intervention in people with diabetes is effective and cost-effective (Li and others 2010; Redmon and others 2010).

Surgical procedures are often used to address obesity and diabetes. Extensive evidence shows that gastric bypass surgery and other approaches to compress the stomach (laparoscopic banding) have benefits, including sustained weight loss, improved cardiometabolic profiles, remission (Gloy and others 2013; Li, Lai, and others 2013; Ricci and others 2015), and possibly even prevention (Merlotti and others 2014) of diabetes. Because of the cost and risk of complications, surgical approaches are reserved for individuals who are morbidly obese or for whom other approaches have not been effective (ADA 2016; IDF 2013; NICE 2013).

More intensive control of blood glucose has been shown to reduce complications such as retinopathy, CKD, and neuropathy in the short term (DCCT Research Group 1993; UKPDS Group 1998a, 1998b) and complications such as coronary heart disease, strokes, and related deaths in the long term (Hayward and others 2015; Holman and others 2008; Nathan and others 2005; UKPDS Group 1998a); these findings related to intensive glycemic control are applicable to both type 1 and type 2 diabetes patients. Meta-analyses and reviews of glucose-lowering trials all show some long-term macrovascular benefit, more so for reducing coronary disease than for reducing cerebrovascular disease (Tandon, Ali, and Narayan 2012). The optimal blood glucose level associated with the greatest benefit remains controversial after major trials have shown no short-term benefit from very aggressive glycemic targets of glycated hemoglobin less than 6 percent (Duckworth and others 2009; Gerstein and others 2008; Patel and others 2008). Still, studies that target less aggressive, but still very good, levels of glycated hemoglobin (7 percent) reduced long-term myocardial infarction and all-cause mortality between 15 percent and 40 percent (Ali, Narayan, and Tandon 2010; Hayward and others 2015; Holman and others 2008). For this reason, experts recommend individualizing glucose targets to the patient's comorbid, psychosocial, and clinical circumstances (Inzucchi and others 2012; Ismail-Beigi and others 2011). In addition, activities that support better glycemic control (like self-management education) may promote patient adherence, encourage better metabolic control, and prevent hypoglycemia (Norris, Engelgau, and Narayan 2001). Culturally appropriate health education has net benefits, especially for glycemic control and possibly for improved lifestyles (Attridge and others 2014). Similarly, self-monitoring of blood glucose, even in patients not using insulin, may improve glycemic control (Farmer and others 2012; Sarol and others 2005), although debates still surround the cost, episodes of hypoglycemia, and quality of life experienced by those adopting self-monitoring (Malanda, Bot, and Nijpels 2013; Polonsky and Fisher 2013).

Lowering blood pressure and lipids also has been shown to reduce microvascular and macrovascular complications, both in RCTs and in large meta-analyses (Kearney and others 2008; Turnbull and others 2005). Still, there is no consensus on the most optimal blood pressure and cholesterol targets, but age- and comorbidity-appropriate treatment goals are advocated. Intensive approaches (behavioral therapies, medications) to decrease or cease tobacco use are unequivocally associated with higher likelihood of sustaining tobacco avoidance and reducing macrovascular events (Critchley and Capewell 2003; Mohiuddin and others 2007).

Strong data support comprehensive control of all risk factors along with provision of protective medications, such as angiotensin-converting enzyme inhibitors (ACEi) and angiotensin-receptor blockers (ARBs). Compared with standard care, comprehensive care implemented among people with diabetes and microalbuminuria (urine albumin greater than or equal to 30 milligrams per 24 hours) was associated with 60 percent fewer complications after eight years of follow-up and 60 percent to 80 percent lower mortality after 13 years in an RCT in Denmark (Gaede and others 2003; Gaede, Lund-Andersen, and others 2008).

Screening for and Preventing Complications

Care guidelines recommend regular screening to detect and treat diabetes complications in their early stages, before irreversible clinical manifestations and disability set in (ADA 2016; IDF 2013; NICE 2013). Because there is a preclinical latent phase before each complication sets in, it is recommended that individuals with diabetes undergo regular eye, foot, and urine checks.

Eye disease, particularly diabetic retinopathy, occurs in all people with diabetes, given sufficient duration of disease (Klein and others 1989a, 1989b). Annual or even biennial retinal screening is recommended—depending on the availability of resources and feasibility—to detect changes early and institute therapy (Echouffo-Tcheugui and others 2013). Once detected, evidence from trials shows conclusively that photocoagulation therapy significantly preserves vision (DRS 1981, 1991).

No treatments exist to reverse diabetic nerve damage. However, because people with diabetes have a 25 percent lifetime risk of experiencing foot ulceration, regular assessments and foot care are considered invaluable for

detecting sensorimotor, autonomic, and vascular abnormalities (Boulton and others 2008). Assessments can be coupled with managing symptoms, educating patients regarding appropriate foot care, and preventing deterioration (ADA 2016). Simple foot care education with periodic assessment and care can reduce the risk of amputation, and efforts are increasing to disseminate resources in LMICs for training health care workers in foot care (McGill 2005; Tulley and others 2009).

To prevent deterioration of kidney function, annual urine screening and use of ACEi and ARB medications are recommended once microalbuminuria sets in (ADA 2016). Early kidney disease increases the risk of CVD and ESRD (Fox and others 2012). Blood glucose and blood pressure management in general, and ACEi/ARB use in particular, have been shown to reduce these major adverse outcomes (Lewis and others 1993) in people with modestly elevated excretion of urinary albumin, as discussed in greater detail in chapter 13 of this volume (Anand and others 2017).

Finally, guidelines encourage annual influenza vaccination and a lifetime pneumococcal vaccination for people with diabetes older than age 60 years. Although there are no RCTs of vaccination among people with diabetes, observational studies show fewer influenza-like illnesses, fewer pneumonia-like illnesses, and fewer hospitalizations among persons with diabetes who were vaccinated compared with those who were not (Colquhoun and others 1997; Heymann and others 2004; Lau and others 2013; Pozzilli and others 1986; Rodriguez-Blanco and others 2012).

TRANSLATING EVIDENCE INTO ACTION

Clinical and epidemiological data have been assimilated into expert preventive and clinical guidelines that are widely accessible (ADA 2016; IDF 2013; NICE 2013), but achieving real health gains requires more than just an accessible compendium of interventions. Complex conditions like diabetes require stakeholders and resources to coalesce at policy, program, clinic, and individual levels. However, because of barriers among policy makers (competing priorities), providers (low accountability, time constraints, lack of incentive schemes), and patients (low motivation), implementation of recommended preventive and care services for diabetes is falling far short of desired goals.

Gaps in Diagnosis and Care

Huge gaps are evident, even in HICs—for example, almost 90 percent of the 86 million people with prediabetes who would be eligible for preventive services

(Li, Geiss, and others 2013) and up to 30 percent of the 29 million people with diabetes in the United States alone (Ali, Bullard, and others 2014) are not aware of their condition, are not engaged in diabetes prevention programs, or are not caring for their diabetes. Because glycated hemoglobin tests are costly and oral glucose tolerance tests are time consuming and disliked by patients, data are lacking to show what proportions of people are at high risk for or have diabetes in LMICs and are aware of their prediabetes or diabetes status; almost no data are representative of entire populations (Narayan and others 2012).

Similar gaps exist with regard to managing diabetes and controlling risk factors. Data from Africa, Asia, Europe, Latin America, and the United States all show that more than half of people with diabetes are not meeting recommended targets to prevent complications (Ali and others 2013; Gakidou and others 2011; Mudaliar and others 2013; Sobngwi and others 2012; Stone and others 2013). Data from eight countries in Europe show that, although 80 percent to 98 percent of people with diabetes had recorded values for glycated hemoglobin, blood pressure, and lipid values in the past 12 months, few had achieved the recommended values (54 percent, 19 percent, and 55 percent, respectively) (Stone and others 2013). For the United States, similar findings were reported using nationally representative surveillance data: only half of all people with diabetes were meeting individual targets, and only 14 percent were controlling all three factors and avoiding tobacco (Ali and others 2013). In Africa, the gaps in care are even larger. In six African countries, fewer than half (47 percent) of all respondents with diabetes had glycated hemoglobin levels recorded in the past year, 29 percent had glycated hemoglobin less than 6.5 percent, and only 13 percent and 65 percent were treated with lipid-lowering or antihypertensive medications, respectively (Sobngwi and others 2012). Systematic reviews of diabetes care in Latin America and Asia show wide variations in risk factor goals, but the findings are similar (Mudaliar and others 2013; Shivashankar and others 2015), suggesting that patient, provider, and system barriers perpetuate gaps in care.

To address these gaps and improve the reach, adoption, effectiveness, and sustainability of diabetes prevention and care interventions, more implementation science (also known as translation research) is needed (Glasgow and others 2001; Jilcott and others 2007). Wider implementation and sustainability of health care and prevention interventions require consistent and strong evidence, adapting the interventions to the context, mobilizing stakeholders and resources, and identifying the processes that permit effective engagement among stakeholders (Brownson, Fielding, and Maylahn 2009).

Implementing Diabetes Prevention

Numerous studies have evaluated the short-term impacts of implementing structured lifestyle interventions to prevent diabetes in different settings. Only a few of these have been in LMICs, largely in South Asia (Iqbal Hydrie and others 2012; Karalliedde and others 2014; Ramachandran and others 2013; Sathish and others 2013; Weber and others 2012). Data from a trial that tested the delivery of lifestyle interventions using mobile phones in India showed a 36 percent reduction in diabetes incidence compared with advice delivered at baseline (Ramachandran and others 2013). Results from a study at clinics in India also showed a 30 percent to 35 percent reduction in diabetes incidence (Weber and others 2016). In the United States, individuals at high risk for diabetes who enrolled in and completed adapted lifestyle intervention programs in clinics, workplaces, places of worship, or community settings achieved an average 4 percent weight loss (Ali, Echouffo-Tcheugui, and Williamson 2012); this amount is considered clinically meaningful, although somewhat lower than the 7 percent weight loss observed in the large Diabetes Prevention Program (DPP) study (Knowler and others 2002). Based on early successes, diabetes prevention programs are being scaled up in countries such as Finland (Saaristo and others 2010), the United States (Albright and Gregg 2013), and parts of Australia (Dunbar and others 2014; Janus and others 2012). These real-world diabetes prevention programs were also associated with meaningful (and quite similar to the DPP study) reductions in other metabolic parameters such as blood pressure and lipids, which lowers the need for medications and lowers overall vascular risk (Mudaliar and others 2016).

Implementing Better Diabetes Care

To improve diabetes management and lower the risk of complications, patient-level, provider-level, and system-level barriers that block achievement of care goals need to be addressed. Several interventions have been tested to address these barriers, either individually or together. The data show that targeted patient-level (reminders, education, motivation by care coordinators), provider-level (reminders, audit and feedback), and system-level (structured team-based care or electronic decision support systems) intervention strategies are promising (Renders and others 2001; Stellefson, Dipnarine, and Stopka 2013; Tricco and others 2012). Empowerment, case management, and task delegation are associated with the greatest effects on risk factors. Although scarce, data in settings outside Europe and the United States—for example, using structured care or peer educators in Cambodia (MoPoTsyo Patient Information Centre 2015); team-based care in Hong Kong SAR, China (Chan and others 2009); or multicomponent interventions (for example, care coordinators and decision-support software) like the chronic care model in India (Ali, Singh, and others 2016)—have shown promise, improving detection, controlling risk factors, lowering ESRD incidence and death, and demonstrating cost-effectiveness (Ko and others 2011). These models may also be of particular relevance as the population of people with comorbidities, such as diabetes and depression or diabetes and HIV/AIDS, grows.

Despite the efforts to adapt interventions to local contexts, two aspects of sustainable implementation warrant further discussion: (1) resources and capacity to implement and (2) context-specific stakeholder perspectives. Our efforts to compile data regarding the value of diabetes interventions and stakeholder perspectives are described in the following sections.

ECONOMIC EVALUATIONS OF DIABETES INTERVENTIONS

To identify and compare the value of different diabetes-focused interventions—that is, the resource inputs required to achieve benefit—we reviewed and synthesized the available literature regarding cost-effectiveness of interventions to detect, prevent, and manage diabetes and its complications. The methodology is described in annex 12B; median and individual study incremental cost-effectiveness ratios (ICER) are provided in annex 12B (table 12B.1) and annex 12C (tables 12C.1–12C.4), respectively.

Cost-Effectiveness

To synthesize the broad findings, we placed all diabetes interventions into four categories:

- Screening for diabetes, prediabetes, or gestational diabetes
- Preventing type 2 diabetes in high-risk individuals
- Managing diabetes (lifestyle interventions; self-management education; self-monitoring of blood glucose; intensive glycemic, blood pressure, and lipid control; case management)
- Screening for and prevention of diabetes-related complications (retinopathy, neuropathy, nephropathy).

Screening for Undiagnosed Diabetes, Prediabetes, or Gestational Diabetes

Cost-effectiveness estimates regarding screening for undiagnosed diabetes, prediabetes, or gestational diabetes were based largely on simulation models because RCTs of screening are neither feasible nor ethical. The modeled estimates are subject to the assumptions defined by each group of investigators. From studies that modeled different scenarios of which patients to screen, when to initiate, and how often to repeat screening, the following themes emerged:

- Screening for undiagnosed diabetes alone is not cost-effective, but screening for both prediabetes and undiagnosed diabetes is.
- Opportunistic screening of entire populations is extremely resource-intensive (CDC 1998; Hoerger and others 2004; Kahn and others 2010), while more targeted screening of individuals at a certain age (45 years) or at any age if risk factors for diabetes already exist is far more cost-effective (Hoerger and others 2004; Kahn and others 2010; Mortaz and others 2012). This finding has led the American Diabetes Association and the National Institute for Health and Care Excellence, among others, to recommend two-stage screening for asymptomatic adults—in other words, asking about risk factors, followed by blood testing.
- Screening is more cost-effective if followed by an intervention than is screening alone, and is both ethically and economically beneficial (Gillies and others 2008; Hoerger and others 2007; Nicholson and others 2005; Schaufler and Wolff 2010).
- Cost-effectiveness of screening also varies depending on the measure used to estimate blood glucose. Although data are limited, oral glucose tolerance and glycated hemoglobin tests are far more expensive than capillary glucose tests. However, cheaper tests need to be assessed for their accuracy and performance (false negative or positive rates).
- Screening all pregnant women can be costly (Nicholson and others 2005; Werner and others 2012), but it may be more cost-effective if followed by postpartum lifestyle management (Lohse, Marseille, and Kahn 2011; Marseille and others 2013) or if the prevalence of gestational diabetes continues to rise. Some HICs advocate screening all pregnant women at 24–28 weeks gestation because of the rising prevalence of gestational diabetes (U.S. Preventive Services Task Force 2014).

Preventing Diabetes among High-Risk Individuals

With respect to diabetes prevention, the findings for high-risk individuals with prediabetes were confirmed by a comprehensive review conducted by the Community

Preventive Services Task Force (Li and others 2015; Pronk and Remington 2015):

- The efficacy, effectiveness, and cost-effectiveness data on diabetes prevention are limited to people with isolated IGT, combined IFG-IGT, or both; there are only extrapolations, but no real data, for people with iIFG.
- Within-trial economic evaluations generally find higher cost per quality-adjusted life year (QALY) gained (DPP Research Group 2003; Irvine and others 2011; van Wier and others 2013) for individual one-on-one lifestyle modification programs than modeled estimates.
- Modeling studies demonstrate that to lower costs, variations of the following could be offered: intervention intensity, number of sessions, type of provider (lay persons vs. medically trained personnel), and delivery format (group vs. one-on-one).
- In pragmatic studies, group-based lifestyle counseling is more feasible and less costly to implement (Absetz and others 2007; Herman and others 2005; Katula and others 2013; Li and others 2015; Segal, Dalton, and Richardson 1998) than interventions delivered to individuals (Eddy, Schlessinger, and Kahn 2005; Lindgren and others 2007; Palmer, Roze, and others 2004).
- Over a longer time horizon, costs per QALY gained for primary prevention drops (DPP Research Group 2012).
- Metformin is not cost-effective in the short term but can be cost saving in the long term (DPP Research Group 2003, 2012). Generic metformin substantially lowers costs (Palmer and Tucker 2012) compared with models based on costs from trials (Herman and others 2005).
- Innovations that lower the costs of delivering primary prevention interventions and that optimize identification, adoption and engagement, adherence, and maintenance will likely be even more cost-effective. This is especially possible in LMICs, as demonstrated in India (Ramachandran and others 2007), but such innovations have not been quantified widely or for different contextual permutations.

Managing Diabetes

Very few economic estimates of lifestyle interventions in individuals with diabetes are available. The prematurely discontinued Look AHEAD study resulted in no reduction in cardiovascular events (Look AHEAD Research Group 2013), but there were other benefits—specifically, reductions in morbidity and other health problems (Gregg, Chen, and others 2012; Redmon and others 2010; Rejeski and others 2012; Wing 2010).

The cost-effectiveness of aerobic and resistance exercises and dietary changes for people with diabetes remains understudied (Coyle and others 2012; Eddy, Schlessinger, and Kahn 2005).

With respect to managing glucose levels through clinical interventions,

- Structured diabetes self-management education programs are cost-effective in studies from Mexico and Nigeria (Adibe, Aguwa, and Ukwe 2013; Diaz de Leon-Castaneda and others 2012) as well as in studies from Europe and the United States (Gillett and others 2010; Gozzoli and others 2001; Shearer and others 2004).
- Self-monitoring of blood glucose is recommended mainly for patients using insulin or oral glucose-lowering drugs who experience fluctuations in blood glucose. Home self-monitoring among non-insulin users is costly and offers low value (Pollock and others 2010; Tunis 2011; Tunis and Minshall 2008).
- The incremental costs to control glycemia intensively (aiming for near-normal glucose levels), compared with conventional treatment, tend to vary according to intensity, number, and costs of the medications used. In general, insulin therapies cost the most and metformin costs the least per QALY gained across all studies (Almbrand and others 2000; CDC Diabetes Cost-Effectiveness Group 2002; Clarke and others 2005; DCCT Research Group 1996; Eastman and others 1997; Palmer and others 2000; Wake and others 2000). The additional resources, patient burden, and risks of hypoglycemia and other potential harms need to be counterbalanced against the potential gains in reducing diabetes complications. This is especially important considering that glycemic control has large benefits in reducing disabling microvascular complications and modest benefits in reducing cardiovascular events over a long period of follow-up (Hayward and others 2015; Holman and others 2008; Nathan and others 2005; UKPDS Group 1998b); moreover, improvements in care, blood pressure control, lipid management, and tobacco cessation are producing the lowest average rates of macrovascular complications ever observed in some HICs (Gregg and others 2014).

With respect to clinical interventions to control CVD risk factors,

- Costs to control blood pressure depend on the target blood pressure. Median costs per QALY gained for blood pressure control are much lower than for glycemic control and likely attributable to a larger effect on CVD morbidity and mortality rather than on a lower cost to implement. Less aggressive targets cost much less per QALY gained than more aggressive targets (CDC Diabetes Cost-Effectiveness Group 2002; Clarke and others 2005; Elliott, Weir, and Black 2000).

- For lipid control, the economic data are largely limited to the use of statins; to our knowledge, there are no data for fibrates or niacin. The type and availability of generic statins as well as the risk level of individuals affect cost-effectiveness: (1) Models based on trial data (using patented medications) show that median costs per QALY gained from using statin therapy vary and can be very high. (2) Often, an intervention has the greatest effect on those at greatest risk. For them, the absolute reduction in incidence of events and mortality is greatest and the number needed to treat or prevent one disease event or death is smaller. As such, the ICER is more favorable. For example, the cost of using a statin per life year saved among people with diabetes and CVD is much lower than among people with diabetes alone (Annemans and others 2010; CDC Diabetes Cost-Effectiveness Group 2002; Grover and others 2000; Jonsson, Cook, and Pedersen 1999; Raikou and others 2007).
- Only one RCT of comprehensive risk factor management in diabetes patients has been conducted (the Steno-II study) (Gaede and others 2003; Gaede, Lund-Anderson, and others 2008). The within-trial ICER indicates a very favorable intervention. Case management in which nurses help patients focus on controlling combined risk factors also seems to provide good value (Gaede, Valentine, and others 2008; Mason and others 2005). More expansive training programs and focused clinics to manage diabetes risks can be much more resource intensive for the health gained (Brownson and others 2009; Gilmer and others 2007; Mason and others 2005).

Screening, Preventing, and Managing Complications

Cost-effectiveness of screening for retinopathy among people with diabetes depends on the equipment used (retinal camera, fundoscopy) and the regularity of screening (annual vs. every two years). Data for retinopathy screening are available for LMICs and HICs (Khan and others 2013; Maberley and others 2003; Tung and others 2008; Vijan, Hofer, and Hayward 2000). Innovations to lower costs, such as smartphone technology, may produce clear enough images, though further testing is needed before they become more mainstream (Blanckenberg, Worst, and Scheffer 2011; Haddock, Kim, and Mukai 2013; Kumar and others 2012; Suto and others 2014).

Of all the interventions to detect and prevent complications, neuropathy screening and foot ulcer prevention have the lowest median ICER and have been shown to be very cost-effective in both HIC and LMIC settings (Habib and others 2010; Ragnarson Tennvall and Apelqvist 2001).

Cost-effectiveness of screening for CKD also varies by the frequency of screening and risk level of persons getting tested:

- Shorter interval and frequent screening (biennial) is more costly than less frequent testing (every five years) (Kessler and others 2012)
- Screening individuals who are free of diabetes or hypertension tends to cost more per QALY gained than targeted screening of higher-risk individuals (Hoerger and others 2010).

The use of angiotensin-modifying agents (ACEi or ARB) to reduce the risk of ESRD among people with diabetes costs a median of US$36,000 per QALY gained in HIC settings (Palmer, Annemans, Roze, Lamotte, Lapuerta, and others 2004; Palmer, Annemans, Roze, Lamotte, Rodby, and Bilous 2004; Palmer and others 2007; Palmer, Valentine, and Ray 2007; Rosen and others 2005; Souchet and others 2003; Szucs, Sandoz, and Keusch 2004). There are no equivalent data in LMICs.

Valuing Interventions

Interpreting the value of investing in different health interventions in a specific context is challenging, especially when the data regarding cost-effectiveness were collected in different settings. The cost to implement interventions differs markedly across settings, as does the purchasing power of individuals and societies. In addition, the effectiveness of interventions may differ slightly in different settings, although there is no reason to believe that biological differences would be striking. Keeping these factors in mind, we compiled and calculated median ceiling ratios, that is, thresholds (of value) for decision makers to benchmark whether the median cost-effectiveness estimates reported fall into very cost-effective or cost saving, cost-effective, or not cost-effective ranges for their respective regions (annex 12D and annex table 12D.1) and even for country-income groups (low income, middle income, and high income) given the heterogeneity within regions. In addition, we used a regional cost index derived from health care input cost data compiled by the WHO to calibrate estimated cost-effectiveness for different LMIC regions (table 12.2). Although imperfect, this approach makes it possible to

Table 12.2 Converted Incremental Cost-Effectiveness Ratios for Interventions to Detect, Prevent, and Manage Diabetes by LMIC Region, 2012 U.S. Dollars

Intervention	Source of estimates	HIC estimates	Region					
			EAP	ECA	LAC	MENA	SA	SSA
Detection								
Screening for undiagnosed diabetes or prediabetes		11,250	820	1,102	1,364	1,158	683	618
Screening with or without intervention		10,908	796	1,069	1,323	1,123	662	599
Screening for gestational diabetes		20,362	1,485	1,995	2,470	2,097	1,236	1,119
Preventing type 2 diabetes among those at high risk								
Individual		17,750	1,295	1,739	2,153	1,828	1,077	975
Group		12,380	903	1,213	1,502	1,275	751	680
Individual	Models	7,582	553	743	920	781	460	417
Diabetes management								
Lifestyle change		48,793	3,559	4,782	5,918	5,025	2,961	2,681
Diabetes self-management education	Within trial	3,882	283	380	471	400	236	213
	Models	9,996	729	980	1,212	1,029	607	549
Self-monitoring of blood glucose		12,262	894	1,202	1,487	1,263	744	674
Intensive glycemic control	Within trial	20,720	1,511	2,030	2,513	2,134	1,257	1,138
	Models	30,304	2,210	2,970	3,676	3,121	1,839	1,665
Intensive blood pressure control	Within trial	1,164	85	114	141	120	71	64
	Models	2,974	217	291	361	306	180	163
Cholesterol control	Within trial	13,180	961	1,292	1,599	1,357	800	724
	Models	73,115	5,332	7,165	8,868	7,529	4,437	4,017
Case management	Within trial	12,944	944	1,268	1,570	1,333	785	711
	Models	23,035	1,680	2,257	2,794	2,372	1,398	1,266
Screening for and preventing diabetes complications								
Retinopathy screening		49,322	3,597	4,833	5,982	5,079	2,993	2,710
Foot care and assessments		25,859	1,886	2,534	3,136	2,663	1,569	1,421
Urine assessments		75,241	5,488	7,373	9,126	7,748	4,566	4,134
Preventing CKD and ESRD		35,817	2,612	3,510	4,344	3,688	2,173	1,968

Note: CKD = chronic kidney disease; EAP = East Asia and Pacific; ECA = Europe and Central Asia; ESRD = end-stage renal disease; HIC = high-income country; LAC = Latin America and the Caribbean; LMIC = low- and middle-income country; MENA = Middle East and North Africa; SA = South Asia; SSA = Sub-Saharan African.

categorize interventions based on their value for LMIC decision makers; however, an important caveat is that these calibrations are linear and would be more accurate if fixed and variable costs, marginal gains, and diminishing returns were accounted for.

Based on benchmarking of ICERs of different diabetes interventions against ceiling thresholds in low-income countries of different regions worldwide

(table 12.2 and annex 12D, table 12D.1), blood pressure control and diabetes self-management education offered the greatest value, and together with screening for dysglycemia and primary prevention interventions, were considered cost-effective or very cost-effective across all regions. Interventions offering the least value were intensive glycemic control, lipid control, and screening for diabetic retinopathy and CKD.

PRIORITY INTERVENTIONS TO ADDRESS DIABETES

To collate stakeholder perspectives regarding appropriateness and priority ranking of interventions for diabetes prevention and management, we performed a systematic two-round Delphi process with a panel of leading experts representing diverse geographic regions characterized by varying levels of financial and human resource constraints. The methodology used is described in detail in annex 12E.

In round 1, respondents were asked to rank an adapted list of interventions identified by Narayan and others (2006) by priority and implementation feasibility in LMICs. They were also asked to rate four components of feasibility:

- *Reach.* Ability to reach the target population
- *Technical complexity.* Level of medical technologies or expertise needed to implement an intervention
- *Capital intensity.* Amount of capital resources required for an intervention
- *Cultural acceptability.* Appropriateness of an intervention based on social norms or religious beliefs in the respondent's geographic region.

Table 12.3 presents the average rankings across experts for both priority and feasibility, and for the four feasibility components.

With regard to average feasibility, the respondents ranked blood pressure control (3.67), preconception care among women with diabetes (3.42), screening for gestational diabetes (3.23), smoking cessation (3.21), and comprehensive foot care (3.19) as the most feasible interventions because they have the greatest reach, lowest technical complexity, and lowest resource needs and are likely to be the most culturally acceptable.

However, scores for feasibility diverged from scores for priority. Notably, only one of the six highest-priority interventions (preconception care among women with diabetes) was also considered highly feasible. Lifestyle interventions to prevent diabetes were considered the least feasible (2.29).

In round 2, respondents were asked to list up to 15 innovative or novel strategies that would facilitate diabetes prevention and control in LMICs and to rank them according to their priority and feasibility. The resulting list of 106 strategies was organized into 15 intervention categories; table 12.4 presents how many times each strategy was mentioned.

KNOWLEDGE GAPS

The effectiveness of interventions to prevent and control diabetes is undisputed. With two exceptions—screening for both prediabetes and diabetes and preventive interventions among persons with iIFGs—all of these interventions have been tested in well-designed, large RCTs. There is no reason to believe that effectiveness will be greatly different across different countries.

Table 12.3 Results of Delphi Surveys: Round 1 Expert Opinions Regarding Intervention Priority and Implementation Feasibility

Average ranking

Intervention	Priority	Implementation feasibility	Feasibility Components		
			Reach	Technical complexity	Capital intensity	Cultural acceptability
Glycemic control in people with glycated hemoglobin above 7 percent	3.75	2.75	2.42	2.67	2.33	3.58
Blood pressure control ACEi therapy for people with diabetes	3.89	3.67	3.42	4.00	3.33	3.92
Statin therapy for secondary prevention of cardiovascular disease in people with dyslipidemia	3.75	2.94	2.50	3.08	2.42	3.75
Smoking cessation	4.31	3.21	3.67	2.67	2.92	3.58
Annual (or biennial) screening for diabetic retinopathy	3.75	2.71	2.83	2.17	2.17	3.67
Comprehensive foot care for those at high risk	4.72	3.19	3.33	2.83	2.83	3.75

table continues next page

Table 12.3 Results of Delphi Surveys: Round 1 Expert Opinions Regarding Intervention Priority and Implementation Feasibility (continued)

Average ranking

Intervention	Priority	Implementation feasibility	Feasibility Components			
			Reach	Technical complexity	Capital intensity	Cultural acceptability
Screening for diabetic nephropathy and ensuring ACEi or ARB therapy in persons with diabetes	3.47	2.98	2.92	2.92	2.42	3.67
Intensive lifestyle intervention in persons with type 2 diabetes using a DPP-type intervention	3.61	2.65	2.58	2.58	2.25	3.17
Preconception care among women with diabetes	3.75	3.42	3.42	3.00	3.33	3.92
Screening for gestational diabetes in women at risk between 24 and 28 weeks gestation	3.75	3.23	3.25	3.08	2.75	3.83
Universal opportunistic screening for undiagnosed type 2 diabetes and multifactorial therapy for screen-detected people	3.47	2.67	2.92	2.67	1.67	3.42
Primary prevention through intensive lifestyle modification using the DPP intervention among those with prediabetes	3.89	2.29	2.08	2.17	1.92	3.00

Note: ACEi = angiotensin-converting enzyme inhibitors; ARB = angiotensin-receptor blocker; DPP = Diabetes Prevention Program. Priority and implementation feasibility are the *average* ranking across all respondents (N = 13). Priority ranking is scored on a scale of 1 to 5, where 1 indicates low priority and 5 indicates high priority. Feasibility is rated based on four criteria, each of which is scored on a scale of 1 to 5, where 1 indicates low feasibility and 5 indicates high feasibility. See text for description of each criterion.

Table 12.4 Number of Mentions for Priority or Feasibility of Innovative Intervention Strategies

Type of intervention	Number of mentions
Macro, environmental, and regulatory policies	
Access to essential medicines (for example, insulin)	9
Creation and implementation of fiscal and regulatory measures (taxing sugar-sweetened beverages)	8
Health promotion (diet and physical activity) in the general population (communities and workplaces)	6
Development of national guidelines and programs and policies	6
Health in all policies or creating environments to facilitate healthy living	5
Human resources development	
Training and sensitizing physicians in diabetes care and management	8
Training and sensitizing community health workers in diabetes education for prevention and control	7
Improve diabetes detection, prevention, and care	
Screening and addressing high-risk individuals	17
Quality-of-care improvement initiatives	7
Education and support programs for people with or at risk for diabetes	6

table continues next page

Table 12.4 Number of Mentions for Priority or Feasibility of Innovative Intervention Strategies (continued)

Type of intervention	Number of mentions
Secondary prevention of complications (foot, leg, and eye care)	4
Set-up and integration of diabetes care for other noncommunicable and infectious diseases	3
Consideration of polypill (and novel therapies) for cardiovascular disease	1
Research priorities	
Development of national surveillance surveys	5
Implementation research	1

Some variation in effectiveness is likely, perhaps because of supply-side differences in reach and implementation or because of demand-side differences in yield, adoption, adherence, and maintenance.

Although the above arguments justify the use of HIC data for LMIC contexts, there is no substitute for local, country-specific data because diabetes prevention and management interventions require sustained behavioral changes, and local social, environmental, cultural, political, and economic conditions affect successful implementation of and adherence to these interventions. Data from LMICs are far overshadowed by data from HICs. Most LMICs still do not have representative surveys that can identify the population-wide prevalence of diabetes, prediabetes, and subtypes of diabetes or the proportion of people with diabetes who are undiagnosed. There are almost no longitudinal data for understanding the natural history of diabetes and whether different ethnic, genotypic, or phenotypic variants of prediabetes and diabetes progress differently. There are also very few, if any, data regarding childhood- or adolescent-onset type 2 diabetes and interventions to address it, even though it appears to be a growing problem. More local observational and experimental data from LMICs are necessary.

In addition, there are key knowledge gaps regarding supply-side aspects of how to implement diabetes detection, prevention, and treatment in LMICs. The understanding of how well-tested diabetes prevention and treatment programs need to be adapted to optimize effectiveness in local LMIC circumstances, or indeed, to address comorbidities (such as diabetes and HIV/AIDS) is very cursory (see chapter 16 in this volume, Magee and others 2017). These aspects, as well as a better understanding of existing infrastructure, resources, and competencies, can help shape how diabetes prevention and treatment interventions will be delivered, by whom, and where. In addition, each country's health care financing varies considerably, and decision makers in payer institutions (ministries, insurance companies, employers) will want to know what up-front, fixed, and variable resource investments are required; what return on investment is possible; and over what time horizon. Indeed, trials of low-cost diagnostics and technologies for detection, prevention, and management hold much promise for lowering supply-side costs, but data are extremely scarce. These factors are important considerations and are relevant to integrating diabetes prevention and management services into routine systems.

There are also large gaps in the availability of qualitative data from LMICs (Hennink and others 2016). In particular, data that inform intervention adaptation, but also marketing, are crucial for generating demand for diabetes services. Intervention programs, tools, and facilities need to be coupled with efforts to optimize adoption, adherence to, and maintenance of the intervention. Generating demand requires effective messaging, communicating the opportunities through appropriate avenues, and using culturally sensitive wording and approaches. Communication needs to convince decision makers that these interventions fit within a context of supportive policies. Diabetes detection, prevention, and control could be facilitated or hindered at employer, insurance, or regulatory levels. For example, employers that support employee efforts to manage their disease risk may encourage better control and be rewarded through employee loyalty and performance.

In comparison with our understanding of individual-focused behavioral interventions, the evidence on societal-level nutrition, agricultural, physical activity, health financing, regulatory, and built-environment policies is weak in design and inconsistent across all countries (Roberto and others 2015). Any policy or program should be accompanied by robust evaluation with an appropriate control group and repeated assessments of exposures and outcomes (Soumerai, Starr, and Majumdar 2015). Evaluations of natural experiments (interventions not introduced or manipulated by researchers) using rigorous methods may provide efficient opportunities to guide future policy (Ackermann and others 2015). Indeed, we also do not know the comparative effectiveness and cost-effectiveness of individual versus population-level interventions.

RECOMMENDATIONS

To recommend priority interventions, we identified interventions for which the data about clinical effectiveness, topical importance, feasibility, and cost-effectiveness were most convergent. In other words, interventions that were, on aggregate, considered effective, important, feasible, and cost-effective were given highest priority. The following interventions to detect, prevent, and manage diabetes should be prioritized in LMICs:

- Blood pressure control among people with diabetes is considered a high priority, most feasible, and very cost-effective.
- Care management as well as aspects of care (self-management education) to support better risk factor control and preventive practices are considered effective and cost-effective and may be delivered by community health workers in practice.
- Lifestyle interventions to prevent diabetes among high-risk individuals are highly effective and cost-effective, but implementing them is challenging, which may reflect our limited understanding of the processes, personnel, financing, and infrastructure needed to deliver and sustain acceptable diabetes prevention services in various LMIC contexts. Yet lifestyle interventions may offer the greatest long-term possibility to slow the growth of diabetes worldwide and warrant further investigation regarding best practices.
- Good glycemic control has important microvascular benefits and may be achievable, but it comes at a fairly high cost. Lipid-lowering medications to prevent CVD events and mortality are also highly efficacious and quite achievable, but they are not universally cost-effective unless cheaper generic versions become widely available. Smoking cessation and foot care are considered important and feasible and have demonstrated value (Li and others 2010).

With respect to the priority actions and approaches to achieving these goals, we recommend pursuing the following supply- and demand-side interventions (in no specific order):

- Targeted (two-step) screening to identify people with prediabetes and diabetes (users of supply-side interventions) is cost-effective and should be a priority, and it should be espoused in guidelines and policy. This step should be complemented by efforts to ensure that the health system has adequate capacity to address the needs identified through screening.
- Purchasers of health care (governments, insurers, employers) should facilitate physical and financial access to essential medicines to treat diabetes and vascular risk factors in diabetes. These medicines should include at least insulin and two classes of oral glucose-lowering medications, at least two classes of blood-pressure-lowering medications, a statin, and possibly a selective serotonin reuptake inhibitor. Access to laboratory testing for periodic monitoring would complement the effectiveness of medications.
- Employers and providers should offer and deliver prevention (health promotion) and care (self-management support) services in clinical and non-clinical settings (workplaces and communities) through trained nonclinical staff (community health workers, lifestyle coaches). Although building capacity and creating infrastructure are expensive up-front costs, health payers, whether government or private, should consider the longer-term benefits and possibilities for financing operational costs sustainably through other means (user fees).
- Researchers should give high priority to addressing important knowledge gaps, especially regarding implementation and scalability.

CONCLUSIONS

The global burden of diabetes is colossal, especially among those least equipped to pay for treatment of end-stage disease. There is general consensus—combining evidence from published sources and expert opinions—that interventions to identify risk and to prevent and manage diabetes are effective, important, and provide value in most settings. There are large gaps in our understanding of how to facilitate implementation, engagement, and sustained success, especially in diverse settings. Governments could consider supporting research to address data gaps with regard to distribution and natural history of disease, implementation sciences, and cost-lowering technologies; building capacity; strengthening infrastructure; and covering up-front costs to catalyze socially valued programs.

Given the pluralistic and evolving needs and priorities in different countries and health care systems—many of which are experiencing changes in disease prevalence, capacity, and financing—ongoing research and evaluation of health system and societal interventions are essential to guide policy makers, donors, communities, and care providers.

ANNEXES

The annexes to this chapter are as follows. They are available at http://www.dcp-3.org/CVRD.

- Annex 12A. Effectiveness and Quality of Evidence Regarding Diabetes Screening, Prevention, and Treatment Interventions
- Annex 12B. Methodology for Cost-Effectiveness Analyses
- Annex 12C. Studies Reporting Cost-Effectiveness of Diabetes Screening, Prevention, and Treatment Interventions
- Annex 12D. Valuing Interventions—Regional Ceiling Ratios for Benchmarking
- Annex 12E. Gathering and Analyzing Stakeholder Perspectives to Prioritize Interventions

NOTE

World Bank Income Classifications as of July 2014 are as follows, based on estimates of gross national income (GNI) per capita for 2013:

- Low-income countries (LICs) = US$1,045 or less
- Middle-income countries (MICs) are subdivided:
  (a) lower-middle-income = US$1,046 to US$4,125
  (b) upper-middle-income (UMICs) = US$4,126 to US$12,745
- High-income countries (HICs) = US$12,746 or more.

REFERENCES

Aalto, A. M., A. Uutela, and T. Kangas. 1996. "Health Behaviour, Social Integration, Perceived Health, and Dysfunction: A Comparison between Patients with Type I and II Diabetes and Controls." *Scandinavian Journal of Public Health* 24 (4): 272–81.

Absetz, P., R. Valve, B. Oldenburg, H. Heinonen, A. Nissinen, and others. 2007. "Type 2 Diabetes Prevention in the 'Real World': One-Year Results of the GOAL Implementation Trial." *Diabetes Care* 30 (10): 2465–70.

Ackermann, R. T., O. Kenrik Duru, J. B. Albu, J. A. Schmittdiel, S. B. Soumerai, and others. 2015. "Evaluating Diabetes Health Policies Using Natural Experiments: The Natural Experiments for Translation in Diabetes Study." *American Journal of Preventive Medicine* 48 (6): 747–54.

ADA (American Diabetes Association). 2016. "Standards of Medical Care in Diabetes—2016." *Diabetes Care* 39 (Suppl 1).

Adibe, M. O., C. N. Aguwa, and C. V. Ukwe. 2013. "Cost-Utility Analysis of Pharmaceutical Care Intervention versus Usual Care in Management of Nigerian Patients with Type 2 Diabetes." *Value in Health Regional Issues* 2: 189–98. doi:10.1016/j.vhri.2013.06.009.

Albright, A. L., and E. W. Gregg. 2013. "Preventing Type 2 Diabetes in Communities across the U.S.: The National Diabetes Prevention Program." *American Journal of Preventive Medicine* 44 (4): S346–51.

Ali, M. K., B. Bhaskarapillai, R. Shivashankar, D. Mohan, Z. A. Fatmi, and others. 2016. "Socioeconomic Status and Cardiovascular Risk in Urban South Asia: The CARRS Study." *European Journal of Preventive Cardiology* 23 (4): 408–19.

Ali, M. K., K. M. Bullard, E. W. Gregg, and C. Del Rio. 2014. "A Cascade of Care for Diabetes in the United States: Visualizing the Gaps." *Annals of Internal Medicine* 161 (10): 681–89.

Ali, M. K., K. M. Bullard, J. B. Saaddine, C. C. Cowie, G. Imperatore, and E. W. Gregg. 2013. "Achievement of Goals in U.S. Diabetes Care, 1999–2010." *New England Journal of Medicine* 368 (17): 1613–24.

Ali, M. K., J. Echouffo-Tcheugui, and D. F. Williamson. 2012. "How Effective Were Lifestyle Interventions in Real-World Settings that Were Modeled on the Diabetes Prevention Program?" *Health Affairs* 31 (1): 67–75.

Ali, M. K., L. M. Jaacks, A. J. Kowalski, K. R. Siegel, and M. Ezzati. 2015. "Noncommunicable Diseases: Three Decades of Global Data Show a Mixture of Increases and Decreases in Mortality Rates." *Health Affairs* 34: 91444–55; doi:10.1377/hlthaff.2015.0570.

Ali, M. K., M. J. Magee, J. A. Dave, I. Ofotokun, M. Tungsiripat, and others. 2014. "HIV and Metabolic, Body, and Bone Disorders: What We Know from Low- and Middle-Income Countries." *Journal of Acquired Immune Deficiency Syndromes* 67 (Suppl 1): S27–39.

Ali, M. K., K. M. Narayan, and N. Tandon. 2010. "Diabetes and Coronary Heart Disease: Current Perspectives." *Indian Journal of Medical Research* 132 (11): 584–97.

Ali, M. K., K. Singh, D. Kondal, R. Devarajan, S. A. Patel, and others. 2016. "Effectiveness of a Multi-Component Quality Improvement Strategy to Improve Achievement of Diabetes Care Goals: A Randomized Controlled Trial." *Annals of Internal Medicine* 165 (6): 399–408. doi: 10.7326/M15-2807.

Almbrand, B., M. Johannesson, B. Sjöstrand, K. Malmberg, and L. Rydén. 2000. "Cost-Effectiveness of Intense Insulin Treatment after Acute Myocardial Infarction in Patients with Diabetes Mellitus; Results from the DIGAMI Study." *European Heart Journal* 21 (9): 733–39.

Anand, S., B. Thomas, G. Remuzzi, M. Riella, M. El Nahas, S. Naicker, and J. Dirks. 2017. "Kidney Disease." In *Disease Control Priorities* (third edition): Volume 5, *Cardiovascular, Respiratory, and Related Disorders*, edited by D. Prabhakaran, S. Anand, T. A. Gaziano, J.-C. Mbanya, Y. Wu, and R. Nugent. Washington, DC: World Bank.

Anjana, R. M., R. Pradeepa, M. Deepa, M. Datta, V. Sudha, and others. 2011. "Prevalence of Diabetes and Prediabetes (Impaired Fasting Glucose and/or Impaired Glucose Tolerance) in Urban and Rural India: Phase I Results of the Indian Council of Medical Research-INdia DIABetes (ICMR-INDIAB) Study." *Diabetologia* 54 (12): 3022–72.

Annemans, L., S. Marbaix, K. Webb, L. Van Gaal, and A. Scheen. 2010. "Cost-Effectiveness of Atorvastatin in Patients with Type 2 Diabetes Mellitus: A Pharmacoeconomic Analysis of the Collaborative Atorvastatin Diabetes Study in the Belgian Population." *Clinical Drug Investigation* 30 (2): 133–42.

Attridge, M., J. Creamer, M. Ramsden, R. Cannings-John, and K. Hawthorne. 2014. "Culturally Appropriate Health

Education for People in Ethnic Minority Groups with Type 2 Diabetes Mellitus." *Cochrane Database of Systematic Reviews* (9): CD006424. doi:10.1002/14651858.CD006424 .pub3.

Bardenheier, B. H., J. Lin, X. Zhuo, M. K. Ali, T. J. Thompson, and others. 2016. "Disability-Free Life-Years Lost among Adults Aged ≥ 50 Years, with and without Diabetes." *Diabetes Care* 39 (7): 1222–29.

Basu, S., C. Millett, S. Vijan, R. A. Hayward, S. Kinra, and others. 2015. "The Health System and Population Health Implications of Large-Scale Diabetes Screening in India: A Microsimulation Model of Alternative Approaches." *PLoS Medicine* 12 (5): e1001827.

Beran, D., and J. S. Yudkin. 2006. "Diabetes Care in Sub-Saharan Africa." *The Lancet* 368 (9548): 1689–95.

Beran, D., J. S. Yudkin, and M. de Courten. 2005. "Access to Care for Patients with Insulin-Requiring Diabetes in Developing Countries: Case Studies of Mozambique and Zambia." *Diabetes Care* 28 (9): 2136–40.

Blanckenberg, M., C. Worst, and C. Scheffer. 2011. "Development of a Mobile Phone Based Ophthalmoscope for Telemedicine." In *Proceedings of the 33rd Annual Conference of the IEEE Engineering in Medicine and Biology Society*, 5236–39. Piscataway, NJ: IEEE.

Boulton, A. J. M., D. G. Armstrong, S. F. Albert, R. G. Frykberg, R. Hellman, and others. 2008. "Comprehensive Foot Examination and Risk Assessment: A Report of the Task Force of the Foot Care Interest Group of the American Diabetes Association, with Endorsement by the American Association of Clinical Endocrinologists." *Diabetes Care* 31 (8): 1679–85.

Brod, M., B. Pohlman, S. Blum, A. Ramasamy, and R. Carson. 2014. "Burden of Illness of Diabetic Peripheral Neuropathic Pain: A Qualitative Study." *Patient* 8 (4): 339–48.

Brownson, C. A., T. J. Hoerger, E. B. Fisher, and K. E. Kilpatrick. 2009. "Cost-Effectiveness of Diabetes Self-Management Programs in Community Primary Care Settings." *Diabetes Educator* 35 (5): 761–69.

Brownson, R. C., J. E. Fielding, and C. M. Maylahn. 2009. "Evidence-Based Public Health: A Fundamental Concept for Public Health Practice." *Annual Review of Public Health* 30: 175–201.

Casagrande, S. S., C. C. Cowie, and J. E. Fradkin. 2013. "Utility of the U.S. Preventive Services Task Force Criteria for Diabetes Screening." *American Journal of Preventive Medicine* 45 (2): 167–74.

CDC (Centers for Disease Control and Prevention). 1998. "The Cost-Effectiveness of Screening for Type 2 Diabetes: CDC Diabetes Cost-Effectiveness Study Group, Centers for Disease Control and Prevention." *Journal of the American Medical Association* 280 (20): 1757–63.

———. 2016. "At a Glance 2016: Diabetes." CDC, Atlanta, GA. http://www.cdc.gov/chronicdisease/resources/publications /aag/diabetes.htm.

CDC Diabetes Cost-Effectiveness Group. 2002. "Cost-Effectiveness of Intensive Glycemic Control, Intensified

Hypertension Control, and Serum Cholesterol Level Reduction for Type 2 Diabetes." *Journal of the American Medical Association* 287 (19): 2542–51.

Chan, J. C., W. Y. So, C. Y. Yeung, G. T. Ko, I. T. Lau, and others. 2009. "Effects of Structured versus Usual Care on Renal Endpoint in Type 2 Diabetes: The SURE Study: A Randomized Multicenter Translational Study." *Diabetes Care* 32 (6): 977–982.

Clarke, P. M., A. M. Gray, A. Briggs, R. J. Stevens, D. R. Matthews, and others. 2005. "Cost-Utility Analyses of Intensive Blood Glucose and Tight Blood Pressure Control in Type 2 Diabetes (UKPDS 72)." *Diabetologia* 48 (5): 868–77.

Colquhoun, A. J., K. G. Nicholson, J. L. Botha, and N. T. Raymond. 1997. "Effectiveness of Influenza Vaccine in Reducing Hospital Admissions in People with Diabetes." *Epidemiology and Infection* 119 (3): 335–41.

Coyle, D., K. Coyle, G. P. Kenny, N. G. Boulé, G. A. Wells, and others. 2012. "Cost-Effectiveness of Exercise Programs in Type 2 Diabetes." *International Journal of Technology Assessment in Health Care* 28 (3): 228–34.

Critchley, J. A., and S. Capewell. 2003. "Mortality Risk Reduction Associated with Smoking Cessation in Patients with Coronary Heart Disease: A Systematic Review." *Journal of the American Medical Association* 290 (1): 86–97.

Danaei, G., C. M. Lawes, S. Vander Hoorn, C. J. Murray, and M. Ezzati. 2006. "Global and Regional Mortality from Ischaemic Heart Disease and Stroke Attributable to Higher-than-Optimum Blood Glucose Concentration: Comparative Risk Assessment." *The Lancet* 368 (9548): 1651–59.

DCCT (Diabetes Control and Complications Trial) Research Group. 1993. "The Effect of Intensive Treatment of Diabetes on the Development and Progression of Long-Term Complications in Insulin-Dependent Diabetes Mellitus." *New England Journal of Medicine* 329 (14): 977–86.

———. 1996. "Lifetime Benefits and Costs of Intensive Therapy as Practiced in the Diabetes Control and Complications Trial." *Journal of the American Medical Association* 276 (17): 1409–15.

Degmecic, D., T. Bacun, V. Kovac, J. Mioc, J. Horvat, and A. Vcev. 2014. "Depression, Anxiety, and Cognitive Dysfunction in Patients with Type 2 Diabetes Mellitus: A Study of Adult Patients with Type 2 Diabetes Mellitus in Osijek, Croatia." *Collegium Antropologicum* 38 (2): 711–16.

Diaz de Leon-Castaneda, C., M. Altagracia-Martínez, J. Kravzov-Jinich, R. Cárdenas-Elizalde Mdel, C. Moreno-Bonett, and J. M. Martínez-Núñez. 2012. "Cost-Effectiveness Study of Oral Hypoglycemic Agents in the Treatment of Outpatients with Type 2 Diabetes Attending a Public Primary Care Clinic in Mexico City." *ClinicoEconomics and Outcomes Research* 4: 57–65.

Dooley, K. E., and R. E. Chaisson. 2009. "Tuberculosis and Diabetes Mellitus: Convergence of Two Epidemics." *The Lancet Infectious Diseases* 9 (12): 737–46.

DPP (Diabetes Prevention Program) Research Group. 2003. "Within-Trial Cost-Effectiveness of Lifestyle Intervention or Metformin for the Primary Prevention of Type 2 Diabetes." *Diabetes Care* 26 (9): 2518–23.

———. 2012. "The 10-Year Cost-Effectiveness of Lifestyle Intervention or Metformin for Diabetes Prevention: An Intent-to-Treat Analysis of the DPP/DPPOS." *Diabetes Care* 35 (4): 723–30.

DRS (Diabetic Retinopathy Study) Research Group. 1981. "Photocoagulation Treatment of Proliferative Diabetic Retinopathy: Clinical Application of Diabetic Retinopathy Study (DRS) Findings, DRS Report Number 8." *Ophthalmology* 88 (7): 583–600.

———. 1991. "Early Photocoagulation for Diabetic Retinopathy: ETDRS Report Number 9." *Ophthalmology* 98 (Suppl 5): 766–85.

Duckworth, W., C. Abraira, T. Moritz, D. Reda, N. Emanuele, and others. 2009. "Glucose Control and Vascular Complications in Veterans with Type 2 Diabetes." *New England Journal of Medicine* 360 (2): 129–39.

Dunbar, J. A., A. Jayawardena, G. Johnson, K. Roger, A. Timoshanko, and others. 2014. "Scaling up Diabetes Prevention in Victoria, Australia: Policy Development, Implementation, and Evaluation." *Diabetes Care* 37 (4): 934–42.

Eastman, R. C., J. C. Javitt, W. H. Herman, E. J. Dasbach, C. Copley-Merriman, and others. 1997. "Model of Complications of NIDDM: II. Analysis of the Health Benefits and Cost-Effectiveness of Treating NIDDM with the Goal of Normoglycemia." *Diabetes Care* 20 (5): 735–44.

Eborall, H. C., R. Davies, A. L. Kinmonth, S. Griffin, and J. Lawton. 2007. "Patients' Experiences of Screening for Type 2 Diabetes: Prospective Qualitative Study Embedded in the ADDITION (Cambridge) Randomised Controlled Trial." *BMJ* 335 (7618): 490.

Eborall, H. C., S. J. Griffin, A. T. Prevost, A.-L. Kinmonth, D. P. French, and S. Sutton. 2007. "Psychological Impact of Screening for Type 2 Diabetes: Controlled Trial and Comparative Study Embedded in the ADDITION (Cambridge) Randomised Controlled Trial." *BMJ* 335 (7618): 486.

Echouffo-Tcheugui, J. B., M. K. Ali, S. J. Griffin, and K. M. Narayan. 2011. "Screening for Type 2 Diabetes and Dysglycemia." *Epidemiologic Reviews* 33 (1): 63–87.

Echouffo-Tcheugui, J. B., M. K. Ali, G. Roglic, R. A. Hayward, and K. M. Narayan. 2013. "Screening Intervals for Diabetic Retinopathy and Incidence of Visual Loss: A Systematic Review." *Diabetic Medicine* 30 (11): 1272–92.

Eddy, D. M., L. Schlessinger, and R. Kahn. 2005. "Clinical Outcomes and Cost-Effectiveness of Strategies for Managing People at High Risk for Diabetes." *Annals of Internal Medicine* 143 (4): 251–64.

Elliott, W. J., D. R. Weir, and H. R. Black. 2000. "Cost-Effectiveness of the Lower Treatment Goal (of JNC VI) for Diabetic Hypertensive Patients. Joint National Committee on Prevention, Detection, Evaluation, and Treatment of High Blood Pressure." *Archives of Internal Medicine* 160 (9): 1277–83.

Engelgau, M. M., and E. W. Gregg. 2012. "Tackling the Global Diabetes Burden: Will Screening Help?" *The Lancet* 380 (9855): 1716–18.

Engelgau, M. M., K. M. Narayan, and W. H. Herman. 2000. "Screening for Type 2 Diabetes." *Diabetes Care* 23 (10): 1563–80.

Farmer, A. J., R. Perera, A. Ward, C. Heneghan, J. Oke, and others. 2012. "Meta-Analysis of Individual Patient Data in Randomised Trials of Self-Monitoring of Blood Glucose in People with Non-Insulin Treated Type 2 Diabetes." *BMJ* 344: e486. doi:http://dx.doi.org/10.1136/bmj.e486.

Fox, C. S., K. Matsushita, M. Woodward, H. J. Bilo, J. Chalmers, and others. 2012. "Associations of Kidney Disease Measures with Mortality and End-Stage Renal Disease in Individuals with and without Diabetes: A Meta-Analysis." *The Lancet* 380 (9854): 1662–73.

Foy, C. G., C. E. Lewis, K. G. Hairston, G. D. Miller, W. Lang, and others. 2011. "Intensive Lifestyle Intervention Improves Physical Function among Obese Adults with Knee Pain: Findings from the Look AHEAD Trial." *Obesity* 19 (1): 83–93.

Franco, O. H., E. W. Steyerberg, F. B. Hu, J. Mackenbach, and W. Nusselder. 2007. "Associations of Diabetes Mellitus with Total Life Expectancy and Life Expectancy with and without Cardiovascular Disease." *Archives of Internal Medicine* 167 (11): 1145–51.

Fu, A. Z., Y. Qiu, L. Radican, and B. J. Wells. 2009. "Health Care and Productivity Costs Associated with Diabetic Patients with Macrovascular Comorbid Conditions." *Diabetes Care* 32 (12): 2187–92.

Gaede, P., H. Lund-Andersen, H. H. Parving, and O. Pedersen. 2008. "Effect of a Multifactorial Intervention on Mortality in Type 2 Diabetes." *New England Journal of Medicine* 358 (6): 580–91.

Gaede, P., W. J. Valentine, A. J. Palmer, D. M. Tucker, M. Lammert, and others. 2008. "Cost-Effectiveness of Intensified versus Conventional Multifactorial Intervention in Type 2 Diabetes: Results and Projections from the Steno-2 Study." *Diabetes Care* 31 (8): 1510–15.

Gaede, P., P. Vedel, N. Larsen, G. V. Jensen, H. H. Parving, and O. Pedersen. 2003. "Multifactorial Intervention and Cardiovascular Disease in Patients with Type 2 Diabetes." *New England Journal of Medicine* 348 (5): 383–93.

Gakidou, E., L. Mallinger, J. Abbott-Klafter, R. Guerrero, S. Villalpando, and others. 2011. "Management of Diabetes and Associated Cardiovascular Risk Factors in Seven Countries: A Comparison of Data from National Health Examination Surveys." *Bulletin of the World Health Organization* 89 (3): 172–83.

Geiss, L. S., W. M. Herman, and P. J. Smith. 1995. "Mortality in Non-Insulin-Dependent Diabetes." In *Diabetes in America*, edited by National Diabetes Data Group, 233–55. 2nd ed. Bethesda, MD: National Institutes of Health and National Institute of Diabetes and Digestive and Kidney Diseases.

Gerstein, H. C., M. E. Miller, R. P. Byington, D. C. Goff Jr., J. T. Bigger, and others. 2008. "Effects of Intensive Glucose

Lowering in Type 2 Diabetes." *New England Journal of Medicine* 358 (24): 2545–59.

Gerstein, H. C., P. Santaguida, P. Raina, K. M. Morrison, C. Balion, and others. 2007. "Annual Incidence and Relative Risk of Diabetes in People with Various Categories of Dysglycemia: A Systematic Overview and Meta-Analysis of Prospective Studies." *Diabetes Research and Clinical Practice* 78 (3): 305–12.

Gillett, M., H. M. Dallosso, S. Dixon, A. Brennan, M. E. Carey, and others. 2010. "Delivering the Diabetes Education and Self-Management for Ongoing and Newly Diagnosed (DESMOND) Programme for People with Newly Diagnosed Type 2 Diabetes: Cost-Effectiveness Analysis." *BMJ* 341 (August 20): c4093.

Gillies, C. L., K. R. Abrams, P. C. Lambert, N. J. Cooper, A. J. Sutton, and others. 2007. "Pharmacological and Lifestyle Interventions to Prevent or Delay Type 2 Diabetes in People with Impaired Glucose Tolerance: Systematic Review and Meta-Analysis." *BMJ* 334 (7588): 299.

Gillies, C. L., P. C. Lambert, K. R. Abrams, A. J. Sutton, N. J. Cooper, and others. 2008. "Different Strategies for Screening and Prevention of Type 2 Diabetes in Adults: Cost-Effectiveness Analysis." *BMJ* 336 (7654): 1180–85.

Gilmer, T. P., S. Roze, W. J. Valentine, K. Emy-Albrecht, J. A. Ray, and others. 2007. "Cost-Effectiveness of Diabetes Case Management for Low-Income Populations." *Health Services Research* 42 (5): 1943–59.

Giovannucci, E., D. M. Harlan, M. C. Archer, R. M. Bergenstal, S. M. Gapstur, and others. 2010. "Diabetes and Cancer: A Consensus Report." *Diabetes Care* 33 (7): 1674–85.

Glasgow, R. E., H. G. McKay, J. D. Piette, and K. D. Reynolds. 2001. "The RE-AIM Framework for Evaluating Interventions: What Can It Tell Us about Approaches to Chronic Illness Management?" *Patient Education and Counseling* 44 (2): 119–27.

Gloy, V. L., M. Briel, D. L. Bhatt, S. R. Kashyap, P. R. Schauer, and others. 2013. "Bariatric Surgery versus Non-Surgical Treatment for Obesity: A Systematic Review and Meta-Analysis of Randomised Controlled Trials." *BMJ* 347: f5934.

Glumer, C., M. Yuyun, S. Griffin, D. Farewell, D. Spiegelhalter, and others. 2006. "What Determines the Cost-Effectiveness of Diabetes Screening?" *Diabetologia* 49 (7): 1536–44.

Gong, Q., E. W. Gregg, J. Wang, Y. An, P. Zhang, and others. 2011. "Long-Term Effects of a Randomised Trial of a 6-Year Lifestyle Intervention in Impaired Glucose Tolerance on Diabetes-Related Microvascular Complications: The China Da Qing Diabetes Prevention Outcome Study." *Diabetologia* 54 (2): 300–7.

Gozzoli, V., A. J. Palmer, A. Brandt, and G. A. Spinas. 2001. "Economic and Clinical Impact of Alternative Disease Management Strategies for Secondary Prevention in Type 2 Diabetes in the Swiss Setting." *Swiss Medical Weekly* 131 (21–22): 303–10.

Gregg, E. W., H. Chen, L. E. Wagenknecht, J. M. Clark, L. M. Delahanty, and others. 2012. "Association of an Intensive Lifestyle Intervention with Remission of Type 2 Diabetes." *Journal of the American Medical Association* 308 (23): 2489–96.

Gregg, E. W., Y. J. Cheng, S. Saydah, C. Cowie, S. Garfield, and others. 2012. "Trends in Death Rates among U.S. Adults with and without Diabetes between 1997 and 2006: Findings from the National Health Interview Survey." *Diabetes Care* 35 (6): 1252–57.

Gregg, E. W., Y. Li, J. Wang, N. Rios Burrows, M. K. Ali, and others. 2014. "Changes in Diabetes-Related Complications in the United States, 1990–2010." *New England Journal of Medicine* 370 (16): 1514–23.

Gregg, E. W., N. Sattar, and M. K. Ali. 2016. "The Changing Face of Diabetes Complications." *The Lancet Diabetes Endocrinology* 4 (6): 537–47.

Grover, S. A., L. Coupal, H. Zowall, and M. Dorais. 2000. "Cost-Effectiveness of Treating Hyperlipidemia in the Presence of Diabetes: Who Should Be Treated?" *Circulation* 102 (7): 722–77.

Habib, S. H., K. B. Biswas, S. Akter, S. Saha, and L. Ali. 2010. "Cost-Effectiveness Analysis of Medical Intervention in Patients with Early Detection of Diabetic Foot in a Tertiary Care Hospital in Bangladesh." *Journal of Diabetes Complications* 24 (4): 259–64.

Haddock, L. J., D. Y. Kim, and S. Mukai. 2013. "Simple, Inexpensive Technique for High-Quality Smartphone Fundus Photography in Human and Animal Eyes." *Journal of Ophthalmology* 3: 518479. doi:10.1155/2013/518479.

Hayward, R. A., P. D. Reaven, W. L. Wiitala, G. D. Bahn, D. J. Reda and others. 2015. "Follow-Up of Glycemic Control and Cardiovascular Outcomes in Type 2 Diabetes." *New England Journal of Medicine* 372 (23): 2197–06.

Hegde, S. V., P. Adhikari, S. Shetty, P. Manjrekar, and V. D'Souza. 2013. "Effect of Community-Based Yoga Intervention on Oxidative Stress and Glycemic Parameters in Prediabetes: A Randomized Controlled Trial." *Complementary Therapies in Medicine* 21 (6): 571–76.

Hempler, N. F., O. Ekholm, and I. Willaing. 2013. "Differences in Social Relations between Persons with Type 2 Diabetes and the General Population." *Scandinavian Journal of Public Health* 41 (4): 340–43.

Hennink, M. M., B. N. Kaiser, S. Sekar, E. P. Griswold, and M. K. Ali. 2016. "How Are Qualitative Methods Used in Diabetes Research? A 30-Year Systematic Review." *Global Public Health* 13: 1–20.

Herman, W. H., T. J. Hoerger, M. Brandle, K. Hicks, S. Sorensen, and others. 2005. "The Cost-Effectiveness of Lifestyle Modification or Metformin in Preventing Type 2 Diabetes in Adults with Impaired Glucose Tolerance." *Annals of Internal Medicine* 142 (5): 323–32.

Heymann, A. D., Y. Shapiro, G. Chodick, V. Shalev, E. Kokia, and others. 2004. "Reduced Hospitalizations and Death Associated with Influenza Vaccination among Patients with and without Diabetes." *Diabetes Care* 27 (11): 2581–84.

Hill, J. O., J. M. Galloway, A. Goley, D. G. Marrero, R. Minners, and others. 2013. "Scientific Statement: Socioecological Determinants of Prediabetes and Type 2 Diabetes." *Diabetes Care* 36 (August): 2430–39.

Hoerger, T. J., R. Harris, K. A. Hicks, K. Donahue, S. Sorensen, and M. Engelgau. 2004. "Screening for Type 2 Diabetes Mellitus: A Cost-Effectiveness Analysis." *Annals of Internal Medicine* 140 (9): 689–99.

Hoerger, T. J., K. A. Hicks, S. W. Sorensen, W. H. Herman, R. E. Ratner, and others. 2007. "Cost-Effectiveness of Screening for Pre-Diabetes among Overweight and Obese U.S. Adults." *Diabetes Care* 30 (11): 2874–79.

Hoerger, T. J., J. S. Wittenborn, J. E. Segel, N. R. Burrows, K. Imai, and others. 2010. "A Health Policy Model of CKD: 2. The Cost-Effectiveness of Microalbuminuria Screening." *American Journal of Kidney Diseases* 55 (3): 463–73.

Holman, R. R., S. K. Paul, M. A. Bethel, D. R. Matthews, H. Andrew, and W. Neil. 2008. "10-Year Follow-Up of Intensive Glucose Control in Type 2 Diabetes." *New England Journal of Medicine* 359 (15): 1577–89.

IDF (International Diabetes Federation). 2013. *Clinical Practice Guidelines.* Brussels: IDF. http://www.idf.org/guidelines.

———. 2015. *IDF Diabetes Atlas.* 7th ed. Brussels: IDF. http://www.idf.org/diabetesatlas.

IDF Europe. Not dated. *Access to Quality Medicines and Devices for Diabetes Care in Europe.* Brussels: IDF. http://www.idf.org/sites/default/files/FULL-STUDY.pdf.

Inzucchi, S. E., R. M. Bergenstal, J. B. Buse, M. Diamant, E. Ferrannini, and others. 2012. "Management of Hyperglycemia in Type 2 Diabetes: A Patient-Centered Approach: Position Statement of the American Diabetes Association (ADA) and the European Association for the Study of Diabetes (EASD)." *Diabetes Care* 35 (6): 1364–79.

Iqbal Hydrie, M. Z., A. Basit, A. S. Shera, and A. Hussain. 2012. "Effect of Intervention in Subjects with High Risk of Diabetes Mellitus in Pakistan." *Journal of Nutrition and Metabolism* 2012: 867604. doi:10.1155/2012/867604.

Irvine, L., G. R. Barton, A. V. Gasper, N. Murray, A. Clark, and others. 2011. "Cost-Effectiveness of a Lifestyle Intervention in Preventing Type 2 Diabetes." *International Journal of Technology Assessment in Health Care* 27 (4): 275–82.

Ismail-Beigi, F., E. Moghissi, M. Tiktin, I. B. Hirsch, S. E. Inzucchi, and S. Genuth. 2011. "Individualizing Glycemic Targets in Type 2 Diabetes Mellitus: Implications of Recent Clinical Trials." *Annals of Internal Medicine* 154 (8): 554–59.

Janus, E., J. D. Best, N. Davis-Lameloise, B. Philpot, A. Hernan, and others. 2012. "Scaling-Up from an Implementation Trial to State-Wide Coverage: Results from the Preliminary Melbourne Diabetes Prevention Study." *Trials* 13 (1): 152.

Jilcott, S., A. Ammerman, S. Sommers, and R. E. Glasgow. 2007. "Applying the RE-AIM Framework to Assess the Public Health Impact of Policy Change." *Annals of Behavioral Medicine* 34 (2): 105–14.

Jonsson, B., J. R. Cook, and T. R. Pedersen. 1999. "The Cost-Effectiveness of Lipid Lowering in Patients with Diabetes: Results from the 4S Trial." *Diabetologia* 42 (11): 1293–301.

Kahn, R., P. Alperin, D. Eddy, K. Borch-Johnsen, J. Buse, and others. 2010. "Age at Initiation and Frequency of Screening to Detect Type 2 Diabetes: A Cost-Effectiveness Analysis." *The Lancet* 375 (9723): 1365–74.

Karalliedde, J., M. Wijesuriya, L. Vasantharajah, M. Gulliford, G. Viberti, and L. Gnudi. 2014. "Effect of Lifestyle Modification on the Prevention of Type 2 Diabetes and Impaired Glucose Tolerance in a Young Healthy Urban South Asian Population." *Diabetologia* 57 (Suppl 1): S34.

Katula, J. A., M. Z. Vitolins, T. M. Morgan, M. S. Lawlor, C. S. Blackwell, and others. 2013. "The Healthy Living Partnerships to Prevent Diabetes Study: 2-Year Outcomes of a Randomized Controlled Trial." *American Journal of Preventive Medicine* 44 (4 Suppl 4): S324–32.

Kearney, P. M., L. Blackwell, R. Collins, A. Keech, J. Simes, and others. 2008. "Efficacy of Cholesterol-Lowering Therapy in 18,686 People with Diabetes in 14 Randomised Trials of Statins: A Meta-Analysis." *The Lancet* 371 (9607): 117–25.

Kessler, R., G. Keusch, T. D. Szucs, J. S. Wittenborn, T. J. Hoerger, and others. 2012. "Health Economic Modelling of the Cost-Effectiveness of Microalbuminuria Screening in Switzerland." *Swiss Medical Weekly* 142: w13508.

Khan, T., M. Y. Bertram, R. Jina, B. Mash, N. Levitt, and K. Hofman. 2013. "Preventing Diabetes Blindness: Cost-Effectiveness of a Screening Programme Using Digital Non-Mydriatic Fundus Photography for Diabetic Retinopathy in a Primary Health Care Setting in South Africa." *Diabetes Research and Clinical Practice* 101 (2): 170–76.

Khunti, K., C. L. Gillies, N. A. Taub, S. A. Mostafa, S. L. Hiles, and others. 2012. "A Comparison of Cost per Case Detected of Screening Strategies for Type 2 Diabetes and Impaired Glucose Regulation: Modelling Study." *Diabetes Research and Clinical Practice* 97 (3): 505–13.

Klein, R., B. E. Klein, S. E. Moss, M. D. Davis, and D. L. DeMets. 1989a. "The Wisconsin Epidemiologic Study of Diabetic Retinopathy: IX. Four-Year Incidence and Progression of Diabetic Retinopathy When Age at Diagnosis Is Less Than 30 Years." *Archives of Ophthalmology* 107 (2): 237–43.

———. 1989b. "The Wisconsin Epidemiologic Study of Diabetic Retinopathy: X. Four-Year Incidence and Progression of Diabetic Retinopathy When Age at Diagnosis Is 30 Years or More." *Archives of Ophthalmology* 107 (2): 244–49.

Knowler, W. C., E. Barrett-Connor, S. E. Fowler, R. F. Hamman, J. M. Lachin, and others. 2002. "Reduction in the Incidence of Type 2 Diabetes with Lifestyle Intervention or Metformin." *New England Journal of Medicine* 346 (6): 393–403.

Knowler, W. C., P. H. Bennett, R. F. Hamman, and M. Miller. 1978. "Diabetes Incidence and Prevalence in Pima Indians: A 19-Fold Greater Incidence Than in Rochester, Minnesota." *American Journal of Epidemiology* 108 (6): 497–505.

Ko, G. T., C. Y. Yeung, W. Y. Leung, K. W. Chan, C. H. Chung, and others. 2011. "Cost Implication of Team-Based Structured versus Usual Care for Type 2 Diabetic Patients with Chronic Renal Disease." *Hong Kong Medical Journal* 17 (Suppl 6): 9–12.

Kosaka, K., M. Noda, and T. Kuzuya. 2005. "Prevention of Type 2 Diabetes by Lifestyle Intervention: A Japanese Trial in IGT Males." *Diabetes Research and Clinical Practice* 67 (2): 152–62.

Kovacs Burns, K., A. Nicolucci, R. I. Holt, I. Willaing, N. Hermanns, and others. 2013. "Diabetes Attitudes, Wishes, and Needs Second Study (DAWN2™): Cross-National Benchmarking Indicators for Family Members Living with People with Diabetes." *Diabetic Medicine* 30 (7): 778–88.

Kumar, S., E. H. Wang, M. J. Pokabla, and R. J. Noecker. 2012. "Teleophthalmology Assessment of Diabetic Retinopathy Fundus Images: Smartphone versus Standard Office Computer Workstation." *Telemedicine and e-Health* 18 (2): 158–62.

Lau, D., D. T. Eurich, S. R. Majumdar, A. Katz, and J. A. Johnson. 2013. "Effectiveness of Influenza Vaccination in Working-Age Adults with Diabetes: A Population-Based Cohort Study." *Thorax* 68 (7): 658–63.

Lavigne, J. E., C. E. Phelps, A. Mushlin, and W. M. Lednar. 2003. "Reductions in Individual Work Productivity Associated with Type 2 Diabetes Mellitus." *PharmacoEconomics* 21 (15): 1123–34.

Levitt, N. S. 2008. "Diabetes in Africa: Epidemiology, Management, and Healthcare Challenges." *Heart* 94 (11): 1376–82.

Lewis, E. J., L. G. Hunsicker, R. P. Bain, and R. D. Rohde. 1993. "The Effect of Angiotensin-Converting-Enzyme Inhibition on Diabetic Nephropathy." *New England Journal of Medicine* 329 (20): 1456–62.

Li, G., P. Zhang, J. Wang, Y. An, Q. Gong, and others. 2014. "Cardiovascular Mortality, All-Cause Mortality, and Diabetes Incidence after Lifestyle Intervention for People with Impaired Glucose Tolerance in the Da Qing Diabetes Prevention Study: A 23-Year Follow-Up Study." *The Lancet Diabetes and Endocrinology* 2 (6): 474–80.

Li, J. F., D. D. Lai, B. Ni, and K. X. Sun. 2013. "Comparison of Laparoscopic Roux-en-Y Gastric Bypass with Laparoscopic Sleeve Gastrectomy for Morbid Obesity or Type 2 Diabetes Mellitus: A Meta-Analysis of Randomized Controlled Trials." *Canadian Journal of Surgery* 56 (6): E158–64.

Li, R., S. Qu, P. Zhang, S. Chattopadhyay, E. W. Gregg, and others. 2015. "Economic Evaluation of Combined Diet and Physical Activity Promotion Programs to Prevent Type 2 Diabetes among Persons at Increased Risk: A Systematic Review for the Community Preventive Services Task Force." *Annals of Internal Medicine* 163 (6): 452–60.

Li, R., P. Zhang, L. E. Barker, F. M. Chowdhury, and X. Zhang. 2010. "Cost-Effectiveness of Interventions to Prevent and Control Diabetes Mellitus: A Systematic Review." *Diabetes Care* 33 (8): 1872–94.

Li, Y., L. S. Geiss, N. R. Burrows, D. B. Rolka, A. Albright, and others. 2013. "Awareness of Prediabetes: United States, 2005–2010." *Morbidity and Mortality Weekly* 62 (11): 209–12.

Lindgren, P., J. Lindström, J. Tuomilehto, M. Uusitupa, M. Peltonen, and others. 2007. "Lifestyle Intervention to Prevent Diabetes in Men and Women with Impaired Glucose Tolerance Is Cost-Effective." *International Journal of Technology Assessment in Health Care* 23 (2): 177–83.

Lipkin, E. W., A. V. Schwartz, A. M. Anderson, C. Davis, K. C. Johnson, and others. 2014. "The Look AHEAD Trial: Bone Loss at Four-Year Follow-Up in Type 2 Diabetes." *Diabetes Care* 37 (10): 2822–29.

Lohse, N., E. Marseille, and J. G. Kahn. 2011. "Development of a Model to Assess the Cost-Effectiveness of Gestational Diabetes Mellitus Screening and Lifestyle Change for the Prevention of Type 2 Diabetes Mellitus." *International Journal of Gynecology and Obstetrics* 115 (Suppl 1): S20–25.

Look AHEAD Research Group. 2006. "The Look AHEAD Study: A Description of the Lifestyle Intervention and the Evidence Supporting It." *Obesity* 14 (5): 737–52.

———. 2013. "Cardiovascular Effects of Intensive Lifestyle Intervention in Type 2 Diabetes." *New England Journal of Medicine* 369 (2): 145–54.

———. 2014. "Impact of Intensive Lifestyle Intervention on Depression and Health-Related Quality of Life in Type 2 Diabetes: The Look AHEAD Trial." *Diabetes Care* 37 (6): 1544–53.

Maberley, D., H. Walker, A. Koushik, and A. Cruess. 2003. "Screening for Diabetic Retinopathy in James Bay, Ontario: A Cost-Effectiveness Analysis." *Canadian Medical Association Journal* 168 (2): 160–64.

Magee, M. J., M. K. Ali, D. Prabhakaran, V. S. Ajay, M. Rabkin, and K. M. V. Narayan. 2017. "Integrated Public Health and Health Service Delivery for Noncommunicable Diseases and Comorbid Infectious Diseases and Mental Health." In *Disease Control Priorities* (third edition): Volume 5, *Cardiovascular, Respiratory, and Related Disorders*, edited by D. Prabhakaran, S. Anand, T. A. Gaziano, J.-C. Mbanya, Y. Wu, and R. Nugent. Washington, DC: World Bank.

Magee, M. J., H. M. Blumberg, and K. M. Narayan. 2011. "Commentary: Co-occurrence of Tuberculosis and Diabetes: New Paradigm of Epidemiological Transition." *International Journal of Epidemiology* 40 (2): 428–31.

Malanda, U. L., S. D. Bot, and G. Nijpels. 2013. "Self-Monitoring of Blood Glucose in Noninsulin-Using Type 2 Diabetic Patients: It Is Time to Face the Evidence." *Diabetes Care* 36 (1): 176–78.

Marseille, E., N. Lohse, A. Jiwani, M. Hod, V. Seshiah, and others. 2013. "The Cost-Effectiveness of Gestational Diabetes Screening Including Prevention of Type 2 Diabetes: Application of a New Model in India and Israel." *Journal of Maternal-Fetal and Neonatal Medicine* 26 (8): 802–10.

Mason, J. M., N. Freemantle, J. M. Gibson, and J. P. New. 2005. "Specialist Nurse-Led Clinics to Improve Control of Hypertension and Hyperlipidemia in Diabetes: Economic Analysis of the SPLINT Trial." *Diabetes Care* 28 (1): 40–46.

McCarthy, M. I. 2010. "Genomics, Type 2 Diabetes, and Obesity." *New England Journal of Medicine* 363 (24): 2339–50.

McDermott, K. 2012. "A Pilot Randomized Controlled Trial of Yoga for Prediabetes." *BMC Complementary and Alternative Medicine* 12 (Suppl 1): P180.

McDermott, K., M. R. Rao, R. Nagarathna, E. J. Murphy, A. Burke, and others. 2014. "A Yoga Intervention for Type 2 Diabetes Risk Reduction: A Pilot Randomized Controlled Trial." *BMC Complementary and Alternative Medicine* 14: 212.

McGill, M. 2005. *Foot-Care Education for People with Diabetes: A Major Challenge.* Brussels: International Diabetes Federation.

https://www.idf.org/sites/default/files/attachments/article_379_en.pdf.

McKellar, J. D., K. Humphreys, and J. D. Piette. 2004. "Depression Increases Diabetes Symptoms by Complicating Patients' Self-Care Adherence." *Diabetes Educator* 30 (3): 485–92.

Mendis, S., K. Fukino, A. Cameron, R. Laing, A. Filipe Jr., and others. 2007. "The Availability and Affordability of Selected Essential Medicines for Chronic Diseases in Six Low- and Middle-Income Countries." *Bulletin of the World Health Organization* 85 (4): 279–88A.

Merlotti, C., A. Morabito, V. Ceriani, and A. E. Pontiroli. 2014. "Prevention of Type 2 Diabetes in Obese at-Risk Subjects: A Systematic Review and Meta-Analysis." *Acta Diabetologica* 51 (5): 853–63.

Mohiuddin, S. M., A. N. Mooss, C. B. Hunter, T. L. Grollmes, D. A. Cloutier, and D. E. Hilleman. 2007. "Intensive Smoking Cessation Intervention Reduces Mortality in High-Risk Smokers with Cardiovascular Disease." *Chest Journal* 131 (2): 446–52.

MoPoTsyo Patient Information Centre. 2015. "Diabetes Network." http://www.mopotsyo.org/diabeticsnetwork.html and http://www.mopotsyo.org/ILR-PEN-24.pdf.

Morgan, C. L., C. J. Currie, and J. R. Peters. 2000. "Relationship between Diabetes and Mortality: A Population Study Using Record Linkage." *Diabetes Care* 23 (8): 1103–07.

Mortaz, S., C. Wessman, R. Duncan, R. Gray, and A. Badawi. 2012. "Impact of Screening and Early Detection of Impaired Fasting Glucose Tolerance and Type 2 Diabetes in Canada: A Markov Model Simulation." *ClinicoEconomics and Outcomes Research* 4: 91–97.

Moss, S. E., R. Klein, and B. E. Klein. 1991. "Cause-Specific Mortality in a Population-Based Study of Diabetes." *American Journal of Public Health* 81 (9): 1158–62.

Mudaliar, U., W. C. Kim, K. Kirk, C. Rouse, K. M. V. Narayan, and M. K. Ali. 2013. "Are Recommended Standards for Diabetes Care Met in Central and South America? A Systematic Review." *Diabetes Research and Clinical Practice* 100 (3): 306–29.

Mudaliar, U., A. Zabetian, M. Goodman, J. B. Echouffo-Tcheugui, A. L. Albright, and others. 2016. "Cardio-Metabolic Risk Factor Changes Observed in Diabetes Prevention Programs in US Settings: A Meta-Analysis." *PLoS Medicine* 13 (7): e1002095. doi:10.1371/journal.pmed.1002095.

Narayan, K. M. V., J. B. Echouffo-Tcheugui, V. Mohan, and M. K. Ali. 2012. "Analysis and Commentary: Global Prevention and Control of Type 2 Diabetes Will Require Paradigm Shifts in Policies within and among Countries." *Health Affairs* 31 (1): 84–92.

Narayan, K. M. V., P. Zhang, A. M. Kanaya, D. E. Williams, M. M. Engelgau, and others. 2006. "Diabetes: The Pandemic and Potential Solutions." In *Disease Control Priorities in Developing Countries* (second edition), edited by D. T. Jamison, J. G. Breman, A. R. Measham, G. Alleyne, M. Claeson, D. B. Evans, P. Jha, A. Mills, and P. Musgrove. Washington, DC: World Bank and Oxford University Press.

Nathan, D. M., P. A. Cleary, J. Y. Backlund, S. M. Genuth, J. M. Lachin, and others. 2005. "Intensive Diabetes Treatment and Cardiovascular Disease in Patients with Type 1 Diabetes." *New England Journal of Medicine* 353 (25): 2643–53.

NCD-RisC (NCD Risk Factor Collaboration). 2016. "Worldwide Trends in Diabetes Since 1980: A Pooled Analysis of 751 Population-Based Studies with 4.4 Million Participants." *The Lancet* 387 (10027): 1513–30.

NICE (National Institute for Health and Care Excellence). 2013. *Preventing Type 2 Diabetes: Risk Identification and Interventions for Individuals at High Risk (PH38).* Public Health Guidance 2013. http://www.nice.org.uk/guidance/index.jsp?action=byID&o=13791.

Nicholson, W. K., L. A. Fleisher, H. E. Fox, and N. R. Powe. 2005. "Screening for Gestational Diabetes Mellitus: A Decision and Cost-Effectiveness Analysis of Four Screening Strategies." *Diabetes Care* 28 (6): 1482–84.

Nicolucci, A., K. Kovacs Burns, R. I. Holt, M. Comaschi, N. Hermanns, and others. 2013. "Diabetes Attitudes, Wishes, and Needs Second Study (DAWN2™): Cross-National Benchmarking of Diabetes-Related Psychosocial Outcomes for People with Diabetes." *Diabetic Medicine* 30 (7): 767–77.

Norris, S. L., K. Donahue, S. S. Rathore, P. Frame, S. H. Woolf, and K. N. Lohr. 2008. "Screening Adults for Type 2 Diabetes: A Review of the Evidence for the U.S. Preventive Services Task Force." *Annals of Internal Medicine* 148 (11): 855–68.

Norris, S. L., M. M. Engelgau, and K. M. Narayan. 2001. "Effectiveness of Self-Management Training in Type 2 Diabetes: A Systematic Review of Randomized Controlled Trials." *Diabetes Care* 24 (3): 561–87.

O'Riordan, M. 2013. "Look AHEAD: No CVD Reduction, but Kidneys, Eyes Benefit." Medscape Cardiology (June). http://www.medscape.com/viewarticle/806816.

Otto, M. H., M. E. Røder, J. B. Prahl, and O. L. Svendsen. 2007. "Diabetic Ketoacidosis in Denmark: Incidence and Mortality Estimated from Public Health Registries." *Diabetes Research and Clinical Practice* 76 (1): 51–56.

Paddison, C. A., H. C. Eborall, D. P. French, A. L. Kinmonth, A. T. Prevost, and others. 2011. "Predictors of Anxiety and Depression among People Attending Diabetes Screening: A Prospective Cohort Study Embedded in the ADDITION (Cambridge) Randomized Control Trial." *British Journal of Health Psychology* 16 (Pt 1): 213–26.

Palmer, A. J., L. Annemans, S. Roze, M. Lamotte, P. Lapuerta, and others. 2004. "Cost-Effectiveness of Early Irbesartan Treatment versus Control (Standard Antihypertensive Medications Excluding ACE Inhibitors, Other Angiotensin-2 Receptor Antagonists, and Dihydropyridine Calcium Channel Blockers) or Late Irbesartan Treatment in Patients with Type 2 Diabetes, Hypertension, and Renal Disease." *Diabetes Care* 27 (8): 1897–903.

Palmer, A. J., L. Annemans, S. Roze, M. Lamotte, R. A. Rodby, and R. W. Bilous. 2004. "An Economic Evaluation of the Irbesartan in Diabetic Nephropathy Trial (IDNT) in a U.K. Setting." *Journal of Human Hypertension* 18 (10): 733–38.

Palmer, A. J., S. Roze, W. J. Valentine, G. A. Spinas, J. E. Shaw, and P. Z. Zimmet. 2004. "Intensive Lifestyle Changes or

Metformin in Patients with Impaired Glucose Tolerance: Modeling the Long-Term Health Economic Implications of the Diabetes Prevention Program in Australia, France, Germany, Switzerland, and the United Kingdom." *Clinical Therapeutics* 26 (2): 304–21.

Palmer, A. J., and D. M. Tucker. 2012. "Cost and Clinical Implications of Diabetes Prevention in an Australian Setting: A Long-Term Modeling Analysis." *Primary Care Diabetes* 6 (2): 109–21.

Palmer, A. J., W. J. Valentine, and J. A. Ray. 2007. "Irbesartan Treatment of Patients with Type 2 Diabetes, Hypertension, and Renal Disease: A U.K. Health Economics Analysis." *International Journal of Clinical Practice* 61 (10): 1626–33.

Palmer, A. J., W. J. Valentine, J. A. Ray, S. Roze, and N. Muszbek. 2007. "Health Economic Implications of Irbesartan Treatment versus Standard Blood Pressure Control in Patients with Type 2 Diabetes, Hypertension, and Renal Disease: A Hungarian Analysis." *European Journal of Health Economics* 8 (2): 161–68.

Palmer, A. J., C. Weiss, P. P. Sendi, K. Neeser, A. Brandt, and others. 2000. "The Cost-Effectiveness of Different Management Strategies for Type I Diabetes: A Swiss Perspective." *Diabetologia* 43 (1): 13–26.

Pan, X. R., G. W. Li, Y. H. Hu, J. X. Wang, and others. 1997. "Effects of Diet and Exercise in Preventing NIDDM in People with Impaired Glucose Tolerance. The Da Qing IGT and Diabetes Study." *Diabetes Care* 20 (4): 537–44.

Park, P., R. K. Simmons, A. T. Prevost, and S. J. Griffin. 2008. "Screening for Type 2 Diabetes Is Feasible, Acceptable, but Associated with Increased Short-Term Anxiety: A Randomised Controlled Trial in British General Practice." *BMC Public Health* 8: 350.

Patel, A., S. MacMahon, J. Chalmers, B. Neal, L. Billot, and others. 2008. "Intensive Blood Glucose Control and Vascular Outcomes in Patients with Type 2 Diabetes." *New England Journal of Medicine* 358 (24): 2560–72.

Pengpid, S., K. Peltzer, and L. Skaal. 2014. "Efficacy of a Church-Based Lifestyle Intervention Programme to Control High Normal Blood Pressure and/or High Normal Blood Glucose in Church Members: A Randomized Controlled Trial in Pretoria, South Africa." *BMC Public Health* 14: 568.

Perreault, L., S. E. Kahn, C. A. Christophi, W. C. Knowler, R. F. Hamman, and others. 2009. "Regression from Pre-Diabetes to Normal Glucose Regulation in the Diabetes Prevention Program." *Diabetes Care* 32 (9): 1583–88.

Piette, J. D., C. Richardson, and M. Valenstein. 2004. "Addressing the Needs of Patients with Multiple Chronic Illnesses: The Case of Diabetes and Depression." *American Journal of Managed Care* 10 (2 Pt 2): 152–62.

Pimentel, G. D., K. C. Portero-McLellan, E. P. Oliveira, A. P. Spada, M. Oshiiwa, and others. 2010. "Long-Term Nutrition Education Reduces Several Risk Factors for Type 2 Diabetes Mellitus in Brazilians with Impaired Glucose Tolerance." *Nutrition Research* 30 (3): 186–90.

Pollock, R. F., W. J. Valentine, G. Goodall, and M. Brändle. 2010. "Evaluating the Cost-Effectiveness of Self-Monitoring of Blood Glucose in Type 2 Diabetes Patients on Oral Anti-Diabetic Agents." *Swiss Medical Weekly* 140: w13103.

Polonsky, W. H., and L. Fisher. 2013. "Self-Monitoring of Blood Glucose in Noninsulin-Using Type 2 Diabetic Patients: Right Answer, but Wrong Question: Self-Monitoring of Blood Glucose Can Be Clinically Valuable for Noninsulin Users." *Diabetes Care* 36 (1): 179–82.

Pozzilli, P., E. A. M. Gale, N. Visallil, M. Baroni, P. Crovari, and others. 1986. "The Immune Response to Influenza Vaccination in Diabetic Patients." *Diabetologia* 29 (12): 850–54.

Pronk, N. P., and P. L. Remington. 2015. "Combined Diet and Physical Activity Promotion Programs for Prevention of Diabetes: Community Preventive Services Task Force Recommendation Statement." *Annals of Internal Medicine* 163 (6): 465–68.

Ragnarson Tennvall, G., and J. Apelqvist. 2001. "Prevention of Diabetes-Related Foot Ulcers and Amputations: A Cost-Utility Analysis Based on Markov Model Simulations." *Diabetologia* 44 (11): 2077–87.

Rahman, M., R. K. Simmons, S. H. Hennings, N. J. Wareham, and S. J. Griffin. 2012. "How Much Does Screening Bring Forward the Diagnosis of Type 2 Diabetes and Reduce Complications? Twelve-Year Follow-Up of the Ely Cohort." *Diabetologia* 55 (6): 1651–59.

Raikou, M., A. McGuire, H. M. Colhoun, D. J. Betteridge, P. N. Durrington, and others. 2007. "Cost-Effectiveness of Primary Prevention of Cardiovascular Disease with Atorvastatin in Type 2 Diabetes: Results from the Collaborative Atorvastatin Diabetes Study (CARDS)." *Diabetologia* 50 (4): 733–40.

Ramachandran, A., C. Snehalatha, S. Mary, B. Mukesh, A. D. Bhaskar, and V. Vijay. 2006. "The Indian Diabetes Prevention Programme Shows That Lifestyle Modification and Metformin Prevent Type 2 Diabetes in Asian Indian Subjects with Impaired Glucose Tolerance (IDPP-1)." *Diabetologia* 49 (2): 289–97.

Ramachandran, A., C. Snehalatha, J. Ram, S. Selvam, M. Simon, and others. 2013. "Effectiveness of Mobile Phone Messaging in Prevention of Type 2 Diabetes by Lifestyle Modification in Men in India: A Prospective, Parallel-Group, Randomised Controlled Trial." *The Lancet Diabetes Endocrinolology* 1 (3): 191–98.

Ramachandran, A., C. Snehalatha, A. Yamuna, S. Mary, and Z. Ping. 2007. "Cost-Effectiveness of the Interventions in the Primary Prevention of Diabetes among Asian Indians: Within-Trial Results of the Indian Diabetes Prevention Programme (IDPP)." *Diabetes Care* 30 (10): 2548–52.

Redmon, J. B., A. G. Bertoni, S. Connelly, P. A. Feeney, S. P. Glasser, and others. 2010. "Effect of the Look AHEAD Study Intervention on Medication Use and Related Cost to Treat Cardiovascular Disease Risk Factors in Individuals with Type 2 Diabetes." *Diabetes Care* 33 (6): 1153–58.

Rejeski, W. J., E. H. Ip, A. G. Bertoni, G. A. Bray, G. Evans, and others. 2012. "Lifestyle Change and Mobility in Obese Adults with Type 2 Diabetes." *New England Journal of Medicine* 366 (13): 1209–17.

Renders, C. M., G. D. Valk, S. Griffin, E. H. Wagner, J. T. Eijk, W. J. Assendelft. 2001. "Interventions to Improve the Management of Diabetes Mellitus in Primary Care, Outpatient, and Community Settings." *Cochrane Database of Systemic Reviews* (1): CD001481.

Ricci, C., M. Gaeta, E. Rausa, E. Asti, F. Bandera, and L. Bonavina. 2015. "Long-Term Effects of Bariatric Surgery on Type II Diabetes, Hypertension, and Hyperlipidemia: A Meta-Analysis and Meta-Regression Study with 5-Year Follow-Up." *Journal of Obesity Surgery* 25 (3): 397–405.

Roberto, C. A., B. Swinburn, C. Hawkes, T. T.-K. Huang, S. A. Costa, and others. 2015. "Patchy Progress on Obesity Prevention: Emerging Examples, Entrenched Barriers, and New Thinking." *The Lancet* 385 (9985): 2400–9.

Rodriguez-Blanco, T., A. Vila-Corcoles, C. de Diego, O. Ochoa-Gondar, E. Valdivieso, and others. 2012. "Relationship between Annual Influenza Vaccination and Winter Mortality in Diabetic People over 65 Years." *Human Vaccines and Immunotherapeutics* 8 (3): 363–70.

Roglic, G., N. Unwin, P. H. Bennett, C. Mathers, J. Tuomilehto, and others. 2005. "The Burden of Mortality Attributable to Diabetes: Realistic Estimates for the Year 2000." *Diabetes Care* 28 (9): 2130–35.

Rosen, A. B., M. B. Hamel, M. C. Weinstein, D. M. Cutler, A. M. Fendrick, and S. Vijan. 2005. "Cost-Effectiveness of Full Medicare Coverage of Angiotensin-Converting Enzyme Inhibitors for Beneficiaries with Diabetes." *Annals of Internal Medicine* 143 (2): 89–99.

Saaristo, T., L. Moilanen, E. Korpi-Hyövälti, M. Vanhala, J. Saltevo, and others. 2010. "Lifestyle Intervention for Prevention of Type 2 Diabetes in Primary Health Care: One-Year Follow-Up of the Finnish National Diabetes Prevention Program (FIN-D2D)." *Diabetes Care* 33 (10): 2146–51.

Sarol, J., Jr., N. Nicodemus, K. Tan, and M. Grava. 2005. "Self-Monitoring of Blood Glucose as Part of a Multi-Component Therapy among Non-Insulin Requiring Type 2 Diabetes Patients: A Meta-Analysis (1966–2004)." *Current Medical Research and Opinion* 21 (2): 173–83.

Sathish, T., E. D. Williams, N. Pasricha, P. Absetz, P. Lorgelly, and others. 2013. "Cluster Randomised Controlled Trial of a Peer-Led Lifestyle Intervention Program: Study Protocol for the Kerala Diabetes Prevention Program." *BMC Public Health* 13: 1035.

Schaufler, T. M., and M. Wolff. 2010. "Cost-Effectiveness of Preventive Screening Programmes for Type 2 Diabetes Mellitus in Germany." *Applied Health Economics and Health Policy* 8 (3): 191–202.

Segal, L., A. C. Dalton, and J. Richardson. 1998. "Cost-Effectiveness of the Primary Prevention of Non-Insulin Dependent Diabetes Mellitus." *Health Promotion International* 13 (3): 197–210.

Selph, S., T. Dana, I. Blazina, C. Bougatsos, H. Patel, and R. Chou. 2015. "Screening for Type 2 Diabetes Mellitus: A Systematic Review for the U.S. Preventive Services Task Force Screening for Type 2 Diabetes Mellitus." *Annals of Internal Medicine* 162 (11): 765–76.

Shearer, A., A. Bagust, D. Sanderson, S. Heller, and S. Roberts. 2004. "Cost-Effectiveness of Flexible Intensive Insulin Management to Enable Dietary Freedom in People with Type 1 Diabetes in the UK." *Diabetic Medicine* 21 (5): 460–67.

Shivashankar, R., K. Kirk, W. C. Kim, C. Rouse, N. Tandon, and others. 2015. "Quality of Diabetes Care in Low- and Middle-Income Asian and Middle Eastern Countries (1993–2012): 20-Year Systematic Review." *Diabetes Research and Clinical Practice* 107 (2): 203–23.

Sobngwi, E., M. Ndour-Mbaye, K. A. Boateng, K. L. Ramaiya, E. W. Njenga, and others. 2012. "Type 2 Diabetes Control and Complications in Specialised Diabetes Care Centres of Six Sub-Saharan African Countries: The Diabcare Africa Study." *Diabetes Research and Clinical Practice* 95 (1): 30–36.

Souchet, T., I. Durand Zaleski, T. Hannedouche, M. Rodier, S. Gaugris, and others. 2003. "An Economic Evaluation of Losartan Therapy in Type 2 Diabetic Patients with Nephropathy: An Analysis of the RENAAL Study Adapted to France." *Diabetes and Metabolism* 29 (1): 29–35.

Soumerai, S. B., D. Starr, and S. R. Majumdar. 2015. "How Do You Know Which Health Care Effectiveness Research You Can Trust? A Guide to Study Design for the Perplexed." *Preventing Chronic Diseases* 12: E101.

Stellefson, M., K. Dipnarine, and C. Stopka. 2013. "The Chronic Care Model and Diabetes Management in U.S. Primary Care Settings: A Systematic Review." *Preventing Chronic Diseases* 10: E26.

Stone, M. A., G. Charpentier, K. Doggen, O. Kuss, U. Lindblad, and others. 2013. "Quality of Care of People with Type 2 Diabetes in Eight European Countries: Findings from the Guideline Adherence to Enhance Care (GUIDANCE) Study." *Diabetes Care* 36 (9): 2628–38.

Stumvoll, M., B. J. Goldstein, and T. W. van Haeften. 2005. "Type 2 Diabetes: Principles of Pathogenesis and Therapy." *The Lancet* 365 (9467): 1333–46.

Suto, S., T. Hiraoka, Y. Okamoto, F. Okamoto, and T. Oshika. 2014. "Photography of Anterior Eye Segment and Fundus with Smartphone." *Nippon Ganka Gakkai Zasshi* 118 (1): 7–14.

Szucs, T. D., M. S. Sandoz, and G. W. Keusch. 2004. "The Cost-Effectiveness of Losartan in Type 2 Diabetics with Nephropathy in Switzerland: An Analysis of the RENAAL Study." *Swiss Medical Weekly* 134 (31–32): 440–47.

Tandon, N., M. K. Ali, and K. M. Narayan. 2012. "Pharmacologic Prevention of Microvascular and Macrovascular Complications in Diabetes Mellitus: Implications of the Results of Recent Clinical Trials in Type 2 Diabetes." *American Journal of Cardiovascular Drugs* 12 (1): 7–22.

Tricco, A. C., N. M. Ivers, J. M. Grimshaw, D. Moher, L. Turner, and others. 2012. "Effectiveness of Quality Improvement Strategies on the Management of Diabetes: A Systematic Review and Meta-Analysis." *The Lancet* 379 (9833): 2252–61.

Tulley, S., A. Foster, M. van Putten, V. Urbancic-Rovan, and K. Bakker. 2009. "Diabetic Foot Care Training in Developing Countries: Addressing the Skills Shortage." *Diabetic Foot Journal* 12 (1): 14–22.

Tunceli, K., C. J. Bradley, J. E. Lafata, M. Pladevall, G. W. Divine, and others. 2007. "Glycemic Control and Absenteeism among Individuals with Diabetes." *Diabetes Care* 30 (5): 1283–85.

Tung, T. H., H. C. Shih, S. J. Chen, P. Chou, C. M. Liu, and J. H. Liu. 2008. "Economic Evaluation of Screening for Diabetic Retinopathy among Chinese Type 2 Diabetics: A Community-Based Study in Kinmen, Taiwan." *Journal of Epidemiology* 18 (5): 225–33.

Tunis, S. L. 2011. "Cost Effectiveness of Self-Monitoring of Blood Glucose (SMBG) for Patients with Type 2 Diabetes and Not on Insulin: Impact of Modelling Assumptions on Recent Canadian Findings." *Applied Health Economics and Health Policy* 9 (6): 351–65.

Tunis, S. L., and M. E. Minshall. 2008. "Self-Monitoring of Blood Glucose in Type 2 Diabetes: Cost-Effectiveness in the United States." *American Journal of Managed Care* 14 (3): 131–40.

Tuomilehto, J., J. Lindström, J. G. Eriksson, T. T. Valle, H. Hämäläinen, and others. 2001. "Prevention of Type 2 Diabetes Mellitus by Changes in Lifestyle among Subjects with Impaired Glucose Tolerance." *New England Journal of Medicine* 344 (18): 1343–50.

Turnbull, F., B. Neal, C. Algert, J. Chalmers, N. Chapman, and others. 2005. "Effects of Different Blood Pressure-Lowering Regimens on Major Cardiovascular Events in Individuals with and without Diabetes Mellitus: Results of Prospectively Designed Overviews of Randomized Trials." *Archives of Internal Medicine* 165 (12): 1410–19.

UKPDS (United Kingdom Prospective Diabetes Study) Group. 1998a. "Effect of Intensive Blood-Glucose Control with Metformin on Complications in Overweight Patients with Type 2 Diabetes (UKPDS 34)." *The Lancet* 352 (9131): 854–65.

———. 1998b. "Intensive Blood-Glucose Control with Sulphonylureas or Insulin Compared with Conventional Treatment and Risk of Complications in Patients with Type 2 Diabetes (UKPDS 33)." *The Lancet* 352 (9131): 837–53.

Unnikrishnan, R. I., M. Rema, R. Pradeepa, M. Deepa, C. Subramaniam Shanthirani, and others. 2007. "Prevalence and Risk Factors of Diabetic Nephropathy in an Urban South Indian Population: The Chennai Urban Rural Epidemiology Study (CURES 45)." *Diabetes Care* 30 (8): 2019–24.

U.S. Preventive Services Task Force. 2014. "Screening for Gestational Diabetes Mellitus: U.S. Preventive Services Task Force Recommendation Statement." *Annals of Internal Medicine* 160 (6): 414–20.

van Wier, M. F., J. Lakerveld, S. D. M. Bot, M. J. M. Chinapaw, G. Nijpels, and M. W. van Tulder. 2013. "Economic Evaluation of a Lifestyle Intervention in Primary Care to Prevent Type 2 Diabetes Mellitus and Cardiovascular Diseases: A Randomized Controlled Trial." *BMC Family Practice* 14 (1): 45.

Vijan, S., T. P. Hofer, and R. A. Hayward. 2000. "Cost-Utility Analysis of Screening Intervals for Diabetic Retinopathy in Patients with Type 2 Diabetes Mellitus." *Journal of the American Medical Association* 283 (7): 889–96.

Vos, T., A. D. Flaxman, M. Naghavi, R. Lozano, C. Michaud, and others. 2012. "Years Lived with Disability (YLDs) for 1160 Sequelae of 289 Diseases and Injuries, 1990–2010: A Systematic Analysis for the Global Burden of Disease Study 2010." *The Lancet* 380 (9859): 2163–96.

Wake, N., A. Hisashige, T. Katayama, H. Kishikawa, Y. Ohkubo, and others. 2000. "Cost-Effectiveness of Intensive Insulin Therapy for Type 2 Diabetes: A 10-Year Follow-Up of the Kumamoto Study." *Diabetes Research and Clinical Practice* 48 (3): 201–10.

Waugh, N., G. Scotland, P. McNamee, M. Gillett, A. Brennan, and others. 2007. "Screening for Type 2 Diabetes: Literature Review and Economic Modelling." *Health Technology Assessment* 11 (17): 1–125.

Weber, M. B., H. Ranjani, G. C. Meyers, V. Mohan, and K. M. V. Narayan. 2012. "A Model of Translational Research for Diabetes Prevention in Low- and Middle-Income Countries: The Diabetes Community Lifestyle Improvement Program (D-CLIP) Trial." *Primary Care Diabetes* 6 (1): 3–9.

Weber, M. B., H. Ranjani, L. R. Staimez, R. M. Anjana, M. K. Ali, and others. 2016. "The Stepwise Approach to Diabetes Prevention: Results from the D-CLIP Randomized Controlled Trial." *Diabetes Care* 39 (10): 1760–67. doi: 10.2337/dc16-1241.

Werner, E. F., C. M. Pettker, L. Zuckerwise, M. Reel, E. F. Funai, and others. 2012. "Screening for Gestational Diabetes Mellitus: Are the Criteria Proposed by the International Association of the Diabetes and Pregnancy Study Groups Cost-Effective?" *Diabetes Care* 35 (3): 529–35.

Wilson, J. G. M., and G. Jungner. 1968. *Principles and Practice of Screening for Disease.* Geneva: World Health Organization.

Wing, R. R. 2010. "Long-Term Effects of a Lifestyle Intervention on Weight and Cardiovascular Risk Factors in Individuals with Type 2 Diabetes Mellitus: Four-Year Results of the Look AHEAD Trial." *Archives of Internal Medicine* 170 (17): 1566–75.

World Health Organization. 2014. "Global Health Estimates 2014 Summary Tables: DALY by Cause, Age and Sex, 2000–2012." WHO, Geneva. http://www.who.int/healthinfo/global_burden_disease/en.

Yang, W., J. Lu, J. Weng, W. Jia, L. Ji, and others. 2010. "Prevalence of Diabetes among Men and Women in China." *New England Journal of Medicine* 362 (12): 1090–101.

Zabetian, A., H. M. Keli, J. B. Echouffo-Tcheugui, K. M. Narayan, and M. K. Ali. 2013. "Diabetes in the Middle East and North Africa." *Diabetes Research and Clinical Practice* 101 (2): 106–22.

Zhang, X., K. McKeever Bullard, E. W. Gregg, G. L. Beckles, D. E. Williams, and others. 2012. "Access to Health Care and Control of ABCs of Diabetes." *Diabetes Care* 35 (7): 1566–71.

Zimmet, P. 2009. "Preventing Diabetic Complications: A Primary Care Perspective." *Diabetes Research and Clinical Practice* 84 (2): 107–16.

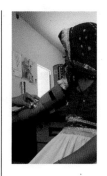

Chapter 13

Kidney Disease

Shuchi Anand, Bernadette Thomas, Giuseppe Remuzzi,
Miguel Riella, Meguid El Nahas, Saraladevi Naicker, and
John Dirks

INTRODUCTION

Deterioration in kidney function, whether acute or chronic, can lead to substantial morbidity and mortality. Acute kidney injury (AKI) is a powerful indicator for in-hospital mortality; those who survive face increased length and cost of hospitalization. Some individuals with chronic kidney disease (CKD) develop progressive renal dysfunction and require costly therapy with dialysis, transplant, or both. Even more often, individuals with CKD face high risks for cardiovascular events, anemia, and fractures.

This chapter reviews current data on the epidemiology and trends in the etiology of AKI, CKD, and end-stage renal disease (ESRD), with a focus on low- and middle-income countries (LMICs). We also review management of these conditions, highlighting several interventions—treatment for AKI, screening for CKD, and modality choice for ESRD—with available data on cost or cost-effectiveness.

ACUTE KIDNEY INJURY

The Condition

Incidence

AKI occurs commonly, although quantifying its exact burden has been challenging. Before 2004, no standardized definition existed. Symptoms do not occur unless severe disease develops. The causes vary widely according to setting—whether AKI is acquired in hospitals or in communities—and establishing practice patterns for

screening is difficult. Community-based studies of prevalence illustrate the wide variation in estimates of AKI that are subject to definition and population; studies report annual incidence rates ranging from 22 to 175 per million population (Himmelfarb and Ikizler 2007).

In the mid-2000s, however, the nephrology community began to establish standardized criteria for a case definition of AKI, and evidence indicates that an increasing number of epidemiology reports rely on this definition (Mehta and others 2015). First released in 2004 (Bellomo and others 2004) and updated in 2007 (Mehta and others 2007) and 2012 (Palevsky and others 2013), these definitions emphasize recognizing early signs of kidney injury, with attention to relatively small changes from baseline serum creatinine or expected urine output—since even these small changes are linked with a substantially increased risk for in-hospital mortality (annex 13A) (Chertow and others 2005).

Standardizing 130 studies to the Kidney Disease: Improving Global Outcomes definition of AKI, an extensive global meta-analysis estimates that one in four adults and one in three children throughout the world suffer from AKI during hospitalized care; about 10 percent of these patients develop AKI severe enough to require dialysis (Hoste and Schurgers 2008; Mehta and others 2015; Susantitaphong and others 2013). The overall AKI incidence rate among adults and children was 23.2 percent (95 percent confidence interval [CI] 21.0 to 25.7 percent), with the highest incidence

Corresponding author: John Dirks, Gairdner Foundation, Toronto, Ontario, Canada; john.dirks@gairdner.org. Shuchi Anand and Bernadette Thomas contributed equally to the work.

rate of 31.7 percent occurring in the critical care setting (95 percent CI 28.6 to 35.0 percent). The severe AKI incidence rate was 2.3 percent. Data available on the incidence rate of community-acquired AKI—that is, patients presenting to the hospital after developing symptoms of kidney dysfunction, rather than presenting with a systemic illness that during its treatment course is associated with AKI (hospital-acquired AKI)—were scarce (only seven studies reported this data); however, the rate was relatively lower than that of hospital-acquired AKI at 8.3 percent (95 percent CI 1.6 to 33.0 percent) (Susantitaphong and others 2013).

This analysis also includes only two studies from LMICs. However, a recent update capturing more data from Africa, Asia, and Latin America reports incidence of AKI in these regions comparable to that in high-income countries (HICs) (Mehta and others 2015).

Mortality

Mortality from AKI in HICs has traditionally been reported to be higher than in LMICs, but a recent report indicates that, at least among patients with severe AKI requiring dialysis, mortality rates in LMICs are equivalent or higher (Bouchard and others 2015). A prospective study

of AKI in patients hospitalized in intensive care units collected data from three middle-income countries (MICs), Brazil, China, and India; findings indicate that patients in MICs experienced twofold higher odds of mortality and nonrecovery of renal function, despite having lower severity of illness, compared with patients in HICs (Bouchard and others 2015). Single-center studies from LMICs have reported large variation in mortality from AKI requiring dialysis, likely reflecting not only the lack of equipment but also variable levels of expertise (table 13.1).

Etiology

Although rigorous registry data are lacking, experts suggest that the incidence of community-acquired AKI is higher in LMICs than in HICs. Severe systemic diseases, such as sepsis or major surgical procedures, cause the majority of cases of AKI in HICs and in urban areas of LMICs. Some community-acquired reasons for AKI are more common in LMICs: obstetric complications; toxins, including snake venom; diarrheal illness; advanced human immunodeficiency virus/acquired immune deficiency syndrome (HIV/AIDS); leptospirosis; and malaria.

In Africa, nephrologists report that major causes of AKI are related to the burden of HIV/AIDS, malaria,

Table 13.1 Selected Studies with Mortality Estimates for Acute Kidney Injury

Study	Study population	Overall mortality (percent of patients with AKI)	Mortality for AKI cases receiving dialysis (percent)
Low- and middle-income countries			
Susantitaphong and others 2013	Pooled global mortality rate	8.0–22.6[a]	—
Mishra and others 2012	Children receiving PD	—	36.8
Ademola and others 2012	Children receiving PD	—	30.0
Bagasha and others 2015	Patients with sepsis at a Ugandan teaching hospital	21	100
Ponce and others 2012	Patients receiving PD for AKI	—	57.3
Trang and others 1992	Patients receiving PD for AKI	—	26.0
Kilonzo and others 2012	PD for AKI in children (20 percent) and adults (80 percent)	—	20.0
Mehta and others 2016	Pooled global mortality rate from community- and hospital-acquired AKI, seven-day mortality	11.5[b]	17.0[b]
High-income countries			
Susantitaphong and others 2013	Pooled global mortality rate	20.9	49.4[c]
Waikar and others 2006	In-hospital mortality, 1998–2002	20.3	28.1
Talabani and others 2014	Community-acquired AKI, three-month mortality	16.5	—

Note: AKI = acute kidney injury; — = not available; PD = peritoneal dialysis.
a. Represents one study from low-income countries and one from low- and middle-income countries.
b. From 1,153 AKI patients from low- and lower-middle-income countries.
c. Of the 31 studies pooled for this estimate, 2 were from low- and middle-income countries.

leptospirosis, and diarrheal diseases (Lameire and others 2013; Naicker, Aboud, and Gharbi 2008; Prakash and others 2015). More than 50 percent of adults with advanced HIV/AIDS or severe malaria develop AKI (Lameire and others 2013). Noninfectious causes specific to LMICs include obstetric and surgical complications, such as severe hemorrhage or late diagnosis of eclampsia, as well as widespread use of traditional herbal remedies or nonsteroidal anti-inflammatory agents (Luyckx and Naicker 2008; Naicker, Aboud, and Gharbi 2008). Such community-acquired AKI more likely afflicts a younger age group and, especially in cases of malaria or diarrheal illness, exhibits seasonal peaks during rainy seasons (Cerda and others 2008; Lameire and others 2013).

Effectiveness of Interventions

AKI management largely depends on etiology and severity. Treatment algorithms in HICs recommend optimizing volume using crystalloid solutions until clinical dehydration is corrected followed by vasopressor support to maintain perfusion pressure (Kellum, Lameire, and KDIGO AKI Guideline Work Group 2013). In conjunction with this approach, treatment of the underlying cause of AKI, such as antibiotics for infection and avoidance of nephrotoxic medications or procedures, often leads to resolution of mild-to-moderate AKI. In HICs, availability of intensive care units, adequate nursing staffing, and rapid-turnaround laboratory facilities allow for frequent and close monitoring of urine output and serum creatinine. Relatively prompt interventions to ameliorate AKI are performed. If AKI progresses to severe renal failure despite these measures, temporary dialysis may be initiated, either to treat volume and electrolyte imbalances or to remove toxins. Continuous hemodiafiltration and intermittent hemodialysis (HD) are the modalities of choice in HICs, although a meta-analysis highlights equivalent survival in patients receiving peritoneal dialysis (PD) versus HD or continuous hemodiafiltration (Chionh and others 2013).

This level of care is not available in most LMICs. The limitations of diagnosis and treatment for advanced AKI are particularly stark in rural areas, but they are also demonstrated in urban university-based hospitals (Bouchard and others 2015; Cerda and others 2008). Data on missed or delayed diagnosis of AKI in LMICs are nonexistent; by their nature, reports on epidemiology of AKI must apply screening criteria that may not be used in standard practice in LMICs. However, studies have confirmed not only a lack of provision of dialysis or transplant but also a lack of intensive care units as crucial gaps in care (Bagasha and others 2015); the infrastructure and budget required to develop renal replacement therapy (RRT) programs to support AKI are often lower priorities in LMICs still struggling with other pressing public health issues, such as infectious diseases, maternal and perinatal health, and nutrition management (Mushi, Marschall, and Flessa 2015). To address such gaps, the International Society of Nephrology has developed an initiative called "0by25." The objective of the initiative is to eliminate preventable deaths from AKI by 2025 by calling for global strategies that permit timely diagnosis and treatment (including dialysis) of potentially reversible AKI, with particular emphasis on LMICs (Mehta and others 2015; Remuzzi and Horton 2013) (see box 13.1 for an example of a dialysis provision program in AKI in LMICs).

Box 13.1

Case Study: Acute Kidney Injury (AKI) Treatment with Peritoneal Dialysis (PD) in Tanzania

An AKI treatment program started in 2007 at Kilimanjaro Christian Medical Centre in Tanzania is a leading example of renal replacement therapy provision for AKI in a low-income country (Burki 2015). The program uses PD.

The program was developed with support from the International Society of Nephrology and the Sustainable Kidney Foundation, which funded training in Brazil for physicians and nurses from Tanzania for PD catheter insertion technique and prescription (Callegari and others 2012; Callegari and others 2013; Kilonzo and others 2012). In a report on the program, directed by Dr. Karen Yeates of Queen's University, Canada, PD was successfully administered to 32 Tanzanian patients with AKI (Burki 2015). The AKI treatment costs were low: approximately US$150–US$400 for the duration of in-hospital treatment, ensuring sustainability once the center assumes total program management.

One of the major lessons has been that nephrologists are not essential for the successful development of such programs. Skilled internists and nurses willing to be trained in PD delivery can achieve satisfactory results (Burki 2015).

Cost and Cost-Effectiveness of Interventions

AKI-related health expenditures reflect costs associated with RRT as well as prolonged hospital stay and increased complexity of care once kidney function has been compromised during illness course, even if compromise of renal function is modest (Chertow and others 2005; Rewa and Bagshaw 2014):

- Prolonged hospitalization
- Intensive care unit services
- Dialysis
- Increased monitoring and intervention
- Increased risk of rehospitalization.

The cost-effectiveness of dialysis provision depends largely on the posthospitalization survival of patients. The SUPPORT study assessed the cost-effectiveness of initiating dialysis in seriously ill hospitalized patients in the United States. Only 27 percent of patients survived after six months; the cost per quality-adjusted life year (QALY) gained was calculated to be US$128,200 (Hamel and others 1997). A study in Finland to assess the cost utility of acute RRT from the societal perspective reported the intervention to be cost-effective only if survival exceeded a year—which occurred only in 43 percent of enrolled patients. Among the first year survivors, mortality was 20 percent over the remaining four years (Laukkanen and others 2013). The study involved a five-year follow-up of patients who received acute RRT in a largely intensive-care-unit-based setting.

Because the demographics of AKI in LMICs skew toward a younger population with lower illness severity, it is likely that the benefits of dialysis provision are greater in LMICs (Anand, Cruz, and Finkelstein 2015; Bouchard and others 2015). However, few cost data are available. One report from Tanzania finds that the cost of one life saved using acute PD was US$370 (Cullis and others 2014). George and others (2011) report that the equipment and solution costs of PD were 3,009 rupees (Rs; US$47), approximately 40 percent of continuous HD filtration costs (Rs 7,184 [US$112]), with equivalent survival.

Recommendations for Policy Makers in LMICs

Although the current understanding of AKI in LMICs is limited, the nephrology community generally agrees on the following (Mehta and others 2015):

- Known incidence is similar to that in HICs.
- Community-acquired causes are more common than in HICs.
- Affected patients are younger than in HICs.
- Lack of intensive care units and access to acute dialysis results in high mortality rates.

This consensus is largely drawn from expert opinions or single-center studies; additional studies are required to estimate the burden, etiology, and mortality of AKI in LMICs.

Based on current consensus, however, the prevention of community-acquired AKI (table 13.2) may play a more crucial role in LMICs. Management algorithms that take the most common region-specific causes into account are crucial in areas with limited staffing of trained physicians. When the need for dialysis arises,

Table 13.2 Prevention and Management of Acute Kidney Injury in LMICs

Recommended intervention	Potential benefit
Prevention or management at the community level	
Improve access to, and quality of, drinking water and sanitation	Prevent AKI related to diarrheal illness, kidney stones, and volume depletion in strenuous working conditions
Educate health care workers, pharmacists, and general populations about nephrotoxic medications and herbs	Reduce AKI related to heavy NSAID, illegal alcohol, or herbal toxin use
Involve local health care workers in the identification of patients at risk of AKI	Prevent or limit exposure to environmental risk factors for AKI, such as parasites, infection-carrying vectors, and obstetric complications
Educate and train nonphysicians, such as nurses or clinical officers, or non–health professionals to locally manage AKI, especially with telemedicine support	Limit the progression of AKI to more severe stages that require dialysis

table continues next page

Table 13.2 Prevention and Management of Acute Kidney Injury in LMICs (continued)

Recommended intervention	Potential benefit
Prevention or management at the hospital level	
Improve perinatal care at first-level hospitals	Reduce AKI related to peripartum hemorrhage or preeclampsia
Enhance region-specific understanding of common causes of AKI at first- and second-level hospitals	Provide rapid treatment of underlying causes of AKI
Implement protocols for intensive or intermediate care at first- and second-level hospitals	Resolve mild-to-moderate AKI via rapid fluid resuscitation, vasopressor support, and antibiotic administration
Provide training in PD provision for AKI at second-level hospitals	Treat severe AKI by training non-nephrology physicians in PD catheter insertion and prescription; enable wider availability of dialysis for severe AKI
Create referral centers for provision of intermittent or continuous HD for patients in whom PD is contraindicated	Select individuals with severe AKI who need specialized care, and efficiently allocate resources for dialysis

Note: AKI = acute kidney injury; HD = hemodialysis; LMICs = low- and middle-income countries; NSAIDs = nonsteroidal anti-inflammatory drugs; PD = peritoneal dialysis.

temporary PD—a less technologically demanding and less costly modality—can be used for both pediatric and adult acute cases. The International Society of Peritoneal Dialysis has published guidelines to standardize the provision of acute PD (Cullis and others 2014). Successful programmatic implementation of PD—training staff, acquiring dialysis equipment, and prescribing dialysis appropriately—has occurred in third-level centers in Benin, Cambodia, Ghana, Sudan, and Tanzania (Finkelstein and others 2014; Wilkie 2014). However, the challenges of scalability and managing patients who do not recover renal function and require long-term dialysis remain (Kilonzo and others 2012).

CHRONIC KIDNEY DISEASE AND END-STAGE RENAL DISEASE

The Condition

Epidemiology of CKD

CKD is diagnosed when an individual has evidence of persistent kidney dysfunction, as reflected by albuminuria, reduction in estimated glomerular filtration rate (eGFR), or both. Identifying individuals with CKD arguably facilitates treatment to reduce cardiovascular events and slow the progression to ESRD (Levey and Coresh 2012).

However, guidelines for streamlining CKD diagnosis have generated controversy because of their reliance on the glomerular filtration rate (GFR) (annex 13B) (Kidney Disease: Improving Global Outcomes Work Group 2012; Levey and others 2003). Older adults who have isolated modest eGFR reductions may have kidney function at the lower end of the normal-for-age range (Wetzels and others 2007), creating the potential for false positives and overutilization of medical resources (Moynihan, Glassock, and Doust 2013; Poggio and Rule 2009). Most cross-sectionally obtained prevalence estimates fail to fulfill the criteria of repeating assessment at three months to determine persistence (Plata and others 1998). Finally, interpretation of albuminuria requires caution in LMICs, where hygiene, malnutrition, and dietary habits may affect urinary excretion of albumin and creatinine.

With these caveats in mind, we make the following interpretation from available population-based prevalence studies (annex 13C):

- CKD prevalence is understudied in LMICs.
- CKD prevalence in LMICs approaches that of HICs.
- Earlier stages of CKD—albuminuria alone—are common in LMICs, unlike HICs, where modest eGFR reductions with or without albuminuria (CKD stage 3) predominate.

At the same time, individuals with CKD in LMICs remain at high risk of adverse events. Notably, albuminuria has been associated with a linear and sizable increase in risk for all-cause mortality and cardiovascular events, starting at urine albumin-to-creatinine ratios above 10 milligrams/gram (Chronic Kidney Disease Prognosis Consortium and others 2010). Risk for ESRD is 4–11 times higher among individuals with albuminuria (Chronic Kidney Disease Prognosis Consortium and others 2010).

Epidemiology of ESRD

ESRD is rare. About 2 million people are undergoing RRT (either dialysis or kidney transplant) worldwide, with a prevalence of 300 per million adult population or 0.03 percent, compared with prevalence estimates in the range of 7 percent to 15 percent for earlier stages of CKD (Anand, Bitton, and Gaziano 2013; Grassman and others 2005; Thomas and others 2015). While the number of people on RRT has nearly doubled since 1990, 80 percent of the individuals receiving RRT live in HICs (Grassmann and others 2005). The latest Global Burden of Disease estimates from the World Health Organization note that 1.8 percent and 1.1 percent to 1.8 percent of deaths in HICs and LMICs, respectively, are attributable to kidney disease; the cause of death is presumably complications of ESRD.

Currently available data only capture information on patients who have access to RRT, not all those who develop ESRD. In HICs, these numbers are roughly equal because most patients who develop ESRD are diagnosed and offered therapy. In LMICs, however, RRT incidence is not a proxy for ESRD incidence, because individuals may die before or immediately after diagnosis, or they may withdraw from therapy because they cannot pay for it (Couser and others 2011).

Two analyses comparing RRT use with projected ESRD prevalence highlight a large disparity (Anand, Bitton, and Gaziano 2013; Liyanage and others 2015); fewer than 5 percent of patients projected to have ESRD actually access therapy in China, India, and Nigeria (Anand, Bitton, and Gaziano 2013). The provision of RRT closely tracks a country's gross national product rather than the prevalence of risk factors.

Trends in Prevalence and Etiology of CKD and ESRD

Despite concerns about accurate diagnosis, most experts agree that CKD is a growing concern worldwide because of the skyrocketing prevalence of its major correlates: diabetes and hypertension. As noted in chapter 2 in this volume (Ajay, Watkins, and Prabhakaran 2017), LMICs are projected to experience the largest percentage increases in the prevalence of diabetes and hypertension (Hossain, Kawar, and El Nahas 2007). Individuals in LMICs are more likely to develop end-organ damage, including progressive CKD, because of delayed diagnosis and poor management of diabetes and hypertension. In a study of individuals with diabetes in Cambodia, more than 50 percent had CKD (Thomas and others 2014), compared with about one-third in the United States (de Boer and others 2011). Not surprisingly, these diseases are an increasingly common cause of ESRD in LMICs. In 2011, 28 percent of cases of ESRD in Brazil were attributed to diabetes, compared with 8 percent in the mid-1990s; 35 percent were attributed to hypertension, compared with 15 percent in 2002 (Oliveira, Romao, and Zatz 2005; Sesso Rde and others 2012).

Although the prevalence of CKD and ESRD related to diabetes and hypertension will increase across the world, HIV nephropathy—a disease of untreated HIV/AIDS resulting in proteinuric kidney disease—will potentially decline. As more individuals with HIV/AIDS have received treatment with antiretroviral drugs, CKD related to side effects of antiretrovirals, comorbid diabetes, or hypertension has already become more common in HICs, a trend that LMICs may follow (Mallipattu, Salem, and Wyatt 2014).

However, kidney diseases related to other infectious diseases—malaria, hepatitis B or C, leptospirosis, and dengue—continue to disproportionately affect individuals in LMICs (Soderland and others 2010). Unusual causes of CKD, including stones and environmental toxins, are also concentrated in LMICs. Stone-related kidney disease is relatively more important in certain regions. In HICs, 3 percent of cases of ESRD are attributed to obstructive uropathy (Jungers and others 2004); in countries along the "stone belt" (a region encompassing North Africa and South and Southeast Asia), up to 6 percent to 11 percent of cases of ESRD are attributed to obstructive uropathy (Jha 2009). Hot climates that predispose individuals to volume depletion or low urine output, low potassium diets, and chewing of calcium hydroxide containing betel leaf all increase the risk for stone formation (Lopez and Hoppe 2010). Limited access to treatment increases the risk for CKD and ESRD.

Individuals in LMICs may experience higher risk for CKD related to environmental toxins, such as lead, arsenic, cadmium, and aristolochic acid. Public health experts from Sri Lanka and the west coast of Central America report that scores of agricultural workers are being diagnosed with CKD unaccompanied by diabetes or hypertension (box 13.2) As yet, there are many unknowns about this phenomenon, including whether the same disease entity is afflicting workers in both regions, and whether strenuous work in high heat may be a major contributing factor.

In summary, while the majority of cases of CKD in both HICs and LMICs is likely to be associated with diabetes or vascular disease, kidney disease from rarer etiologies—from HIV/AIDS to environmental toxins—is much more likely to occur in LMICs than in HICs. It is increasingly apparent that CKD in LMICs is a multifactorial condition caused by interacting factors such as poverty and social deprivation, poor sanitation and hygiene, exposure to water- and food-borne toxins, pollution, and infectious diseases. Accordingly, the epidemiology and treatment of CKD

Case Study: Investigating Kidney Disease in Farm Workers

Since the early 2000s a form of chronic disease unaccompanied by diabetes or significant hypertension has been reported primarily in rice paddy farmers in the dry zone of Sri Lanka (Chandrajith and others 2011) and sugarcane workers in the lowlands of Nicaragua and El Salvador (Weiner and others 2013). Estimates of mortality are high. In 2009, kidney disease was the second-largest cause of death among men in El Salvador (Wesseling and others 2013). Some distinguishing features of the disease have been described: it afflicts middle-age men more than women, lacks heavy proteinuria, and tends to progress to end-stage renal disease. On kidney biopsy, pathologists note tubulointerstitial nephritis (Nanayakkara and others 2012; Wijkstrom and others 2013).

A rural lowland community in Nicaragua is referred to as "La Isla de las Viudas" (the Island of Widows) because of the high rates of death among men in the village from renal failure. One of the nongovernmental organizations working to address this problem, La Isla Foundation, is based in this region. La Isla Foundation has extended its efforts beyond activism to generate media attention and to support collaborative research in the field. In addition, scientists from a variety of institutions, including Boston University, the National Autonomous University of Nicaragua at León, and the University of Colorado at Denver, are investigating potential triggers for kidney disease. The Consortium for the Epidemic of Nephropathy in Central America and Mexico has been formed to help researchers communicate and coordinate.

One prevailing hypothesis for the cause of this epidemic is recurrent dehydration resulting from strenuous work in high heat conditions (Roncal Jimenez and others 2013). However, there is widespread belief among local populations in Meso-America and in Sri Lanka that exposure to agrochemicals is at least partly responsible for the occupational nature of this form of CKD (Jayasumana and others 2015). An as-yet undefined infection also remains an important consideration (Murray and others 2015).

Most of those afflicted by the disease earn their livelihoods from agricultural work; a diagnosis of progressive CKD is disabling for them and their families. There is little to no provision of dialysis therapy in these regions, lending great urgency to identifying an etiology and preventing the disease.

---

should be studied in LMICs as an entity separate from the end-organ consequence of diabetes or vascular disease.

Effectiveness of Interventions

Screening for CKD

Major primary care and nephrology guidelines in HICs do not advocate universal screening for CKD. The National Kidney Foundation Kidney Disease Outcomes Quality Initiative recommends first evaluating individuals for risk factors for CKD during routine clinical encounters; if risk is determined, individuals should be further evaluated for serum creatinine and urine abnormalities. The risk factors include age; diabetes; hypertension; autoimmune disease, such as lupus; urinary tract abnormalities, such as infections, stones, and neoplasia; low birth weight; and exposure to toxins, such as drugs, environmental agents, or infections.

In practice, physicians target screening to individuals with diabetes or hypertension. Because serum creatinine and automated reporting of eGFR are often part of routine studies in primary care, even individuals without specific risk factors for CKD are recognized at an early stage (Wyatt and others 2007).

The adoption of a targeted screening strategy in LMICs needs to be reassessed, given the lack of self-awareness of underlying risk factors for CKD. For example, in a community-based sample from urban India, individuals with and without knowledge of diabetes had similar prevalence of CKD (Anand and others 2015). Accordingly, selecting high-risk individuals for CKD screening may not be feasible.

Prevention of ESRD

Pharmacotherapy for CKD associated with diabetes or hypertension. Nephrologists use angiotensin-converting enzyme (ACE) inhibitors and angiotensin II receptor blockers (ARBs) as the primary medical therapies for delaying the progression to ESRD. Data from several randomized clinical trials have shown that these medications can slow the progression of CKD among individuals with proteinuric (diabetic and nondiabetic) kidney disease, with risk reduction approaching 40 percent for a composite endpoint of doubling of serum creatinine or ESRD (Kshirsagar and others 2000). A trial in China replicated these findings for individuals with proteinuria and advanced renal disease (Hou and others 2006). Some evidence indicates that even among individuals with CKD and hypertension without significant proteinuria, the use of ACE inhibitors may delay the progression of CKD beyond the effects achieved by other standard antihypertensive agents (Wright and others 2002). Whether the effect of ACE inhibitors is totally independent of improved blood pressure control has been debated. These medications, which are relatively inexpensive in their generic form, are well tolerated but require laboratory monitoring for hyperkalemia or significant change in serum creatinine among older patients and those with advanced CKD because of associated risk for AKI.

Pharmacotherapy for glomerular diseases. CKD associated with diabetes or renovascular disease is often diagnosed only with screening. Individuals with glomerulonephritis, in contrast, often have classic symptoms, such as edema, hematuria, or arthralgias, and are referred to nephrologists for immunotherapy. Steroids are the initial choice of therapy for many glomerular processes: minimal change disease, membranous nephropathy, focal segmental glomerulonephritis, and IgA nephropathy. Newer steroid-sparing therapies, such as calcineurin inhibitors, are used in individuals at serious risk for adverse events related to steroids or for maintenance therapy. Cyclophosphamide had been the mainstay of therapy for severe glomerulonephritis resulting from lupus or vasculitis. Mycophenolate mofetil (Ginzler and others 2005) and rituximab (Stone and others 2010) have been shown to be equally efficacious in treating severe glomerulonephritis resulting from lupus or vasculitis, respectively.

Race or ethnicity may affect the efficacy of immunotherapy. African-American and Hispanic individuals with lupus reportedly respond better to mycophenolate mofetil than to cyclophosphamide (Isenberg and others 2010). Initial clinical trials from China report the efficacy of mycophenolate mofetil in individuals with IgA nephropathy, but these results have not been replicated in clinical trials in Belgium and the United States (Floege and Eitner 2011).

Data on availability and appropriate use of these pharmacotherapies in LMICs are limited. One study from Mexico reports that one-third of primary care physicians working in the public sector scored in the "very low knowledge" category in a competence evaluation of diabetic kidney disease (Martinez-Ramirez and others 2006). Only 50 percent of patients with diabetes underwent simple screening for kidney disease; fewer than 20 percent of patients with proteinuria had been placed on ACE inhibitors in a third-level center in Nigeria (Agaba and others 2009).

CKD-specific programs in LMICs. We conducted a PUBMED and EMBASE systematic search to capture any programs designed specifically to improve care of patients with CKD or ESRD in LMICs. Of the 292 articles captured by the search, we culled 18 with available full text in English for further review; articles were excluded if they were not applicable to LMICs, if they were presented in abstract only at conferences, or if they did not describe a specific intervention. After excluding reports that were too general or did not capture any outcomes, we found 11 studies that described CKD care programs in LMICs (table 13.3). Although the data on evaluation of these programs were of poor to fair quality, an emerging theme in these reports is the importance of education of primary care physicians in identifying and treating patients at risk for CKD progression.

Treatment of ESRD
Survival on dialysis. Survival on dialysis—equivalent for HD and PD—is generally poor in HICs, with annual mortality rates nearing 20 percent to 25 percent (van Dijk and others 2001). Many LMICs report equivalent, if not better, survival on dialysis (Anand, Bitton, and Gaziano 2013). At the same time, several studies have noted poorer provision of long-term care in LMICs: late referral to nephrologists, greater reliance on twice-weekly HD (Bieber and others 2013), less frequent laboratory draws and use of ancillary medications (Bieber and others 2013), and lack of enforcement of standards for water treatment for HD (Braimoh and others 2012). Patient selection factors may explain this incongruity between better survival despite reported poorer quality of care. In South Africa, where government-sponsored dialysis is offered to patients who fulfill the criteria for eventual transplantation, patients older than age 60 years and patients with diabetes are significantly less likely to receive dialysis (Moosa and Kidd 2006). Thus, a rationing process—whether at a societal or familial level—may create artificially better outcomes in LMICs, because a younger, healthier population is most likely to be able to access expensive dialysis therapy; see chapter 21 in this volume (Sakuma and others 2017) for a more detailed discussion.

Survival on transplantation. Compared with dialysis, first-year post–kidney transplant mortality is less than 10 percent in most HICs (van Dijk and others 2001). Better survival after a kidney transplant reflects a combination of selection factors—a healthier group of patients receiving transplants, and greater efficacy of therapy (Wolfe and others 1999). Most individuals in HICs receive cadaveric transplants.

In LMICs, reported outcomes for living donor transplantation are similar to those in HICs (Anand, Bitton, and Gaziano 2013). Cadaveric donation is much less common in LMICs because of the lack of deceased-donor registries; in one center's report, cadaveric donation was associated with poorer outcomes than in HICs (Medina-Pestana 2006). Reasons behind the poorer transplant outcomes in LMICs should be

Table 13.3 Summary of Programs Targeted to Caring for Patients with CKD in LMICs

Authors	Country	Intervention	Level	Outcomes
Mastroianni-Kirsztajn, Bastos, and Burdmann 2011	Brazil	Previna-se: A campaign by the Brazilian Society of Nephrology to increase awareness of CKD among health professionals and the public	National	• In 2009, 700 local programs registered for educational campaigns • Generated pamphlets and videos for PCPs and public • Attempted to standardize reporting of GFR • Undertook several screening campaigns in São Paulo
Zhang and others 2008	China	Established a renal management clinic study at Peking University that incorporated nephrologists, dieticians, and nurses	Third-level hospital	• Challenges in follow-up, with 10 percent of patients with advanced CKD not returning for follow-up • Despite creation of multidisciplinary clinic, lack of involvement of nurses or dieticians
Jiang and Yu 2011	China	Created 12 satellite PD clinics to an academic hospital Used standardized protocols for training staff	Third-level and first-level care partners	• Increased capacity • Decline in peritonitis rate (from 1 episode/39.4 to 1 episode/46.2 patient months) • Fewer patient drop outs, from 28 percent to 18 percent per year
Wong, Chow, and Chan 2010	China	Randomized PD patients to renal and general nephrology nurse follow-up versus usual care (physicians only)	Third-level hospital	• With involvement of nurses, improved diet adherence, symptom control, and quality of life
Mani 2010	India	Developed a protocol for titration of ACEi/ARB among patients with CKD who lived remotely from the specialists; instructions were faxed after patients relayed results of protocol labs	Community	• Among patients who were able to follow the protocol, rate of decline in kidney function was significantly slower • Able to perform titration despite only 6 or 12 months of follow-up from patients
Cortes-Sanabria and others 2008	Mexico	Randomized PCPs to usual care versus six months of CKD education in patients with type 2 diabetes	Primary care	• Improved PCP clinical competence • Better controlled BP and albuminuria, with higher doses of ACEi/ARB used among patients of educated PCPs
Cueto-Manzano, Martinez-Ramirez, and Cortes-Sanabria 2013	Mexico	Prospective study of patients with type 2 diabetes and early CKD assigned to participate in multidisciplinary (educated PCP, dietician, physical therapist, and social worker) versus usual care	Primary care	• Improved medication compliance • Improved BP, hemoglobin A1c, and waist circumference in patients with multidisciplinary care
Garcia-Garcia and others 2013; Murray and others 2015	Mexico	Created a multidisciplinary clinic (nurse, physician, dietician, and social worker) to care for patients without insurance, referred from community or via screening	Third-level hospital	• Compared with baseline intake, patients seen in the clinic improved in several parameters, including in meeting targets for blood pressure and ACEi/ARB use (90 percent)

table continues next page

Table 13.3 Summary of Programs Targeted to Caring for Patients with CKD in LMICs (continued)

Authors	Country	Intervention	Level	Outcomes
Edefonti and others 2010	Nicaragua	Partnership between Milanese and Nicaraguan hospitals to create a pediatric nephrology program	National	• Trained three pediatric nephrologists and two pathologists • Created a network of PCPs in six other regions; these PCPs have access to basic diagnostics and could streamline referral to main hospital • Covers 61 percent of pediatric population
Schwedt and others 2010	Uruguay	A national renal health care program that focused on education of both PCPs and nephrologists, with referral to nephrologists recommended at advanced CKD	National	• Post implementation, patients getting care from PCPs and from nephrologists demonstrated improved BP and lipid control
Sharma and others 2014	Nepal	An intervention program in resource-poor setting of eastern Nepal with cheap antihypertensive, antidiabetic, or renoprotective (ACE) drugs	Rural communities of eastern Nepal	• 76 percent on active monitoring after three-year follow-up • Improved BP and glycemic control • 63 percent of participants with dipstick proteinuria >1+ at baseline decreased to normal values • 48 percent of participants with eGFR <60 ml/min/ 1.73 m² at baseline improved renal function

Note: ACE = angiotensin-converting enzyme; ACEi/ARB = angiotensin-converting enzyme inhibitors/angiotensin II receptor blocker; BP = blood pressure; CKD = chronic kidney disease; eGFR = estimated glomerular filtration rate; GFR = glomerular filtration rate; LMICs = low- and middle-income countries; PCP = primary care physician; PD = peritoneal dialysis.

further studied, especially considering that recipients tend to have fewer comorbidities and are younger. In most LMICs with flourishing transplant centers—such as Brazil, India, the Islamic Republic of Iran, Pakistan, South Africa, and Tunisia—the technical training of surgeons and nephrologists is comparable to that in HICs. However, two factors specific to LMICs may be at play:

• Funding of immunosuppression medication varies; some governments, such as Brazil, pay the full costs; others expect a majority of patients to self-pay. Because immunosuppression medications are expensive, patients might minimize or discontinue use if asked to self-pay.

• Risks for serious posttransplant infection are likely to be higher in LMICs. An estimated 10 percent to 15 percent of individuals with kidney transplants develop tuberculosis in endemic regions (Malhotra 2007; Rizvi and others 2003). Among those who have a co-infection, the mortality rate has been reported to be 75 percent (Chen and others 2008).

Use of modality. Kidney transplant offers the best survival rates and quality of life for individuals with

ESRD when transplantation is performed using optimal practice standards. In HICs, kidney transplants meet the needs of 30 percent to 40 percent of prevalent ESRD patients (Grassmann and others 2005). Advances in patient selection, organ suitability, and organ availability have increased transplantation rates. National and regional organ donation chains can maximize adequate donor-recipient pairing over a large geographical area to ensure maximal chance of transplantation rate and allograft survival (Gentry, Montgomery, and Segev 2011). Recent changes to the deceased-donor system in the United States are anticipated to allocate organs more efficiently.

As in HICs, HD is the most commonly used therapy in LMICs. Transplants are relatively more commonly used in the Middle East and North Africa and in South Asia, compared with other LMIC regions (figure 13.1). In the Islamic Republic of Iran, compensation for organ donation may drive this trend (Ghods and Savaj 2006). PD is relatively more commonly used in Latin America and the Caribbean.

In addition to limits to organ availability, many LMICs struggle with inadequate infrastructure for safe transplantation and postsurgical care (Rizvi and others 2011). Deceased-donor registries do not exist in most countries. Practices such as black market trade and financial compensation are more prevalent and often disproportionally target poorer members of the population as donors (Mendoza 2010).

The preponderance of efficacy data demonstrate equivalent survival for patients on HD compared with PD, but HD predominates as the primary mode of therapy. Approximately 20 percent of patients who receive RRT in HICs receive PD (Anand, Bitton, and Gaziano 2013). Some reasons for this low uptake include skewed provider incentives toward in-center care, lack of patient education about alternate modalities, and patient fear of self-care.

PD, a relatively low-technology technique that requires neither a high ratio of trained nurses and nephrologists nor specialized facilities with water treatment capabilities, can have greater uptake in LMICs. Mexico and Thailand are exceptions to the generally low use of PD. Historically, Mexican clinicians have been trained in PD and disseminated the technique (Riella and Locatelli 2007); internists have been able to prescribe PD (Pecoits-Filho and others 2007). Following the model of Hong Kong SAR, China, the Ministry of Health in Thailand has tied use of PD first (before other interventions) to reimbursement and has supported expansion of PD; see chapter 21 in this volume (Sakuma and others 2017) for a detailed discussion.

Cost and Cost-Effectiveness of Interventions

Screening for CKD

The cost-effectiveness of screening for CKD has been extensively studied in HICs. The accuracy of creatinine-based eGFR alone in predicting outcomes and progression has remained questionable; not surprisingly, its use in the general population resulted in incremental cost-effectiveness ratios (ICERs) exceeding US$100,000 per QALY gained (Komenda and others 2014). Narrowing to the diabetic population, however, the ICER for screening was US$23,680 per QALY gained.

Assessment of proteinuria via urine albumin-to-creatinine ratio is generally considered to be a more reliable test, although Jafar and others (2007) have shown high specificity but moderate sensitivity (46 percent to 60 percent) in an Indo-Asian population. The cost of testing for urine albumin-to-creatinine ratio is significantly higher than that of serum creatinine, but more acceptable ICERs were noted for its application to those ages 50 years and older: US$73,000 per QALY gained if performed annually, to US$22,000 per QALY gained if performed every 10 years, compared with no screening (Hoerger and others 2010). ICERs for individuals with diabetes or hypertension were US$15,000 per

Figure 13.1 Use of Renal Replacement Therapy by Modality

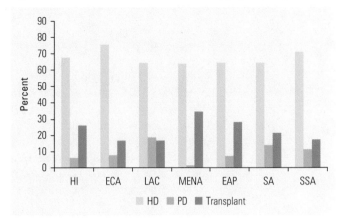

Source: Anand, Bitton, and Gaziano 2013.
Note: EAP = East Asia and Pacific; ECA = Europe and Central Asia; HD = hemodialysis; HI = high income; LAC = Latin America and the Caribbean; MENA = Middle East and North Africa; PD = peritoneal dialysis; SA = South Asia; SSA = Sub-Saharan Africa.

QALY gained if urine albumin-to-creatinine testing is performed every 10 years.

Targeted screening may be the most cost-effective strategy for HICs, but identifying high-risk individuals in LMICs is difficult, and the cost of and utility loss from the development of ESRD is higher, given the restrictions on RRT. Two-stage screening may be a strategy worth investigating (box 13.3). When Howard and others (2010) modeled the use of annual dipstick screening for proteinuria in all Australians ages 50–69 years, followed by confirmatory urine protein-to-creatinine ratio and initiation of treatment, the resulting ICERs were US$5,298 per QALY gained. Similarly, a study of elderly patients at Veterans Administration hospitals in the United States finds that the number needed to treat to prevent a case of ESRD over a three-year period was substantially lower among individuals with dipstick proteinuria, compared with those without proteinuria and modest reductions in eGFR (O'Hare and others 2014).

Renal Replacement Therapy Program and Modality Choice

No recent studies from HICs have evaluated the cost-effectiveness of supporting an individual's decision to pursue RRT rather than palliative care. Most HICs include RRT as part of universal health care packages or government-sponsored insurance programs. In 2011, the U.S. Medicare agency paid US$87,945 per patient for HD, US$71,630 for PD, US$99,826 for first year of transplant, and US$12,019 for ongoing post-transplant care (U.S. Renal Data System 2013). Other HICs report similar ranking of costs across modalities.

Case Study: Integrated Screening Program in Tamil Nadu

A low-cost integrated screening program can be radically effective (Mani 2003, 2005). Working with the Kidney Help Trust of Chennai, M. K. Mani has implemented a program in rural Tamil Nadu in which lay health workers perform a urine test for protein and glucose, and record blood pressure in individuals over age five years (N = 25,000). Any abnormalities are further investigated with more specific laboratory tests after physician evaluation; treatment with low-cost drugs is initiated.

The program cost was US$0.27 cents per capita. After two years, compared to an area with similar demographics, the proportion of individuals with eGFR < 80 ml/min/1.73m² was significantly lower in the treatment area.

Figure 13.2 Association of HD/PD Cost Ratio to the Human Developmental Index

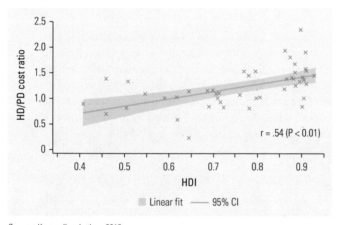

Sources: Karopadi and others 2013.
Note: Countries with higher Human Developmental Indexes had cost ratios favoring use of PD. CI = confidence interval; HD = hemodialysis; HDI = Human Development Index; PD = peritoneal dialysis.

Despite the high upfront procedural costs, transplantation is the most cost-effective form of therapy in the long term because of its efficacy and low maintenance costs (Winkelmayer and others 2002). Data from LMICs are limited, but these results are likely to be confirmed even in resource-limited settings. However, transplantation has several unmodifiable limitations: it can rarely be preemptive; it is contraindicated in patients with serious comorbidity, such as cardiovascular disease, cancer, or infection; and most important, it faces a limited supply of organs.

PD offers similar survival and quality of life compared with HD; based on its cost rankings in HICs, PD could be hypothesized to be more cost-effective than HD (Karopadi and others 2013). Uptake remains low. Efforts to rein in costs related to ESRD led to the 2011 implementation of bundling rules in the United States, which require that several ancillary services be packaged into a fixed payment to dialysis facilities. Although the impact of bundling on patient outcomes has yet to be studied in detail, these measures provide incentives for home-based PD or HD. After only two years of implementation, the number of prevalent individuals on PD had risen by 30 percent for two of the largest dialysis providers in the United States (Golper 2013).

Despite its lower requirements for specialized treatment facilities and nephrology-trained staff, costs associated with PD in LMICs are estimated to be equivalent to or higher than those of HD (figure 13.2) (Karopadi and others 2013). Although further study is required to determine the reason for these cost differences, economies of scale and costs of importing PD solutions and equipment likely play a substantial role. Local manufacturing of PD solutions and equipment in India and Mexico, for example, has resulted in PD costs being lower than those for HD.

Recommendations for Policy Makers in LMICs

Although the data on caring for patients with CKD and ESRD in LMICs are limited, some cornerstones of management—such as educating primary care physicians to recognize diabetic CKD or prioritizing kidney transplants in RRT programs—will translate directly, even in low-resource settings (table 13.4). However, others—in particular, CKD screening and innovative ways of maximizing dialysis provision—require research specific to LMICs.

Table 13.4 Recommendations for CKD and ESRD care in LMICs

Intervention	Platform	Potential benefit	Evidence
CKD			
Consider two-step screening in chronic disease surveillance programs	Government	Identify high-risk individuals for further testing or referral	Limited: Economic modeling based on two observational studies in HICs
Educate physicians about diabetic CKD, the most common form of progressive CKD	Primary care	Prevent ESRD and CV events among patients with diabetes	Strong: RCT evidence from HICs and LMICs
Ensure availability of ACEi or ARBs	Primary care	Delay progression of ESRD for a majority of patients with CKD (particularly proteinuric CKD)	Strong: RCT evidence from HICs and LMICs
ESRD			
Develop deceased-donor registries	Government	Increase organ availability for kidney transplant, the most efficacious and cost-effective therapy	Strong: Large observational studies and economic modeling from HICs
Create high-throughput transplantation centers	Third-level hospital	Take advantage of volumes to develop surgical expertise and standardized immunosuppression protocols	Limited: Observational studies from one LMIC
If not able to provide transplantation, create relationships with middle-income countries with high-throughput transplantation centers	Government	Increase worldwide accessibility for kidney transplant	Expert opinion
Provide incentives for the use of PD	Government	Use economies of scale to decrease costs associated with dialysis provision; create wider access to dialysis using a less-specialized work force	Modest: One meta-analysis and a real-life implementation in Thailand
Create palliative care programs for patients unable to sustainably afford dialysis	Government or community level		Expert opinion

Note: ACEi = angiotensin-converting enzyme inhibitors; ARBs = angiotensin II receptor blockers; CKD = chronic kidney disease; CV = cardiovascular; ESRD = end-stage renal disease; HICs = high-income countries; LMICs = low- and middle-income countries; PD = peritoneal dialysis; RCT = randomized controlled trial.

CONCLUSIONS

Overall, care provision for patients with either AKI or CKD is limited in LMICs, especially since the severe forms of each require the use of expensive RRT. However, several current gaps can be addressed with careful policy consideration.

For AKI, gathering more data on its true incidence and risk factors is crucial. Because the community-based form of AKI may be more prevalent in LMICs, if we can identify the most common etiologies, we can work to prevent them. In addition to identifying regional centers that can accommodate patients who acutely require RRT, protocols that optimize intensive care at first- or second-level hospitals are an initial first step in its management. Use of PD for AKI may be achievable even at second-level hospitals but requires further study.

LMICs are likely to face a growing burden of individuals with CKD and ESRD. Current data indicate that screening a high-risk, older population for CKD is cost-effective, but identifying such a population in countries without first-level health care systems is a key challenge. Low-cost strategies, such as the use of a urine dipstick, can be readily integrated into programs for chronic disease surveillance but also require further study. Most patients with proteinuric and, to a modest extent, hypertensive CKD benefit from initiation of ACE inhibitor and ARB therapy, which are available as low-cost generics.

Finally, although ESRD is rare, large gaps remain between LMICs and HICs in the provision of therapy. Efforts to increase access to RRT need to first focus on increasing the provision of transplantation—the most effective and cost-effective form of RRT. Because transplantation is not appropriate for all individuals with

ESRD, dialysis is required for any RRT program. PD—while not clearly more cost-effective in LMICs—holds the most promise in its ability to reach a larger swath of individuals without intensive technical and equipment requirements.

ANNEXES

The annexes to this chapter are as follows. They are available at http://www.dcp-3.org/CVRD.

- Annex 13A. Kidney Disease Improving Global Outcomes: Criteria for AKI Severity
- Annex 13B. Kidney Disease Improving Global Outcomes: Stages of Chronic Kidney Disease
- Annex 13C. Selected Population-Based Studies Reporting Prevalence of Chronic Kidney Disease

NOTE

World Bank Income Classifications as of July 2014 are as follows, based on estimates of gross national income (GNI) per capita for 2013:

- Low-income countries (LICs) = US$1,045 or less
- Middle-income countries (MICs) are subdivided:
  (a) lower-middle-income = US$1,046 to US$4,125
  (b) upper-middle-income (UMICs) = US$4,126 to US$12,745
- High-income countries (HICs) = US$12,746 or more.

REFERENCES

Ademola, A. D., A. O. Asinobi, O. O. Ogunkunle, B. N. Yusuf, and O. E. Ojo. 2012. "Peritoneal Dialysis in Childhood Acute Kidney Injury: Experience in Southwest Nigeria." *Peritoneal Dialysis International* 32 (3): 267–72. doi:10.3747/pdi.2011.00275.

Agaba, E. I., F. H. Puepet, S. O. Ugoya, P. A. Agaba, R. Adabe, and others. 2009. "Chronic Kidney Disease Screening and Renoprotection in Type 2 Diabetes." *Annals of African Medicine* 8 (1): 52–54.

Ajay, V. S., D. A. Watkins, and D. Prabhakaran. 2017. "Relationships among Major Risk Factors and the Burden of Cardiovascular Diseases, Diabetes, and Chronic Lung Disease." In *Disease Control Priorities* (third edition): Volume 5, *Cardiovascular, Respiratory, and Related Diseases*, edited by D. Prabhakaran, S. Anand, T. A. Gaziano, J.-C. Mbanya, Y. Wu, and R. Nugent. Washington, DC: World Bank.

Anand, S., A. Bitton, and T. A. Gaziano. 2013. "The Gap between Estimated Incidence of End-Stage Renal Disease and Use of Therapy." *PLoS One* 8 (8): e72860. doi:10.1371/journal.pone.0072860.

Anand, S., D. N. Cruz, and F. O. Finkelstein. 2015. "Understanding Acute Kidney Injury in Low Resource Settings: A Step Forward." *BMC Nephrology* 16: 5. doi:10.1186/1471-2369-16-5.

Anand, S., R. Shivashankar, M. K. Ali, D. Kondal, B. Binukumar, and others. 2015. "Prevalence of Chronic Kidney Disease in Two Major Indian Cities and Projections for Associated Cardiovascular Disease." *Kidney International* 88 (1): 178–85. doi:10.1038/ki.2015.58.

Bagasha, P., F. Nakwagala, A. Kwizera, E. Ssekasanvu, and R. Kalyesubula. 2015. "Acute Kidney Injury among Adult Patients with Sepsis in a Low-Income Country: Clinical Patterns and Short-Term Outcomes." *BMC Nephrology* 16: 4. doi:10.1186/1471-2369-16-4.

Bellomo, R., C. Ronco, J. A. Kellum, R. L. Mehta, P. Palevsky, and the Workgroup Acute Dialysis Quality Initiative. 2004. "Acute Renal Failure: Definition, Outcome Measures, Animal Models, Fluid Therapy and Information Technology Needs: The Second International Consensus Conference of the Acute Dialysis Quality Initiative (ADQI) Group." *Critical Care* 8 (4): R204–12. doi:10.1186/cc2872.

Bieber, B., J. Qian, S. Anand, Y. Yan, N. Chen, and others. 2013. "Two-Times Weekly Hemodialysis in China: Frequency, Associated Patient and Treatment Characteristics and Quality of Life in the China Dialysis Outcomes and Practice Patterns Study." *Nephrology Dialysis Transplantation* 29 (9): 1770–77. doi:10.1093/ndt/gft472.

Bouchard, J., A. Acharya, J. Cerda, E. R. Maccariello, R. C. Madarasu, and others. 2015. "A Prospective International Multicenter Study of AKI in the Intensive Care Unit." *Clinical Journal of the American Society of Nephrology* 10 (8): 1324–31. doi:10.2215/CJN.04360514.

Braimoh, R. W., M. O. Mabayoje, C. O. Amira, and H. Coker. 2012. "Quality of Hemodialysis Water in a Resource-Poor Country: The Nigerian Example." *Hemodialysis International* 16 (4): 532–38. doi:10.1111/j.1542-4758.2012.00682.x.

Burki, T. 2015. "Tanzania's Model Peritoneal Dialysis Programme." *The Lancet* 385 (9981): 1935–36. doi:10.1016/S0140-6736(15)60946-1.

Callegari, J. G., S. Antwi, G. Wystrychowski, E. Zukowska-Szczechowska, N. W. Levin, and M. Carter. 2013. "Peritoneal Dialysis as a Mode of Treatment for Acute Kidney Injury in Sub-Saharan Africa." *Blood Purification* 36 (3–4): 226–30. doi:10.1159/000356627.

Callegari, J. G., K. G. Kilonzo, K. E. Yeates, G. J. Handelman, F. O. Finkelstein, and others. 2012. "Peritoneal Dialysis for Acute Kidney Injury in Sub-Saharan Africa: Challenges Faced and Lessons Learned at Kilimanjaro Christian Medical Centre." *Kidney International* 81 (4): 331–33. doi:10.1038/ki.2011.408.

Cerda, J., N. Lameire, P. Eggers, N. Pannu, S. Uchino, and others. 2008. "Epidemiology of Acute Kidney Injury." *Clinical Journal of the American Society of Nephrology* 3 (3): 881–86. doi:10.2215/CJN.04961107.

Chandrajith, R., S. Nanayakkara, K. Itai, T. N. Aturaliya, C. B. Dissanayake, and others. 2011. "Chronic Kidney Diseases of Uncertain Etiology (CKDUE) in Sri Lanka: Geographic Distribution and Environmental Implications."

Environmental Geochemistry and Health 33 (3): 267–78. doi:10.1007/s10653-010-9339-1.

Chen, S. Y., C. X. Wang, L. Z. Chen, J. G. Fei, S. X. Deng, and others. 2008. "Tuberculosis in Southern Chinese Renal-Transplant Recipients." *Clinical Transplantation* 22 (6): 780–84. doi:10.1111/j.1399-0012.2008.00878.x.

Chertow, G. M., E. Burdick, M. Honour, J. V. Bonventre, and D. W. Bates. 2005. "Acute Kidney Injury, Mortality, Length of Stay, and Costs in Hospitalized Patients." *Journal of the American Society of Nephrology* 16 (11): 3365–70. doi:10.1681/ASN.2004090740.

Chionh, C. Y., S. S. Soni, F. O. Finkelstein, C. Ronco, and D. N. Cruz. 2013. "Use of Peritoneal Dialysis in AKI: A Systematic Review." *Clinical Journal of the American Society of Nephrology* 8 (10): 1649–60. doi:10.2215/CJN.01540213.

Chronic Kidney Disease Prognosis Consortium, K. Matsushita, M. van der Velde, B. C. Astor, M. Woodward, and others. 2010. "Association of Estimated Glomerular Filtration Rate and Albuminuria with All-Cause and Cardiovascular Mortality in General Population Cohorts: A Collaborative Meta-Analysis." *The Lancet* 375 (9731): 2073–81. doi:10.1016/S0140-6736(10)60674-5.

Cortes-Sanabria, L., C. E. Cabrera-Pivaral, A. M. Cueto-Manzano, E. Rojas-Campos, G. Barragan, and others. 2008. "Improving Care of Patients with Diabetes and CKD: A Pilot Study for a Cluster-Randomized Trial." *American Journal of Kidney Disease* 51 (5): 777–88. doi:10.1053/j.ajkd.2007.12.039.

Couser, W. G., G. Remuzzi, S. Mendis, and M. Tonelli. 2011. "The Contribution of Chronic Kidney Disease to the Global Burden of Major Noncommunicable Diseases." *Kidney International* 80 (12): 1258–70. doi:10.1038/ki.2011.368.

Cueto-Manzano, A. M., H. R. Martinez-Ramirez, and L. Cortes-Sanabria. 2013. "Comparison of Primary Health-Care Models in the Management of Chronic Kidney Disease." *Kidney International Supplements* (2011) 3 (2): 210–14. doi:10.1038/kisup.2013.16.

Cullis, B., M. Abdelraheem, G. Abrahams, A. Balbi, D. N. Cruz, and others. 2014. "Peritoneal Dialysis for Acute Kidney Injury." *Peritoneal Dialysis International* 34 (5): 494–517. doi:10.3747/pdi.2013.00222.

de Boer, I. H., T. C. Rue, Y. N. Hall, P. J. Heagerty, N. S. Weiss, and others. 2011. "Temporal Trends in the Prevalence of Diabetic Kidney Disease in the United States." *Journal of the American Medical Association* 305 (24): 2532–39. doi:10.1001/jama.2011.861.

Edefonti, A., G. Marra, M. C. Perez, M. S. Diaz, F. Sereni, and others. 2010. "A Comprehensive Cooperative Project for Children with Renal Diseases in Nicaragua." *Clinical Nephrology* 74: S119–25.

Finkelstein, F. O., W. E. Smoyer, M. Carter, A. Brusselmans, and J. Feehally. 2014. "Peritoneal Dialysis, Acute Kidney Injury, and the Saving Young Lives Program." *Peritoneal Dialysis International* 34 (5): 478–80. doi:10.3747/pdi.2014.00041.

Floege, J., and F. Eitner. 2011. "Current Therapy for IgA Nephropathy." *Journal of the American Society of Nephrology* 22 (10): 1785–94. doi:10.1681/ASN.2011030221.

Garcia-Garcia, G., Y. Martinez-Castellanos, K. Renoirte-Lopez, A. Barajas-Murguia, L. de la Torre-Campos, and others. 2013. "Multidisciplinary Care for Poor Patients with Chronic Kidney Disease in Mexico." *Kidney International Supplements* (2011) 3 (2): 178–83. doi:10.1038/kisup.2013.9.

Gentry, S. E., R. A. Montgomery, and D. L. Segev. 2011. "Kidney Paired Donation: Fundamentals, Limitations, and Expansions." *American Journal of Kidney Disease* 57 (1): 144–51. doi:10.1053/j.ajkd.2010.10.005.

George, J., S. Varma, S. Kumar, J. Thomas, S. Gopi, and R. Pisharody. 2011. "Comparing Continuous Venovenous Hemofiltration and Peritoneal Dialysis in Critically Ill Patients with Acute Kidney Injury: A Pilot Study." *Peritoneal Dialysis* 31 (4): 422–29.

Ghods, A. J., and S. Savaj. 2006. "Iranian Model of Paid and Regulated Living-Unrelated Kidney Donation." *Clinical Journal of the American Society of Nephrology* 1 (6): 1136–45. doi:10.2215/CJN.00700206.

Ginzler, E. M., M. A. Dooley, C. Aranow, M. Y. Kim, J. Buyon, and others. 2005. "Mycophenolate Mofetil or Intravenous Cyclophosphamide for Lupus Nephritis." *New England Journal of Medicine* 353 (21): 2219–28. doi:10.1056/NEJMoa043731.

Golper, T. A. 2013. "The Possible Impact of the US Prospective Payment System ('Bundle') on the Growth of Peritoneal Dialysis." *Peritoneal Dialysis International* 33 (6): 596–99. doi:10.3747/pdi.2013.00212.

Grassmann, A., S. Gioberge, S. Moeller, and G. Brown. 2005. "ESRD Patients in 2004: Global Overview of Patient Numbers, Treatment Modalities and Associated Trends." *Nephrology Dialysis Transplantation* 20 (12): 2587–93. doi:10.1093/ndt/gfi159.

Hamel, M. B., R. S. Phillips, R. B. Davis, N. Desbiens, A. F. Connors, Jr., and others. 1997. "Outcomes and Cost-Effectiveness of Initiating Dialysis and Continuing Aggressive Care in Seriously Ill Hospitalized Adults. SUPPORT Investigators. Study to Understand Prognoses and Preferences for Outcomes and Risks of Treatments." *Annals of Internal Medicine* 127 (3): 195–202.

Himmelfarb, J., and T. A. Ikizler. 2007. "Acute Kidney Injury: Changing Lexicography, Definitions, and Epidemiology." *Kidney International* 71 (10): 971–76. doi:10.1038/sj.ki.5002224.

Hoerger, T. J., J. S. Wittenborn, J. E. Segel, N. R. Burrows, K. Imai, and others. 2010. "A Health Policy Model of CKD: 2. The Cost-Effectiveness of Microalbuminuria Screening." *American Journal of Kidney Disease* 55 (3): 463–73. doi:10.1053/j.ajkd.2009.11.017.

Hossain, P., B. Kawar, and M. El Nahas. 2007. "Obesity and Diabetes in the Developing World: A Growing Challenge." *New England Journal of Medicine* 356 (3): 213–15. doi:10.1056/NEJMp068177.

Hoste, E. A., and M. Schurgers. 2008. "Epidemiology of Acute Kidney Injury: How Big Is the Problem?" *Critical Care Medicine* 36 (Suppl 4): S146–51. doi:10.1097/CCM.0b013e318168c590.

Hou, F. F., X. Zhang, G. H. Zhang, D. Xie, P. Y. Chen, and others. 2006. "Efficacy and Safety of Benazepril for Advanced

Chronic Renal Insufficiency." *New England Journal of Medicine* 354 (2): 131–40. doi:10.1056/NEJMoa053107.

Howard, K., S. White, G. Salkeld, S. McDonald, J. C. Craig, and others. 2010. "Cost-Effectiveness of Screening and Optimal Management for Diabetes, Hypertension, and Chronic Kidney Disease: A Modeled Analysis." *Value in Health* 13 (2): 196–208.

Isenberg, D., G. B. Appel, G. Contreras, M. A. Dooley, E. M. Ginzler, and others. 2010. "Influence of Race/Ethnicity on Response to Lupus Nephritis Treatment: The ALMS Study." *Rheumatology (Oxford)* 49 (1): 128–40. doi:10.1093/rheumatology/kep346.

Jafar, T. H., N. Chaturvedi, J. Hatcher, and A. S. Levey. 2007. "Use of Albumin Creatinine Ratio and Urine Albumin Concentration as a Screening Test for Albuminuria in an Indo-Asian Population." *Nephrology Dialysis Transplantation* 22 (8): 2194–200.

Jayasumana, C., P. Paranagama, S. Agampodi, C. Wijewardane, S. Gunatilake, and others. 2015. "Drinking Well Water and Occupational Exposure to Herbicides Is Associated with Chronic Kidney Disease, in Padavi-Sripura, Sri Lanka." *Environmental Health* 14 (1): 6. doi:10.1186/1476-069X-14-6.

Jha, V. 2009. "Current Status of Chronic Kidney Disease Care in Southeast Asia." *Seminars in Nephrology* 29 (5): 487–96. doi:10.1016/j.semnephrol.2009.06.005.

Jiang, Z., and X. Yu. 2011. "Advancing the Use and Quality of Peritoneal Dialysis by Developing a Peritoneal Dialysis Satellite Center Program." *Peritoneal Dialysis International* 31 (2): 121–26. doi:10.3747/pdi.2010.00041.

Jungers, P., D. Joly, F. Barbey, G. Choukroun, and M. Daudon. 2004. "ESRD Caused by Nephrolithiasis: Prevalence, Mechanisms, and Prevention." *American Journal of Kidney Disease* 44 (5): 799–805.

Karopadi, A. N., G. Mason, E. Rettore, and C. Ronco. 2013. "Cost of Peritoneal Dialysis and Haemodialysis across the World." *Nephrology Dialysis Transplantation* 28 (10): 2553–69. doi:10.1093/ndt/gft214.

Kellum, J. A., N. Lameire, and KDIGO AKI Guideline Work Group. 2013. "Diagnosis, Evaluation, and Management of Acute Kidney Injury: A KDIGO Summary (Part 1)." *Critical Care* 17 (1): 204. doi:10.1186/cc11454.

Kidney Disease: Improving Global Outcomes Work Group. 2012. "KDIGO 2012 Clinical Practice Guideline for the Evaluation and Management of Chronic Kidney Disease." *Kidney International Supplements* 2013 (3): 1–150.

Kilonzo, K. G., S. Ghosh, S. A. Temu, V. Maro, J. G. Callegari, and others. 2012. "Outcome of Acute Peritoneal Dialysis in Northern Tanzania." *Peritoneal Dialysis International* 32 (3): 261–66. doi:10.3747/pdi.2012.00083.

Komenda, P., T. W. Ferguson, K. Macdonald, C. Rigatto, C. Koolage, and others. 2014. "Cost-Effectiveness of Primary Screening for CKD: A Systematic Review." *American Journal of Kidney Disease* 63 (5): 789–97. doi:10.1053/j.ajkd.2013.12.012.

Kshirsagar, A. V., M. S. Joy, S. L. Hogan, R. J. Falk, and R. E. Colindres. 2000. "Effect of ACE Inhibitors in Diabetic and Nondiabetic Chronic Renal Disease: A Systematic Overview of Randomized Placebo-Controlled Trials." *American Journal of Kidney Disease* 35 (4): 695–707.

Lameire, N. H., A. Bagga, D. Cruz, J. De Maeseneer, Z. Endre, and others. 2013. "Acute Kidney Injury: An Increasing Global Concern." *The Lancet* 382 (9887): 170–79. doi:10.1016/S0140-6736(13)60647-9.

Laukkanen, A., L. Emaus, V. Pettila, and K. M. Kaukonen. 2013. "Five-Year Cost-Utility Analysis of Acute Renal Replacement Therapy: A Societal Perspective." *Intensive Care Medicine* 39 (3): 406–13. doi:10.1007/s00134-012-2760-4.

Levey, A. S., and J. Coresh. 2012. "Chronic Kidney Disease." *The Lancet* 379 (9811): 165–80. doi:10.1016/S0140-6736(11)60178-5.

Levey, A. S., J. Coresh, E. Balk, A. T. Kausz, A. Levin, and others. 2003. "National Kidney Foundation Practice Guidelines for Chronic Kidney Disease: Evaluation, Classification, and Stratification." *Annals of Internal Medicine* 139 (2): 137–47.

Liyanage, T., T. Ninomiya, V. Jha, B. Neal, H. M. Patrice, and others. 2015. "Worldwide Access to Treatment for End-Stage Kidney Disease: A Systematic Review." *The Lancet* 385 (9981): 1975–82. doi:10.1016/S0140-6736(14)61601-9.

Lopez, M., and B. Hoppe. 2010. "History, Epidemiology and Regional Diversities of Urolithiasis." *Pediatric Nephrology* 25 (1): 49–59. doi:10.1007/s00467-008-0960-5.

Luyckx, V. A., and S. Naicker. 2008. "Acute Kidney Injury Associated with the Use of Traditional Medicines." *Nature Clinical Practice. Nephrology* 4 (12): 664–71. doi:10.1038/ncpneph0970.

Malhotra, K. K. 2007. "Challenge of Tuberculosis in Renal Transplantation." *Transplant Proceedings* 39 (3): 756–58. doi:10.1016/j.transproceed.2007.01.062.

Mallipattu, S. K., F. Salem, and C. M. Wyatt. 2014. "The Changing Epidemiology of HIV-Related Chronic Kidney Disease in the Era of Antiretroviral Therapy." *Kidney International* 86 (2): 259–65. doi:10.1038/ki.2014.44.

Mani, M. K. 2003. "Prevention of Chronic Renal Failure at the Community Level." *Kidney International Supplements* (83): S86–89.

———. 2005. "Experience with a Program for Prevention of Chronic Renal Failure in India." *Kidney International Supplements* (94): S75–78. doi:10.1111/j.1523-1755.2005.09419.x.

———. 2010. "Treating Renal Disease in India's Poor: The Art of the Possible." *Seminars in Nephrology* 30 (1): 74–80. doi:http://dx.doi.org/10.1016/j.semnephrol.2009.10.012.

Martinez-Ramirez, H. R., B. Jalomo-Martinez, L. Cortes-Sanabria, E. Rojas-Campos, G. Barragan, and others. 2006. "Renal Function Preservation in Type 2 Diabetes Mellitus Patients with Early Nephropathy: A Comparative Prospective Cohort Study between Primary Health Care Doctors and a Nephrologist." *American Journal of Kidney Disease* 47 (1): 78–87. doi:10.1053/j.ajkd.2005.09.015.

Mastroianni-Kirsztajn, G., M. G. Bastos, and E. A. Burdmann. 2011. "Strategies of the Brazilian Chronic Kidney Disease Prevention Campaign (2003–2009)." *Nephron Clinical Practice* 117 (3): c259–65. doi:10.1159/000320741.

Medina-Pestana, J. O. 2006. "Organization of a High-Volume Kidney Transplant Program: The 'Assembly Line' Approach."

Transplantation 81 (11): 1510–20. doi:10.1097/01.tp.000021 4934.48677.e2.

Mehta, R. L., E. A. Burdmann, J. Cerda, J. Feehally, F. Finkelstein, and others. 2016. "Current Practice for Recognition and Management of Acute Kidney Injury: The International Society of Nephrology 0by25 Global Snapshot Study: A multinational cross-sectional." *The Lancet* 387 (10032): 2017–25.

Mehta, R. L., J. Cerda, E. A. Burdmann, M. Tonelli, G. Garcia-Garcia, and others. 2015. "International Society of Nephrology's 0by25 Initiative for Acute Kidney Injury (Zero Preventable Deaths by 2025): A Human Rights Case for Nephrology." *The Lancet* 385 (9987): 2616–43. doi:10.1016 /S0140-6736(15)60126-X.

Mehta, R. L., J. A. Kellum, S. V. Shah, B. A. Molitoris, C. Ronco, and others. 2007. "Acute Kidney Injury Network: Report of an Initiative to Improve Outcomes in Acute Kidney Injury." *Critical Care* 11 (2): R31. doi:10.1186/cc5713.

Mendoza, R. L. 2010. "Kidney Black Markets and Legal Transplants: Are They Opposite Sides of the Same Coin?" *Health Policy* 94 (3): 255–65. doi:10.1016/j.healthpol.2009.10.005.

Mishra, O. P., A. K. Gupta, V. Pooniya, R. Prasad, N. K. Tiwary, and others. 2012. "Peritoneal Dialysis in Children with Acute Kidney Injury: A Developing Country Experience." *Peritoneal Dialysis International* 32 (4): 431–36. doi:10.3747 /pdi.2012.00118.

Moosa, M. R., and M. Kidd. 2006. "The Dangers of Rationing Dialysis Treatment: The Dilemma Facing a Developing Country." *Kidney International* 70 (6): 1107–14. doi:5001750 [pii] 10.1038/sj.ki.5001750.

Moynihan, R., R. Glassock, and J. Doust. 2013. "Chronic Kidney Disease Controversy: How Expanding Definitions Are Unnecessarily Labelling Many People as Diseased." *British Medical Journal* 347: f4298. doi:10.1136/bmj.f4298.

Murray, K. O., R. S. Fischer, D. Chavarria, C. Duttmann, M. N. Garcia, and others. 2015. "Mesoamerican Nephropathy: A Neglected Tropical Disease with an Infectious Etiology?" *Microbes and Infection* 17 (10): 671–75. doi:10.1016/j.micinf .2015.08.005.

Mushi, L., P. Marschall, and S. Flessa. 2015. "The Cost of Dialysis in Low and Middle-Income Countries: A Systematic Review." *BMC Health Services Research* 15: 506. doi:10.1186 /s12913-015-1166-8.

Naicker, S., O. Aboud, and M. B. Gharbi. 2008. "Epidemiology of Acute Kidney Injury in Africa." *Seminars in Nephrology* 28 (4): 348–53. doi:10.1016/j.semnephrol.2008.04.003.

Nanayakkara, S., T. Komiya, N. Ratnatunga, S. T. Senevirathna, K. H. Harada, and others. 2012. "Tubulointerstitial Damage as the Major Pathological Lesion in Endemic Chronic Kidney Disease among Farmers in North Central Province of Sri Lanka." *Environmental Health and Preventive Medicine* 17 (3): 213–21. doi:10.1007/s12199-011-0243-9.

O'Hare, A. M., J. R. Hotchkiss, M. Kurella Tamura, E. B. Larson, B. R. Hemmelgarn, and others. 2014. "Interpreting Treatment Effects from Clinical Trials in the Context of Real-World Risk Information: End-Stage Renal Disease Prevention in Older Adults." *JAMA Internal Medicine* 174 (3): 391–97. doi:10.1001/jamainternmed.2013.13328.

Oliveira, M. B., J. E. Romao, Jr., and R. Zatz. 2005. "End-Stage Renal Disease in Brazil: Epidemiology, Prevention, and Treatment." *Kidney International Supplements* (97): S82–86. doi:10.1111/j.1523-1755.2005.09714.x.

Palevsky, P. M., K. D. Liu, P. D. Brophy, L. S. Chawla, C. R. Parikh, and others. 2013. "KDOQI US Commentary on the 2012 KDIGO Clinical Practice Guideline for Acute Kidney Injury." *American Journal of Kidney Disease* 61 (5): 649–72. doi:10.1053/j.ajkd.2013.02.349.

Pecoits-Filho, R., H. Abensur, A. M. Cueto-Manzano, J. Dominguez, J. C. Divino Filho, and others. 2007. "Overview of Peritoneal Dialysis in Latin America." *Peritoneal Dialysis International* 27 (3): 316–21. doi:27/3/316 [pii].

Plata, R., C. Silva, J. Yahuita, L. Perez, A. Schieppati, and others. 1998. "The First Clinical and Epidemiological Programme on Renal Disease in Bolivia: A Model for Prevention and Early Diagnosis of Renal Diseases in the Developing Countries." *Nephrology Dialysis Transplantation* 13 (12): 3034–36.

Poggio, E. D., and A. D. Rule. 2009. "A Critical Evaluation of Chronic Kidney Disease: Should Isolated Reduced Estimated Glomerular Filtration Rate Be Considered a 'Disease'?" *Nephrology Dialysis Transplantation* 24 (3): 698–700. doi:10.1093/ndt/gfn704.

Ponce, D., J. T. Caramori, P. Barretti, and A. L. Balbi. 2012. "Peritoneal Dialysis in Acute Kidney Injury: Brazilian Experience." *Peritoneal Dialysis International* 32 (3): 242–46. doi:0.3747/pdi.2012.00089.

Prakash, J., T. Gupta, S. Prakash, S. S. Rathore, Usha, and others. 2015. "Acute Kidney Injury in Patients with Human Immunodeficiency Virus Infection." *Indian Journal of Nephrology* 25 (2): 86–90. doi:10.4103/0971-4065.138696.

Remuzzi, G., and R. Horton. 2013. "Acute Renal Failure: An Unacceptable Death Sentence Globally." *The Lancet* 382 (9910): 2041–42. doi:10.1016/S0140-6736(13)62193-5.

Rewa, O., and S. M. Bagshaw. 2014. "Acute Kidney Injury: Epidemiology, Outcomes and Economics." *Nature Reviews Nephrology* 10 (4): 193–207. doi:10.1038/nrneph.2013.282.

Riella, M. C., and A. J. Locatelli. 2007. "History of Peritoneal Dialysis in Latin America." *Peritoneal Dialysis International* 27 (3): 322–72. doi:27/3/322 [pii].

Rizvi, S. A., S. A. Naqvi, Z. Hussain, A. Hashmi, F. Akhtar, and others. 2003. "Renal Transplantation in Developing Countries." *Kidney International Supplements* (83): S96–100.

Rizvi, S. A., S. A. Naqvi, M. N. Zafar, Z. Hussain, A. Hashmi, and others. 2011. "A Renal Transplantation Model for Developing Countries." *American Journal of Transplantation* 11 (11): 2302–7. doi:10.1111/j.1600-6143.2011.03712.x.

Roncal Jimenez, C. A., T. Ishimoto, M. A. Lanaspa, C. J. Rivard, T. Nakagawa, and others. 2013. "Fructokinase Activity Mediates Dehydration-Induced Renal Injury." *Kidney International* 86 (2): 294–302. doi:10.1038/ki.2013.492.

Sakuma, Y., A. Glassman, and C. Vacca. 2017. "Priority-Setting Processes for Expensive Treatments for Chronic Diseases." In *Disease Control Priorities* (third edition): Volume 5, *Cardiovascular, Respiratory, and Related Diseases,* edited by D. Prabhakaran, S. Anand, T. A. Gaziano, J.-C. Mbanya, Y. Wu, and R. Nugent. Washington, DC: World Bank.

Schwedt, E., L. Sola, P. G. Rios, N. Mazzuchi, and National Renal Healthcare Program. 2010. "Improving the Management of Chronic Kidney Disease in Uruguay: A National Renal Healthcare Program." *Nephron Clinical Practice* 114 (1): c47–59. doi:10.1159/000245069.

Sesso Rde, C., A. A. Lopes, F. S. Thome, J. R. Lugon, Y. Watanabe, and others. 2012. "[Chronic Dialysis in Brazil: Report of the Brazilian Dialysis Census, 2011]." *Brazilian Journal of Nephrology* 34 (3): 272–77.

Sharma, S. K., A. Ghimire, S. Carminati, G. Remuzzi, and N. Perico. 2014. "Management of Chronic Kidney Disease and Its Risk Factors in Eastern Nepal." *The Lancet Global Health* 2 (9): e506–7. doi:10.1016/S2214-109X(14)70281-5.

Soderland, P., S. Lovekar, D. E. Weiner, D. R. Brooks, and J. S. Kaufman. 2010. "Chronic Kidney Disease Associated with Environmental Toxins and Exposures." *Advances in Chronic Kidney Disease* 17 (3): 254–64. doi:10.1053/j.ackd.2010.03.011.

Stone, J. H., P. A. Merkel, R. Spiera, P. Seo, C. A. Langford, and others, for the Rave-ITN Research Group. 2010. "Rituximab versus Cyclophosphamide for ANCA-Associated Vasculitis." *New England Journal of Medicine* 363 (3): 221–32. doi:10.1056/NEJMoa0909905.

Susantitaphong, P., D. N. Cruz, J. Cerda, M. Abulfaraj, F. Alqahtani, and others. 2013. "World Incidence of AKI: A Meta-Analysis." *Clinical Journal of the American Society of Nephrology* 8 (9): 1482–93. doi:10.2215/CJN.00710113.

Talabani, B., S. Zouwail, R. D. Pyart, S. Meran, S. G. Riley, and others. 2014. "Epidemiology and Outcome of Community-Acquired Acute Kidney Injury." *Nephrology (Carlton)* 19 (5): 282–87. doi:10.1111/nep.12221.

Thomas, B., M. van Pelt, R. Mehrotra, C. Robinson-Cohen, and J. LoGerfo. 2014. "An Estimation of the Prevalence and Progression of Chronic Kidney Disease in a Rural Diabetic Cambodian Population." *PLoS One* 9 (1): e86123. doi:10.1371/journal.pone.0086123.

Thomas, B., S. Wulf, B. Bikbov, N. Perico, M. Cortinovis, and others. 2015. "Maintenance Dialysis throughout the World in Years 1990 and 2010." *Journal of the American Society of Nephrology* 26 (11): 2621–33. doi:10.1681/ASN.2014101017.

Trang, T. T., N. H. Phu, H. Vinh, T. T. Hien, B. M. Cuong, and others. 1992. "Acute Renal Failure in Patients with Severe *Falciparum* Malaria." *Clinical Infectious Diseases* 15 (5): 874–80.

U.S. Renal Data System. 2013. *2013 Annual Data Report: Atlas of Chronic Kidney Disease and End-Stage Renal Disease in the United States.* Bethesda, MD: National Institutes of Health, NIDDK.

van Dijk, P. C., K. J. Jager, F. de Charro, F. Collart, R. Cornet, and others. 2001. "Renal Replacement Therapy in Europe: The Results of a Collaborative Effort by the ERA-EDTA Registry and Six National or Regional Registries." *Nephrology Dialysis Transplantation* 16 (6): 1120–09.

Waikar, S. S., G. C. Curhan, R. Wald, E. P. McCarthy, and G. M. Chertow. 2006. "Declining Mortality in Patients with Acute Renal Failure, 1988 to 2002." *Journal of the American Society of Nephrology* 17 (4): 1143–50. doi:10.1681/ASN.2005091017.

Weiner, D. E., M. D. McClean, J. S. Kaufman, and D. R. Brooks. 2013. "The Central American Epidemic of CKD." *Clinical Journal of the American Society of Nephrology* 8 (3): 504–11. doi:10.2215/CJN.05050512.

Wesseling, C., J. Crowe, C. Hogstedt, K. Jakobsson, R. Lucas, and others. 2013. "The Epidemic of Chronic Kidney Disease of Unknown Etiology in Mesoamerica: A Call for Interdisciplinary Research and Action." *American Journal of Public Health* 103 (11): 1927–30. doi:10.2105/AJPH.2013.301594.

Wetzels, J. F., L. A. Kiemeney, D. W. Swinkels, H. L. Willems, and M. den Heijer. 2007. "Age- and Gender-Specific Reference Values of Estimated GFR in Caucasians: The Nijmegen Biomedical Study." *Kidney International* 72 (5): 632–37. doi:10.1038/sj.ki.5002374.

Wijkstrom, J., R. Leiva, C. G. Elinder, S. Leiva, Z. Trujillo, and others. 2013. "Clinical and Pathological Characterization of Mesoamerican Nephropathy: A New Kidney Disease in Central America." *American Journal of Kidney Disease* 62 (5): 908–18. doi:10.1053/j.ajkd.2013.05.019.

Wilkie, M. 2014. "The Role of Peritoneal Dialysis in Saving Young Lives from Acute Kidney Injury." *Peritoneal Dialysis International* 34 (5): 476–77. doi:10.3747/pdi.2014.00185.

Winkelmayer, W. C., M. C. Weinstein, M. A. Mittleman, R. J. Glynn, and J. S. Pliskin. 2002. "Health Economic Evaluations: The Special Case of End-Stage Renal Disease Treatment." *Medical Decision Making* 22 (5): 417–30.

Wolfe, R. A., V. B. Ashby, E. L. Milford, A. O. Ojo, R. E. Ettenger, L. Y. Agodoa, and others. 1999. "Comparison of Mortality in All Patients on Dialysis, Patients on Dialysis Awaiting Transplantation, and Recipients of a First Cadaveric Transplant." *New England Journal of Medicine* 341 (23): 1725–30. doi:10.1056/NEJM199912023412303.

Wong, F. K., S. K. Chow, and T. M. Chan. 2010. "Evaluation of a Nurse-Led Disease Management Programme for Chronic Kidney Disease: A Randomized Controlled Trial." *International Journal of Nursing Studies* 47 (3): 268–78. http://onlinelibrary.wiley.com/o/cochrane/clcentral/articles/848/CN-00743848/frame.html.

Wright, J. T., Jr., G. Bakris, T. Greene, L. Y. Agodoa, L. J. Appel, and others. 2002. "Effect of Blood Pressure Lowering and Antihypertensive Drug Class on Progression of Hypertensive Kidney Disease: Results from the AASK Trial." *Journal of the American Medical Association* 288 (19): 2421–31.

Wyatt, C., V. Konduri, J. Eng, and R. Rohatgi. 2007. "Reporting of Estimated GFR in the Primary Care Clinic." *American Journal of Kidney Diseases* 49 (5): 634–41.

Zhang, A. H., H. Zhong, W. Tang, S. Y. Chen, L. He, and others. 2008. "Establishing a Renal Management Clinic in China: Initiative, Challenges, and Opportunities." *International Urology and Nephrology* 40 (4): 1053–58. doi:10.1007/s11255-008-9450-8.

Chapter 14

Peripheral Artery Disease

Uchechukwu K. A. Sampson, F. Gerald R. Fowkes, Nadraj G. Naidoo, and Michael H. Criqui

INTRODUCTION

The term *peripheral artery disease* (PAD) classically encompasses the various diseases that affect noncardiac, nonintracranial arteries. The most common cause of PAD is atherosclerosis; less common causes include inflammatory disorders of the arterial wall (vasculitis) and noninflammatory arteriopathies, such as fibromuscular dysplasia (Kullo and Rooke 2016). Lower extremity PAD is a leading cause of atherosclerotic vascular morbidity and is only surpassed by coronary artery disease and stroke (Caro and others 2005; Criqui and others 1992; Dormandy and Rutherford 2000).

The global importance of PAD is rising because the number of people living with PAD has increased in the past decade; causes of the increase include aging populations and increased exposure to risk factors, particularly in low- and middle-income countries (LMICs) (Fowkes and others 2013). Consequently, assessing the need for coordinated and cost-effective responses to the burden of PAD is important.

This chapter discusses the global epidemiology of PAD based on recent evidence that provides updated comparisons of age- and gender-specific prevalence between high-income countries (HICs) and LMICs, risk factors for PAD in HICs and LMICs, and robust estimates of PAD deaths and the number of people living with PAD regionally and globally. The chapter provides insights into the implications of current PAD epidemiology for potential cost-effective approaches to prevention and treatment in LMICs.

CAUSE AND DIAGNOSIS

Atherosclerosis is plaque buildup in the arteries, which leads to stenosis (narrowing or blockage) of the vessels that deliver blood from the heart to the legs. Although most patients may be asymptomatic, the classic symptom is claudication, defined as pain, cramp, or ache in the legs (hip, buttock, thigh, or calf) due to exertion and relieved by rest. Patients may also present with critical limb ischemia or, occasionally, acute limb ischemia. Potential findings on examination include the presence of nonhealing wounds, decreased or absent pulses, hair loss, and muscle atrophy.

The diagnosis of PAD is usually made in symptomatic patients using clinical signs alone, including appropriate typical symptoms, absence of peripheral pulses, presence of ischemic skin changes, and presence of necrosis. However, diagnosis is usually aided by the use of resting ankle-brachial index (ABI), particularly to quantify symptomatic disease, evaluate atypical symptoms, and find asymptomatic disease. ABI is a noninvasive test that measures the systolic blood pressure (SBP) in the ankle and compares it with SBP in the arm. SBP is determined with a pneumatic cuff, which is first inflated

Corresponding author: Uchechukwu K. A. Sampson, National Heart, Lung, and Blood Institute, National Institutes of Health, Bethesda, Maryland, United States; Uchechukwu.Sampson@nih.gov.

until flow ceases and then deflated slowly until the flow signal reappears, usually detected by Doppler ultrasound or oscillometric methods (Aboyans and others 2012; Rooke and others 2011). Normal ABI ranges between 1.00 and 1.40; abnormal values are defined as those less than 0.90. ABI values of 0.91–0.99 are considered borderline; values greater than 1.40 indicate stiff or noncompressible arteries (Rooke and others 2011).

Additional information for the assessment of PAD may be derived from examination of treadmill exercise testing with and without ABI assessments; a six-minute walk test; and imaging tests such as ultrasound, magnetic resonance angiography, contrast angiography, and computed tomographic angiography (Rooke and others 2011). Patients with PAD have high coprevalence of other atherosclerotic conditions such as coronary and carotid artery disease (getABI Study Group 2002; Saw and others 2006). Consequently, patients have a high risk of adverse cardiovascular events, particularly myocardial infarctions. Death among PAD patients is usually not a direct effect of the disease but is due to associated atherosclerotic complications such as myocardial infarction or stroke, or attendant problems such as infectious or surgical complications.

Recent evidence indicates that the risk of PAD progression is higher than previously expected (Sigvant, Lundin, and Wahlberg 2016). Therefore, although the prevention of PAD has not been formally evaluated, PAD is likely to be ameliorated by typical cardiovascular prevention strategies (Pande and others 2011). Recommendations for the management of patients with PAD focus on cardiovascular risk reduction and treatment of claudication and critical limb ischemia. Recommended cardiovascular risk reduction strategies include the use of lipid-lowering drugs such as statins; antihypertensives such as angiotensin-converting enzyme inhibitors and beta blockers; antiplatelet and antithrombotic drugs such as aspirin and clopidogrel; and smoking cessation efforts aided by pharmacological agents such as nicotine and bupropion therapy. Interventions for claudication include exercise rehabilitation, use of medical and pharmacological agents, and endovascular or surgical treatment for lifestyle-limiting disability. The main approaches to the treatment of limb ischemia include thrombolysis for acute cases and endovascular and surgical interventions.

EPIDEMIOLOGY

Prevalence

According to a study of the global estimates of prevalence and risk factors for PAD, prevalence has increased across all ages in HICs and LMICs (Fowkes and others 2013). Four models of PAD prevalence by age and gender in HICs and LMICs are shown in figure 14.1. The prevalence of PAD in HICs is not meaningfully different between men and women. Prevalence at ages 40–44 years was 4.6 percent (95 percent confidence interval [CI] 2.6–7.9 percent) in men and 4.5 percent (95 percent CI 2.6–7.6 percent) in women; at ages 80–84 years, prevalence was 16.3 percent (95 percent CI 11.2–23.2 percent) in men and 15.9 percent (95 percent CI 10.4–23.6 percent) in women.

In LMICs, the prevalence of PAD was consistently higher in women than in men, although the differences were attenuated with increasing age. At ages 40–45 years, prevalence was 5.6 percent (95 percent CI 4.1–7.7 percent) in women and 2.3 percent (95 percent CI 1.5–3.5 percent) in men; at ages 80–84 years, it was 13.7 percent (95 percent CI 10.2–18.1 percent) in women and 12.3 percent (95 percent CI 8.4–17.7 percent) in men. At all ages up to 60–64 years prevalence was consistently higher in HICs compared with LMICs.

The number of people with PAD increased by 23.5 percent from 164 million in 2000 to 202 million in 2010. The proportional increase was higher in LMICs than in HICs (28.7 percent versus 13.1 percent). In LMICs, gender differences in the increase in PAD cases paralleled noted differences in prevalence. In Sub-Saharan Africa, more women in 2010 had PAD than did men (9.9 million versus 4.4 million); the estimated prevalence in women was twice the prevalence in men for all ages younger than 60 years. Overall, in 2010 the largest number of people with PAD were in the Southeast Asia and Western Pacific regions; most cases in these regions were in people younger than age 55 years (figure 14.2).

Risk Factors for PAD

In addition to age, the risk factors significantly associated with PAD in HICs and LMICs were smoking and history of cardiovascular disease, diabetes, hypertension, and hypercholesterolemia (Fowkes and others 2013).

- *Current smoking.* The estimates were meta–odds ratio (meta-OR) 2.7 (95 percent CI 2.4–3.1) in HICs and 1.4 (1.3–1.6) in LMICs; those for former smoking were 2.0 (1.7–2.4) and 1.5 (1.1–1.9), respectively.
- *History of cardiovascular disease.* The estimates were 2.6 (2.2–3.0) and 1.8 (1.4–2.2) in HICs and LMICs, respectively.
- *Diabetes.* The estimates were 1.9 (1.7–2.1) and 1.5 (1.3–1.7) in HICs and LMICs, respectively.

Figure 14.1 Prevalence of Peripheral Artery Disease by Age in Men and Women in High-Income and Low- and Middle-Income Countries

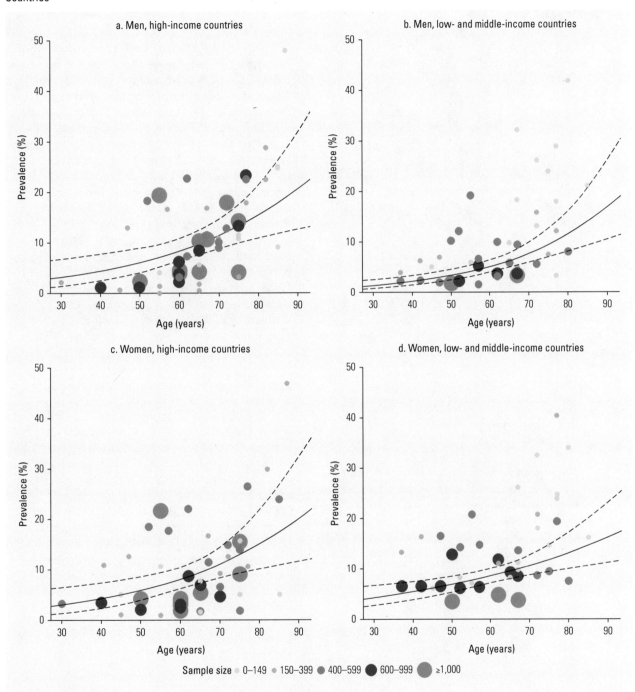

a. Men, high-income countries

b. Men, low- and middle-income countries

c. Women, high-income countries

d. Women, low- and middle-income countries

Sample size ● 0–149 ● 150–399 ● 400–599 ● 600–999 ● ≥1,000

Source: Fowkes and others 2013.
Note: Size and color of circles equivalent to sample size of population from which datapoint was derived. At younger (< 40 years) and older (> 80 years) ages, regression lines are based on projection only or on very few datapoints. Akaike Information Criterion for model goodness of fit: male high-income countries 1,974.72; male low-income or middle-income countries 838.36; female high-income countries 1,971.59; female low-income or middle-income countries 1,115.09.

Figure 14.2 Estimate of the Number of Cases of PAD and Contributing Age Groups in Eight High-Income and Low- and Middle-Income Regions, 2010

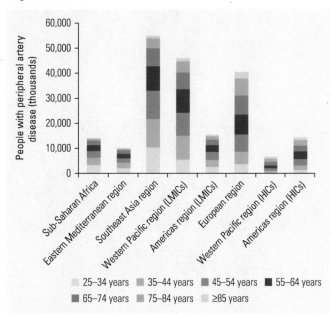

Source: Fowkes and others 2013.
Note: HICs = high-income countries; LMICs = low- and middle-income countries; PAD = peripheral artery disease.

- *Hypertension.* The estimates were 1.6 (1.4–1.7) and 1.4 (1.2–1.5) in HICs and LMICs, respectively.
- *Hypercholesterolemia.* The estimates were 1.2 (1.1–1.3) and 1.1 (1.0–1.3) in HICs and LMICs, respectively.

Globally, there was a statistically significant association between gender and PAD, with observed decreased risk for men compared with women (meta-OR 0.8, 95 percent CI 0.7–0.9). However, men were at increased risk in HICs but at much decreased risk in LMICs: meta-OR 1.4 (95 percent CI 1.2–1.7) versus meta-OR 0.5 (95 percent CI 0.4–0.6).

Trends in Burden by Age and Gender

The age-specific death rates per 100,000 population associated with PAD in 1990 ranged from 0.05 (95 percent CI 0.03–0.09) among those ages 40–44 years to 16.6 (95 percent CI 10.5–25.3) in ages 80 years and older (Sampson and others 2014). The corresponding estimates in 2010 were 0.07 (95 percent CI 0.04–0.13) and 28.7 (95 percent CI 18.3–43.1). In both 1990 and 2010, the death rate consistently increased with increasing age; in all age categories, the 2010 rates exceeded the 1990 rates.

Regional estimates of PAD death rates are shown in figure 14.3. The highest death rates in 1990 and 2010 were in Australasia; North America, high income; and

Western Europe. The Caribbean, Central Europe, southern Sub-Saharan Africa, tropical Latin America, and East Asia regions also ranked high. The death rates increased from 0.07 (95 percent CI 0.04–0.13) in 1990 to 0.44 (95 percent CI 0.18–0.69) in 2010 in the Asia Pacific high-income region (figure 14.3). However the relative change in median death rate was +6.03 (95 percent CI 1.5–11.8) and was largely driven by women: +17.4 (95 percent CI 1.8–32.0) versus +1.3 (95 percent CI 0.1–2.4) in men. Similarly, a remarkable relative change in median death rate of +3.7 (95 percent CI 1.7–7.6) was observed in Oceania and was driven by a relative change of +4.8 (95 percent CI 2.1–9.7) in women versus +1.6 (95 percent CI 0.7–3.6) in men. The overall relative change in median death rate in HICs was higher in women than men (figure 14.4).

Generally, the changes in regional death rates were more striking among women compared with men between 1990 and 2010 (panels a and b of figure 14.5). Figure 14.6 provides estimates of age-specific death rates attributed to PAD for all regions, demonstrating increases in death rates by age in all regions between 1990 and 2010.

EFFECTIVENESS OF INTERVENTIONS

The main goals in treating patients with PAD are to reduce the risks of adverse cardiovascular outcomes, improve functional capacity, and preserve limb viability. Patients with atherosclerotic PAD in the lower limbs typically present to clinicians with intermittent claudication. Less commonly, they may present with critical limb ischemia, which is more severe and involves pain at rest, ulceration, or gangrene. The management of intermittent claudication and critical limb ischemia may be quite different, and the effectiveness of treatments needs to be considered separately. There are reasons for the different treatment approaches: The risk of limb loss in patients with functional ischemia is low, and the primary goal of treatment is the quality of life. In patients with critical ischemia, the primary goal is limb salvage.

Intermittent Claudication

In assessing the effectiveness of treatments for intermittent claudication, the main outcome measure is the additional distance that patients can walk. This measure may be pain-free walking distance (PFWD) until the onset of claudication or maximum walking distance until stopping walking because of pain. For many years, a large number of medications were advocated for improving walking distance. Now, however, only three—cilostazol, naftidrofuryl, and pentoxifylline—tend to be used in clinical practice; this approach may vary by country because of guidelines, availability, and resource limitations. In recent Cochrane reviews, cilostazol compared with placebo was found to increase PFWD by a mean of 31 meters (95 percent CI 22–40) (Bedenis and others 2014) and naftidrofuryl increased PFWD by 48 meters (95 percent CI 36–61) (de Backer and others 2012). A meta-analysis of trials of pentoxifylline showed an increase in maximum walking distance of 59 meters (95 percent CI 37–81) (Momsen and others 2009).

Regular exercise, in which patients undergo a supervised training program, has been evaluated as a method of improving walking distance (Fakhry and others 2012). The training programs and methods of supervision vary in approach and intensity. A meta-analysis of trials found a mean improvement of 109 meters (95 percent CI 38–180) (Lane and others 2014), suggesting that exercise therapy is more effective than pharmacotherapy. However, such programs are resource intensive. Unsupervised exercise regimes have been evaluated, but they were not as effective as supervised programs (Fokkenrood and others 2013). Although the long-term durability favors supervised exercise, the uptake for such exercise programs is variable and the drop-out rate is high.

In specialist vascular centers, endovascular therapy may be used for more intractable cases of claudication. Among the many techniques of endovascular therapy, balloon angioplasty is one of the simplest and most commonly used. The results are comparable to exercise therapy (Liu and others 2014); however, following angioplasty, restenosis is a frequent occurrence within a few years. Open bypass surgery is not commonly used for the treatment of claudication, and its effectiveness compared with endovascular therapy is not clearly known.

Critical Limb Ischemia

Critical limb ischemia is a very serious condition, which, if untreated, can lead to limb loss with associated significant disabilities; it can also lead to death. The principal outcomes of treatment are survival and limb salvage to avoid amputation. The two treatment options are bypass surgery and endovascular therapy; to date, only one major comparative trial has been conducted in an HIC (Adam and others 2005). Amputation-free survival did not differ significantly between the two approaches after six months of follow-up (hazard ratio 0.73, 95 percent CI 0.49–1.07).

If open surgery or endovascular therapy is unavailable, primary amputation may be the preferred treatment.

Figure 14.3 Death Rates per 100,000 Population Attributed to Peripheral Artery Disease and Relative Change in Median Death Rates, by GBD 2010 Region, 1990 and 2010

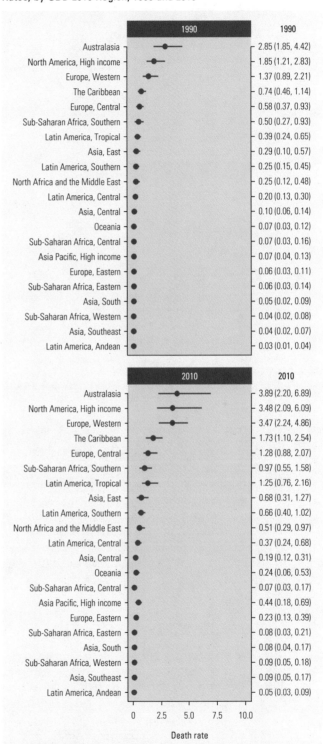

Source: © Global Heart. Reproduced, with permission, from Sampson and others 2014; further permission required for reuse.

Note: GBD 2010 = Global Burden of Disease study 2010. The dots denote estimates of mean death rates attributed to peripheral artery disease in all GBD regions. The parenthetical numbers are the corresponding 95 percent confidence intervals.

Figure 14.4 Relative Change in Median Death Rates per 100,000 Population, by Country Development Status, 1990 and 2010

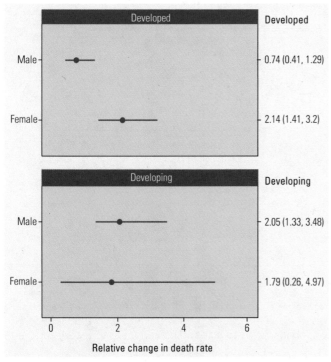

Source: © *Global Heart.* Reproduced with permission from Sampson and others 2014; further permission required for reuse.
Note: The dots denote the relative change in median death rates attributed to peripheral artery disease in developed and developing countries by gender. The parenthetical numbers are the corresponding 95 percent confidence intervals.

In patients deemed high risk for endovascular therapy or surgery, prostanoid medications may be tried. A systematic review of trials of prostanoids, compared with other pharmacological preparations or placebo, found no differences in rates of amputation or mortality; it did find some improvements in pain relief (relative risk 1.3, 95 percent CI 1.1–1.6) and ulcer healing (relative risk 1.5, 95 percent CI 1.2–2.0) (Ruffolo, Romano, and Ciapponi 2010).

COST-EFFECTIVENESS OF INTERVENTIONS

Very little research has been conducted on the cost-effectiveness of treatments for PAD; the research conducted has primarily focused on HICs. In treating claudication, medications to improve walking distance are moderately expensive in LMICs (approximately US$3 per day), have limited effectiveness, and need to be continued throughout life. Exercise therapy has been shown to be more cost-effective than endovascular treatment; however, the cost per quality-adjusted life year gained of approximately US$8,000 in 2013 (Mazari and

others 2013) makes it too expensive for most LMICs. Furthermore, the feasibility of establishing suitable programs is difficult. For LMICs, the treatment of claudication needs to rely instead on the simple, well-established advice to patients to "stop smoking and keep walking" (Housley 1988).

In treating critical limb ischemia, the cost-effectiveness of the two key treatments of bypass surgery and angioplasty have been compared in one randomized controlled trial; the cost of angioplasty per quality-adjusted life year gained was found to be less than for bypass surgery (Forbes and others 2010). However, the two treatments need to be carried out in specialized vascular centers, which are not available in most LMICs. The high costs of the procedures—US$25,000–US$35,000 in the United Kingdom in 2010—may not justify their use in most LMICs.

The range of PAD treatments in HICs may not be justified for most LMICs. If the critical limb ischemia is life threatening, amputation may be more appropriate in these settings; this procedure can usually be provided in a first-level hospital. Otherwise, conservative medical therapy to relieve pain and infection is likely to be the most feasible approach. The high cost of prostanoid drugs and their limited benefits make them inappropriate in this setting. The emphasis is better placed instead on secondary prevention of major cardiovascular events. Smoking cessation, lipid lowering, diabetic control, antihypertensives, and antiplatelets are relatively inexpensive; the costs and substantial benefits in patients with PAD are similar to those for other cardiovascular diseases (see chapter 19 in this volume, Gaziano and others 2017).

Rationale of Interventions

The observed trends in global PAD epidemiology indicate a rising burden in LMICs with increasing involvement of younger adults and women, raising concerns and requiring targeted cost-effective responses. An array of interventions for PAD is available, including comprehensive control of risk factors and resource-intensive interventions such as endovascular and other surgical treatments for claudication and critical limb ischemia. The resource challenges in LMICs preclude reliance on surgical and emergency services to handle the increases in the number of patients with chronic claudication who may require elective or emergency revascularization procedures or limb amputation. In these settings, prevention and early disease management through risk factor control may be the most realistic strategies. The observed trends suggesting that increased exposure to PAD risk factors is occurring at relatively young ages

Figure 14.5 Death Rates per 100,000 Population Attributed to Peripheral Artery Disease, by GBD 2010 Region, 1990 and 2010

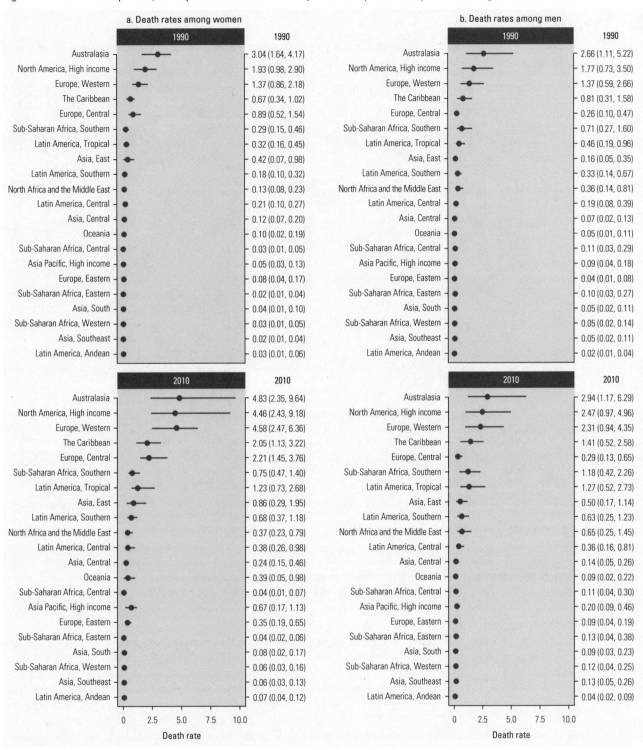

Source: © *Global Heart.* Reproduced, with permission, from Sampson and others 2014; further permission required for reuse.
Note: GBD 2010 = Global Burden of Disease study 2010. The dots denote estimates of mean death rates attributable to peripheral artery disease in all GBD regions. The parenthetical numbers are the corresponding 95 percent confidence intervals.

Figure 14.6 Death Rates Attributed to Peripheral Artery Disease by GBD Region and Age Group, 1990 and 2010

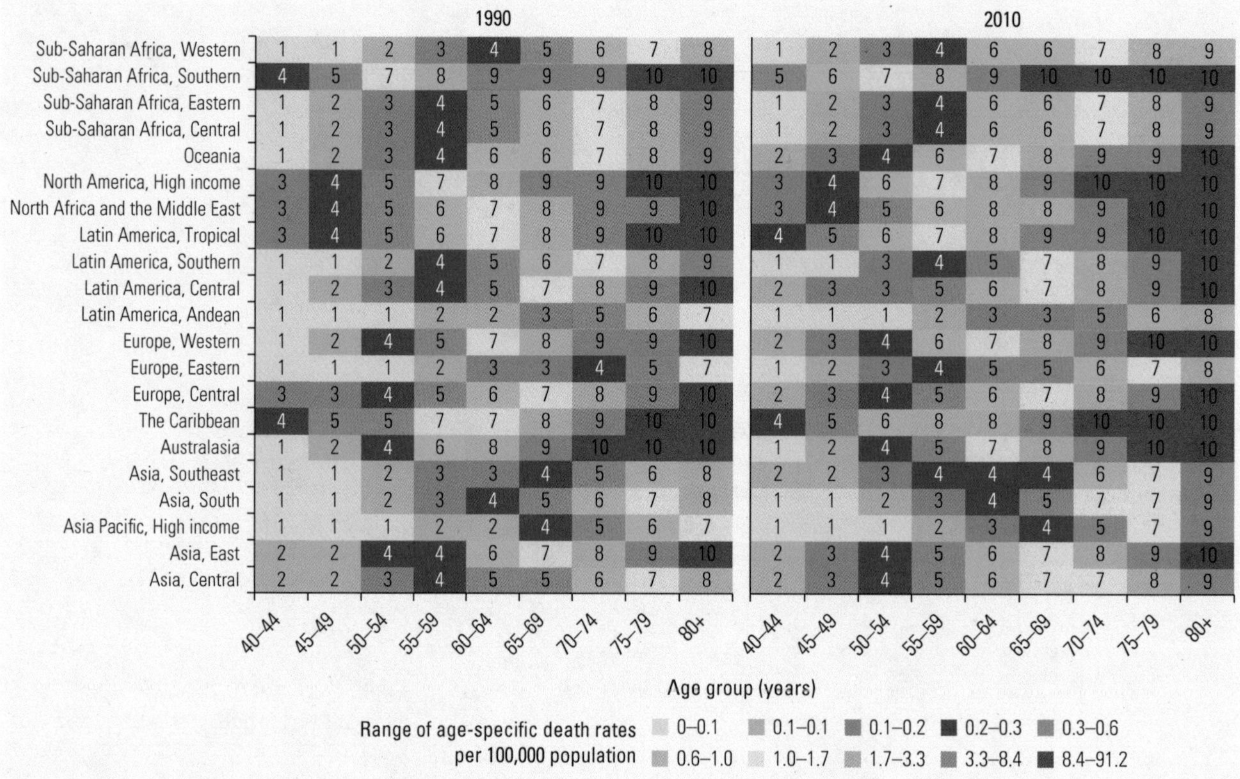

Source: © Global Heart. Reproduced, with permission, from Sampson and others 2014; further permission required for reuse.
Note: GBD = Global Burden of Disease. The figure provides estimates of age-specific death rates attributed to peripheral artery disease for all GBD regions. Each color-coded box represents a range of age-specific death rates for a GBD region. Color gradations (also delineated by numbers within the color-coded boxes) represent different tiers of death rates. The color gradient from blue to green to orange to red (or increasing numbers) observed with increasing age indicates increases in death rates by age in all regions in 1990 and 2010. Age groups are in years, and the rates are per 100,000 population.

underscores the merits of risk factor control (Fowkes and others 2013).

Targeting risk factors may be the most cost-effective approach for both prevention and early disease management and may yield good return on investment. The potential gain from this approach is amplified by the fact that the risk factors for PAD are common to other cardiovascular diseases that have emerged as leading causes of morbidity and mortality in both HICs and LMICs.

CONCLUSIONS

PAD is a global problem, evidenced by increased associated disability and mortality and a striking relative increase in the burden of disease in LMICs. The rising disease burden among women and increased involvement of young adults indicate that PAD is no longer limited to men or elderly persons.

Governments, nongovernmental organizations, and private sectors in LMICs need to address the social and economic impacts and evaluate the best strategies for optimal treatment and prevention (Papia and others 2015). Risk factor control could be a key part of a coordinated response to the increased PAD burden, especially in LMICs where health systems are not sufficiently robust to handle an increased number of patients with chronic PAD. In these settings, the scarcity of surgical services, especially emergency services, will lead to unmet need for elective or emergency peripheral artery revascularization procedures or limb amputations. Potential response approaches may include the combination of environmental, policy, and legislative interventions for health promotion and primary prevention, coupled with improved access to evaluation, diagnosis, and treatment, as well as control of major risk factors using evidence-based treatments that are affordable in low-resource settings.

NOTE

World Bank Income Classifications as of July 2014 are as follows, based on estimates of gross national income (GNI) per capita for 2013:

- Low-income countries (LICs) = US$1,045 or less
- Middle-income countries (MICs) are subdivided:
  (a) lower-middle-income = US$1,046 to US$4,125
  (b) upper-middle-income (UMICs) = US$4,126 to US$12,745
- High-income countries (HICs) = US$12,746 or more.

REFERENCES

Aboyans, V., M. H. Criqui, P. Abraham, M. A. Allison, M. A. Creager, and others. 2012. "Measurement and Interpretation of the Ankle-Brachial Index: A Scientific Statement from the American Heart Association." *Circulation* 126 (24): 2890–909.

Adam, D. J., J. D. Beard, T. Cleveland, J. Bell, A. W. Bradbury, and others. 2005. "Bypass versus Angioplasty in Severe Ischaemia of the Leg (BASIL): Multicentre, Randomised Controlled Trial." *The Lancet* 366 (9501): 1925–34.

Bedenis, R., M. Stewart, M. Cleanthis, P. Robless, D. P. Mikhailidis, and G. Stansby. 2014. "Cilostazol for Intermittent Claudication." *Cochrane Database of Systematic Reviews* 10: CD003748. doi:10.1002/14651858.CD003748 .pub4.

Caro, J., K. Migliaccio-Walle, K. J. Ishak, and I. Proskorovsky. 2005. "The Morbidity and Mortality Following a Diagnosis of Peripheral Arterial Disease: Long-Term Follow-up of a Large Database." *BMC Cardiovascular Disorders* 5: 14.

Criqui, M. H., R. D. Langer, A. Fronek, H. S. Feigelson, M. R. Klauber, and others. 1992. "Mortality over a Period of 10 Years in Patients with Peripheral Arterial Disease." *New England Journal of Medicine* 326 (6): 381–86.

de Backer, T. L. M., R. Vander Stichele, P. Lehert, and L. Van Bortel. 2012. "Naftidrofuryl for Intermittent Claudication." *Cochrane Database of Systematic Reviews* 12: CD001368. doi:10.1002/14651858.CD001368.pub4.

Dormandy, J. A., and R. B. Rutherford. 2000. "Management of Peripheral Arterial Disease (PAD). TASC Working Group. TransAtlantic Inter-Society Consensus (TASC)." *Journal of Vascular Surgery* 31 (1 Pt 2): S1–296.

Fakhry, F., K. M. van de Luijtgaarden, L. Bax, P. T. den Hoed, M. G. Hunink, and others. 2012. "Supervised Walking Therapy in Patients with Intermittent Claudication." *Journal of Vascular Surgery* 56 (4): 1132–42.

Fokkenrood, H. J. P., B. L. W. Bendermacher, G. J. Lauret, E. M. Willigendael, M. H. Prins, and others. 2013. "Supervised Exercise Therapy versus Non-Supervised Exercise Therapy for Intermittent Claudication." *Cochrane Database of Systematic Reviews* 8: CD005263. doi:10.1002/14651858.CD005263.pub3.

Forbes, J. F., D. J. Adam, J. Bell, F. G. Fowkes, I. Gillespie, and others. 2010. "Bypass versus Angioplasty in Severe Ischaemia of the Leg (BASIL) Trial: Health-Related Quality of Life Outcomes, Resource Utilization, and Cost-Effectiveness Analysis." *Journal of Vascular Surgery* 51 (Suppl 5): S43S–51.

Fowkes, F. G., D. Rudan, I. Rudan, V. Aboyans, J. O. Denenberg, and others. 2013. "Comparison of Global Estimates of Prevalence and Risk Factors for Peripheral Artery Disease in 2000 and 2010: A Systematic Review and Analysis." *The Lancet* 382 (9901): 1329–40.

Gaziano, T. A., M. Suhrcke, E. Brouwer, C. Levin, I. Nikolic, and R. Nugent. 2017. "Costs and Cost-Effectiveness of Interventions and Policies to Prevent and Treat Cardiovascular and Respiratory Diseases." In *Disease Control Priorities* (third edition): Volume 5, *Cardiovascular, Respiratory, and Related Disorders*, edited by D. Prabhakaran, S. Anand, T. A. Gaziano, J.-C. Mbanya, Y. Wu, and R. Nugent. Washington, DC: World Bank.

getABI Study Group. 2002. "getABI: German Epidemiological Trial on Ankle Brachial Index for Elderly Patients in Family Practice to Detect Peripheral Arterial Disease, Significant Marker for High Mortality." *Vasa* 31 (4): 241–48.

Housley, E. 1988. "Treating Claudication in Five Words." *British Medical Journal (Clinical Research Edition)* 296 (6635): 1483–84.

Kullo, I. J., and T. W. Rooke. 2016. "Clinical Practice: Peripheral Artery Disease." *New England Journal of Medicine* 374 (9): 861–71.

Lane, R., B. Ellis, L. Watson, and G. C. Leng. 2014. "Exercise for Intermittent Claudication." *Cochrane Database of Systematic Reviews* 7: CD000990. doi:10.1002/14651858 .CD000990.pub3.

Liu, J., Y. Wu, Z. Li, W. Li, and S. Wang. 2014. "Endovascular Treatment for Intermittent Claudication in Patients with Peripheral Arterial Disease: A Systematic Review." *Annals of Vascular Surgery* 28 (4): 977–82.

Mazari, F. A., J. A. Khan, D. Carradice, N. Samuel, R. Gohil, and others. 2013. "Economic Analysis of a Randomized Trial of Percutaneous Angioplasty, Supervised Exercise or Combined Treatment for Intermittent Claudication due to Femoropopliteal Arterial Disease." *British Journal of Surgery* 100 (9): 1172–79.

Momsen, A. H., M. B. Jensen, C. B. Norager, M. R. Madsen, T. Vestersgaard-Andersen, and others. 2009. "Drug Therapy for Improving Walking Distance in Intermittent Claudication: A Systematic Review and Meta-Analysis of Robust Randomised Controlled Studies." *European Journal of Vascular and Endovascular Surgery* 38 (4): 463–74.

Pande, R. L., T. S. Perlstein, J. A. Beckman, and M. A. Creager. 2011. "Secondary Prevention and Mortality in Peripheral Artery Disease: National Health and Nutrition Examination Study, 1999 to 2004." *Circulation* 124 (1): 17–23.

Papia, G., P. Mayer, D. Kelton, D. Queen, J. A. Elliott, and J. L. Kuhnke. 2015. "Just Leg Pain? Think Again: What Health Leaders Must Know about Peripheral Arterial Disease." *Healthcare Management Forum* 28 (Suppl 6): S5–9.

Rooke, T. W., A. T. Hirsch, S. Misra, A. N. Sidawy, J. A. Beckman, and others. 2011. "2011 ACCF/AHA Focused Update of the Guideline for the Management of Patients with Peripheral Artery Disease (Updating the 2005 Guideline): A Report of the American College of Cardiology Foundation/American Heart Association Task Force on Practice Guidelines." *Journal of the American College of Cardiology* 58 (19): 2020–45.

Ruffolo, A. J., M. Romano, and A. Ciapponi. 2010. "Prostanoids for Critical Limb Ischaemia." *Cochrane Database of Systematic Reviews* 1: CD006544. doi:10.1002/14651858 .CD006544.pub2.

Sampson, U. K., F. G. Fowkes, M. M. McDermott, M. H. Criqui, V. Aboyans, and others. 2014. "Global and Regional Burden of Death and Disability from Peripheral Artery Disease: 21 World Regions, 1990 to 2010." *Global Heart* 9 (1): 145–58 e121.

Saw, J., D. L. Bhatt, D. J. Moliterno, S. J. Brener, S. R. Steinhubl, and others. 2006. "The Influence of Peripheral Arterial Disease on Outcomes: A Pooled Analysis of Mortality in Eight Large Randomized Percutaneous Coronary Intervention Trials." *Journal of the American College of Cardiology* 48 (8): 1567–72.

Sigvant, B., F. Lundin, and E. Wahlberg. 2016. "The Risk of Disease Progression in Peripheral Arterial Disease Is Higher than Expected: A Meta-Analysis of Mortality and Disease Progression in Peripheral Arterial Disease." *European Journal of Vascular and Endovascular Surgery* 51 (3): 395–403.

Chapter 15

Chronic Lower Respiratory Tract Diseases

Peter Burney, Rogelio Perez-Padilla, Guy Marks, Gary Wong,
Eric Bateman, and Deborah Jarvis

INTRODUCTION

Chronic respiratory diseases are common and increasing in relative terms as causes of disability and death. They refer to noninfectious conditions of the lung and respiratory tract, excluding cancers and trauma. In the *International Classification of Diseases*, they are covered mostly in chapter X (table 15.1) (WHO 2010). This chapter focuses on the more common of these conditions, but we have been influenced by the availability of data. Not addressed are two common conditions of the upper respiratory tract—allergic and chronic rhinosinusitis—that cause considerable disability but are not associated with substantial mortality. Smoking cessation and reduction or elimination of other harmful exposures is an important component of the management of any chronic respiratory disease. Tobacco cessation is addressed in chapter 4 in this volume (Roy and others 2017) and in chapter 10 of volume 3 (Jha and others 2015).

The two main conditions contributing to death and disability are asthma and chronic obstructive pulmonary disease (COPD). Both are clinical diagnoses and are associated with narrowed airways and difficulty exhaling. Asthma has become more common in many countries in parallel with increasing prevalence of allergic sensitization. COPD, in particular, is an increasing burden as the world's population ages and tobacco smoking increases in many low- and middle-income countries (LMICs), especially among women. The effects of both diseases and mortality from all causes tend to be greater in persons with smaller lungs, and smaller lung volumes are more common in LMICs.

Although these diseases are rarely curable, effective treatments to reduce both disability and death are available and affordable.

DISTRIBUTION OF DISEASE, DISEASE BURDEN, RISK FACTORS, AND PRIMARY PREVENTION

Asthma

Asthma is a common cause of morbidity in children and adults; it is generally amenable to treatment with effective low-cost medications that have minimal long-term adverse side effects. An estimated 300 million people worldwide suffer from asthma; more than 250,000 asthma-related deaths occur annually. Asthma ranks forty-second in the list of diseases and conditions that cause death globally (Lozano and others 2013), but fourteenth in the list of causes of years lived with disability (Salomon and others 2012; Vos and others 2012). The disease generally has an early onset and tends to persist throughout life; deaths among young people with asthma are rare.

The prevalence of asthma has been increasing, although this increase may be slowing or even reversing in some countries. In LMICs, very low prevalence has been recorded in rural compared with urban environments (Calvert and Burney 2005; Keeley and Gallivan 1991;

Corresponding author: P. G. J. Burney, National Heart and Lung Institute, Imperial College, London, United Kingdom; P.burney@imperial.ac.uk.

Table 15.1 Principal Rubrics of the International Classification of Diseases, 10th Revision, Covered in This Chapter

J40–J47 Chronic lower respiratory diseases:

- J40 Bronchitis, not specified as acute or chronic
- J41 Simple and mucopurulent chronic bronchitis
- J42 Unspecified chronic bronchitis
- J43 Emphysema
- J44 Other chronic obstructive pulmonary disease
- J45 Asthma
- J46 Status asthmaticus
- J47 Bronchiectasis

J60–J70 Lung diseases due to external agents:

- J60 Coalworker's pneumoconiosis
- J61 Pneumoconiosis due to asbestos and other mineral fibres
- J62 Pneumoconiosis due to dust containing silica
- J63 Pneumoconiosis due to other inorganic dusts
- J64 Unspecified pneumoconiosis
- J65 Pneumoconiosis associated with tuberculosis
- J66 Airway disease due to specific organic dust
- J67 Hypersensitivity pneumonitis due to organic dust
- J68 Respiratory conditions due to inhalation of chemicals, gases, fumes and vapours
- J69 Pneumonitis due to solids and liquids
- J70 Respiratory conditions due to other external agents

J80–J84 Other respiratory diseases principally affecting the interstitium:

- J84 Other interstitial pulmonary diseases

Source: WHO 2010.

Perzanowski and others 2002), but the prevalence in LMICs is likely to rise as they become more urbanized. The increased prevalence in urban populations is associated with an increase in positive skin tests to allergens, which is explained in part by increases in body mass index (Calvert and Burney 2005) and in part by the quality of the urban diet (Hooper and others 2008). Within urban communities, socioeconomic deprivation is associated with more frequent symptoms and exacerbations of asthma, use of emergency services, hospitalizations, and mortality, likely due to lower access to effective therapy and health services (Poyser and others 2002).

Consistent with these findings, prevalence rates vary widely for children and adults. The first phase of the International Study of Asthma and Allergies in Childhood provided findings for 463,801 children ages 13–14 years (155 centers in 56 countries) and 257,800 children ages 6–7 years (91 centers in 38 countries) (Asher and others 1998). The prevalence of asthma

symptoms was based on a positive response to the question, "Have you had wheezing or whistling in the chest in the last 12 months?" For younger and older children, there was an approximate 20-fold range of prevalence, with the highest rates generally in countries with high gross national income (GNI) as defined by the World Bank, but severe asthma was proportionally more common in low-income areas of Africa and South and South-East Asia (Lai and others 2009).

The World Health Survey interviewed adults older than age 18 years on six continents using questions derived from the European Community Respiratory Health Survey on wheezing and on diagnosed asthma (Sembajwe and others 2010). The prevalence of diagnosed asthma ranged from 2 percent in Vietnam to 33 percent in Australia. The lowest mean prevalence was found in middle-income countries; however, the percentage of sites with prevalence greater than 10 percent rose from 19 percent (4 of 21) in the countries with the lowest income (less than US$3,000) to 59 percent (10 of 17) in countries with intermediate incomes (US$7,999) and to 73 percent (22 of 30) in countries with per capita incomes greater than US$8,000 per year.

Asthma runs in families, but the basis for inheritance is complex; the observation that up to 30 percent of childhood asthma is related to genetics needs further study (Moffatt and others 2010), but evidence for heritability is less strong for adults. Asthma is associated with allergy, and both allergy and allergic asthma are less common in poorer countries (Weinmayr and others 2010); nonallergic wheeze is distributed fairly evenly by levels of poverty. Many risk factors have been associated with the onset of disease and with disease exacerbations. Risk factors for disease onset that are potentially remediable include parental (and even grandparental) smoking, obesity, poor diet, and workplace exposure to allergens. Evidence for dietary factors preventing asthma is inconclusive; studies with improved design are needed (Nurmatov, Devereux, and Sheikh 2011). Adult-onset asthma caused by occupational exposures are preventable by appropriate measures to limit exposures in the workplace and by screening of exposed workers to detect early signs of disease. Exacerbations are associated with viral upper respiratory tract infections, especially in children, and with exposure to airborne allergens in the outdoor environment; these factors are more difficult to avoid.

Most people with asthma develop symptoms in childhood. During adolescence, symptoms of the disease remit in up to 40 percent of cases; however, in approximately 50 percent of these cases, for unknown reasons, symptoms return during adult life. Asthma that begins in adult life tends to be more severe and is more common in women; exposure to cigarette smoke and an inadequate intake of antioxidants may play a role (Larkin and others 2015).

Death rates from asthma are relatively low, but are higher in older adults than in children or young adults (Lozano and others 2013). In countries with efficient programs for diagnosing and treating asthma, death rates of less than 1 per 1 million population are being achieved. Accordingly, from a public health perspective, asthma deaths need to be viewed as preventable. Poorly controlled asthma is also a risk factor for the development of fixed airway obstruction in later life (Obaseki and others 2014).

Chronic Airway Obstruction and COPD

Chronic airway obstruction is defined as the ratio of one-second forced expiratory volume (FEV_1) to vital capacity (VC). FEV_1 is the volume of air that can be blown out with maximum force from a full inspiration in one second. VC is the maximum volume of air that can be expired from a full inspiration in one breath and is generally measured as forced vital capacity (FVC) in the same maneuver as FEV_1. VC and FVC are measures of lung size, and FEV_1 is a measure of flow over the first second of expiration; the FEV_1/FVC ratio is a measure of flow adjusted for lung size.

This section focuses on irreversible obstruction: the presence of a low FEV_1/FVC ratio following administration of a bronchodilator. There has been debate about the best index for measuring irreversible obstruction. The Global Initiative for Chronic Obstructive Lung Disease (GOLD 2014) has recommended a single index for all ages—a fixed FEV_1/FVC ratio of 0.7. However, because this ratio declines universally with age, an alternative approach is to define a low ratio as being a value below the lower limit of normal (Miller and others 2005; Swanney and others 2008). The lower limit of normal is the level of FEV_1/FVC exceeded in 95 percent of the normal population, generally defined as persons who have never smoked and have no respiratory diagnosis and (sometimes) no respiratory symptoms. This measure takes account of the person's age. The ratio is affected by age and disease, but does not seem to be affected by other factors, such as height, gender, and ethnicity (Hankinson, Odencrantz, and Fedan 1999).

COPD is the most common cause of chronic airflow limitation. In COPD, obstruction arises because the small airways either are narrowed or are obstructed by inflammation (small airway disease) or because, as in emphysema, lung tissue is destroyed and loses elasticity, which is required for keeping airways open during exhalation. In chronic asthma, bronchoconstriction, that is, thickening of airway walls due to predominantly allergic inflammation, edema, an increase in smooth muscle, and some subtle scar tissue, narrows the airways.

Lung function may be tested before or after inhalation of a bronchodilator to increase the caliber of the airway. Prebronchodilator obstruction that reverses after a bronchodilator is administered is described as reversible obstruction, and demonstrating this at some stage is considered necessary for the diagnosis of asthma. Up to two-thirds of patients with COPD show evidence of improvement of obstruction, but it is generally of a lesser magnitude. Increases of more than 400 milliliters (ml) suggest a diagnosis of asthma. Among the normal population, 95 percent have an increase of FEV_1 of less than 12 percent of baseline value following administration of 200 micrograms inhaled salbutamol (Tan and others 2012).

Although family studies suggest that approximately 50 percent of the variation in lung function is due to genetic factors, only a very small part of this variation has been attributed to specific genes (Loth and others 2014). Globally, the most common reason for a low postbronchodilator FEV_1/FVC ratio is smoking. Smoking in adolescence prevents FEV_1 from developing to its full potential (Jaakkola and others 1991); continuing smokers have a dose-related decline in FEV_1 of about 10–15 ml per year greater than that of never smokers, former smokers, or quitters (U.S. Surgeon General 1984). Lung function returns to normal rates on cessation of smoking, but FEV_1 does not recover more than about 200 ml (Dockery and others 1988). Passive smoking is also associated with loss of FEV_1/FVC ratio (Hooper and others 2012). Figure 15.1 shows the prevalence of a low FEV_1/FVC ratio in the Burden of Obstructive Lung Disease study, defined as the lower limit of normal for men and women plotted against the mean pack years of cigarettes smoked (Burney and others 2014). The two measures are strongly associated, as are the ratio and the prevalence of ratios below the lower limit of normal. Where smoking is rare, the prevalence of a low FEV_1/FVC ratio is close to 5 percent, the value expected, by definition, in a normal population without known respiratory disease.

Other associations with chronic airway obstruction include a history of tuberculosis (Allwood, Myer, and Bateman 2013), occupational exposures to dust, a low body mass index, and age (Hooper and others 2012). A history of tuberculosis is more strongly associated with airway obstruction than it is with restrictive spirometry (low FVC) (Hooper and others 2012; Hwang and others 2014; Lam and others 2010; Menezes and others 2007). Studies have found a protective effect

Figure 15.1 Prevalence of a Low FEV$_1$/FVC Ratio (below the Lower Limit of Normal) in the BOLD Study Plotted against the Mean Pack Years of Cigarettes Smoked

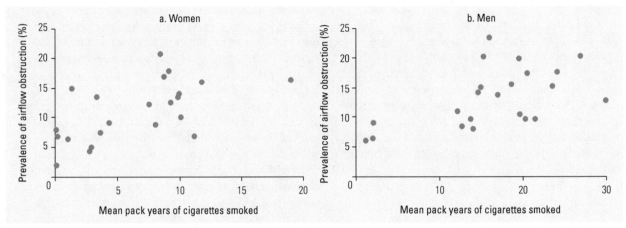

Source: Burney and others 2014.
Note: BOLD = Burden of Obstructive Lung Disease; FEV$_1$ = one-second forced expiratory volume; FVC = forced vital capacity.

on lung function from a healthy diet, characterized by high intake of fiber, fruits, and vegetables and low intake of simple sugars and saturated fats (Root and others 2014; Shaheen and others 2001). An adverse effect of processed meats has also been described (Varraso and others 2007). There is an association with age after adjustment of lung function for age and for years smoking (Hooper and others 2012). Because the evidence of an association with age comes largely from cross-sectional studies, there are two possible explanations: another environmental risk that is associated with cumulative reduction in FEV$_1$ and an effect associated with year of birth rather than with age, that is, a birth-cohort effect. The latter effect implies the appearance of a risk factor in early life that has a persistent effect over the life course and that may affect succeeding generations differently.

Two risk factors commonly associated with obstruction are air pollution, particularly indoor air pollution, and occupational exposures, but evidence that these risk factors are important is less convincing. They are associated with increased symptoms of bronchitis, frequency of acute exacerbations (lung attacks), and even effects on mortality when lifetime exposures are considered (Hansell and others 2016), but evidence of an effect on the FEV$_1$/FVC ratio has been less consistent, at least in studies of the general population (Hooper and others 2012; Schikowski and others 2014; Smith and others 2014). It has, however, been argued that a coherence in the evidence relating to different sources of particulate pollution from cigarette smoking, indoor sources, and outdoor sources suggests that all of these factors play a part (Burnett and others 2014).

Idiopathic Low FVC

Low FEV$_1$ is associated with several comorbidities and an increase in overall mortality. This condition is associated with low total lung capacity (Pedone and others 2012) and low FVC (Burney and Hooper 2011; Fried and others 1998; Kannel and others 1980); it is not associated with airflow obstruction. In clinical medicine, low FVC is generally linked to specific restrictive lung diseases associated with fibrosis, which are relatively rare. A low FVC, however, is common, particularly in poor populations, and rates are strongly associated with annual GNI per capita of less than US$15,000. Figure 15.2 shows the prevalence of low FVC (below the lower limit of normal in the U.S. National Health and Nutrition Examination Survey white population [Hankinson, Odencrantz, and Fedan 1999]) plotted against GNI per capita (Burney and others 2014).

A similar pattern is seen for the distribution of mortality from COPD (figure 15.3), suggesting that the distribution of low FVC is strongly associated with death attributed to COPD. It seems that high mortality rates attributed to COPD are associated more strongly with low lung volumes (FVC) than with obstruction (a low FEV$_1$/FVC ratio). This observation fits with the evidence on survival among people with a low FEV$_1$/FVC ratio, which is more or less normal, when adjusted for the other effects of cigarette smoking, whereas people with low FVC have poor survival rates (Burney and Hooper 2011).

Figure 15.2 Prevalence of a Spirometric Restriction (FVC < LLN) Plotted against Annual per Capita Gross National Income

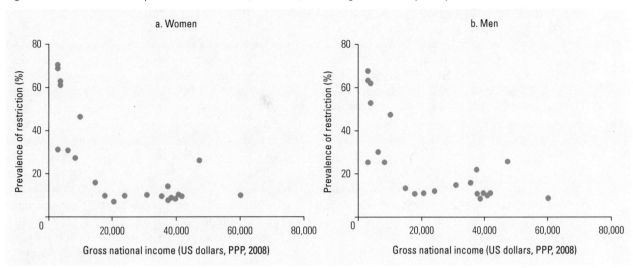

Source: Burney and others 2014.
Note: All participants were ages 40 years or older. FVC = forced vital capacity; LLN = lower limit of normal; PPP = purchasing power parity.

Figure 15.3 Age-Standardized National Chronic Obstructive Pulmonary Disease Mortality (Ages 15 Years and Older), by Gender and Annual per Capita Gross National Income

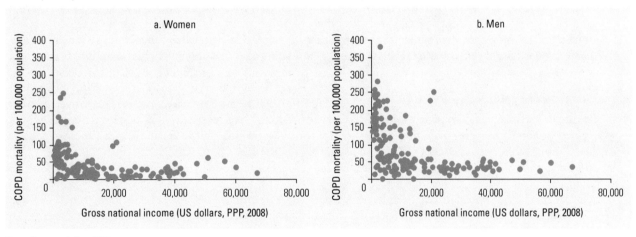

Source: Burney and others 2014.
Note: COPD = chronic obstructive pulmonary disease; PPP = purchasing power parity.

Historically, the association between low lung volumes and mortality also fits with the association between social class and death from COPD in high-income countries (HICs), where the gradient across social classes has been even greater than that for tuberculosis and far greater than that for lung cancer (U.K. Office of Population Censuses and Surveys 1986), another condition strongly associated with cigarette smoking.

The risk factors for low FVC, apart from poverty, are not well established. A consistent association has been made with low birth weight, confirming that this is at least in part a developmental condition determined early in life (Barker and others 1991; Lawlor, Ebrahim, and Davey 2005). Nutrition might also play a role. In one study, children randomized to receive vitamin A in early life had higher FVCs than those randomized to receive a placebo (Checkley and others 2010), a finding that may be relevant in populations with low intake of vitamin A. A second randomized trial used a much lower dose of vitamin A as part of a multinutrient supplement during pregnancy. No effect on lung function was seen at age eight years (Devakumar and others 2015). Some evidence indicates lower FVC in those exposed to higher levels of air pollution early in life (Schultz and others 2016), but the evidence has been inconsistent (Fuertes and others 2015). Although the evidence is so far inconclusive, ongoing trials reducing exposure to high levels of particulate pollution in children in low-income settings will be important. Other risk factors for low FVC are even more speculative, but any factors associated with low birth weight could, in theory, also be important.

The influence of ethnicity or race on FVC has been a topic of debate. African Americans have lower FVCs than white Americans of the same age, gender, and height (Hankinson, Odencrantz, and Fedan 1999). This is also true for African, Caribbean, and other ethnic minorities in the United Kingdom (Hooper and Burney 2013) and for Aboriginal Australians (Cooksley and others 2015). However, the common assumption that low FVC is explained by race alone is unwarranted at this time (Lundy Braun, Wolfgang, and Dickersin 2013) for two reasons. First, ethnic minorities in all countries have poorer backgrounds, and because social deprivation has been strongly associated with low FVC, this is a potential confounder (Menezes and others 2015; Sonnappa and others 2015). Second, the mortality for persons with a given FVC, age, height, and gender is the same irrespective of ethnicity, at least in the United States (Burney and Hooper 2012). This finding suggests that, whether the origins are genetic or environmental, the effects are similarly detrimental (Burney and Hooper 2012).

Restrictive Lung Disease and Fibrosis

Reduced maximal lung inflation (restriction) can be caused by chest wall stiffness, respiratory muscle weakness, or one of the many causes of widespread disease of the lung parenchyma that may result in diffuse lung scarring, called *fibrosis*. These diseases, termed idiopathic interstitial pneumonias, have recently been classified by an American Thoracic Society/European Respiratory Society Working Group (Travis and others 2013) and are also collectively referred to as *diffuse parenchymal lung disease* (Antoniou and others 2015). They are relatively uncommon and are further classified into those of known and unknown causes. Known causes include exposure to known fibrosing agents like inorganic or organic dusts. Unknown causes include sarcoidosis and idiopathic pulmonary fibrosis (IPF) (Antoniou and others 2015); IPF is the most common. Best estimates of mortality from IPF are 5–10 cases per 100,000 population (age standardized), and its prevalence appears to be increasing (Hutchinson and others 2014). Adding occupational causes or causes secondary to systemic disease may double or triple the prevalence of diffuse parenchymal fibrotic lung disease (Behr 2009). IPF has a relentless course until death ensues in three to five years, often from acute exacerbation (Travis and others 2013).

The clinical presentation of fibrosing lung diseases is shortness of breath and widespread inspiratory crackles in the lung bases that become more widespread as disease progresses. The chest roentgenogram usually shows diffuse nodular, or linear, opacities of varying size and combinations, depending on the cause; lung function testing shows reduced lung volumes and, in more advanced cases, impairment of gas exchange (respiratory failure). Finger clubbing is a common sign in established disease. Patients presenting with these features require referral because the diagnosis may require specialized procedures and even lung biopsies. High-resolution computed tomography scans of the chest provide useful information and may be sufficient to confirm the diagnosis of IPF in cases in which other clinical features (including history) suggest this diagnosis. Lung biopsies are obtained through a limited thoracotomy or by use of minimally invasive thoracoscopic methods (Aziz and others 2004; Travis and others 2013). In some cases, biopsies can be avoided; the diagnosis can be confirmed by bronchoscopic means that can be combined with use of bronchoalveolar lavage (washings from bronchi), which may provide confirmatory evidence of lung malignancy, hemorrhage into lung tissue, an eosinophilic lung condition, or a chronic infection such as tuberculosis. Transbronchial or endobronchial biopsies are useful when sarcoidosis, an organizing pneumonia, or hypersensitivity pneumonitis is suspected to be IPF. Because the treatments for these different conditions vary widely, definitive diagnosis, sometimes by exclusion, is essential.

Hypersensitivity pneumonitis usually has a benign course, especially with antigen avoidance. Corticosteroids are recommended for severely symptomatic patients with important functional and radiologic abnormalities. In some patients, however, especially those with bird fancier's or pigeon-breeder's lung, the prognosis is worse; some individuals develop severe and progressive fibrosis and cor pulmonale (Glazer 2015).

Lung fibrosis secondary to rheumatic diseases, for which blood tests are usually confirmatory, has a slightly better prognosis than IPF, but its presence worsens the prognosis of the diseases themselves (Castelino and Varga 2010).

Chronic Bronchitis and Bronchiectasis

Chronic bronchitis is defined as chronic cough, usually occurring in the winter months, that lasts for three months or more, occurs in two successive years, and is associated with the production of phlegm.

Acute exacerbations of COPD are more common in patients with chronic bronchitis and are commonly associated with bacterial infections in the bronchi (GOLD 2014). Because exacerbations are thought to lead to more rapid loss of lung function and progression of COPD, preventing them is an important goal of COPD management (Vestbo and Hogg 2006).

However, the symptoms of chronic bronchitis are nonspecific, meaning that other lung conditions, particularly asthma and bronchiectasis, may present with similar symptoms. Inhalation of irritants in outdoor and indoor air pollution (Ehrlich and others 2004; Holland and Reid 1965; Jindal and others 2006) and in the workplace may also produce similar symptoms (Blanc and Torén 2007; Ehrlich and others 2004). There is little evidence that chronic bronchitis not associated with advanced COPD is associated with increased mortality (Peto and others 1983).

In bronchiectasis, increased sputum production is commonly associated with chronic bacterial colonization of the abnormal airways by one or more varieties of pathogenic organism. Infective flare-ups are common, often as a result of the appearance of more virulent organisms, and are marked by an increase in the volume or change in the color of sputum, with or without systemic features of infection, such as malaise and a temperature. The pathology in bronchiectasis involves local thinning and weakening of the bronchial wall, leading to areas of dilatation. In addition, the chronic infection leads to scarring of bronchi beyond the dilated areas that may cause airflow obstruction resembling COPD. Likewise, weakened collapsible bronchi and damage to the lining of bronchi result in ineffective cough and clearance of secretions, favoring persistence and recurrence of infections. Bronchiectasis has become less common in HICs, but remains common in LMICs because of the continuing burden of infectious diseases and lung infections—tuberculosis, human immunodeficiency virus/acquired immunodeficiency syndrome (HIV/AIDS), pertussis, measles, and adenoviral infections—particularly those occurring in childhood. Other factors, such as malnutrition, that compromise the immune system also play a role (Chalmers, Aliberti, and Blasi 2015).

PRIMARY PREVENTION OF CHRONIC LUNG DISEASES

The clear association between respiratory mortality and socioeconomic conditions strongly suggests that poverty reduction will lead to a lowering of the burden from respiratory disease (Burney and others 2015), although the mechanisms are unknown. The most important specific measure for primary prevention of COPD is smoking cessation, including the reduction of exposure to environmental tobacco smoke, addressed in chapter 4 of this volume (Roy and others 2017) (see box 15.1). Improved prevention and management of tuberculosis are also likely to reduce the prevalence of chronic airway obstruction significantly in some regions, as will improvement of work environments. Other preventive measures for airflow obstruction are less well established; the use of cleaner fuels or improved biomass stoves is expected to reduce at least the symptoms of chronic respiratory diseases.

There is little evidence on the causes of low lung volume (low FVC) or on how low FVC may be prevented. It is reasonable to speculate that improving birth weights through dietary measures and supplements for mothers or children (or both) might be beneficial. Encouraging mothers not to smoke during pregnancy might also be effective. Current large-scale trials of the reduction of biomass exposure will quantify the benefits to be derived from this effort.

The primary prevention of chronic bronchitis also involves reducing the use of tobacco products and exposure to air pollutants. For bronchiectasis, the main strategy is to prevent the spread of infection either by prophylactic treatment (for HIV/AIDS in newborns) or immunization against tuberculosis, measles, and pertussis, in combination with adequate and prompt treatment of infections. Annual influenza and five-yearly polyvalent pneumococcal vaccination may reduce serious morbidity in persons at risk of pneumonia, including the elderly and persons with chronic heart, lung, renal, or liver disease. The role of smoking in increasing the risk of most pulmonary infections, including tuberculosis, provides further grounds for public health measures to target this addiction.

Box 15.1

Common Preventable Causes of Chronic Airflow Obstruction

- Stronger evidence of link to COPD
  - Smoking
  - Tuberculosis
  - Occupational exposure.
- Weaker evidence of link to COPD
  - Indoor air pollution
  - Outdoor air pollution
  - Diet high in oxidants, low in antioxidant content.

PRINCIPLES OF CARE

The aims of disease management for patients with chronic respiratory disease vary according to the nature and stage of the disease. Principal objectives in all cases are early detection to limit the progression and severity of disease, and implementation of secondary preventive measures. Early identification of persons susceptible to the effects of harmful exposures permits a more targeted approach to risk reduction and may be relevant to their family members, for example, by identifying persons with rare genetic conditions that render them susceptible to developing emphysema. At-risk persons need to be given clear instructions on how to avoid potentially harmful smoke and other pollutants.

Proposed treatments need to be evaluated for their efficacy, acceptability, effectiveness, value for money, and scalability (box 15.2). The attributes of an intervention or treatment are not necessarily the same in all environments; most research on the treatment of lung diseases has been performed in HICs, and recommendations may not be applicable in other settings. Nevertheless, the evidence from HICs may be the only evidence available.

Box 15.2

Principles of Care

- *Efficacy of the treatment.* Efficacy is the ability of the treatment to achieve an objective under experimental conditions. Efficacy is best tested in randomized controlled trials (RCTs); the findings may be combined in systematic reviews to arrive at more reliable assessments from which recommendations may be made. A regularly updated source of such reviews can be found at http://www.cochranelibrary.com/app/content/browse/page/?context=topic/Lungs%20%26%20airways. Even this evidence, however, is limited by several factors: the context in which the trials have been conducted; the selection of patients, which is generally more restricted than the use of the treatment in practice; the heterogeneity of patients, who may not all have the same response to treatment; and the selection of the medication with which the medication being studied has been compared. These limitations are particularly relevant to lung diseases in low- and middle-income countries, where few RCTs have been performed and results from high-income countries do not necessarily apply.
- *Effectiveness of the impact of the intervention on a population.* Efficacious remedies may not be used because they are unavailable, unaffordable, or unacceptable to the patients, or they may be prescribed or used inappropriately. Inhaled drugs have a very good ratio of efficacy to side effects. However, acceptability of the inhalation route for treatment delivery is a barrier in some countries; adherence is poor unless there is a concerted effort to promote this form of treatment. Other barriers to use include high costs relative to other treatments; fear of taking corticosteroids; diverse cultural views about treatment of disease; and poor inhaler technique, particularly with pressurized metered dose inhalers, which require coordination of actuation with inhalation (GINA 2014; Masoli and others 2004).
- *Value for money.* Value for money is a comparative judgment generally made by the party paying for the treatment—patients, health authorities, or third-party payers. It involves comparing the relative benefit from the treatment to the benefit that could be derived from all other uses of the available resources. These judgments are not easily transferred from one person or one country to another, and relative costs and available resources may vary markedly.
- *Scalability.* Scalability is the ability to provide a good service to the whole population. Scalability requires simple algorithms (care pathways) to guide the assessment and treatment of patients (Graham and others 2006), access to quality-assured and affordable essential medicines, and inclusion of algorithms in guidelines customized both for the end users (primary care physicians, nurses) and for practice settings (country, facility, human and health resources, prevalent diseases, and health needs) (Ottmani and others 2005).

MANAGEMENT OF CHRONIC LUNG DISEASES

Every effort should be made to reduce all harmful exposures linked to any respiratory disease: tobacco, occupational dusts, and indoor and outdoor pollution. The availability of nicotine replacement therapy is beneficial.

Asthma

Despite the development of many regional and international asthma guidelines that have reduced the burden of disease and death in most countries (Haahtela and others 2006), the level of asthma control is poor in a large proportion of patients in other regions (Ayuk and others 2014; Masoli and others 2004; Price, Fletcher, and van der Molen 2014; Vietri, Burslem, and Su 2014; Zemedkun, Woldemichael, and Tefera 2014). The success in reducing asthma-related death rates in HICs has highlighted the disparity with LMICs.

Diagnosis

Asthma as a heterogeneous disease, usually characterized by chronic airway inflammation and its diagnosis, involves the recognition of characteristic symptoms of periodic respiratory airflow obstruction. The Global Initiative for Asthma (GINA) recommends that the clinical diagnosis should in all cases be confirmed by measurements of reversible airflow at some time, either in the past or currently. Characteristic symptoms are wheeze, shortness of breath, chest tightness, and cough that vary over time and in intensity and are relieved, at least partially, by use of a rapid-acting inhaled bronchodilator (GINA 2014). Heterogeneity refers to the varying patterns of disease with respect to onset, time course (Martinez and others 1995), associations with allergic diseases, and severity (Boudier and others 2013). This heterogeneity has important implications for selection of treatment, particularly in severe asthma.

A multidimensional view of asthma that aids diagnosis, assessment, and therapy has been proposed (Gibson, McDonald, and Marks 2010). This multidimensionality includes airway pathology, symptoms, lung function abnormalities, body mass and nutrition, gas exchange abnormalities, exercise capacity, and comorbidity. Other features that may be present are variability of symptoms from day to day and from season to season, onset during early childhood, almost immediate relief from the use of a short-acting bronchodilator, and periods when symptoms disappear, particularly as associated with a trial of inhaled corticosteroids.

Airflow limitation is demonstrated by the use of peak flow meters or spirometers, which measure airflow during forced expiration either as peak expiratory flow or FEV_1 (GINA 2014). These measures are compared with the predicted value for the patient's gender, age, and height. Measurements taken before and after a dose (four puffs are recommended) of a short-acting beta2-agonist confirms reversible airflow limitation, which should be interpreted in the context of the syndromic diagnosis. The pathophysiology of asthma in most cases involves hyperresponsiveness of airway smooth muscle and bronchospasm. Several other respiratory conditions may present with some of these features, and these conditions vary according to the patient's age. The use of alternative diagnostic terms like *recurrent bronchitis* or *wheezy bronchitis* may delay diagnosis and appropriate treatment (Speight, Lee, and Hey 1983).

Assessment

Proper management of the disease involves assessing both day-to-day control (also called *impairment*) and the likelihood of longer-term problems, including asthma exacerbations (also referred to as *risk*) (GINA 2014; National Asthma Education and Prevention Program 2007).

Satisfactory control of asthma symptoms (day-to-day control) is defined as infrequent symptoms during the day (fewer than twice a week) and infrequent need for a short-acting beta2-agonist to relieve symptoms (fewer than twice a week), absence of any night waking due to asthma symptoms, and the achievement of normal or near-normal lung function (if measured). These measures are combined in a single score, and the asthma is described as controlled, partly controlled, or uncontrolled.

A second component of satisfactory asthma control (also called future risk, because these features are usually the result of ongoing poor asthma symptom control, or complications of treatment) includes the following: freedom from attacks of asthma (exacerbations) that require emergency treatment (usually with oral corticosteroids and administration of additional bronchodilators); chronically reduced or declining lung function; and the side-effects caused by long-term or repeated short courses of oral or systemic corticosteroids, a common situation in LMICs without access to safer but more costly asthma medications.

There has been intense research interest in finding simple and accurate ways of measuring predictors of response to therapy to assist in targeting therapy most appropriately, as well as response to therapy to evaluate success. Measurement of the fraction of nitric oxide in exhaled breath (Powell and others 2011), sputum (Siva and others 2007), and blood eosinophils (Bafadhel and others 2012) are the most promising predictors of response to inhaled corticosteroids and new biologicals such as anti-interleukin-5.

Further implementation research on biomarker-based targeted approaches to therapy for asthma is ongoing. Biomarkers have limited value in diagnosing asthma in routine practice, but they are used in specialized centers. The limited availability and high cost of these tests and of the targeted treatments will restrict their use, even in severe asthma (Chung and others 2014). The great majority of patients with asthma are adequately diagnosed and managed using predominantly symptom-based clinical algorithms that target asthma control alone (GINA 2014).

Pharmacological Management

Control-based asthma management, as recommended in the GINA strategy, is a stepwise approach in which treatment is escalated and de-escalated to establish the lowest level of treatment intensity that maintains symptom control with the absence of asthma attacks (exacerbations). Satisfactory asthma control is defined as infrequent symptoms and need for a short-acting beta2-agonist during the day (fewer than twice per week), night waking due to asthma symptoms, the achievement of normal or near normal lung function (if measured), and freedom from attacks of asthma (exacerbations) that require emergency treatment (usually with oral corticosteroids and administration of additional bronchodilators).

In the GINA strategy, Treatment Step 1 is as-needed use of a rapid- and short-acting beta2-agonist (for example, salbutamol) alone. For persisting symptoms and to reduce exacerbation risk, Step 2 is the addition of regular (once or twice daily) low-dose inhaled corticosteroids *or* leukotriene receptor antagonists. If symptom control is not achieved or exacerbations recur, the next step (Step 3) involves an increase in the dose of inhaled corticosteroids to either a medium dose (the preferred step in children) or a switch to once- or twice-daily use of the combination of a low-dose inhaled corticosteroid and long acting beta2-agonist (for example, formoterol). If this treatment fails to achieve satisfactory symptom control, the next step (Step 4) involves increasing to a medium- or high-dose inhaled corticosteroid combined with a long-acting beta2-agonist. At Step 4, the addition of other controller medications is considered. These include tiotropium (a long-acting inhaled anticholinergic, previously used only for COPD) and theophylline. For patients being considered for Step 4 treatments, referral to a specialist in asthma management is recommended. In Step 5, options include tiotropium, a daily dose of oral corticosteroids (adjusted to the lowest dose that maintains

freedom from exacerbations and maximal achievable daily freedom from symptoms), anti-immunoglobulin E therapy (administered as a monthly injection), or the biological agent anti-interleukin-5 (anti-IL5), recently approved for use in severe asthma.

Additional measures are recommended before escalating treatment:

• Check both adherence and inhaler technique
• Treat or avoid modifiable risk or exacerbating factors
• Manage any side effects of treatment.

Long-acting beta2-agonist therapy should never be used without inhaled corticosteroid in patients with asthma; this mode of treatment has been associated with increased risk of death (Durham and others 1999). Only inhaled corticosteroid alone or inhaled corticosteroid plus long-acting beta2-agonist combination inhalers should be prescribed for patients with asthma (U.S. FDA 2010). Relatively low-cost generic versions of all of these classes of drugs are available.

Barriers to Care

The efficacy and safety of inhaled corticosteroids in the management of patients with asthma is well established (Adams, Bestall, and Jones 2009; Adams and others 2008; Adams and others 2009). The use of inhaled corticosteroids is associated with reduced risk of asthma-related death (Suissa and others 2000).

However, many barriers to effective implementation of treatment result in suboptimal outcomes. The most significant barrier in LMICs is access to inhaled corticosteroids, usually because of lack of affordability of the medication (GINA 2014). The ratio of inhaled corticosteroid to rescue inhaler use (bronchodilator) has a strong inverse correlation with hospitalizations for asthma attacks and asthma mortality. The higher the population coverage with inhaled corticosteroid, the lower the asthma morbidity (Phui, Tan, and Lim 2008). The next most important barrier is patient nonadherence to controller treatments, a factor shared with other chronic diseases that require regular daily treatment. Other barriers include delayed diagnosis, ineffective patient education, poor inhaler technique, low expectations of control, and lack of appreciation of inadequate control by physicians and patients. Other barriers are cultural values, preferences, and priorities.

Health system barriers include poor training of health care workers, lack of availability of quality-controlled products, and lack of affordability (Aït-Khaled and others 2000). If good-quality medication is locally available and affordable, the major barrier is the need for patients to take this medication using either inhaled dry powder or pressurized inhalers with spacers. Poor inhalation technique reduces the efficacy of the medication; poor adherence results in suboptimal control of the disease.

In general, regular follow-up by health care workers may represent the most cost-effective way to improve adherence and ensure correct inhaler techniques. The Finnish asthma program has shown that a community approach to setting up a network of support for practitioners may be a very cost-effective way to improve asthma control (Erhola and others 2003; GINA 2014; Haahtela and others 2001; Haahtela and others 2006; Kauppi and others 2013).

Many asthma educational programs have been developed by national health agencies, such as the Finnish Asthma Program; by individual hospitals; and by patient organizations and nongovernmental organizations. There is no doubt that a combined effort in diagnosis and early use of and easy access to anti-inflammatory therapy, along with periodic assessment of asthma control, will reduce asthma-related morbidity and mortality. Despite the best care, however, approximately 5–10 percent of patients still have significant symptomatic asthma. Alternative approaches to managing these patients, who are responsible for a substantial burden of costs and poor outcomes, are needed (Bousquet and others 2010; Chung and others 2014).

Chronic Airway Obstruction

Diagnosis

COPD typically presents in a person older than age 40 years with breathlessness on exertion that is persistent and progressive. Wheezing and chest tightness and an intermittent or persistent cough that may be associated with the production of sputum may also be present (GOLD 2014). Exacerbations—that is, episodes of worsening of symptoms (breathlessness, cough, or sputum production) beyond the normal day-to-day variation—are an important feature of the history of chronic airway obstruction. The diagnosis is confirmed by spirometry and is defined as FEV_1/FVC ratio below the lower limit of normal following inhalation of a short-acting bronchodilator. This definition of normal is specific to a given age, gender, and height; however, because almost all spirometers can be programmed to show the normal value, the lower limit of normal should be used to define the presence of an abnormality rather than the fixed cutoff of 70 percent.

Not all primary care facilities have access to spirometry, and a peak flow meter can be used to exclude the diagnosis with reasonable accuracy. Moderate obstruction is unlikely if the prebronchodilator peak expiratory flow rate is greater than 2.2 liters per second per square meter ($l/sec/m^2$); severe disease is unlikely if it is greater than 1.8 $l/sec/m^2$ postbronchodilator or 1.3 $l/sec/m^2$ prebronchodilator (Jithoo and others 2013).

Peak flow meters are inexpensive and should be widely available. Spirometers are more expensive, but at least the cheaper of the spirometers need to be available for secondary care. The main limitation of spirometers is lack of training in the use and interpretation of findings.

Clinical Course and Management

Patients with COPD generally experience a slow but progressive cycle of worsening exertional dyspnea, which leads to lack of exercise and muscle deconditioning and reduces both work capacity and quality of life. Exercise programs can, to some extent, slow this cycle, improve effort tolerance, relieve dyspnea and fatigue, and improve quality of life (Lacasse and others 2006). Such programs do not need to be expensive or complex; they are best incorporated into a lifestyle of regular exercise four or more times a week, involving both endurance and muscle strengthening (Iepsen and others 2015). A simple physical activity enhancement program using pedometers can effectively improve physical activity level and quality of life in COPD patients in low-resource settings (Mendoza and others 2015). Aerobic exercise training also reduces disease exacerbations (Güell and others 2000).

Some patients with severe COPD, but not necessarily in respiratory failure, lose body weight. This weight loss is not entirely explained by reduced dietary intake and relates to the systemic effects of chronic lung disease and to deconditioning and loss of muscle mass. This process has an impact on functional ability and quality of life and is associated with increased mortality. Nutritional supplements, coupled with an exercise program, can improve but not reverse this process; they can increase body weight, respiratory muscle strength, walking ability, and quality of life (Ferreira and others 2009). Anabolic steroids have no lasting effect (Pan and others 2014).

For hypoxemic patients with COPD, the long-term use of supplemental oxygen improves survival (Medical Research Council Working Party 1981) and may improve quality of life (Eaton and others 2002). Long-term domiciliary oxygen therapy at a flow rate determined by measurement of blood oxygen saturation may delay the onset of pulmonary hypertension. Its benefit for chronic pulmonary diseases other than COPD has not been demonstrated (Jindal and Agarwal 2012). This therapy should be used for a minimum of 12 hours per day, and it is usually restricted to patients with COPD who have stopped smoking. Ambulatory oxygen therapy, even if it does not improve survival, facilitates independence, lessens restrictions on physical and social activities, and improves quality of life.

Annual influenza vaccination reduces the incidence of exacerbations, particularly those due to influenza virus, and is recommended for patients with COPD (Poole and others 2006). Although it is not effective against the majority of viruses that cause upper respiratory tract infections, vaccination may reduce morbidity and mortality in these susceptible patients during the annual influenza season. Most of the exacerbations of asthma, especially in children, and COPD are precipitated by a viral upper respiratory tract infection and are accompanied by secondary bacterial bronchial infection. Rhinoviruses, for which no vaccine is available, are the most common viruses responsible for these events; antibiotics are indicated for the bacterial component and when purulent sputum becomes evident (Poole and others 2006). Pneumococcal vaccines are effective in preventing the more severe forms of infection caused by the pneumococcus organism, the most important cause of pneumonia in patients of all ages (Walters and others 2010). Five-yearly administration of polyvalent pneumococcal vaccine is advised for patients with chronic lung disease (Walters and others 2010).

Common comorbid conditions, including heart disease, diabetes, cancer, lower respiratory tract infections, musculoskeletal conditions, and psychiatric disorders, should be treated or controlled to improve outcomes in patients with chronic respiratory disease (Gershon and others 2015).

Pharmacological Management of Stable Disease
Most patients with COPD respond to inhaled short-acting bronchodilators, which are the first line of treatment for symptomatic disease and provide temporary relief of symptoms in most people. Two pharmacological classes of short-acting bronchodilators are available: beta2-agonists and anti-muscarinics. Neither class has a clear advantage (Chong, Karner, and Poole 2012). They may be given either alone or in combination; combination inhalers containing both are available. They are generally administered for use as needed; if symptoms are more persistent, they are administered for use every four to six hours. Their duration of action is less than six hours, which explains their failure to improve patients' quality of life or prevent COPD exacerbations.

Inhaled long-acting beta2-agonists (LABAs) (Kew, Mavergames, and Walters 2013) or long-acting muscarinic antagonists (Karner, Chong, and Poole 2014) are taken once or twice daily and provide sustained bronchodilation.

They are recommended for patients with persistent daily symptoms that limit activity, especially those who have experienced at least one COPD exacerbation in the past year. Used alone or in combination, they have been shown to result in sustained bronchodilation, improved symptoms and quality of life, reduced activity limitation, improved endurance for rehabilitation programs, and reduced exacerbations. A short-acting beta2-agonist or short-acting muscarinic antagonist is usually provided for as-needed use. Long-acting formulations are generally well tolerated and are recommended when symptoms are not adequately controlled with inhaled short-acting beta2-agonists.

Short-acting bronchodilators, taken regularly or as required, are cheaper and more widely available; long-acting bronchodilators, taken once or twice daily, are generally more convenient and provide more sustained benefit (GOLD 2014). The U.S. Food and Drug Administration has expressed concern about the occurrence of severe exacerbations by some patients using LABAs (U.S. FDA 2010). This concern seems to be limited to patients who take this class of medication without inhaled corticosteroids.

Oral beta2-agonists and oral theophylline are cheaper alternatives to inhaled bronchodilators. However, they have more systemic side effects and are less effective than inhaled medications. Accordingly, they are not recommended.

The use of inhaled corticosteroids in patients with COPD is controversial. Although these agents are not as effective for COPD as for asthma, they do reduce the frequency of exacerbations in people with a history of frequent exacerbations and severe disease; they also reduce the rate of decline in quality of life (Yang and others 2012). They have not been shown to have any effect on decline in lung function or mortality (GOLD 2014). Their use in COPD has been associated with an increased risk of pneumonia, leading to caution except when specifically indicated (Suissa and others 2013). High doses are contraindicated because the risk of pneumonia is dose related. Other side effects include candidiasis, skin bruising, cataracts, and possibly reactivation of previous pulmonary tuberculosis.

Several combination inhaler devices are available that contain either two long-acting bronchodilators (beta2-adrenergic agonists and muscarinic antagonists) or a long-acting bronchodilator and an inhaled steroid. The effect of these combination inhalers is probably similar to that of the addition of their individual components, but a single inhaler is generally more convenient and may lead to enhanced adherence to treatment regimens.

Evidence about the effectiveness of long-term oral corticosteroids in people with stable chronic airway obstruction is lacking. Their adverse effects, including myopathy, are well established; they are probably best avoided, if possible, or otherwise administered in the smallest feasible dose.

Management of Exacerbations

First-line management of exacerbations of COPD includes the use of repeated inhaled beta2-agonists by the most efficient route; supplemental oxygen if the patient is hypoxemic (the presence of cyanosis, preferably confirmed by oximeter); and either oral corticosteroids or antibiotics, or both. Administration of systemic corticosteroids (usually oral) to patients presenting with acute exacerbations of COPD reduces the risk of treatment failure and early relapse, causes more rapid improvement in lung function (FEV_1), and is associated with shorter length of hospital stay (Walters and others 2014). However, it is also associated with an increased risk of adverse effects (Walters and others 2014). Administration of antibiotics to patients with acute exacerbations of COPD probably reduces the risk of treatment failure; the evidence is strongest for people with severe exacerbations requiring hospitalization (Vollenweider and others 2012).

Supplemental oxygen therapy should be administered to patients with acute exacerbations of COPD who are hypoxemic with low-flow (1–2 liters per minute) oxygen administered via nasal cannulas. In patients with acute or acute-on-chronic respiratory failure (low blood oxygen content) due to an acute exacerbation of COPD, the administration of noninvasive positive pressure ventilation, also known as bi-level positive airway pressure, via a nasal or face mask reduces length of hospital stay, avoids the need for intubation and invasive mechanical ventilation, and may improve survival (Ram and others 2009).

Self-management with prescription drugs to be taken in the event of a subsequent exacerbation reduces the delay in commencing treatment and may reduce the risk of hospitalization. Active rehabilitation following hospitalization reduces mortality and rehospitalization. Methylxanthines are not recommended (GOLD 2014).

Idiopathic Low FVC

There is no recognized treatment for patients with idiopathic low FVC, but careful assessment should be made for comorbidities, including diabetes and cardiovascular disease. Treatment options may be available for patients with low FVC associated with the conditions identified in the next section.

Restrictive and Fibrosing Lung Diseases

Diagnosis

The diagnosis of interstitial lung diseases is generally made following referral to specialists. However, the diagnosis is frequently delayed for several months, and patients are misdiagnosed and wrongly treated for congestive cardiac failure, pneumonia, asthma, COPD, or tuberculosis. The most important clues to the correct diagnosis are a typical chest roentgenogram and the presence of inspiratory crackles and clubbing.

Owing to their rarity, no strategy for screening in the general population is warranted except in populations with a higher risk of developing specific forms of fibrosing lung diseases, such as workers exposed to inhaled agents (fibrogenic dusts such as asbestos or silica or a variety of organic antigens). These categories of worker should be reviewed periodically by radiography with or without spirometric studies. Patients with rheumatoid arthritis, scleroderma, systemic lupus erythematosus, mixed connective tissue disease, and dermatomyositis or polymyositis are also at risk, and their respiratory status should be reviewed regularly by their physicians. Lung involvement in these diseases often dominates the clinical course of the disease and may be fatal.

Treatment

General support measures are appropriate. Reducing or avoiding further exposure to the offending agents in secondary fibrotic lung disease, such as hypersensitivity pneumonitis or pneumoconiosis, is important. The presence of gastroesophageal reflux should be considered in all patients, and appropriate investigations performed; if present, the condition should be treated. The presence of gastroesophageal reflux leads to faster deterioration in lung function and produces more respiratory symptoms (Raghu 2013). Effective treatment of gastroesophageal reflux is possible even in low-resource settings.

No treatment for IPF has improved survival or quality of life sufficiently to be recommended widely in individuals with active and progressive disease. Several drugs and combinations of drugs, predominantly immunosuppressants and corticosteroids, have been used unsuccessfully to treat IPF (Davies, Richeldi, and Walters 2003; Richeldi 2012). Although pirfenidone has not demonstrated a reduction in mortality, it may slow the decline in lung function (FVC, diffusing capacity of carbon monoxide [DL_{CO}], or six-minute walking distance) (Azuma and others 2005; Noble and others 2011; Spagnolo and others 2010; Taniguchi and others 2010). However, its use is associated with significant side effects (Jiang and others 2012). Other drugs investigated in randomized controlled trials in IPF patients include cotrimoxazole (Shulgina and others 2013), sildenafil (preserves exercise capacity in patients with right-ventricular hypertrophy or systolic dysfunction [Han and others 2013]), and high-dose tyrosine-kinase inhibitor (nintedanib) (Richeldi and others 2011). Confirmation of these findings in other trials is awaited. The more specialized medications are unlikely to be widely available in low-resource settings or outside of third-level facilities.

Exacerbations of IPF have many causes, such as pulmonary thromboembolism, respiratory infection, and heart failure; an idiopathic acute exacerbation has been described, consisting of diffuse alveolar damage. In general, acute exacerbations of IPF are treated with antibiotics, systemic corticosteroids, and, at times, immunosuppressive drugs, although the prognosis remains poor despite these measures (Agarwal and Jindal 2008).

Hypersensitivity pneumonitis (for example, bird fancier's or pigeon-breeder's lung) generally responds to antigen avoidance, but corticosteroids are recommended for highly symptomatic patients with important functional and radiologic abnormalities. Some individuals develop severe fibrosis.

In patients with progressive systemic sclerosis with deteriorating lung function and high-resolution computed tomography abnormalities suggesting inflammation, a modest response to cyclophosphamide was found after one year of treatment, although with significant toxicity (Tashkin and others 2006). This benefit had largely waned at the second year of follow-up (Khanna and others 2007). Patients with progressive interstitial lung disease in rheumatoid arthritis or systemic lupus erythematosus may warrant treatment with corticosteroids, with or without immunosuppressive drugs, although there is little evidence from clinical trials to support the use of this therapy.

Patients with advanced disease or with more aggressive IPF require evaluation for lung transplantation.

Bronchiectasis

Evidence-based guidelines for the management of bronchiectasis have been prepared for HICs (Chang and others 2010; Hill and others 2011), but the quality of the available evidence is low. Management is directed to improving mucus clearance and preventing and treating infections to limit the long-term consequences of repeated episodes of lower respiratory tract infections.

Limited evidence exists for nonpharmacological interventions. Inspiratory muscle training (Bradley, Moran, and Greenstone 2002) is moderately helpful; airway

clearance techniques (Lee, Burge, and Holland 2013) are safe and improve quality of life. Moderate evidence supports the use of pneumococcal vaccine (Chang and others 2009) in chronic lung diseases, including bronchiectasis. However, no evidence is available to indicate that influenza vaccine is beneficial, but this void may reflect the small size of studies (Chang, Morris, and Chang 2007).

Inhalation of nebulized mannitol increases the time between exacerbations (Hart and others 2014); mucolytics, such as acetylcysteine, that reduce the tenacity of sputum (Wilkinson and others 2014) may be helpful in conjunction with other therapies. Prolonged antibiotics, particularly macrolides, may be beneficial in reducing purulent sputum and preventing episodes of clinical infection, possibly through their effect on local defense mechanisms rather than their antibiotic properties (Evans, Bara, and Greenstone 2007). Their long-term or even intermittent use is, however, associated with the development of bacterial resistance to antibiotics and colonization of the bronchi with a sequence of more virulent treatment-sensitive organisms like *Moraxella catarrhalis* and streptococcal strains, through *Haemophilus influenzae*, then *Staphylococcus aureus*, and finally, less pathogenic but relatively treatment-resistant organisms, such as *Pseudomonas aeruginosa*. This march of organisms can be reduced by using antibiotics judiciously and using principles and regimens recommended for patients with cystic fibrosis (Chalmers, Aliberti, and Blasi 2015).

SYSTEMS AND ORGANIZATION OF CARE

The system of care for patients with respiratory diseases is as important as the treatments. Chronic respiratory diseases are often overlooked or poorly managed in outmoded health systems that focus on treating exacerbations or acute events rather than relying on effective chronic care to prevent such events. Similarly, a reliable source of continuing care and a clear management plan are as important as the correct diagnosis and initial treatment. The plan most appropriate for a given population depends on the access to care and the available resources, but the principles are similar. Effective management programs for patients with chronic lung disease have improved quality of life and exercise tolerance and reduced hospitalizations; the introduction of national programs has been associated with reduced hospitalization, drug costs, and disabilities associated with asthma (Haahtela and others 2006) as well as hospitalizations and disabilities associated with COPD (Pietinalho and others 2007). In LMICs, the Practical Approach to Lung Health has reduced prescribing costs per patient (Hamzaoui and Ottmani 2012). Costs of medications remain high in many LMICs, often many times the guide price for essential medicines (Beran and others 2015). Where available at or close to the guide price (table 15.2), however, medications are affordable in most places, particularly among those in paid employment where they may reduce absence due to sickness (Burney and others 2008).

Several key issues in planning health services warrant consideration:

- The importance of ensuring continuity of care, particularly with asthma, has been studied extensively and confirmed in HICs and LMICs.
- Integration ensures that the correct treatment is given at the lowest level capable of delivering it effectively and appropriately and that patients are referred promptly to higher levels of care when appropriate. In most cases, staff members with basic training and adequate supervision can provide care for common conditions.
- Financing arrangements vary substantially; patients in poorer countries are more likely to bear the costs of treatment at the point of service. Financial constraints limit the services that can be offered, particularly for chronic diseases; methods of payment may pose separate barriers. Simple insurance schemes that are affordable, whether individual or financed through taxes or payroll levies, help spread the costs across time and risk groups and make it more likely that uptake of services will be continuous; these schemes may reduce overall costs in the long term.

- Selecting appropriate treatments is inevitably a local decision. The affordable care packages and costs of treatments and staff vary. The cost of importing medications may not vary greatly, but the availability of foreign exchange does.
- The purchasing and security of supply of medications are challenging in some LMICs. The costs are often higher, and the quality is often poor, a consequence of underdeveloped and unregulated markets. The provision of inhalers that have the correct specification for good penetration into the airway is technically difficult. If the supply chain does not deliver affordable and high-quality medications on a regular basis without repeated stockouts, effective management of these conditions is impossible.

The World Health Organization (WHO) programs of integrated care for adults can serve as a model for LMICs. An example is Practical Approach to Lung Health, developed by the Stop TB Partnership, which includes care pathways for the diagnosis and management of asthma and COPD alongside those for screening and treating tuberculosis (WHO 2008). The approach has been implemented and audited in many countries and has provided consistent benefits, even achieving cost savings for health systems. Another example is the Integrated Management of Adolescent and Adult Illness (IMAI), which describes care pathways for acute and chronic diseases, with a strong focus on integrating patient care with care for HIV/AIDS and tuberculosis. IMAI has been implemented in several countries, but its length and density of recommendations present barriers to its use in poorly

Table 15.2 Guide Price for Medicines Commonly Used in COPD and Asthma

Drug	Dose	Median unit price for buyer (US$)	Typical dosage	Indicative cost per month (US$)
Prednisolone	25 mg	0.039	10 tablets	0.39[a]
Salbutamol	100 mcg inhaler	0.0078	2 puffs qds	1.87
Ipratropium	20 mcg inhaler	0.0328	2 puffs qds	7.87
Beclometasone	50 mcg inhaler	0.0131	2 puffs bd	1.57
	100 mcg inhaler	0.0160	2 puffs bd	1.92
	250 mcg inhaler	0.0170	2 puffs bd	2.04
Budesonide	100 mcg inhaler	0.007	2 puffs bd	0.84
	200 mcg inhaler	0.0272	2 puffs bd	3.26
Salmeterol/fluticasone	25/250 mcg inhaler	0.0568	2 puffs bd	6.82

Source: Data extracted from MSH 2015.
Note: bd = two times a day; COPD = chronic obstructive pulmonary disease; mcg = microgram; mg = milligram; qds = four times a day.
a. Cost per course.

resourced countries. However, it may serve as a useful resource for health departments seeking to develop locally applicable integrated models of care (WHO 2013b). A third example is the WHO package of essential noncommunicable disease interventions for primary health care, which includes evidence-based guidelines on diabetes, chronic respiratory disease, cancer, heart disease, and stroke. Pilot implementation projects are ongoing in several countries (box 15.3; WHO 2013a).

Box 15.3

Case Study: Practical Approach to Lung Health in South Africa/Primary Care 101/Practical Approach to Care Kit

A further example of integrated care is the Practical Approach to Lung Health in South Africa/Primary Care 101/Practical Approach to Care Kit (PALSA/PC101/PACK) program. This program, developed in South Africa, began with a local version of Practical Approach to Lung Health (English and others 2006; English and others 2008). After development and testing, the first version of the guideline and training program, called the Practical Approach to Lung Health in South Africa (PALSA), was revised and expanded. The first revision included the chronic care of patients with HIV/AIDS (PALSA PLUS) (Barton and others 2013; Stein and others 2008).

The second revision included the management of approximately 80 percent of the conditions for which adult patients attend primary care clinics, including asthma, COPD, pneumonia, tuberculosis, hypertension, diabetes, and several other common diseases. This program has been developed for international use as the Practical Approach to Care Kit (PACK); it has been introduced in South Africa and is being piloted in Brazil. Versions of PALSA/PACK have been piloted or implemented in Botswana, Brazil, Malawi, and Mexico (Schull and others 2011; Sodhi and others 2014).

This program is based on the following principles:

- *Integration.* Silo management results in prioritization of some diseases; integration ensures their inclusion, which is particularly important for respiratory diseases that have had a low priority, with little provision of resources. Integration ensures that clinicians are led through processes that consider all relevant contributing or comorbid diseases.
- *Localization.* Integrated guidelines are context specific, designed around locally available resources—personnel, facilities, equipment, medications, and local or national health guidelines and prescribing provisions. In many instances, integrated

guidelines help guide policy based on review of the evidence and best-buy principles in each country. Annual updates are essential, especially for disease areas where treatment policies change frequently.
- *Clarity.* Integration seeks to strengthen health services by removing inconsistencies in different guidelines and providing clear recommendations for the levels and tasks of health workers. Clarity optimizes work flows, especially in resource-poor settings with heavy workloads, and facilitates task sharing (Fairall and others 2012; Georgeu and others 2012).
- *Effective training.* Training uses modern adult learning techniques. The guideline serves as the curriculum for case-based, onsite continuing education for nurses and physicians. This training has been introduced in nursing colleges and medical schools, replacing the didactic, lecture-based, off-site training that has a poor record for changing the behavior of clinicians (Stein and others 2008; Zwarenstein and others 2011). The results of these programs have been reported in several papers, including four pragmatic cluster randomized controlled trials. These studies have confirmed consistent improvements in clinician behavior and outcomes, including screening, prescribing, and referral. They have further demonstrated that the approach is highly acceptable to all categories of health teams and that users find it empowering and effective. It has resulted in concurrent improvements in the care of patients with communicable and noncommunicable diseases (Fairall and others 2005), improvements in some health outcomes (Fairall and others 2008; Fairall and others 2010), and more appropriate referrals and reductions in the length and duration of hospital admissions. Reports indicate a dose-response effect of the clinical training, confirming the effectiveness of continuing onsite education.

CONCLUSIONS

LMICs typically have a high burden of disease associated with chronic respiratory conditions, yet the information on which to formulate policy is negligible when compared with the information in HICs. The lack of reliable information is compounded by generally poor infrastructure for commissioning, providing, and monitoring services and training and supporting staff members.

The highest mortality attributed to COPD occurs in South-East Asia. This region has very high age-specific mortality from the condition. An understanding of the nature of the problem is only emerging with the completion of large-scale descriptive surveys with good-quality spirometry. The descriptive epidemiology of chronic respiratory diseases remains sketchy in many low-income areas. The studies in these areas clearly do not replicate findings in the more affluent regions. Extrapolating from high- to low-income contexts is not warranted.

Information on the efficacy and safety of different medications is also largely drawn from studies in HICs. Relatively little information specifically addresses the assessment of these medications in other populations. The lack of clarity on the safety of LABAs in some ethnic groups makes it difficult to optimize health care for these groups.

Infrastructure for effective implementation is inadequate. Health services require a reliable and secure supply of diagnostic services, as well as medications and other treatments, to function well. These elements need to be linked to well-supported staff members with the skills to deploy these services optimally.

Examples of effective primary care and tuberculosis control programs in LMICs provide encouraging evidence. Quality of care—diagnosis, treatment, and appropriate referral to higher levels of care—can be achieved through customized integrated programs that educate, empower, and support frontline clinicians, even in severely resource-constrained settings. Such programs can prompt changes in policies and positive resources necessary for managing these common but currently neglected chronic respiratory diseases.

NOTE

World Bank Income Classifications as of July 2014 are as follows, based on estimates of gross national income (GNI) per capita for 2013:

- Low-income countries (LICs) = US$1,045 or less
- Middle-income countries (MICs) are subdivided:
  (a) lower-middle-income = US$1,046 to US$4,125
  (b) upper-middle-income (UMICs) = US$4,126 to US$12,745
- High-income countries (HICs) = US$12,746 or more.

REFERENCES

Adams, N. P., J. C. Bestall, and P. Jones. 2009. "Budesonide versus Placebo for Chronic Asthma in Children and Adults." *Cochrane Database of Systematic Reviews* 4: CD003274.

Adams, N. P., J. C. Bestall, T. J. Lasserson, P. Jones, and C. J. Cates. 2008. "Fluticasone versus Placebo for Chronic Asthma in Adults and Children." *Cochrane Database of Systematic Reviews* 4: CD003135.

Adams, N. P., J. C. Bestall, R. Malouf, T. J. Lasserson, and P. Jones. 2009. "Beclomethasone versus Placebo for Chronic Asthma." *Cochrane Database of Systematic Reviews* 1: CD002738.

Agarwal, R., and S. K. Jindal. 2008. "Acute Exacerbation of Idiopathic Pulmonary Fibrosis: A Systematic Review." *European Journal of Internal Medicine* 19 (4): 227–35.

Aït-Khaled, N., G. Auregan, N. Bencharif, L. Camara Mady, E. Dagli, and others. 2000. "Affordability of Inhaled Corticosteroids as a Potential Barrier to Treatment of Asthma in Some Developing Countries." *International Journal of Tuberculosis and Lung Disease* 4 (3): 268–71.

Allwood, B. W., L. Myer, and E. D. Bateman. 2013. "A Systematic Review of the Association between Pulmonary Tuberculosis and the Development of Chronic Airflow Obstruction in Adults." *Respiration* 86 (1): 76–85.

Antoniou, K. M. M., S. Tomassetti, F. Bonella, U. Costabel, and V. Poletti. 2015. "Interstitial Lung Disease." *European Respiratory Review* 23: 40–54.

Asher, M. I., P. K. Pattermore, A. C. Harrison, E. A. Mitchell, H. H. Rea, and others. 1998. "International Comparison of the Prevalence of Asthma Symptoms and Bronchial Hyperresponsiveness." *American Review of Respiratory Disease* 138 (3): 524–29.

Ayuk, A. C., T. Oguonu, A. N. Ikefuna, and B. C. Ibe. 2014. "Asthma Control and Quality of Life in School-Age Children in Enugu South East, Nigeria." *Nigerian Postgraduate Medical Journal* 21 (2): 160–64.

Aziz, Z. A., A. U. Wells, D. M. Hansell, G. A. Bain, S. J. Copley, and others. 2004. "HRCT Diagnosis of Diffuse Parenchymal Lung Disease: Inter-Observer Variation." *Thorax* 59 (6): 506–11.

Azuma, A., T. Nukiwa, E. Tsuboi, M. Suga, S. Abe, and others. 2005. "Double-Blind, Placebo-Controlled Trial of Pirfenidone in Patients with Idiopathic Pulmonary Fibrosis." *American Journal of Respiratory and Critical Care Medicine* 171 (9): 1040–47.

Bafadhel, M., S. McKenna, S. Terry, V. Mistry, M. Pancholi, and others. 2012. "Blood Eeosinophils to Direct Corticosteroid Treatment of Exacerbations of Chronic Obstructive Pulmonary Disease: A Randomized Placebo-Controlled Trial." *American Journal of Respiratory and Critical Care Medicine* 186 (1): 48–55.

Barker, D. J. P., K. M. Godfrey, C. Fall, C. Osmond, P. D. Winter, and others. 1991. "Relation of Birth Weight and Childhood Respiratory Infection to Adult Lung Function and Death from Chronic Obstructive Airways Disease." *British Medical Journal* 303 (6804): 671–75.

Barton, G. R., L. Fairall, M. O. Bachmann, K. Uebel, V. Timmerman, and others. 2013. "Cost-Effectiveness of Nurse-Led versus Doctor-Led Antiretroviral Treatment in

South Africa: Pragmatic Cluster Randomised Trial." *Tropical Medicine and International Health* 18 (6): 769–77.

Behr, J. T. V. 2009. "Update in Diffuse Parenchymal Lung Disease 2008." *American Journal of Respiratory and Critical Care Medicine* 179 (6): 439–44.

Beran, D., H. J. Zar, C. Perrin, A. M. Menezes, P. G. J. Burney, and others. 2015. "Burden of Asthma and Chronic Obstructive Pulmonary Disease and Access to Essential Medicines in Low-Income and Middle-Income Countries." *The Lancet Respiratory Medicine* 3 (2): 159–70.

Blanc, P. D., and K. Torén. 2007. "Occupation in Chronic Obstructive Pulmonary Disease and Chronic Bronchitis: An Update." *International Journal of Tuberculosis and Lung Disease* 11 (3): 251–57.

Boudier, A., I. Curjuric, X. Basagana, H. Hazgui, J. M. Anto, and others. 2013. "Ten-Year Follow-Up of Cluster-Based Asthma Phenotypes in Adults: A Pooled Analysis of Three Cohorts." *American Journal of Respiratory and Critical Care Medicine* 188 (5): 550–60.

Bousquet, J., E. Mantzouranis, A. A. Cruz, N. Aït-Khaled, C. E. Baena-Cagnani, and others. 2010. "Uniform Definition of Asthma Severity, Control, and Exacerbations: Document Presented for the World Health Organization Consultation on Severe Asthma." *Journal of Allergy and Clinical Immunology* 126 (5): 926–38.

Bradley, J. M., F. Moran, and M. Greenstone. 2002. "Physical Training for Bronchiectasis." *Cochrane Database of Systematic Reviews* 2 (July): CD002166.

Burnett, R. T., C. A. Pope III, M. Ezzati, C. Olives, S. S. Lim, and others. 2014. "An Integrated Risk Function for Estimating the Global Burden of Disease Attributable to Ambient Fine Particulate Matter Exposure." *Environmental Health Perspectives* 122 (4): 397–403.

Burney, P. G. J., A. Jithoo, B. Kato, C. Janson, D. Mannino, and others. 2014. "Chronic Obstructive Pulmonary Disease Mortality and Prevalence: The Associations with Smoking and Poverty—A BOLD Analysis." *Thorax* 69 (5): 465–73.

Burney, P. G. J., and R. Hooper. 2011. "Forced Vital Capacity, Airway Obstruction, and Survival in a General Population Sample from the USA." *Thorax* 66 (1): 49–54.

———. 2012. "The Use of Ethnically Specific Norms for Ventilatory Function in African-American and White Populations." *International Journal of Epidemiology* 41 (3): 782–90.

Burney, P. G. J., J. Patel, R. Newson, C. Minelli, and M. Naghavi. 2015. "Global and Regional Trends in COPD Mortality, 1990–2010." *European Respiratory Journal* 45 (5): 1239–47.

Burney, P. G. J., J. Potts, N. Aït-Khaled, R. M. D. Sepulveda, N. Zidouni, and others. 2008. "A Multinational Study of Treatment Failures in Asthma Management." *International Journal of Tuberculosis and Lung Disease* 12 (1): 13–18.

Calvert, J., and P. G. J. Burney. 2005. "Effect of Body Mass on Exercise Induced Bronchoconstriction and Atopy in African Children." *Journal of Allergy and Clinical Immunology* 116 (4): 773–79.

Castelino, F. V., and J. Varga. 2010. "Interstitial Lung Disease in Connective Tissue Diseases: Evolving Concepts of Pathogenesis and Management." *Arthritis Research and Therapy* 12 (4): 213.

Chalmers, J. D., S. Aliberti, and F. Blasi. 2015. "State of the Art Review: Management of Bronchiectasis in Adults." *European Respiratory Journal* 45 (5): 1446–62.

Chang, A. B., S. C. Bell, C. A. Byrnes, K. Grimwood, P. W. Holmes, and others. 2010. "Chronic Suppurative Lung Disease and Bronchiectasis in Children and Adults in Australia and New Zealand: A Position Statement from the Thoracic Society of Australia and New Zealand and the Australian Lung Foundation." *Medical Journal of Australia* 193 (6): 356–65.

Chang, C. C., P. S. Morris, and A. B. Chang. 2007. "Influenza Vaccine for Children and Adults with Bronchiectasis." *Cochrane Database of Systematic Reviews* 3 (July): CD006218.

Chang, C. C., R. J. Singleton, P. S. Morris, and A. B. Chang. 2009. "Pneumococcal Vaccines for Children and Adults with Bronchiectasis." *Cochrane Database of Systematic Reviews* 2 (April): CD006316.

Checkley, W., J. K. P. West, R. A. Wise, M. R. Baldwin, L. Wu, and others. 2010. "Maternal Vitamin A Supplementation and Lung Function in Offspring." *New England Journal of Medicine* 362 (19): 1784–94.

Chong, J., C. Karner, and P. Poole. 2012. "Tiotropium versus Long-Acting Beta-Agonists for Stable Chronic Obstructive Pulmonary Disease." *Cochrane Database of Systematic Reviews* 9: CD009157.

Chung, K. F., S. E. Wenzel, J. L. Brozek, A. Bush, M. Castro, and others. 2014. "International ERS/ATS Guidelines on Definition, Evaluation, and Treatment of Severe Asthma." *European Respiratory Journal* 43 (2): 343–73.

Cooksley, N. A., D. Atkinson, G. B. Marks, B. G. Toelle, D. Reeve, and others. 2015. "Prevalence of Airflow Obstruction and Reduced Forced Vital Capacity in an Aboriginal Australian Population: The Cross-Sectional BOLD Study." *Respirology* 20 (5): 766–74.

Davies, H. R., L. Richeldi, and E. H. Walters. 2003. "Immunomodulatory Agents for Idiopathic Pulmonary Fibrosis." *Cochrane Database of Systematic Reviews* 3: CD003134.

Devakumar, D., J. Stocks, J. G. Ayres, J. Kirkby, S. K. Yadav, and others. 2015. "Effects of Antenatal Multiple Micronutrient Supplementation on Lung Function in Mid-Childhood: Follow-Up of a Double-Blind Randomised Controlled Trial in Nepal." *European Respiratory Journal* 45 (6): 1566–75.

Dockery, D. W., F. E. Speizer, B. G. Ferris, J. H. Ware, T. A. Louis, and others. 1988. "Cumulative and Reversible Effects of Lifetime Smoking on Simple Tests of Lung Function in Adults." *American Review of Respiratory Disease* 137 (2): 286–92.

Durham, S. R., S. M. Walker, E. M. Varga, M. R. Jacobson, F. O'Brien, and others. 1999. "Long-Term Clinical Efficacy of Grass-Pollen Immunotherapy." *New England Journal of Medicine* 341 (August): 468–75.

Eaton, T., J. E. Garrett, P. Young, W. Fergusson, J. Kolbe, and others. 2002. "Ambulatory Oxygen Improves Quality of Life of COPD Patients: A Randomised Controlled Study." *European Respiratory Journal* 20 (2): 306–12.

Ehrlich, R. I., N. White, R. Norman, R. Laubscher, K. Steyn, and others. 2004. "Predictors of Chronic Bronchitis in South African Adults." *International Journal of Tuberculosis and Lung Disease* 8 (3): 369–76.

English, R. G., M. O. Bachmann, E. D. Bateman, M. Zwarenstein, L. R. Fairall, and others. 2006. "Diagnostic Accuracy of an Integrated Respiratory Guideline in Identifying Patients with Respiratory Symptoms Requiring Screening for Pulmonary Tuberculosis: A Cross-Sectional Study." *BioMed Central Pulmonary Medicine* 6 (August): 22.

English, R. G., E. D. Bateman, M. F. Zwarenstein, L. R. Fairall, A. Bheekie, and others. 2008. "Development of a South African Integrated Syndromic Respiratory Disease Guideline for Primary Care." *Primary Care Respiratory Journal* 17 (3): 156–63.

Erhola, M., R. Mäkinen, K. Koskela, V. Bergman, T. Klaukka, and others. 2003. "The Asthma Programme of Finland: An Evaluation Survey in Primary Health Care." *International Journal of Tuberculosis and Lung Disease* 7 (6): 592–98.

Evans, D. J., A. Bara, and M. Greenstone. 2007. "Prolonged Antibiotics for Purulent Bronchiectasis in Children and Adults." *Cochrane Database of Systematic Reviews* 2 (August): CD001392.

Fairall, L. R., M. O. Bachmann, C. Lombard, V. Timmerman, K. Uebel, and others. 2012. "Task Shifting of Antiretroviral Treatment from Doctors to Primary-Care Nurses in South Africa (STRETCH): A Pragmatic, Parallel, Cluster-Randomised Trial." *The Lancet* 380 (9845): 889–98.

Fairall, L. R., M. O. Bachmann, G. M. Louwagie, C. van Vuuren, P. Chikobvu, and others. 2008. "Effectiveness of Antiretroviral Treatment in the South African Public-Sector Programme: Cohort Study." *Archives of Internal Medicine* 168 (1): 86–93.

Fairall, L. R., M. O. Bachmann, M. Zwarenstein, E. D. Bateman, L. W. Niessen, and others. 2010. "Cost-Effectiveness of Educational Outreach to Primary Care Nurses to Increase Tuberculosis Case Detection and Improve Respiratory Care: Economic Evaluation Alongside a Randomised Trial." *Tropical Medicine and International Health* 15 (3): 277–86.

Fairall, L. R., M. Zwarenstein, E. D. Bateman, M. Bachmann, C. Lombard, and others. 2005. "Effect of Educational Outreach to Nurses on Tuberculosis Case Detection and Primary Care of Respiratory Illness: Pragmatic Cluster Randomised Controlled Trial." *British Medical Journal* 331 (7519): 750–54.

Ferreira, A., C. Garvey, G. L. Connors, L. Hilling, J. Rigler, and others. 2009. "Pulmonary Rehabilitation in Interstitial Lung Disease: Benefits and Predictors of Response." *Chest* 135 (2): 442–47.

Fried, L. P., R. A. Kronmal, A. B. Newman, D. E. Bild, M. B. Mittelmark, and others. 1998. "Risk Factors for 5-Year Mortality in Older Adults: The Cardiovascular Health Study." *Journal of the American Medical Association* 279 (8): 585–92.

Fuertes, E., J. Bracher, C. Flexeder, I. Markevych, C. Klümper, and others. 2015. "Long-Term Air Pollution Exposure and Lung Function in 15 Year-Old Adolescents Living in an Urban and Rural Area in Germany: The GINIplus and LISAplus Cohorts." *International Journal of Hygiene and Environmental Health* 218 (7): 656–65.

Georgeu, D., C. J. Colvin, S. Lewin, L. R. Fairall, M. O. Bachmann, and others. 2012. "Implementing Nurse-Initiated and Managed Antiretroviral Treatment (NIMART) in South Africa: Qualitative Process Evaluation of the STRETCH Trial." *Implementation Science* 7 (July): 66.

Gershon, A. S., G. C. Mecredy, J. Guan, J. C. Victor, R. Goldstein, and others. 2015. "Quantifying Comorbidity in Individuals with COPD: A Population Study." *European Respiratory Journal* 45 (1): 51–59.

Gibson, P. G., V. M. McDonald, and G. B. Marks. 2010. "Asthma in Older Adults." *The Lancet* 376 (9743): 803–13.

GINA (Global Initiative for Asthma). 2014. *Global Strategy for Asthma Management and Prevention.* GINA. http://www.ginasthma.com.

Glazer, C. S. 2015. "Chronic Hypersensitivity Pneumonitis: Important Considerations in the Work-Up of This Fibrotic Lung Disease." *Current Opinion in Pulmonary Medicine* 21 (2): 171–77.

GOLD (Global Initiative for Chronic Obstructive Lung Disease). 2014. "Global Strategy for the Diagnosis, Management, and Prevention of Chronic Obstructive Pulmonary Disease." GOLD.

Graham, I. D., J. Logan, M. B. Harrison, S. E. Straus, J. Tetroe, and others. 2006. "Lost in Knowledge Translation: Time for a Map?" *Journal of Continuing Education in the Health Professions* 26 (1): 13–24.

Güell, R., P. Casan, J. Belda, M. Sangenis, F. Morante, and others. 2000. "Long-Term Effects of Outpatient Rehabilitation of COPD: A Randomized Trial." *Chest* 117 (4): 976–83.

Haahtela, T., T. Klaukka, K. Koskela, M. Erhola, L. A. Laitinen, and others. 2001. "Asthma Programme in Finland: A Community Problem Needs Community Solutions." *Thorax* 56 (10): 806–14.

Haahtela, T., L. E. Tuomisto, A. Pietinalho, T. Klaukka, M. Erhola, and others. 2006. "A 10-Year Asthma Programme in Finland: Major Change for the Better." *Thorax* 61 (8): 663–70.

Hamzaoui, A., and S. Ottmani. 2012. "Practical Approach to Lung Health: Lung Health for Everyone?" *European Respiratory Review* 21 (125): 186–95.

Han, M. K., D. S. Bach, P. G. Hagan, E. Yow, K. R. Flaherty, and others. 2013. "Sildenafil Preserves Exercise Capacity in Patients with Idiopathic Pulmonary Fibrosis and Right-Sided Ventricular Dysfunction." *Chest* 143 (6): 1699–708.

Hankinson, J. L., J. R. Odencrantz, and F. B. Fedan. 1999. "Spirometric Reference Values from a Sample of the General U.S. Population." *American Journal of Respiratory and Critical Care Medicine* 159 (1): 179–87.

Hansell, A., R. E. Ghosh, M. Blangiardo, C. Perkins, D. Vienneau, and others. 2016. "Historic Air Pollution Exposure and Long-Term Mortality Risks in England and Wales: Prospective Longitudinal Cohort Study." *Thorax* 71 (4): 330–38.

Hart, A., K. Sugumar, S. J. Milan, S. J. Fowler, and I. Crossingham. 2014. "Inhaled Hyperosmolar Agents for Bronchiectasis." *Cochrane Database of Systematic Reviews* 5: CD002996.

Hill, A. T., M. Pasteur, C. Cornford, S. Welham, and D. Bilton. 2011. "Primary Care Summary of the British Thoracic Society Guideline on the Management of Non-Cystic Fibrosis Bronchiectasis." *Primary Care Respiratory Journal* 20 (2): 135–40.

Holland, W. W., and D. D. Reid. 1965. "The Urban Factor in Chronic Bronchitis." *The Lancet* 40 (7383): 445–48.

Hooper, R., and P. G. J. Burney. 2013. "Cross-Sectional Relation of Ethnicity to Ventilatory Function in a West London Population." *International Journal of Tuberculosis and Respiratory Disease* 17 (3): 400–5.

Hooper, R., P. G. J. Burney, W. Vollmer, M. McBurnie, T. Gislason, and others. 2012. "Risk Factors for COPD Spirometrically Defined from the Lower Limit of Normal in the BOLD Project." *European Respiratory Journal* 39 (6): 1343–53.

Hooper, R., J. Calvert, R. L. Thompson, M. E. Deetlefs, and P. G. J. Burney. 2008. "Urban/Rural Differences in Diet and Atopy in South Africa." *Allergy* 63 (4): 425–31.

Hutchinson, J. P., T. M. McKeever, A. W. Fogarty, V. Navaratnam, and R. B. Hubbard. 2014. "Increasing Global Mortality from Idiopathic Pulmonary Fibrosis in the Twenty-First Century." *Annals of the American Thoracic Society* 11 (8): 1176–85.

Hwang, Y. I., J. H. Kim, C. Y. Lee, S. Park, Y. B. Park, and others. 2014. "The Association between Airflow Obstruction and Radiologic Change by Tuberculosis." *Journal of Thoracic Disease* 6 (5): 471–76.

Iepsen, U. W., K. J. Jørgensen, T. Ringbæk, H. Hansen, C. Skrubbeltrang, and others. 2015. "A Combination of Resistance and Endurance Training Increases Leg Muscle Strength in COPD: An Evidence-Based Recommendation Based on Systematic Review with Meta-Analyses." *Chronic Respiratory Disease* 12 (2): 132–45.

Jaakkola, M. S., P. Ernst, J. J. K. Jaakkola, L. W. N'Gan'ga, and M. Becklake. 1991. "Effect of Cigarette Smoking on Evolution of Ventilatory Lung Function in Young Adults: An Eight Year Longitudinal Study." *Thorax* 46 (12): 907–13.

Jha, P., M. MacLennon, F. J. Chaloupka, A. Yurekli, C. Ramasundarahettige, and others. 2015. "Global Hazards of Tobacco and the Benefits of Smoking Cessation and Tobacco Taxes." In *Disease Control Priorities* (third edition): Volume 3, *Cancer*, edited by H. Gelband, P. Jha, R. Sankaranarayanan, and S. Horton. Washington, DC: World Bank.

Jiang, C., H. Huang, J. Liu, Y. Wang, Z. Lu, and others. 2012. "Adverse Events of Pirfenidone for the Treatment of Pulmonary Fibrosis: A Meta-Analysis of Randomized Controlled Trials." *PLoS One* 7 (10): e47024.

Jindal, S. K., and R. Agarwal. 2012. "Long-Term Oxygen Therapy." *Expert Review of Respiratory Medicine* 6 (6): 639–49.

Jindal, S. K., A. N. Aggarwal, K. Chaudhry, S. K. Chhabra, G. A. D'Souza, and others. 2006. "A Multicentric Study on Epidemiology of Chronic Obstructive Pulmonary Disease and Its Relationship with Tobacco Smoking and Environmental Tobacco Smoke Exposure." *Indian Journal of Chest Diseases and Allied Sciences* 48 (1): 23–29.

Jithoo, A., P. L. Enright, P. G. J. Burney, A. S. Buist, E. D. Bateman, and others. 2013. "Case-Finding Options for COPD: Results from the Burden of Obstructive Lung Disease Study." *European Respiratory Journal* 41 (3): 548–55.

Kannel, W. B., E. A. Lew, H. B. Hubert, and W. P. Castelli. 1980. "The Value of Measuring Vital Capacity for Prognostic Purposes." *Transactions of the Association of Life Insurance Medical Directors of America* 64: 66–83.

Karner, C., J. Chong, and P. Poole. 2014. "Tiotropium versus Placebo for Chronic Obstructive Pulmonary Disease." *Cochrane Database of Systematic Reviews* 7 (July 21): CD009285.

Kauppi, P., M. Linna, J. Martikainen, M. J. Mäkelä, and T. Haahtela. 2013. "Follow-Up of the Finnish Asthma Programme 2000–2010: Reduction of Hospital Burden Needs Risk Group Rethinking." *Thorax* 68 (3): 292–93.

Keeley, D. J., and S. Gallivan. 1991. "Comparison of the Prevalence of Reversible Airways Obstruction in Rural and Urban Zimbabwean Children." *Thorax* 46 (8): 549–53.

Kew, K. M., C. Mavergames, and A. E. J. Walters. 2013. "Long-Acting Beta-2-Agonists for Chronic Obstructive Pulmonary Disease." *Cochrane Database of Systematic Reviews* 10 (October): CD010177.

Khanna, D., X. Yan, D. P. Tashkin, D. E. Furst, R. Elashoff, and others. 2007. "Impact of Oral Cyclophosphamide on Health-Related Quality of Life in Patients with Active Scleroderma Lung Disease: Results from the Scleroderma Lung Study." *Arthritis and Rheumatism* 56 (5): 1676–84.

Lacasse, Y., R. A. Goldstein, T. Lasserson, and S. Martin. 2006. "Pulmonary Rehabilitation for Chronic Obstructive Pulmonary Disease." *Cochrane Database of Systematic Reviews* 4 (February): CD003793.

Lai, C. K. W., R. Beasley, J. Crane, S. Foliaki, J. Shah, and others. 2009. "Global Variation in the Prevalence and Severity of Asthma Symptoms: Phase Three of the International Study of Asthma and Allergies in Childhood (ISAAC)." *Thorax* 64 (6): 476–83.

Lam, H. K.-B., C. Q. Jiang, R. E. Jordan, M. R. Miller, W. S. Zhang, and others. 2010. "Prior TB, Smoking, and Airflow Obstruction: A Cross-Sectional Analysis of the Guangzhou Biobank Cohort Study." *Chest* 137 (3): 593–600.

Larkin, E. K., Y.-T. Gao, T. Gebretsadik, T. J. Hartman, P. Wu, and others. 2015. "New Risk Factors for Adult-Onset Incident Asthma: A Nested Case-Control Study of Host Antioxidant Defence." *American Journal of Respiratory and Critical Care Medicine* 191 (1): 45–53.

Lawlor, D. A., S. Ebrahim, and S. G. Davey. 2005. "Association of Birth Weight with Adult Lung Function: Findings from the British Women's Heart and Health Study and a Meta-Analysis." *Thorax* 60 (10): 851–58.

Lee, A. L., A. Burge, and A. E. Holland. 2013. "Airway Clearance Techniques for Bronchiectasis." *Cochrane Database of Systematic Reviews* 5 (May): CD008351.

Loth, D. W., M. Soler Artigas, S. A. Gharib, L. V. Wain, N. Franceschini, and others. 2014. "Genome-Wide Association Analysis Identifies Six New Loci Associated with Forced Vital Capacity." *Nature Genetics* 46 (7): 669–77.

Lozano, R., M. Naghavi, K. Foreman, S. Lim, K. Shibuya, and others. 2013. "Global and Regional Mortality from 235 Causes of Death for 20 Age Groups in 1990 and 2010:

A Systematic Analysis for the Global Burden of Disease Study 2010." *The Lancet* 380 (9859): 2095–128.

Lundy Braun, L., M. Wolfgang, and K. Dickersin. 2013. "Defining Race/Ethnicity and Explaining Difference in Research Studies on Lung Function." *European Respiratory Journal* 41 (6): 1362–70.

Martinez, F. D., A. L. Wright, L. M. Taussig, C. J. Holberg, M. Halonen, and others. 1995. "Asthma and Wheezing in the First Six Years of Life." *New England Journal of Medicine* 332 (3): 133–38.

Masoli, M., D. Fabian, S. Holt, and R. Beasley. 2004. "The Global Burden of Asthma: Executive Summary of the GINA Dissemination Committee Report." *Allergy* 59 (5): 469.

Medical Research Council Working Party. 1981. "Long-Term Domiciliary Oxygen Therapy in Chronic Hypoxic Cor Pulmonale Complicating Chronic Bronchitis and Emphysema." *The Lancet* 1 (8222): 681–86.

Mendoza, L., P. Horta, J. Espinoza, M. Aguilera, N. Balmaceda, and others. 2015. "Pedometers to Enhance Physical Activity in COPD: A Randomised Controlled Trial." *European Respiratory Journal* 45 (2): 347–54.

Menezes, A. M. B., P. C. Hallal, R. Perez-Padilla, J. R. B. Jardim, A. Muiño, and others. 2007. "Tuberculosis and Airflow Obstruction: Evidence from the PLATINO Study in Latin America." *European Respiratory Journal* 30 (6): 1180–85.

Menezes, A. M. B., F. C. Wehrmeister, F. P. Hartwig, R. Perez-Padilla, D. P. Gigante, and others. 2015. "African Ancestry, Lung Function, and the Effect of Genetics." *European Respiratory Journal* 45 (6): 1582–89.

Miller, M. R., J. Hankinson, V. Brusasco, F. Burgos, R. Casaburi, and others. 2005. "Standardisation of Spirometry." *European Respiratory Journal* 26 (2): 153–61.

Moffatt, M., I. Gut, F. Demenais, D. Strachan, E. Bouzigon, and others. 2010. "A Large-Scale, Consortium-Based Genomewide Association Study of Asthma." *New England Journal of Medicine* 363 (13): 1211.

MSH (Management Sciences for Health). 2015. *International Drug Indicator Guide, 2014 Edition.* Updated annually. Medford, MA: MSH.

National Asthma Education and Prevention Program. 2007. *Expert Panel Report 3: Guidelines for the Diagnosis and Management of Asthma.* Bethesda, MD: National Institutes of Health, National Heart, Lung, and Blood Institute.

Noble, P. W., C. Albera, W. Z. Bradford, U. Costabel, M. K. Glassberg, and others. 2011. "Pirfenidone in Patients with Idiopathic Pulmonary Fibrosis (CAPACITY): Two Randomised Trials." *The Lancet* 377 (9779): 1760–69.

Nurmatov, U., G. Devereux, and A. Sheikh. 2011. "Nutrients and Foods for the Primary Prevention of Asthma and Allergy: Systematic Review and Meta-Analysis." *Journal of Allergy and Clinical Immunology* 127 (3): 724–33.

Obaseki, D., J. Potts, G. Joos, J. Baelum, T. Haahtela, and others. 2014. "The Relation of Airway Obstruction to Asthma, Chronic Rhinosinusitis, and Age: Results from a Population Survey of Adults." *Allergy* 69 (9): 1205–14.

Ottmani, S. E., R. Scherpbier, A. Pio, P. Chaulet, and N. A. Khaled. 2005. *Practical Approach to Lung Health (PAL): A Primary Health Care Strategy for Integrated Management of Respiratory Conditions in People Five Years of Age and Over.* Geneva: World Health Organization.

Pan, L., M. Wang, X. Xie, C. Du, and Y. Guo. 2014. "Effects of Anabolic Steroids on Chronic Obstructive Pulmonary Disease: A Meta-Analysis of Randomised Controlled Trials." *PLoS One* 10 (9): e84855.

Pedone, C., S. Scarlata, D. Chiurco, M. E. Conte, F. Forastiere, and others. 2012. "Association of Reduced Total Lung Capacity with Mortality and Use of Health Services." *Chest* 141 (4): 1025–30.

Perzanowski, M. S., P. Ngari, T. A. E. Platts-Mills, J. Odhiambo, M. D. Chapman, and others. 2002. "Atopy, Asthma, and Antibodies to *Ascaris* among Rural and Urban Children in Kenya." *Journal of Pediatrics* 140 (5): 582–88.

Peto, R., F. E. Speizer, A. L. Cochrane, F. Moore, C. M. Fletcher, and others. 1983. "The Relevance in Adults of Air-Flow Obstruction, but Not of Mucus Hypersecretion, to Mortality from Chronic Lung Disease: Results from 20 Years of Prospective Observation." *American Review of Respiratory Disease* 128 (3): 491–500.

Phui, N. C., N. C. Tan, and T. K. Lim. 2008. "Impact of the Singapore National Asthma Program (SNAP) on Preventor-Reliever Prescription Ratio in Polyclinics." *Annals of the Academy of Medicine, Singapore* 37 (2): 114–17.

Pietinalho, A., V. L. Kinnula, A. R. A. Sovijärvi, S. Vilkman, O. Säynäjäkangas, and others. 2007. "Chronic Bronchitis and Chronic Obstructive Pulmonary Disease: The Finnish Action Programme, Interim Report." *Respiratory Medicine* 101 (7): 1419.

Poole, P., E. E. Chacko, R. Wood-Baker, and C. J. Cates. 2006. "Influenza Vaccine for Patients with Chronic Obstructive Pulmonary Disease." *Cochrane Database of Systematic Reviews* 1: CD002733

Powell, H., V. E. Murphy, D. R. Taylor, M. J. Hensley, K. McCaffery, and others. 2011. "Management of Asthma in Pregnancy Guided by Measurement of Fraction of Exhaled Nitric Oxide: A Double-Blind, Randomised Controlled Trial." *The Lancet* 378 (9795): 983–90.

Poyser, M. A., H. Nelson, R. I. Ehrlich, E. D. Bateman, S. Parnell, and others. 2002. "Socioeconomic Deprivation and Asthma Prevalence and Severity in Young Adolescents." *European Respiratory Journal* 19 (5): 892–98.

Price, D., M. Fletcher, and T. van der Molen. 2014. "Asthma Control and Management in 8,000 European Patients: The REcognise Asthma and LInk to Symptoms and Experience (REALISE) Survey." *Nature Partner Journals Primary Care Respiratory Medicine* 24: 14009.

Raghu, G. 2013. "Anti-Acid Treatment and Disease Progression in Idiopathic Pulmonary Fibrosis: An Analysis of Data from Three Randomised Controlled Trials." *The Lancet Respiratory Medicine* 1 (5): 369–76.

Ram, S. F. F., J. Picot, J. Lightowler, and J. A. Widzicha. 2009. "Non-Invasive Positive Pressure Ventilation for Treatment of Respiratory Failure due to Exacerbations of Chronic Obstructive Pulmonary Disease." *Cochrane Database of Systematic Reviews* 4: CD004104.

Richeldi, L. 2012. "Assessing the Treatment Effect from Multiple Trials in Idiopathic Pulmonary Fibrosis." *European Respiratory Review* 21 (124): 147–51.

Richeldi, L., U. Costabel, M. Selman, D. S. Kim, D. M. Hansell, and others. 2011. "Efficacy of a Tyrosine Kinase Inhibitor in Idiopathic Pulmonary Fibrosis." *New England Journal of Medicine* 365 (12): 1079–87.

Root, M. M., S. M. Houser, J. J. Anderson, and H. R. Dawson. 2014. "Healthy Eating Index 2005 and Selected Macronutrients Are Correlated with Improved Lung Function in Humans." *Nutrition Research* 34 (4): 77–84.

Roy, A., I. Rawal, S. Jabbour, and D. Prabhakaran. 2017. "Tobacco and Cardiovascular Disease: A Summary of Evidence." In *Disease Control Priorities* (third edition): Volume 5, *Cardiovascular, Respiratory, and Related Disorders*, edited by D. Prabhakaran, S. Anand, T. A. Gaziano, J.-C. Mbanya, Y. Wu, and R. Nugent. Washington, DC: World Bank.

Salomon, J., H. Wang, M. Freeman, T. Vos, A. Flaxman, and others. 2012. "Healthy Life Expectancy for 187 Countries, 1990–2010: A Systematic Analysis for the Global Burden of Disease Study 2010." *The Lancet* 380 (9859): 2144–62.

Schikowski, T., M. Adam, A. Marcon, Y. Cai, A. Vierkötter, and others. 2014. "Association of Ambient Air Pollution with the Prevalence and Incidence of COPD." *European Respiratory Journal* 44 (3): 614–26.

Schull, M. J., R. Cornick, S. Thompson, G. Faris, L. Fairall, and others. 2011. "From PALSA PLUS to PALM PLUS: Adapting and Developing a South African Guideline and Training Intervention to Better Integrate HIV/AIDS Care with Primary Care in Rural Health Centers in Malawi." *Implementation Science* 6 (July): 82.

Schultz, E., J. Hallberg, T. Bellander, A. Bergström, M. Bottai, and others. 2016. "Early-Life Exposure to Traffic-Related Air Pollution and Lung Function in Adolescence." *American Journal of Respiratory and Critical Care Medicine* 193 (2): 171–77.

Sembajwe, G., M. Cifuentes, S. W. Tak, D. Kriebel, R. Gore, and others. 2010. "National Income, Self-Reported Wheezing, and Asthma Diagnosis from the World Health Survey." *European Respiratory Journal* 35 (2): 279–86.

Shaheen, S. O., J. A. C. Sterne, R. L. Thompson, C. E. Songhurst, B. M. Margetts, and others. 2001. "Dietary Antioxidants and Asthma in Adults: Population-Based Case-Control Study." *American Journal of Respiratory and Critical Care Medicine* 164 (10, Pt 1): 1823–28.

Shulgina, L., A. P. Cahn, E. R. Chilvers, H. Parfrey, A. B. Clark, and others. 2013. "Treating Idiopathic Pulmonary Fibrosis with the Addition of Co-Trimoxazole: A Randomised Controlled Trial." *Thorax* 68 (2): 155–62.

Siva, R., R. H. Green, C. E. Brightling, M. Shelley, B. Hargadon, and others. 2007. "Eosinophilic Airway Inflammation and Exacerbations of COPD: A Randomised Controlled Trial." *European Respiratory Journal* 29 (5): 906.

Smith, M., L. Li, M. Augustyn, O. Kurmi, J. Chen, and others. 2014. "Prevalence and Correlates of Airflow Obstruction in 317,000 Never-Smokers in China." *European Respiratory Journal* 44 (1): 66–77.

Sodhi, S., H. Banda, D. Kathyola, M. Joshua, F. Richardson, and others. 2014. "Supporting Middle-Cadre Health Care Workers in Malawi: Lessons Learned during Implementation of the PALM PLUS Package." *BioMed Central Health Services Research* 14 (Suppl 1): S8.

Sonnappa, S., S. Lum, J. Kirkby, R. Bonner, A. M. Wade, and others. 2015. "Disparities in Pulmonary Function in Healthy Children across the Indian Urban-Rural Continuum." *American Journal of Respiratory and Critical Care Medicine* 191 (1): 79–86.

Spagnolo, P., C. Del Giovane, F. Luppi, S. Cerri, S. Balduzzi, and others. 2010. "Non-Steroid Agents for Idiopathic Pulmonary Fibrosis." *Cochrane Database of Systematic Reviews* 9: CD003134.

Speight, A. N., D. A. Lee, and E. N. Hey. 1983. "Underdiagnosis and Undertreatment of Asthma in Childhood." *British Medical Journal* 286 (6373): 1253–56.

Stein, J., S. Lewin, L. R. Fairall, P. Mayers, R. English, and others. 2008. "Building Capacity for Antiretroviral Delivery in South Africa: A Qualitative Evaluation of the PALSA PLUS Nurse Training Programme." *BioMed Central Health Services Research* 8 (November): 240.

Suissa, S., P. Ernst, S. Benayoun, M. Baltzan, and B. Cai. 2000. "Low-Dose Inhaled Corticosteroids and the Prevention of Death from Asthma." *New England Journal of Medicine* 343 (5): 332–36.

Suissa, S., V. Patenaude, F. Lapi, and P. Ernst. 2013. "Inhaled Corticosteroids in COPD and the Risk of Serious Pneumonia." *Thorax* 68 (11): 1029–36.

Swanney, M. P., G. Ruppel, P. L. Enright, O. F. Pedersen, R. O. Crapo, and others. 2008. "Using the Lower Limit of Normal for the FEV_1/FVC Ratio Reduces the Misclassification of Airway Obstruction." *Thorax* 63 (12): 1046–51.

Tan, W., W. Vollmer, B. Lamprecht, D. Mannino, A. Jithoo, and others. 2012. "Worldwide Patterns of Bronchodilator Responsiveness: Results from the Burden of Obstructive Lung Disease Study." *Thorax* 67 (8): 718–26.

Taniguchi, H., M. Ebina, Y. Kondoh, T. Ogura, A. Azuma, and others. 2010. "Pirfenidone in Idiopathic Pulmonary Fibrosis." *European Respiratory Journal* 35 (4): 821–29.

Tashkin, D. P., R. Elashoff, P. J. Clements, J. Goldin, M. D. Roth, and others. 2006. "Cyclophosphamide versus Placebo in Scleroderma Lung Disease." *New England Journal of Medicine* 354 (25): 2655–66.

Travis, W. D., U. Costabel, D. M. Hansell, T. E. King, D. A. Lynch, and others. 2013. "An Official American Thoracic Society/European Respiratory Society Statement: Update of the International Multidisciplinary Classification of the Idiopathic Interstitial Pneumonias." *American Journal of Respiratory and Critical Care Medicine* 188 (6): 733–48.

U.K. Office of Population Censuses and Surveys. 1986. *Occupational Mortality: The Registrar General's Decennial Supplement for Great Britain, 1979–80, 1982–83.* London: H.M. Stationery Office.

U.S. FDA (U.S. Food and Drug Administration). 2010. *Questions and Answers: New Safety Requirements for Long-Acting Asthma Medications Called Long-Acting Beta Agonists (LABAs).* Rockville, MD: U.S. FDA. http://www.fda.gov /Drugs/DrugSafety/InformationbyDrugClass/ucm200719 .htm#_Ref252367488.

U.S. Surgeon General. 1984. *Surgeon General: The Health Consequences of Smoking—Chronic Obstructive Lung Disease.* Rockville, MD: U.S. Department of Health and Human Services.

Varraso, R., R. Jiang, R. G. Barr, W. Willett, and C. A. Camargo Jr. 2007. "Prospective Study of Cured Meats Consumption and Risk of Chronic Obstructive Pulmonary Disease in Men." *American Journal of Epidemiology* 166 (12): 1438–45.

Vestbo, J., and J. Hogg. 2006. "Convergence of the Epidemiology and Pathology of COPD." *Thorax* 61 (1): 86–88.

Vietri, J., K. Burslem, and J. Su. 2014. "Poor Asthma Control among U.S. Workers: Health-Related Quality of Life, Work Impairment, and Health Care Use." *Journal of Occupational and Environmental Medicine* 56 (4): 425–30.

Vollenweider, D. J., H. Jarrett, C. A. Steurer-Stey, J. Garcia-Aymerich, and M. A. Puhan. 2012. "Antibiotics for Exacerbations of Chronic Obstructive Pulmonary Disease." *Cochrane Database of Systematic Reviews* 12: CD010257.

Vos, T., A. D. Flaxman, M. Naghavi, R. Lozano, C. Michaud, and others. 2012. "Years Lived with Disability (YLDs) for 1160 Sequelae of 289 Diseases and Injuries 1990–2010: A Systematic Analysis for the Global Burden of Disease Study 2010." *The Lancet* 380 (9859): 2163–96.

Walters, J. A. E., S. Smith, P. Poole, R. H. Granger, and R. Wood-Baker. 2010. "Injectable Vaccines for Preventing Pneumococcal Infection in Patients with Chronic Obstructive Pulmonary Disease." *Cochrane Database of Systematic Reviews* 11 (November): CD001390.

Walters, J. A., D. J. Tan, C. J. White, P. G. Gibson, R. Wood-Baker, and others. 2014. "Systemic Corticosteroids for Acute Exacerbations of Chronic Obstructive Pulmonary Disease." *Cochrane Database of Systematic Reviews* 1 (January): CD001288.

Weinmayr, G., J. Genuneit, G. Nagel, B. Bjorksten, M. van Hage, and others. 2010. "International Variations in Associations of Allergic Markers and Diseases in Children: ISAAC Phase Two." *Allergy* 65 (6): 766.

WHO (World Health Organization). 2008. *Practical Approach to Lung Health: Manual on Initiating PAL Implementation.* Geneva: WHO.

———. 2010. "International Statistical Classification of Diseases and Related Health Problems, 10th Revision (ICD-10) Version for 2010." WHO, Geneva. http://apps.who.int/classifications/icd10/browse/2010/en#/X.

———. 2013a. *Implementation Tools Package of Essential Non-Communicable (PEN) Disease Interventions for Primary Health Care in Low-Resource Settings.* Geneva: WHO.

———. 2013b. *Integrated Management of Adolescent and Adult Illness (IMAI) Modules.* Geneva: WHO. http://www.who.int/hiv/pub/imai/en/index.html.

Wilkinson, M., K. Sugumar, S. J. Milan, A. Hart, A. Crockett, and others. 2014. "Mucolytics for Bronchiectasis." *Cochrane Database of Systematic Reviews* 1 (May): CD001289.

Yang, I. A., M. S. Clarke, E. H. Sim, and K. M. Fong. 2012. "Inhaled Corticosteroids for Stable Chronic Obstructive Pulmonary Disease." *Cochrane Database of Systematic Reviews* 7 (July): CD002991.

Zemedkun, K., K. Woldemichael, and G. Tefera. 2014. "Assessing Control of Asthma in Jush, Jimma, South West Ethiopia." *Ethiopian Journal of Health Sciences* 24 (1): 49–58.

Zwarenstein, M., L. R. Fairall, C. Lombard, P. Mayers, A. Bheekie, and others. 2011. "Outreach Education for Integration of HIV/AIDS Care, Antiretroviral Treatment, and Tuberculosis Care in Primary Care Clinics in South Africa: PALSA PLUS Pragmatic Cluster Randomised Trial." *British Medical Journal* 342 (April): d2022.

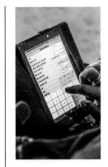

Chapter 16

Integrated Public Health and Health Service Delivery for Noncommunicable Diseases and Comorbid Infectious Diseases and Mental Health

Matthew Magee, Mohammed Ali, Dorairaj Prabhakaran, Vamadevan S. Ajay, and K. M. Venkat Narayan

INTRODUCTION

The co-occurrence of noncommunicable diseases and communicable diseases raises important challenges to the integration of public health and care delivery for more than one morbidity. Effective integration requires assessing needs, designing integrated systems, leveraging existing infrastructure, and addressing resource challenges through creative organizational and technological strategies.

This chapter uses the example of diabetes as a prototypical noncommunicable disease and highlights the urgent need for integrated approaches to addressing three key comorbidities in patients with diabetes: mental health disorders, tuberculosis, and human immunodeficiency virus/acquired immune deficiency syndrome (HIV/AIDS). We explore the epidemiology of joint burdens, risk factors, and prognoses of these co-occurring conditions. We summarize the available evidence and address the challenges of integrating public health and health services for persons jointly affected by diabetes and the three comorbidities. We focus on a case study for integrating care for diabetes and mental health disorders. Finally, we address gaps in data regarding combined

burdens and effectiveness and cost-effectiveness of integrated interventions and make recommendations for closing those gaps.

GLOBAL BURDEN OF COEXISTING DIABETES WITH DEPRESSION, TUBERCULOSIS, AND HIV/AIDS

Diabetes and Mental Health

Joint Burdens

Mental illnesses, especially depression, occur more commonly in people with other chronic illnesses (Patel, Chatterji, and others 2011; Poongothai and others 2010; Poongothai and others 2011; Raval and others 2010). A study of 245,404 participants from 60 countries showed that, although one-year prevalence of depression based on codes in the 10th edition of the *International Statistical Classification of Diseases and Related Heath Problems* was 3.2 percent, between 9.3 percent and 23.0 percent of participants with one or more chronic illnesses had comorbid depression. Adjusting for all other socioeconomic conditions and comorbidities, depression remained the most important contributor to

Corresponding author: Matthew Magee, Division of Epidemiology and Biostatistics, School of Public Health, Georgia State University, Atlanta, Georgia, United States; mjmagee@gsu.edu.

self-reported poor health scores in these persons (Moussavi and others 2007). In a large meta-analysis, depression was twice as common in people with diabetes than in those without the disease (Anderson and others 2001); up to 50 percent of patients with cancer suffer from depression or anxiety (Massie 2004).

Mental illnesses may be risk factors for the development of chronic diseases. Depression has been shown to be a risk factor for type 2 diabetes (Carnethon and others 2007; Golden and others 2004; Knol and others 2006; Llorente and Urrutia 2006). Depression increases the risk independent of smoking, physical activity, alcohol intake, C-reactive protein, and other factors associated with both depression and diabetes (Carnethon and others 2007). Depression may induce hypothalamic-pituitary-adrenal axis dysregulation and adverse autonomic nervous system dysfunction (Carnethon and others 2003). Both short- and long-term activation of sympathetic nervous systems suppress beta-cell function and insulin secretion, which may contribute to the increased risk for type 2 diabetes (Everson-Rose and others 2004). This bidirectional relationship makes comorbid diabetes-depression challenging to prevent and treat.

Individual and Societal Risk Factors

Mental illnesses are generally multifactorial. Mood disorders such as depression are related to different demographic, economic, contextual, psychological, and biological factors (Patel and others 1999; Patel and others 2009). In many cases, the confluence of vulnerabilities, stressors, and timing results in psychological distress and illness.

Prognosis and Outcomes

People with comorbid chronic and mental illnesses report worse health status and more burdensome symptoms; they have a higher risk of end-organ complications, relapse of depression (Lustman, Griffith, Freedland, and Clouse 1997), disability, and mortality.

Biologically, depression is linked to systemic inflammatory (Frohlich and others 2000; Konsman, Parnet, and Dantzer 2002) and endothelial (Laghrissi-Thode and others 1997; Musselman and others 1996) processes that perpetuate atherosclerosis and heighten the risk for cardiovascular disease (Joynt, Whellan, and O'Connor 2003; Rugulies 2002). A meta-analysis of depression and cardiovascular disease reported that persons with clinical depression had 2.7 (95 percent confidence interval [CI] 1.6–4.4) times the risk of coronary heart disease compared with those without depression (Rugulies 2002).

These poor outcomes may be mediated by behavioral or pathophysiological processes. For example, depression adversely affects self-care for diabetes (Beverly and others 2012; Gonzalez and others 2008; Llorente and Urrutia 2006; Sridhar and Madhu 2002) and worsens glycemic control (Lustman, Anderson, and others 2000) and quality of life (Egede, Grubaugh, and Ellis 2010; Sridhar 2007). People with depression are twice as likely to smoke (Lasser and others 2000) and are less likely to engage in protective physical activity (Roshanaei-Moghaddam, Katon, and Russo 2009).

Mental illnesses, particularly depression, are the leading risk factors for suicide (Whiteford and others 2013); mental illnesses also increase the risk for other health outcomes and mortality. People with diabetes and depression have twice the risk of intensive care unit admissions and longer hospital stays than do those without depression (Davydow and others 2011). Comorbid depression is associated with up to three times higher risk of mortality in people with diabetes or chronic kidney disease (Bot and others 2012; Lin and others 2009; Sullivan and others 2012; Young and others 2010).

Diabetes and Tuberculosis

Each year, nearly 9 million people develop active tuberculosis; nearly 2 million die from tuberculosis-related causes, accounting for 2 percent of deaths from infectious diseases (WHO 2012). More than 95 percent of all tuberculosis cases occur in low- and middle-income countries (LMICs); an estimated 2 billion people have *Mycobacterium tuberculosis* complex infection and are at risk for developing the active disease (Nelson and Williams 2007). Diabetes prevalence (currently 366 million and estimated to reach 570 million by 2030) and diabetes cause-specific mortality (1.3 million deaths in 2010) are expanding (IDF 2013). The anticipated increases in diabetes-associated burdens will occur disproportionately in LMICs, where tuberculosis is likely to remain endemic for the foreseeable future (Magee, Blumberg, and Narayan 2011).

The increasing coprevalence has heightened public health interest in the intersection of diabetes and tuberculosis in individuals. Diabetes increases the chance of developing active tuberculosis by approximately threefold (Jeon and Murray 2008). Both in vivo and in vitro studies suggest that diabetes may affect vulnerability to *Mycobacterium tuberculosis* infection by altering cytokine signaling related to both innate and adaptive immune responses (figure 16.1) (Martinez and Kornfeld 2014; Restrepo and Schlesinger 2013).

Tuberculosis may increase the risk of diabetes. Chronic inflammation that results from major infections such as tuberculosis can induce stress-related hyperglycemia (Kapur and Harries 2013), and active tuberculosis disease can worsen existing hyperglycemia and insulin resistance. However, older studies that have documented changes in

Figure 16.1 Tuberculosis Infection and Disease States and Effects of Diabetes Mellitus

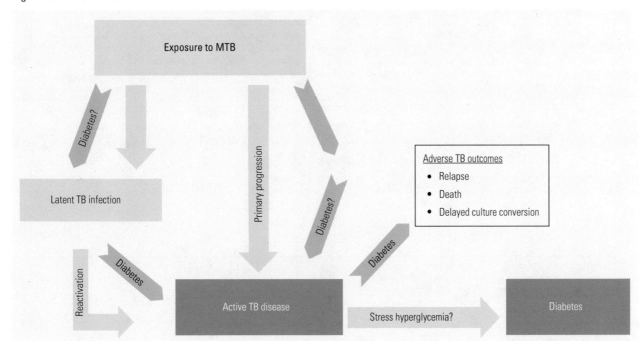

Note: MTB = *Mycobacterium tuberculosis*; TB = tuberculosis. Arrows including "diabetes" indicate a hypothesized increased risk due to diabetes; "?" indicates a hypothesis without substantial epidemiologic data.

glucose tolerance during and after tuberculosis treatment report that a high proportion of newly diagnosed tuberculosis patients with hyperglycemia or diabetes return to normal blood glucose levels after tuberculosis treatment (WHO 2011). Additional research is needed to differentiate the impact of tuberculosis on the risk of incident diabetes (versus new diagnosis of previous diabetes) and to describe glycemic trajectories before, during, and after tuberculosis treatment.

An increased proportion of new tuberculosis cases is attributed to diabetes—an estimated 15 percent or 1.4 million annual cases (Lonnroth, Roglic, and Harries 2014). The struggle to reduce the incidence of tuberculosis and diabetes has resulted in an increased global burden of people experiencing both diseases. The co-occurrence of these two pandemics illustrates a new epidemiological phenomenon in which chronic diseases occur simultaneously with infectious diseases not only in the same population but also in the same individuals (Magee, Blumberg, and Narayan 2011).

Joint Burdens

The annual global incidence of tuberculosis is concentrated among 22 high-burden countries, all LMICs. In 2011, an estimated 82 percent (7.1 million) of all incident tuberculosis cases (8.7 million) occurred in these countries; 37 percent (3.2 million) were in China and India (WHO 2012). Historically, national programs in the high-tuberculosis-burden countries have not routinely conducted surveillance of diabetes among patients with tuberculosis. Similarly, diabetes care guidelines have not traditionally incorporated recommendations for tuberculosis screening in diabetic patients.

In 2009, the International Union Against Tuberculosis and Lung Disease and the World Health Organization (WHO) recognized the need for bidirectional screening and initiated pilot screening programs in China and India. In India, more than 8,000 tuberculosis patients from third-level clinics and tuberculosis units were screened for fasting blood glucose; 13.4 percent had diabetes by the WHO standard classification (table 16.1) (Kumar and others 2013). The prevalence of diabetes in patients with tuberculosis was consistently higher in South India than in North India; this difference partially reflects the geographic and age distribution of diabetes in India, but it is also likely attributable to increased screening in South India (Kumar and others 2013). A similar pilot screening program in 2011 in China detected 12.3 percent prevalence of diabetes among 8,886 patients with tuberculosis who were screened in urban and rural regions (Li and others 2012). Although data are not widely available and considerable geographic variation exists, the prevalence of

Table 16.1 Prevalence of Tuberculosis, Diabetes Mellitus, and Co-Occurring Tuberculosis and Diabetes Mellitus in Select High-Burden Countries

Location	Study	2011 National Tuberculosis Incidence[a] Number (thousands)	2011 National Diabetes Prevalence[b] Number (thousands)	2011 National Diabetes Prevalence[b] %	Diabetes Prevalence in Patients with Tuberculosis Number	Diabetes Prevalence in Patients with Tuberculosis %
India	Kumar and others 2013	2,200	61,258	8.3	1,084/8,109	13.4
China	Li and others 2012	1,000	90,045	9.3	1,090/8,886	12.3
Indonesia	Alisjahbana and others 2007	450	7,293	4.7	94/634	14.8
Pakistan	Jawad and others 1995	410	6,349	6.7	21/106	19.8
South Africa	—	500	1,947	6.5	—	—

Source: Based on WHO 2012.
Note: — = not available.
a. Unadjusted estimates in adults ages 20–79 years (IDF 2011).
b. IDF 2013.

diabetes among tuberculosis patients in most LMICs is likely to be greater than the prevalence of diabetes in the nontuberculosis population.

Individual and Societal Risk Factors

In LMICs, especially in regions where the prevalence of HIV/AIDS is low, diabetes may be responsible for a large proportion of incident tuberculosis cases, and this proportion is projected to increase. Using standard attributable fraction formulas, Stevenson, Forouhi, and others (2007) estimated that 15.1 percent of adult incident tuberculosis cases (141,548 cases) in India in 2000 could be attributed to diabetes. Even though the increased risk of developing active tuberculosis is much lower in diabetic patients than in HIV/AIDS patients, the high prevalence of diabetes is an important factor that inhibits global progress in reducing tuberculosis incidence.

Prognosis and Outcomes

The burden of diabetes on tuberculosis control extends beyond an increased risk of active tuberculosis. Observational studies that compared patients with both conditions to tuberculosis patients without diabetes have reported important differences in clinical manifestations of tuberculosis. Although standardized measures of clinical tuberculosis severity are not widely used in epidemiology, studies reported clinical symptoms of tuberculosis among tuberculosis-diabetes patients that are characteristic of greater severity. Examples of important measures of clinical severity at baseline include positive acid-fast bacilli (AFB) sputum smear grade

(Mac Kenzie and others 2011; Wallis and others 2000), cough with blood (hemoptysis), extent of bacterial involvement according to chest radiographs (Holtz and others 2006; Ralph and others 2010; Stout and others 2010; Wallis and others 2000), and presence of multidrug-resistant tuberculosis (Holtz and others 2006). Greater initial disease severity among tuberculosis-diabetes patients may increase the duration of treatment, require more human and financial resources, and lead to poor tuberculosis treatment outcomes.

More studies that have compared AFB smear status and grade characteristics of tuberculosis patients at the time of diagnosis demonstrated an association between diabetes and the more infectious, smear-positive forms of tuberculosis (table 16.2) (Stevenson, Critchley, and others 2007). Previous studies comparing tuberculosis symptoms at time of presentation also reported more cough (Restrepo and others 2007; Singla and others 2006) and hemoptysis (Restrepo and others 2007; Singla and others 2006; Wang and others 2009) in tuberculosis patients with diabetes than in tuberculosis patients without diabetes. Studies that examined radiographic findings in tuberculosis-diabetes patients and in tuberculosis patients without diabetes have documented important differences (Dooley and Chaisson 2009). Several studies have demonstrated that tuberculosis-diabetes patients had greater lower-lung involvement and more cavitary lesions compared with tuberculosis patients without diabetes (table 16.3); these radiographic characteristics are associated with misdiagnosis of tuberculosis and treatment failure.

Table 16.2 Acid-Fast Bacilli Smear Positivity among Tuberculosis Patients with and without Diabetes Mellitus at Time of Tuberculosis Diagnosis

Location	Study	Tuberculosis-diabetes patients (N)	Tuberculosis-only patients (N)	AFB smear + tuberculosis-diabetes (%)	AFB smear + tuberculosis only (%)
Turkey	Bacakoglu and others 2001	92	92	72.8	91.3
Saudi Arabia	Singla and others 2006	187	505	65.2	54.1
Indonesia	Alisjahbana and others 2007	94	540	29.8	38.9
Mexico	Restrepo and others 2007	607	2,804	96.8	94.9
Texas, United States	Restrepo and others 2007	401	1,040	64.9	50.9
Taiwan, China	Wang and others 2009	74	143	68.9	53.8
Baltimore, MD, United States	Dooley and others 2009	42	255	54.8	41.2
Taiwan, China	Chang and others 2011	60	132	88.3	59.1

Source: Based on Ruslami and others 2010.
Note: AFB = acid-fast bacilli.

Table 16.3 Chest X-Ray Findings among Tuberculosis Patients with and without Diabetes Mellitus

Location	Study	Diabetes-tuberculosis patients (N)	Tuberculosis-only patients (N)	More lower-lung involvement among diabetes-tuberculosis patients	More cavitary lesions among diabetes-tuberculosis patients
Turkey	Bacakoglu and others 2001	92	92	No	No
Mexico	Perez-Guzman and others 2003	192	130	Yes	Yes
Saudi Arabia	Singla and others 2006	187	505	Yes	—
Indonesia	Alisjahbana and others 2007	94	540	—	No
Texas, United States	Restrepo and others 2007	401	1,040	—	Yes
Saudi Arabia	Al-Tawfiq and Saadeh 2009	57	78	—	No
Taiwan, China	Wang and others 2009	74	143	Yes	Yes
Baltimore, MD, United States	Dooley and others 2009	42	255	—	Yes
Taiwan, China	Chang and others 2011	60	132	—	Yes
Portugal	Carreira and others 2012	123	123	Yes	No
Mexico	Jimenez-Corona and others 2013	313	758	—	Yes

Sources: Based on Dooley and others 2009; Ruslami and others 2010.
Note: — = not available.

The prevalence of multidrug-resistant tuberculosis among tuberculosis-diabetes patients has not been extensively examined. In general, studies examining multidrug-resistant tuberculosis in patients with and without diabetes have not reported an association between diabetes and drug-resistant tuberculosis (Alisjahbana and others 2007; Chang and others 2011; Singla and others 2006; Stevenson, Critchley, and others 2007), although important exceptions exist (Bashar and others 2001; Fisher-Hoch and others 2008). Several studies have found consistent associations with clinical manifestations in tuberculosis-diabetes patients, but previously mentioned studies were all observational in design, and the quality of key study metrics, such as diabetes status, was highly variable.

Increased risk of poor clinical outcomes among tuberculosis-diabetes patients is an additional burden conferred by the confluence of the two diseases. Most observational studies that compare tuberculosis treatment outcomes in patients with and without diabetes indicate slower sputum culture conversion time (Guler and others 2007; Restrepo and others 2008) and increased risk of treatment failure (Ponce-de-Leon and others 2004), death (Faurholt-Jepsen and others 2013), or relapse (Zhang, Xiao, and Sugawara 2009) among tuberculosis-diabetes patients.

A meta-analysis estimated that, compared with tuberculosis patients without diabetes, the effect of diabetes on the risk ratio (RR) for death among tuberculosis-diabetes patients was 1.89 (95 percent CI 1.52–2.36) (Baker and others 2011); however, this RR estimate was not adjusted for important confounders such as age and HIV/AIDS status (Baker and others 2011). The same meta-analysis also estimated a greater risk of tuberculosis relapse among tuberculosis-diabetes patients than among tuberculosis patients without diabetes (RR 3.89; 95 percent CI 2.43–6.23). Studies examining the effect of tuberculosis on diabetes outcomes are notably lacking.

Diabetes and HIV/AIDS

Joint Burdens

As a result of longer life expectancy, persons living with HIV/AIDS experience prolonged exposure to traditional and HIV/AIDS-specific risk factors for metabolic disorders, including diabetes.

The prevalence of diabetes among persons with treatment-naive HIV/AIDS (patients who previously have not received care for HIV/AIDS) varies considerably by geographic region and is distributed similarly to trends in diabetes prevalence in general populations. In high-income countries (HICs), the prevalence of diabetes in patients with HIV/AIDS ranges from 1.9 percent to 14.9 percent (table 16.4) (Brown and others 2005; Butt and others 2009; Mondy and others 2007), similar to the national prevalence of diabetes among those ages 20 years or older (11.3 percent). The prevalence of diabetes is lower in LMICs than in HICs. A study from South Africa found that 3.4 percent of HIV/AIDS treatment-naive patients had diabetes (Dave and others 2011); a multicountry study from South America reported diabetes prevalence from 0.8 percent to 6.5 percent in patients with HIV/AIDS (Cahn and others 2010). Although diabetes prevalence is lower in LMICs than in HICs, the absolute number of persons with both diabetes and HIV/AIDS is greater in LMICs because of the higher burden of HIV/AIDS.

Few studies have compared the incidence of diabetes among patients with HIV/AIDS to the incidence of diabetes in HIV-negative persons. A study in the United States from 1999 to 2003 reported that the adjusted incidence of diabetes was 4.1 times greater among patients with HIV/AIDS than among patients without HIV/AIDS (Brown and others 2005). However, a study in Denmark from 1999 to 2009 found no differences in diabetes incidence when comparing patients with and without HIV/AIDS (Rasmussen and others 2012).

Individual and Societal Risk Factors

The same well-established risk factors for diabetes mellitus in the general population are also associated with increased risk of diabetes in patients with HIV/AIDS. Older age; obesity (both body mass index and waist circumference); lifestyle factors; close relatives with a history of diabetes; hypertension; low levels of high-density lipoprotein cholesterol; and, for women, a history of gestational diabetes are all associated with diabetes in persons both with and without HIV/AIDS (Kalra and Agrawal 2013; Tebas 2008). Patients with HIV/AIDS who have lipodystrophy and recently had CD4 counts below 200 cells per microliter are at increased risk of developing diabetes (Petoumenos and others 2012).

Among patients with HIV/AIDS, certain antiretroviral medications are associated with the development of diabetes. Many of the agents associated with diabetes incidence were part of earlier generations of antiretrovirals and are no longer commonly used. Protease inhibitors—specifically indinavir, ritonavir, and amprenavir—are associated with increased risk of diabetes. Protease inhibitors directly affect glucose uptake by inhibiting the transport function of insulin in adipose tissue and lead to hyperglycemia (Murata, Hruz, and Mueckler 2000).

Cumulative exposure to reverse transcriptase inhibitors, specifically stavudine and efavirenz, is associated with increased dysglycemia in HIV-infected persons. A large Danish population-based cohort study reported

Table 16.4 Incidence and Prevalence of Diabetes Mellitus in Patients with and without HIV/AIDS from Large Observational Cohort Studies

Study	Study	Study years	Location	HIV-positive diabetes prevalence (%)[a]	HIV-positive diabetes incidence[b]	HIV-negative diabetes incidence[c]	Adjusted incidence ratio	Antiretroviral treatment and diabetes association[d]
MACS	Brown and others 2005	1999–2003	United States	13.9	4.7	1.4	4.1 (1.9–9.2)	Ritonavir
WIHS	Tien and others 2007	2000–06	United States	11.2	2.9	2.0	1.2 (0.7–1.9)[e]	Lamivudine
DHCS	Rasmussen and others 2012	1996–98	Denmark	—	0.5	0.2	3.2 (1.4–7.4)	Stavudine
DHCS	Rasmussen and others 2012	1999–2009	Denmark	—	0.4	0.4	1.0 (0.8–1.3)	Stavudine
NTUH	Lo and others 2009	1993–2007	Taiwan, China	2.5	1.3	—	—	Zidovudine
SHCS	Ledergerber and others 2007	2000–06	Switzerland	1.9	0.4	—	—	Stavudine and didanosine, stavudine and lamivudine, and didanosine and tenofovir
D:A:D	De Wit and others 2008	1999–2007	Multiple	2.9	0.6	—	—	Stavudine, zidovudine, and didanosine
VACS	Butt and others 2009	2002–04	United States	14.9	—	—	—	—

Note: — = not available; D:A:D = Data Collection on Adverse Events of Anti-HIV Drugs study; DHCS = Danish HIV Cohort Study; HIV/AIDS = human immunodeficiency virus/acquired immune deficiency syndrome; MACS = Multicenter AIDS Cohort Study; NTUH = National Taiwan University Hospital study; SHCS = Swiss HIV Cohort Study; VACS = Veterans Aging Cohort Study; WIHS = Women's Interagency HIV Study.

a. Prevalence of diabetes mellitus at cohort baseline unless otherwise noted.
b. Unadjusted rate per 100 person-years for HIV-positive persons on antiretroviral treatment.
c. Unadjusted rate per 100 person-years for HIV-negative persons from study's comparison group.
d. Among HIV-infected persons, any antiretroviral drugs associated with increased risk of incident diabetes.
e. Hazard ratio.

higher diabetes incidence (RR 1.8, 95 percent CI 1.2–2.8) in patients with HIV/AIDS who were ever exposed to stavudine compared with those who were never exposed to stavudine (Rasmussen and others 2012). A study of 849 patients with HIV/AIDS in South Africa showed that exposure to efavirenz was associated with dysglycemia (odds ratio 1.7, 95 percent CI 1.2–2.5) even after controlling for age, gender, and CD4 count (Dave and others 2011).

Globally, infection with hepatitis C virus (HCV) is frequently prevalent in persons who inject drugs. Unsterile injection of drugs is also a common transmission route for HIV; many persons with HIV/AIDS also have coprevalent HCV. Chronic HCV infection is associated with increased risk of diabetes. A meta-analysis of 10 cohort studies, mainly retrospective studies from Italy and the United States, reported a 67 percent increase in the rate of incident diabetes in persons with HCV compared with persons without HCV (White, Ratziu, and El-Serag 2008).

Prognosis and Outcomes

Few studies have examined the prognosis or treatment outcomes of patients with HIV/AIDS and diabetes. Among patients with HIV/AIDS, having diabetes increases the risk of peripheral lipoatrophy and greater waist-hip ratio; these are likely to be intermediate factors on the causal path to poor HIV/AIDS treatment outcomes, including cardiovascular disease, renal disease, and mortality (Kalra and Agrawal 2013; Tebas 2008).

Among patients with HIV/AIDS, coprevalent diabetes is predictive of cardiovascular disease. In the Data Collection on Adverse Effects of Anti-HIV Drugs study, a large multinational prospective cohort study, diabetes was associated with increased hazards of cardiovascular disease (hazard ratio [HR] 1.9, 95 percent CI 1.6–2.4), coronary heart disease (HR 1.9, 95 percent CI 1.5–2.4), and myocardial infarction (HR 2.3, 95 percent CI 1.7–3.0) (Friis-Moller and others 2010). Chronic kidney disease, including progression to end-stage renal failure, is also more common among patients with HIV/AIDS and diabetes than among patients with diabetes alone.

A study from Malawi compared kidney function in patients with HIV/AIDS and diabetes to patients with diabetes alone. Those with co-occurring HIV/AIDS and diabetes were significantly more likely to have albuminuria than patients with diabetes alone (48.0 percent and 33.3 percent, respectively) (Cohen and others 2010). In the United States, a cohort of veterans was followed to determine rates of progression to chronic kidney disease. Compared with patients without HIV/AIDS or diabetes, the rate of progression to chronic kidney disease was greater in patients with diabetes only (HR 2.48, 95 percent CI 2.19–2.80) and with HIV/AIDS only (HR 2.80, 95 percent CI 2.50–3.15) and greatest among those with both HIV/AIDS and diabetes (HR 4.47, 95 percent CI 3.87–5.17) (Medapalli and others 2012). Acute renal failure is also associated with diabetes among patients with HIV/AIDS. A 2003 cohort of hospitalized patients in New York was analyzed to determine risk factors for the development of acute renal failure. The study reported that patients with HIV/AIDS and diabetes were more likely to have acute renal failure (odds ratio 1.3, 95 percent CI 1.1–1.5) than patients with HIV/AIDS only (Wyatt and others 2006).

OPPORTUNITIES AND CHALLENGES TO INTEGRATION

Integration of Care

The rise of chronic noncommunicable diseases worldwide has presented new challenges for most health systems, particularly in LMICs. Vertical approaches alone that have proved quite successful in combating communicable diseases may not be feasible and cost-effective in treating noncommunicable diseases, given their chronic nature and the continued long-term care required. Insufficient empirical evidence exists to estimate the efficacy or cost-effectiveness of applying communicable disease approaches to noncommunicable disease care.

A search of existing literature on collaborative care returned 1,097 published studies, of which 246 were related to integration. Only seven studies reviewed were related to integration of diabetes care with care for HIV/AIDS, tuberculosis, or depression. Table 16.5 summarizes the observational and case studies of integrated care; table 16.6 summarizes the randomized trials.

Although efficacious and cost-effective preventive and curative solutions exist, timely and sustained

Table 16.5 Examples of Integrated Service Programs from Low- and Middle-Income Countries

Location	Study	Integrated services	Objective	Outcome
Siem Reap and Takeo, Cambodia	Janssens and others 2007	• HIV: HAART • Diabetes: metformin and glibenclamide • Hypertension: antihypertensive protocol	• Drug adherence • Lifestyle changes • Self-management of diseases	• HIV/NCD integration feasible • Services gained efficiency • Low patient loss to follow-up
Rural Rwanda	van Olmen 2011	• Chronic renal disease screening in patients with HIV/AIDS, hypertension, and diabetes	• Screening for serum creatinine or proteinuria in high-risk patients at noncommunicable disease clinics	• Algorithms for outpatient management of kidney disease and mild hyperkalemia
Manzini, Swaziland	Church and others 2015	• Counseling and testing integrated with family planning, pregnancy counseling, and promotion of condom use	• Improved efficiency of two-care systems in high HIV/AIDS-prevalence setting	• Integration not fully achieved • Organizational factors limited capacity to implement integration
Western Kenya	Ouma and Pastakia 2010	• Shared electronic medical records systems for patients with HIV/AIDS, tuberculosis, and diabetes • Home glucose monitoring	• Enhanced diabetes care in rural setting with high HIV/AIDS and tuberculosis burden	• Observed reductions in glycated hemoglobin • Insulin doses adjusted based on standardized protocols

Note: HAART = highly active antiretroviral therapy; HIV/AIDS = human immunodeficiency virus/acquired immune deficiency syndrome; NCD = noncommunicable disease.

Table 16.6 Randomized Controlled Trials of Integrated Care for Diabetes and Depression

Location	Study	Design	Integration summary
Hong Kong SAR, China, public hospital	Chan and others 2014	Randomized trial JADE+PEARL	After one year, patients with type 2 diabetes receiving integrated care with peer support had similar proportions achieving glycated hemoglobin targets and self-reported depression scores compared with controls.
Washington, United States, primary care clinic	Katon and others 2010b	Randomized trial with medically supervised nurse	After one year, patients with type 2 diabetes and coexisting depression receiving care in coordination with primary care nurses had better glycated hemoglobin and depression scores compared with controls.
Washington, United States, primary care clinic	Katon and others 2004	Randomized trial Pathways case management	After one year, patients with type 2 diabetes and coexisting depression receiving care in coordination with case management had improved depression scores but similar glycated hemoglobin levels compared with controls.

Note: JADE = Joint Asia Diabetes Evaluation; PEARL = Peer Support, Empowerment, and Remote Communication Linked by Information Technology.

delivery of these interventions is a major challenge. Meeting this challenge requires concurrently strengthening the health systems and integrating efforts to address both communicable and noncommunicable diseases synergistically under the umbrella of primary health care (Atun and others 2010). Given the increased global prevalence of several noncommunicable diseases and the health system burdens they have created, the WHO and the United Nations High-level Meeting on Non-Communicable Diseases have called for health system strengthening and integration as essential pathways.

Noncommunicable diseases often have shared risks or coexist with communicable diseases, thereby increasing the risk or adverse impact of each other. Such interconnections provide a clear rationale for implementing common prevention, screening, management, and follow-up strategies within health systems. Table 16.5 presents examples of three programs that have integrated health services in LMICs to improve the efficiency of care.

Proposed Pathways for Integration

A potential framework for conceptualizing integration includes engaging civil society groups to meet the supply of and demand for public health systems (figure 16.2). Inputs into this framework include standardized guidelines, workforce development, quality assurance, financial protection, technology, and disease surveillance.

The information, education, and communication strategies used by communicable disease programs could be expanded to include messages about preventing and controlling noncommunicable diseases. Bidirectional screening (Jeon and others 2010) with common management guidelines could be another potential pathway

Figure 16.2 Macrolevel Framework for Integration of Noncommunicable and Communicable Disease Health Systems

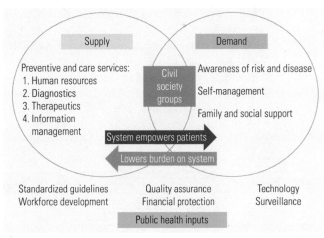

to integrating health care services. Maternal and child health programs could be similarly engaged, using existing structures and personnel to assess blood pressure, blood glucose, and cardiovascular risk, as well as to promote risk reduction measures and management. Simple nonlaboratory risk assessment could be promoted across programs, particularly those that entail multiple contacts with health personnel.

Optimizing available human resources by sharing tasks and shifting care to community health workers is another pathway that merits consideration for strengthening health systems and integrating communicable and noncommunicable disease services. Data on the effectiveness of nonphysician health care workers in chronic disease care, although limited, are summarized in chapter 17 of this volume (Joshi and others 2017).

Strategies for Integration

Integration requires multiple strategies:

- *Diverting health workers from redundant programs.* This approach requires reassessing the continuing relevance of existing health programs from which health workers could be diverted. For example, where control programs for guinea worm, leprosy, or other neglected tropical diseases have eradicated diseases, the trained manpower from these control programs may be redeployed.
- *Retraining and imparting multiple skills to the workforce in existing health programs.* In many countries, health care professionals encounter patients with noncommunicable diseases who are more proactive in their health-seeking behavior than patients with existing diseases. Patient management requires coordinated care, which demands teamwork and skills. The health care workforce needs to be up to date with the explosive growth of knowledge and technologies and with their application to care delivered in health facilities, homes, and communities (Frenk and others 2010). Training approaches need to be restructured to include a new set of core competencies for noncommunicable disease care that includes patient-centered care, partnering, quality improvement, information and communication technology, and public health perspectives (Pruitt and Epping-Jordan 2005).
- *Expanding and reorienting the health system to prevent, detect, and care for chronic diseases, with particular focus on nonphysicians.* The existing health system needs to be expanded and reoriented to deliver chronic disease care. An integrated chronic care model includes multiple components, such as patient self-management support, delivery system design, decision support, clinical information systems, community resources, and multisector collaboration (WHO 2013). Of these components, self-management support, delivery system design, and decision support have been shown to be effective. However, large-scale population-based studies in LMICs that attempt to implement such models are essential. For cost-effectiveness, early results are inconclusive; costs, savings, and benefits need to be studied in more detail (Busse, Schreyögg, and Smith 2008). Integrated chronic care models need to be built around nonphysician health cadres that are also adapted to the resource constraints in LMICs (Katon and others 2010a, 2010b).

The most effective integration mechanisms will likely depend on the structure of the health system in each setting. For example, in some countries the provision of clinical care for diabetes or mental health may be outsourced to nongovernmental agencies or private service providers, whereas in other countries integrated care coordination could be used by government health systems.

CASE STUDIES OF SUCCESSFUL MODELS OR MODELS WORTHY OF EVALUATION

Prevention

Addressing societal risk factors to prevent depression will be important, but the literature and empirical data in this area are extremely limited (Lund and others 2011). General goals in trying to prevent depression include the following:

- Increasing engagement in health promotion activities
- Increasing self-efficacy in the areas of decision making, conflict management, and positive thinking
- Increasing resilience and self-esteem.

These goals may be achieved through a variety of approaches (for example, education, mental health promotion, violence prevention) and settings (for example, schools, homes, workplaces). However, more robust and context-specific data are needed before those approaches can be recommended widely.

Treatment and Barriers

Strong evidence indicates that management of depression with pharmacotherapy, psychotherapy, or both is effective and cost-effective. However, most LMICs have barriers to care in both the supply of and the demand for mental health services (Collins and others 2011; Wang, Simon, and Kessler 2003).

Many similarities exist between mental illnesses and chronic diseases with regard to treatment approaches and barriers to care. For example, mental health and cardiometabolic diseases are chronic, complex, progressive, and costly (Unutzer and others 2009); identification is a key step toward initiating clinical care and self-care; and for both conditions, behavioral activation and motivation are critical for adherence to management plans. Care for both conditions is hampered by major patient- (Egede and Osborn 2010), provider-, and system-level barriers, all of which interact (Balabanova and others 2009). These similarities, as well as the synergistic effects of these conditions (Golden and others 2008; Mezuk and others 2008; Pan and others 2012), offer opportunities to identify and integrate care platforms that efficiently address both sets of conditions.

Integrated care models address barriers to care by leveraging existing facilities, infrastructure, and human resources.

Integrated care can be based in primary care settings or specialist care settings. In primary care, the approach involves decentralizing management of mental illnesses and chronic diseases through structured, collaborative care, and using nonmedical personnel to augment care (Gilbody and others 2006). The goal is to leverage common infrastructure to detect and manage all diseases, whether comorbid or single, in the same location with the same resources (Kolappa, Henderson, and Kishore 2013).

Comprehensive care requires targeting symptoms of depression and hopelessness with medications and behavioral therapies, improving self-management through empowerment, helping patients adopt health-promoting behaviors, and optimizing treatment intensification by health care providers to improve chronic disease care. Integrated care may offer synergistic benefits by managing depression and chronic diseases together. Optimizing therapy for control of depression, glucose, blood pressure, and cholesterol together is associated with better depressive outcomes than focusing on depression alone (Katon and others 2004; Katon and others 2010a; Lustman, Freedland, and others 2000; Lustman, Griffith, Clouse, and others 1997; Lustman and others 1998); exercise, weight loss, and better glycemic control decrease depressive symptoms in people with both diabetes and depression (Blumenthal and others 1999; Testa and Simonson 1998; Wing, Phelan, and Tate 2002).

Studies evaluating models of care that incorporate structured, collaborative care approaches to managing patients with comorbid diseases have shown significantly enhanced responses to treatment of depression, as well as enhanced medical control of diabetes. Randomized controlled trials demonstrated that interventions that included collaborative care with primary health care via enhanced education or nurse case management lead to improvements in adherence and follow-up, reductions in depressive symptoms, and better control of diabetes and cardiovascular risk factors (Katon and others 2004; Katon and others 2010a; Simon and others 2007).

These complex care delivery interventions require resource investments, and studies evaluating the cost-effectiveness of these interventions have noted that the investment costs are offset by savings for future medical care (Shidhaye, Lund, and Chisholm 2015; Simon and others 2001; Simon and others 2007). In HICs, collaborative care models have been adopted by health care providers, payers, and some health agencies (Kates and Craven 2002; Meadows 1998).

There are, however, few or no data regarding collaborative care models from LMICs. Models of care that have been evaluated in LMICs involve using nonmedical personnel to deliver mental health services, particularly depression care, in primary care settings. In India (Patel and others 2010; Patel, Weiss, and others 2011), lay counselors were trained to manage cases and deliver psychotherapy, with step-up to antidepressant drugs provided by primary care physicians under the supervision of mental health specialists. Compared with usual care, this intervention was associated with a 30 percent reduction in the prevalence of mental health disorders, 36 percent reduction in suicidal attempts or plans, fewer days missed from work, and less psychological morbidity among public facility attendees over the year. In Chile (Araya and others 2003; Araya and others 2006), nonmedical health workers helped deliver patient care that included psychoeducation in groups, structured follow-up, and antidepressant medications, where indicated. After a six-month follow-up, 70 percent of intervention participants experienced a significant reduction in depressive symptoms, compared with 30 percent of usual care participants. However, these interventions were focused on mental illness and not on coexisting chronic and mental illnesses.

CONCLUSIONS

Longer life expectancy and growing prevalence of chronic diseases are associated with an increase in coexisting mental and physical morbidities—particularly chronic diseases and comorbid depression. This coexistence exacerbates health and economic impacts on patients, families, communities, and countries.

Given the similarities in the course of disease and barriers to care, as well as the adverse interactions, integrated care that combines mental health management with cardiometabolic risk reduction may provide efficient opportunities to reduce morbidity and to improve physical and social functioning (Katon and others 2010b; McGregor, Lin, and Katon 2011). The goals of collaborative care are to improve patient-centered self-care and adherence, provider accountability, teamwork in clinical settings, and relapse prevention. Achieving all of these goals will help strengthen health systems.

At least four important gaps in knowledge and information regarding the co-occurrence of diseases need to be addressed:

- Expanding current global disease surveillance systems for collection of information on comorbid conditions to enhance the ability to prioritize which co-occurring diseases should be addressed with greatest intensity
- Providing additional studies to clarify the effects of co-occurring diseases on the prognosis of each illness

Table 16.7 Public Health Integration Recommendations

Health system recommendations	Research recommendations
• Establish disease surveillance for comorbid conditions	• Expand research on etiologic prognosis of comorbid diseases
• Implement bidirectional screening programs	• Identify efficacious therapies for patients with co-occurring diseases
• Retrain health care workers for multiple disease skill sets	• Evaluate intervention cost-effectiveness
• Reorient systems to the prevention of comorbid conditions	

- Providing data to determine the effectiveness of interventions to address the confluence of diseases and effective management of two diseases simultaneously
- Determining the cost-effectiveness of interventions to improve disease outcomes for individuals with co-occurring diabetes and HIV/AIDS.

National health programs and public health agencies need to address the emerging co-occurring diseases. However, funding gaps are likely to arise, and identifying additional resources will be a challenge. Funding agencies historically committed to the control of infectious diseases also need to promote efforts to gather data, implement interventions, and test integrated prevention and treatment programs for both communicable and noncommunicable diseases (table 16.7). Expanding the growing list of global health priorities to include the integration of care is likely to lead to primary prevention, improved disease prognosis, and enhanced knowledge regarding implementation sciences and health care delivery.

NOTE

World Bank Income Classifications as of July 2014 are as follows, based on estimates of gross national income (GNI) per capita for 2013:

- Low-income countries (LICs) = US$1,045 or less
- Middle-income countries (MICs) are subdivided:
  (a) lower-middle-income = US$1,046 to US$4,125
  (b) upper-middle-income (UMICs) = US$4,126 to US$12,745
- High-income countries (HICs) = US$12,746 or more.

REFERENCES

Alisjahbana, B., E. Sahiratmadja, E. J. Nelwan, A. M. Purwa, Y. Ahma, and others. 2007. "The Effect of Type 2 Diabetes Mellitus on the Presentation and Treatment Response of Pulmonary Tuberculosis." *Clinical Infectious Disease* 45 (4): 428–35.

Al-Tawfiq, J. A., and B. M. Saadeh. 2009. "Radiographic Manifestations of Culture-Positive Pulmonary Tuberculosis: Cavitary or Non-Cavitary?" *International Journal of Tuberculosis and Lung Disease* 13 (3): 367–70.

Anderson, R. J., K. E. Freedland, R. E. Clouse, and P. J. Lustman. 2001. "The Prevalence of Comorbid Depression in Adults with Diabetes: A Meta-Analysis." *Diabetes Care* 24 (6): 1069–78.

Araya, R., T. Flynn, G. Rojas, R. Fritsch, and G. Simon. 2006. "Cost-Effectiveness of a Primary Care Treatment Program for Depression in Low-Income Women in Santiago, Chile." *American Journal of Psychiatry* 163 (8): 1379–87.

Araya, R., G. Rojas, R. Fritsch, J. Gaete, M. Rojas, and others. 2003. "Treating Depression in Primary Care in Low-Income Women in Santiago, Chile: A Randomised Controlled Trial." *The Lancet* 361 (9362): 995–1000.

Atun, R., T. de Jongh, F. Secci, K. Ohiri, and O. Adeyi. 2010. "Integration of Targeted Health Interventions into Health Systems: A Conceptual Framework for Analysis." *Health Policy and Planning* 25 (2): 104–11.

Bacakoglu, F., O. K. Basoglu, G. Cok, A. Sayiner, and M. Ates. 2001. "Pulmonary Tuberculosis in Patients with Diabetes Mellitus." *Respiration* 68 (6): 595–600.

Baker, M. A., A. D. Harries, C. Y. Jeon, J. E. Hart, A. Kapur, and others. 2011. "The Impact of Diabetes on Tuberculosis Treatment Outcomes: A Systematic Review." *BMC Medicine* 9 (July): 81.

Balabanova, D., M. McKee, N. Koroleva, I. Chikovani, K. Goguadze, and others. 2009. "Navigating the Health System: Diabetes Care in Georgia." *Health Policy and Planning* 24 (1): 46–54.

Bashar, M., P. Alcabes, W. N. Rom, and R. Condos. 2001. "Increased Incidence of Multidrug-Resistant Tuberculosis in Diabetic Patients on the Bellevue Chest Service, 1987 to 1997." *Chest* 120 (5): 1514–19.

Beverly, E. A., O. P. Ganda, M. D. Ritholz, Y. Lee, K. M. Brooks, and others. 2012. "Look Who's (Not) Talking." *Diabetes Care* 35 (7): 1466–72.

Blumenthal, J. A., M. A. Babyak, K. A. Moore, W. E. Craighead, S. Herman, and others. 1999. "Effects of Exercise Training on Older Patients with Major Depression." *Archives of Internal Medicine* 159 (19): 2349–56.

Bot, M., F. Pouwer, M. Zuidersma, J. P. van Melle, and P. de Jonge. 2012. "Association of Coexisting Diabetes and Depression with Mortality after Myocardial Infarction." *Diabetes Care* 35 (3): 503–9.

Brown, T. T., S. R. Cole, X. Li, L. A. Kingsley, F. J. Palella, and others. 2005. "Antiretroviral Therapy and the Prevalence and Incidence of Diabetes Mellitus in the Multicenter AIDS Cohort Study." *Archives of Internal Medicine* 165 (10): 1179–84.

Busse, R., J. Schreyögg, and P. C. Smith. 2008. "Variability in Healthcare Treatment Costs amongst Nine EU Countries—Results from the HealthBASKET Project." *Health Economics* 17 (1 Suppl): S1–S8. doi:10.1002/hec.1330.

Butt, A. A., K. McGinnis, M. C. Rodriguez-Barradas, S. Crystal, M. Simberkoff, and others. 2009. "HIV Infection and the Risk of Diabetes Mellitus." *AIDS* 23 (10): 1227–34.

Cahn, P., O. Leite, A. Rosales, R. Cabello, C. A. Alvarez, and others. 2010. "Metabolic Profile and Cardiovascular Risk Factors among Latin American HIV-Infected Patients Receiving HAART." *Brazilian Journal of Infectious Diseases* 14 (2): 158–66.

Carnethon, M. R., M. L. Biggs, J. I. Barzilay, N. L. Smith, V. Vaccarino, and others. 2007. "Longitudinal Association between Depressive Symptoms and Incident Type 2 Diabetes Mellitus in Older Adults: The Cardiovascular Health Study." *Archives of Internal Medicine* 167 (8): 802–7.

Carnethon, M. R., D. R. Jacobs Jr., S. Sidney, and K. Liu. 2003. "Influence of Autonomic Nervous System Dysfunction on the Development of Type 2 Diabetes: The CARDIA Study." *Diabetes Care* 26 (11): 3035–41.

Carreira, S., J. Costeira, C. Gomes, J. M. Andre, and N. Diogo. 2012. "Impact of Diabetes on the Presenting Features of Tuberculosis in Hospitalized Patients." *Revista Portuguesa de Pneumologia* 18 (5): 239–43.

Chan, J. C., Y. Sui, B. Oldenburg, Y. Zhang, H. H. Chung, and others. 2014. "Effects of Telephone-Based Peer Support in Patients with Type 2 Diabetes Mellitus Receiving Integrated Care: A Randomized Clinical Trial." *JAMA Internal Medicine* 174 (6): 972–81.

Chang, J. T., H. Y. Dou, C. L. Yen, Y. H. Wu, R. M. Huang, and others. 2011. "Effect of Type 2 Diabetes Mellitus on the Clinical Severity and Treatment Outcome in Patients with Pulmonary Tuberculosis: A Potential Role in the Emergence of Multidrug-Resistance." *Journal of the Formosan Medical Association* 110 (6): 372–81.

Church, K., A. Wringe, S. Lewin, G. B. Ploubidis, P. Fakudze, and others. 2015. "Exploring the Feasibility of Service Integration in a Low-Income Setting: A Mixed Methods Investigation into Different Models of Reproductive Health and HIV Care in Swaziland." *PLoS One* 10 (5): e0126144.

Cohen, D. B., T. J. Allain, S. Glover, D. Chimbayo, H. Dzamalala, and others. 2010. "A Survey of the Management, Control, and Complications of Diabetes Mellitus in Patients Attending a Diabetes Clinic in Blantyre, Malawi, an Area of High HIV Prevalence." *American Journal of Tropical Medicine and Hygiene* 83 (3): 575–81.

Collins, P. Y., V. Patel, S. S. Joestl, D. March, T. R. Insel, and others. 2011. "Grand Challenges in Global Mental Health." *Nature* 475 (7354): 27–30.

Dave, J. A., E. V. Lambert, S. Badri, S. West, G. Maartens, and others. 2011. "Effect of Nonnucleoside Reverse Transcriptase Inhibitor–Based Antiretroviral Therapy on Dysglycemia and Insulin Sensitivity in South African HIV-Infected Patients." *Journal of Acquired Immune Deficiency Syndromes* 57 (4): 284–89.

Davydow, D. S., J. E. Russo, E. Ludman, P. Ciechanowski, E. H. Lin, and others. 2011. "The Association of Comorbid Depression with Intensive Care Unit Admission in Patients with Diabetes: A Prospective Cohort Study." *Psychosomatics* 52 (2): 117–26.

De Wit, S., C. A. Sabin, R. Weber, S. W. Worm, P. Reiss, and others. 2008. "Incidence and Risk Factors for New-Onset Diabetes in HIV-Infected Patients: The Data Collection on Adverse Events of Anti-HIV Drugs (D:A:D) Study." *Diabetes Care* 31 (6): 1224–29.

Dooley, K. E., and R. E. Chaisson. 2009. "Tuberculosis and Diabetes Mellitus: Convergence of Two Epidemics." *The Lancet Infectious Diseases* 9 (12): 737–46.

Dooley, K. E., T. Tang, J. E. Golub, S. E. Dorman, and W. Cronin. 2009. "Impact of Diabetes Mellitus on Treatment Outcomes of Patients with Active Tuberculosis." *American Journal of Tropical Medicine and Hygiene* 80 (4): 634–39.

Egede, L. E., A. L. Grubaugh, and C. Ellis. 2010. "The Effect of Major Depression on Preventive Care and Quality of Life among Adults with Diabetes." *General Hospital Psychiatry* 32 (6): 563–69.

Egede, L. E., and C. Y. Osborn. 2010. "Role of Motivation in the Relationship between Depression, Self-Care, and Glycemic Control in Adults with Type 2 Diabetes." *Diabetes Education* 36 (2): 276–83.

Everson-Rose, S. A., P. M. Meyer, L. H. Powell, D. Pandey, J. I. Torrens, and others. 2004. "Depressive Symptoms, Insulin Resistance, and Risk of Diabetes in Women at Midlife." *Diabetes Care* 27 (12): 2856–62.

Faurholt-Jepsen, D., N. Range, G. Praygod, K. Jeremiah, M. Faurholt-Jepsen, and others. 2013. "Diabetes Is a Strong Predictor of Mortality during Tuberculosis Treatment: A Prospective Cohort Study among Tuberculosis Patients from Mwanza, Tanzania." *Tropical Medicine and International Health* 18 (7): 822–29.

Fisher-Hoch, S. P., E. Whitney, J. B. McCormick, G. Crespo, B. Smith, and others. 2008. "Type 2 Diabetes and Multidrug-Resistant Tuberculosis." *Scandinavian Journal of Infectious Diseases* 40 (11–12): 888–93.

Frenk, J., L. Chen, Z. A. Bhutta, J. Cohen, N. Crisp, and others. 2010. "Health Professionals for a New Century: Transforming Education to Strengthen Health Systems in an Interdependent World." *The Lancet* 376 (9756): 1923–58. doi:10.1016/S0140-6736(10)61854-5.

Friis-Moller, N., R. Thiebaut, P. Reiss, R. Weber, A. D. Monforte, and others. 2010. "Predicting the Risk of Cardiovascular Disease in HIV-Infected Patients: The Data Collection on Adverse Effects of Anti-HIV Drugs Study." *European Journal of Cardiovascular Prevention and Rehabilitation* 17 (5): 491–501.

Frohlich, M., A. Imhof, G. Berg, W. L. Hutchinson, M. B. Pepys, and others. 2000. "Association between C-Reactive Protein and Features of the Metabolic Syndrome: A Population-Based Study." *Diabetes Care* 23 (12): 1835–39.

Gilbody, S., P. Bower, J. Fletcher, D. Richards, and A. J. Sutton. 2006. "Collaborative Care for Depression: A Cumulative

Meta-Analysis and Review of Longer-Term Outcomes." *Archives of Internal Medicine* 166 (21): 2314–21.

Golden, S. H., M. Lazo, M. Carnethon, A. G. Bertoni, P. J. Schreiner, and others. 2008. "Examining a Bidirectional Association between Depressive Symptoms and Diabetes." *Journal of the American Medical Association* 299 (23): 2751–59.

Golden, S. H., J. E. Williams, D. E. Ford, H. C. Yeh, C. Paton Sanford, and others. 2004. "Depressive Symptoms and the Risk of Type 2 Diabetes: The Atherosclerosis Risk in Communities Study." *Diabetes Care* 27 (2): 429–35.

Gonzalez, J. S., S. A. Safren, L. M. Delahanty, E. Cagliero, D. J. Wexler, and others. 2008. "Symptoms of Depression Prospectively Predict Poorer Self-Care in Patients with Type 2 Diabetes." *Diabetic Medicine* 25 (9): 1102–7.

Guler, M., E. Unsal, B. Dursun, O. Aydln, and N. Capan. 2007. "Factors Influencing Sputum Smear and Culture Conversion Time among Patients with New Case Pulmonary Tuberculosis." *International Journal of Clinical Practice* 61 (2): 231–35.

Holtz, T. H., M. Sternberg, S. Kammerer, K. F. Laserson, V. Riekstina, and others. 2006. "Time to Sputum Culture Conversion in Multidrug-Resistant Tuberculosis: Predictors and Relationship to Treatment Outcome." *Annals of Internal Medicine* 144 (9): 650–59.

IDF (International Diabetes Federation). 2013. *Diabetes Atlas*, 6th edition. Brussels: International Diabetes Federation.

Janssens, B., W. Van Damme, B. Raleigh, J. Gupta, S. Khem, and others. 2007. "Offering Integrated Care for HIV/AIDS, Diabetes, and Hypertension within Chronic Disease Clinics in Cambodia." *Bulletin of the World Health Organization* 85 (11): 880–85.

Jawad, F., A. S. Shera, R. Memon, and G. Ansari. 1995. "Glucose Intolerance in Pulmonary Tuberculosis." *Journal of the Pakistan Medical Association* 45 (September): 237–38.

Jeon, C. Y., A. D. Harries, M. A. Baker, J. E. Hart, A. Kapur, and others. 2010. "Bi-Directional Screening for Tuberculosis and Diabetes: A Systematic Review." *Tropical Medicine and International Health* 15 (11): 1300–1314.

Jeon, C. Y., and M. B. Murray. 2008. "Diabetes Mellitus Increases the Risk of Active Tuberculosis: A Systematic Review of 13 Observational Studies." *PLoS Medicine* 5 (7): e152.

Jimenez-Corona, M. E., L. P. Cruz-Hervert, L. Garcia-Garcia, L. Ferreyra-Reyes, G. Delgado-Sanchez, and others. 2013. "Association of Diabetes and Tuberculosis: Impact on Treatment and Post-Treatment Outcomes." *Thorax* 68 (3): 214–20.

Joshi, R., A. P. Kengne, F. Hersch, M. B. Weber, H. McGuire, and A. Patel. 2017. "Innovations in Community-Based Health Care for Cardiometabolic and Respiratory Diseases." In *Disease Control Priorities* (third edition): Volume 5, *Cardiovascular, Respiratory, and Related Disorders,* edited by D. Prabhakaran, S. Anand, T. A. Gaziano, J.-C. Mbanya, Y. Wu, and R. Nugent. Washington, DC: World Bank.

Joynt, K. E., D. J. Whellan, and C. M. O'Connor. 2003. "Depression and Cardiovascular Disease: Mechanisms of Interaction." *Biological Psychiatry* 54 (3): 248–61.

Kalra, S., and N. Agrawal. 2013. "Diabetes and HIV: Current Understanding and Future Perspectives." *Current Diabetes Reports* 13 (3): 419–27.

Kapur, A., and A. D. Harries. 2013. "The Double Burden of Diabetes and Tuberculosis: Public Health Implications." *Diabetes Research and Clinical Practice* 101 (1): 10–19.

Kates, N., and M. Craven. 2002. "Shared Mental Health Care: Update from the Collaborative Working Group of the College of Family Physicians of Canada and the Canadian Psychiatric Association." *Canadian Family Physician* 48 (May): 936.

Katon, W. J., E. H. Lin, M. Von Korff, P. Ciechanowski, E. J. Ludman, and others. 2010a. "Collaborative Care for Patients with Depression and Chronic Illnesses." *New England Journal of Medicine* 363 (27): 2611–20.

———. 2010b. "Integrating Depression and Chronic Disease Care among Patients with Diabetes and/or Coronary Heart Disease: The Design of the TEAMcare Study." *Contemporary Clinical Trials* 31 (4): 312–22.

Katon, W. J., M. Von Korff, E. H. Lin, G. Simon, E. Ludman, and others. 2004. "The Pathways Study: A Randomized Trial of Collaborative Care in Patients with Diabetes and Depression." *Archives of General Psychiatry* 61 (10): 1042–49.

Knol, M., J. Twisk, A. Beekman, R. Heine, F. Snoek, and others. 2006. "Depression as a Risk Factor for the Onset of Type 2 Diabetes Mellitus: A Meta-Analysis." *Diabetologia* 49 (5): 837–45.

Kolappa, K., D. C. Henderson, and S. P. Kishore. 2013. "No Physical Health without Mental Health: Lessons Unlearned?" *Bulletin of the World Health Organization* 91 (1): 3–3A.

Konsman, J. P., P. Parnet, and R. Dantzer. 2002. "Cytokine-Induced Sickness Behaviour: Mechanisms and Implications." *Trends in Neurosciences* 25 (3): 154–59.

Kumar, A., D. C. Jain, D. Gupta, S. Satyanarayana, A. M. Kumar, and others. 2013. "Screening of Patients with Tuberculosis for Diabetes Mellitus in India." *Tropical Medicine and International Health* 18 (5): 636–45.

Laghrissi-Thode, F., W. R. Wagner, B. G. Pollock, P. C. Johnson, and M. S. Finkel. 1997. "Elevated Platelet Factor 4 and Beta-Thromboglobulin Plasma Levels in Depressed Patients with Ischemic Heart Disease." *Biological Psychiatry* 42 (4): 290–95.

Lasser, K., J. W. Boyd, S. Woolhandler, D. U. Himmelstein, D. McCormick, and others. 2000. "Smoking and Mental Illness: A Population-Based Prevalence Study." *Journal of the American Medical Association* 284 (20): 2606–10.

Ledergerber, B., H. Furrer, M. Rickenbach, R. Lehmann, L. Elzi, and others. 2007. "Factors Associated with the Incidence of Type 2 Diabetes Mellitus in HIV-Infected Participants in the Swiss HIV Cohort Study." *Clinical Infectious Diseases* 45 (1): 111–19.

Li, L., Y. Lin, F. Mi, S. Tan, B. Liang, and others. 2012. "Screening of Patients with Tuberculosis for Diabetes Mellitus in China." *Tropical Medicine and International Health* 17 (10): 1294–301.

Lin, E. H., S. R. Heckbert, C. M. Rutter, W. J. Katon, P. Ciechanowski, and others. 2009. "Depression and

Increased Mortality in Diabetes: Unexpected Causes of Death." *Annals of Family Medicine* 7 (5): 414–21.

Llorente, M. D., and V. Urrutia. 2006. "Diabetes, Psychiatric Disorders, and the Metabolic Effects of Antipsychotic Medications." *Clinical Diabetes* 24 (1): 18–24.

Lo, Y. C., M. Y. Chen, W. H. Sheng, S. M. Hsieh, H. Y. Sun, and others. 2009. "Risk Factors for Incident Diabetes Mellitus among HIV-Infected Patients Receiving Combination Antiretroviral Therapy in Taiwan: A Case-Control Study." *HIV Medicine* 10 (5): 302–9.

Lonnroth, K., G. Roglic, and A. D. Harries. 2014. "Improving Tuberculosis Prevention and Care through Addressing the Global Diabetes Epidemic: From Evidence to Policy and Practice." *The Lancet Diabetes and Endocrinology* 2 (9): 730–39.

Lund, C., M. De Silva, S. Plagerson, S. Cooper, D. Chisholm, and others. 2011. "Poverty and Mental Disorders: Breaking the Cycle in Low-Income and Middle-Income Countries." *The Lancet* 378 (9801): 1502–14.

Lustman, P. J., R. J. Anderson, K. E. Freedland, M. de Groot, R. M. Carney, and others. 2000. "Depression and Poor Glycemic Control: A Meta-Analytic Review of the Literature." *Diabetes Care* 23 (7): 934–42.

Lustman, P. J., K. E. Freedland, L. S. Griffith, and R. E. Clouse. 2000. "Fluoxetine for Depression in Diabetes: A Randomized Double-Blind Placebo-Controlled Trial." *Diabetes Care* 23 (5): 618–23.

Lustman, P. J., L. S. Griffith, R. E. Clouse, K. E. Freedland, S. A. Eisen, and others. 1997. "Effects of Nortriptyline on Depression and Glycemic Control in Diabetes: Results of a Double-Blind, Placebo-Controlled Trial." *Psychosomatic Medicine* 59 (3): 241–50.

Lustman, P. J., L. S. Griffith, K. E. Freedland, and R. E. Clouse. 1997. "The Course of Major Depression in Diabetes." *General Hospital Psychiatry* 19 (2): 138–43.

Lustman, P. J., L. S. Griffith, K. E. Freedland, S. S. Kissel, and R. E. Clouse. 1998. "Cognitive Behavior Therapy for Depression in Type 2 Diabetes Mellitus: A Randomized, Controlled Trial." *Annals of Internal Medicine* 129 (8): 613–21.

Mac Kenzie, W. R., C. M. Heilig, L. Bozeman, J. L. Johnson, G. Muzanye, and others. 2011. "Geographic Differences in Time to Culture Conversion in Liquid Media: Tuberculosis Trials Consortium Study 28; Culture Conversion Is Delayed in Africa." *PLoS One* 6 (4): e18358.

Magee, M. J., H. M. Blumberg, and K. M. Narayan. 2011. "Commentary: Co-Occurrence of Tuberculosis and Diabetes: New Paradigm of Epidemiological Transition." *International Journal of Epidemiology* 40 (2): 428–31.

Martinez, N., and H. Kornfeld. 2014. "Diabetes and Immunity to Tuberculosis." *European Journal of Immunology* 44 (3): 617–26.

Massie, M. J. 2004. "Prevalence of Depression in Patients with Cancer." *Journal of the National Cancer Institute Monographs* 32: 57–71.

McGregor, M., E. H. Lin, and W. J. Katon. 2011. "TEAMcare: An Integrated Multicondition Collaborative Care Program for Chronic Illnesses and Depression." *Journal of Ambulatory Care Management* 34 (2): 152–62.

Meadows, G. N. 1998. "Establishing a Collaborative Service Model for Primary Mental Health Care." *Medical Journal of Australia* 168 (4): 162–65.

Medapalli, R. K., C. R. Parikh, K. Gordon, S. T. Brown, A. A. Butt, and others. 2012. "Comorbid Diabetes and the Risk of Progressive Chronic Kidney Disease in HIV-Infected Adults: Data from the Veterans Aging Cohort Study." *Journal of Acquired Immune Deficiency Syndromes* 60 (4): 393–99.

Mezuk, B., W. Eaton, S. Albrecht, and S. Golden. 2008. "Depression and Type 2 Diabetes over the Lifespan: A Meta-Analysis." *Diabetes Care* 31 (December): 2383–90.

Mondy, K., E. T. Overton, J. Grubb, S. Tong, W. Seyfried, and others. 2007. "Metabolic Syndrome in HIV-Infected Patients from an Urban, Midwestern U.S. Outpatient Population." *Clinical Infectious Disease* 44 (5): 726–34.

Moussavi, S., S. Chatterji, E. Verdes, A. Tandon, V. Patel, and others. 2007. "Depression, Chronic Diseases, and Decrements in Health: Results from the World Health Surveys." *The Lancet* 370 (9590): 851–58.

Murata, H., P. W. Hruz, and M. Mueckler. 2000. "The Mechanism of Insulin Resistance Caused by HIV Protease Inhibitor Therapy." *Journal of Biological Chemistry* 275 (27): 20251–54.

Musselman, D. L., A. Tomer, A. K. Manatunga, B. T. Knight, M. R. Porter, and others. 1996. "Exaggerated Platelet Reactivity in Major Depression." *American Journal of Psychiatry* 153 (10): 1313–17.

Nelson, K., and C. Williams. 2007. *Infectious Disease Epidemiology: Theory and Practice.* Sudbury, MA: Jones and Bartlett.

Ouma, M. N., and S. D. Pastakia. 2010. "A Comprehensive Collaborative Enhanced Diabetes Care Program in the Rural Resource Constrained Setting of Eldoret, Kenya." Prepared for the American Diabetes Association 70th Conference Scientific Sessions, Orlando, June 25–29.

Pan, A., N. Keum, O. I. Okereke, Q. Sun, M. Kivimaki, and others. 2012. "Bidirectional Association between Depression and Metabolic Syndrome." *Diabetes Care* 35 (5): 1171–80.

Patel, V., R. Araya, M. de Lima, A. Ludermir, and C. Todd. 1999. "Women, Poverty, and Common Mental Disorders in Four Restructuring Societies." *Social Science and Medicine* 49 (11): 1461–71.

Patel, V., S. Chatterji, D. Chisholm, S. Ebrahim, G. Golapakrishna, and others. 2011. "Chronic Diseases and Injuries in India." *The Lancet* 377 (January): 413–28.

Patel, V., C. Lund, S. Heatherill, S. Plagerson, J. Corrigal, and others. 2009. "Social Determinants of Mental Disorders." In *Priority Public Health Conditions: From Learning to Action on Social Determinants of Health*, edited by E. Blas and A. S. Kurup. Geneva: World Health Organization.

Patel, V., H. A. Weiss, N. Chowdhary, S. Naik, S. Pednekar, and others. 2010. "Effectiveness of an Intervention Led by Lay Health Counsellors for Depressive and Anxiety Disorders in Primary Care in Goa, India (MANAS): A Cluster Randomised Controlled Trial." *The Lancet* 376 (9758): 2086–95.

———. 2011. "Lay Health Worker Led Intervention for Depressive and Anxiety Disorders in India: Impact on

Clinical and Disability Outcomes over 12 Months." *British Journal of Psychiatry* 199 (6): 459–66.

Perez-Guzman, C., M. H. Vargas, A. Torres-Cruz, J. R. Perez-Padilla, M. E. Furuya, and others. 2003. "Diabetes Modifies the Male:Female Ratio in Pulmonary Tuberculosis." *International Journal of Tuberculosis and Lung Disease* 7 (4): 354–58.

Petoumenos, K., S. W. Worm, E. Fontas, R. Weber, S. De Wit, and others. 2012. "Predicting the Short-Term Risk of Diabetes in HIV-Positive Patients: The Data Collection on Adverse Events of Anti-HIV Drugs (D:A:D) Study." *Journal of the International AIDS Society* 15 (2): 17426.

Ponce-de-Leon, A., L. Garcia-Garcia, M. C. Garcia-Sancho, F. J. Gomez-Perez, J. L. Valdespino-Gomez, and others. 2004. "Tuberculosis and Diabetes in Southern Mexico." *Diabetes Care* 27 (7): 1584–90.

Poongothai, S., R. M. Anjana, R. Pradeepa, A. Ganesan, N. Umapathy, and others. 2010. "Prevalence of Depression in Relation to Glucose Intolerance in Urban South Indians: The Chennai Urban Rural Epidemiology Study (CURES-76)." *Diabetes Technology and Therapy* 12 (12): 989–94.

Poongothai, S., R. M. Anjana, R. Pradeepa, A. Ganesan, R. Unnikrishnan, and others. 2011. "Association of Depression with Complications of Type 2 Diabetes: The Chennai Urban Rural Epidemiology Study (CURES-102)." *Journal of the Association of Physicians of India* 59 (October): 640–44.

Pruitt, S. D., and J. E. Epping-Jordan. 2005. "Preparing the 21st Century Global Healthcare Workforce." *BMJ* 330 (7492): 637–39.

Ralph, A. P., M. Ardian, A. Wiguna, G. P. Maguire, N. G. Becker, and others. 2010. "A Simple, Valid, Numerical Score for Grading Chest X-Ray Severity in Adult Smear-Positive Pulmonary Tuberculosis." *Thorax* 65 (10): 863–69.

Rasmussen, L. D., E. R. Mathiesen, G. Kronborg, C. Pedersen, J. Gerstoft, and others. 2012. "Risk of Diabetes Mellitus in Persons with and without HIV: A Danish Nationwide Population-Based Cohort Study." *PLoS One* 7 (9): e44575.

Raval, A., E. Dhanaraj, A. Bhansali, S. Grover, and P. Tiwari. 2010. "Prevalence and Determinants of Depression in Type 2 Diabetes Patients in a Tertiary Care Centre." *Indian Journal of Medical Research* 132 (August): 195–200.

Restrepo, B. I., S. P. Fisher-Hoch, J. G. Crespo, E. Whitney, A. Perez, and others. 2007. "Type 2 Diabetes and Tuberculosis in a Dynamic Bi-National Border Population." *Epidemiology and Infection* 135 (3): 483–91.

Restrepo, B. I., S. P. Fisher-Hoch, B. Smith, S. Jeon, M. H. Rahbar, and others. 2008. "Mycobacterial Clearance from Sputum Is Delayed during the First Phase of Treatment in Patients with Diabetes." *American Journal of Tropical Medicine and Hygiene* 79 (4): 541–44.

Restrepo, B. I., and L. S. Schlesinger. 2013. "Host-Pathogen Interactions in Tuberculosis Patients with Type 2 Diabetes Mellitus." *Tuberculosis* 93 (Suppl): S10–S14.

Roshanaei-Moghaddam, B., W. J. Katon, and J. Russo. 2009. "The Longitudinal Effects of Depression on Physical Activity." *General Hospital Psychiatry* 31 (4): 306–15.

Rugulies, R. 2002. "Depression as a Predictor for Coronary Heart Disease: A Review and Meta-Analysis." *American Journal of Preventive Medicine* 23 (1): 51–61.

Ruslami, R., R. E. Aarnoutse, B. Alisjahbana, A. J. van der Ven, and R. van Crevel. 2010. "Implications of the Global Increase of Diabetes for Tuberculosis Control and Patient Care." *Tropical Medicine and International Health* 15 (11): 1289–99.

Shidhaye, R., C. Lund, and D. Chisholm. 2015. "Closing the Treatment Gap for Mental, Neurological, and Substance Use Disorders by Strengthening Existing Health Care Platforms: Strategies for Delivery and Integration of Evidence-Based Interventions." *International Journal of Mental Health Systems* 9 (December): 40.

Simon, G. E., W. J. Katon, E. H. Lin, C. Rutter, W. G. Manning, and others. 2007. "Cost-Effectiveness of Systematic Depression Treatment among People with Diabetes Mellitus." *Archives of General Psychiatry* 64 (1): 65–72.

Simon, G. E., W. G. Manning, D. J. Katzelnick, S. D. Pearson, H. J. Henk, and others. 2001. "Cost-Effectiveness of Systematic Depression Treatment for High Utilizers of General Medical Care." *Archives of General Psychiatry* 58 (2): 181–87.

Singla, R., N. Khan, N. Al-Sharif, M. O. Ai-Sayegh, M. A. Shaikh, and others. 2006. "Influence of Diabetes on Manifestations and Treatment Outcome of Pulmonary TB Patients." *International Journal of Tuberculosis and Lung Disease* 10 (1): 74–79.

Sridhar, G. R. 2007. "Psychiatric Co-Morbidity and Diabetes." *Indian Journal of Medical Research* 125: 311–20.

Sridhar, G. R., and K. Madhu. 2002. "Psychosocial and Cultural Issues in Diabetes Mellitus." *Current Science* 83 (12): 1556–64.

Stevenson, C. R., J. A. Critchley, N. G. Forouhi, G. Roglic, B. G. Williams, and others. 2007. "Diabetes and the Risk of Tuberculosis: A Neglected Threat to Public Health?" *Chronic Illness* 3 (3): 228–45.

Stevenson, C. R., N. G. Forouhi, G. Roglic, B. G. Williams, J. A. Lauer, and others. 2007. "Diabetes and Tuberculosis: The Impact of the Diabetes Epidemic on Tuberculosis Incidence." *BMC Public Health* 7 (September): 234.

Stout, J. E., A. S. Kosinski, C. D. Hamilton, P. C. Goodman, A. Mosher, and others. 2010. "Effect of Improving the Quality of Radiographic Interpretation on the Ability to Predict Pulmonary Tuberculosis Relapse." *Academic Radiology* 17 (2): 157–62.

Sullivan, M. D., P. O'Connor, P. Feeney, D. Hire, D. L. Simmons, and others. 2012. "Depression Predicts All-Cause Mortality." *Diabetes Care* 35 (8): 1708–15.

Tebas, P. 2008. "Insulin Resistance and Diabetes Mellitus Associated with Antiretroviral Use in HIV-Infected Patients: Pathogenesis, Prevention, and Treatment Options." *Journal of Acquired Immune Deficiency Syndromes* 49 (Suppl 2): S86–92.

Testa, M. A., and D. C. Simonson. 1998. "Health Economic Benefits and Quality of Life during Improved Glycemic Control in Patients with Type 2 Diabetes Mellitus: A Randomized,

Controlled, Double-Blind Trial." *Journal of the American Medical Association* 280 (17): 1490–96.

Tien, P. C., M. F. Schneider, S. R. Cole, A. M. Levine, M. Cohen, and others. 2007. "Antiretroviral Therapy Exposure and Incidence of Diabetes Mellitus in the Women's Interagency HIV Study." *AIDS* 21 (13): 1739–45.

Unutzer, J., M. Schoenbaum, W. J. Katon, M. Y. Fan, H. A. Pincus, and others. 2009. "Healthcare Costs Associated with Depression in Medically Ill Fee-for-Service Medicare Participants." *Journal of the American Geriatrics Society* 57 (3): 506–10.

van Olmen, J. 2011. *The Partners in Health Guide to Chronic Care Integration for Endemic Non-Communicable Diseases: Rwanda Edition.* Boston, MA: Partners in Health.

Wallis, R. S., M. D. Perkins, M. Phillips, M. Joloba, A. Namale, and others. 2000. "Predicting the Outcome of Therapy for Pulmonary Tuberculosis." *American Journal of Respiratory and Critical Care Medicine* 161 (4 Pt 1): 1076–80.

Wang, C. S., C. J. Yang, H. C. Chen, S. H. Chuang, I. W. Chong, and others. 2009. "Impact of Type 2 Diabetes on Manifestations and Treatment Outcome of Pulmonary Tuberculosis." *Epidemiology and Infection* 137 (2): 203–10.

Wang, P. S., G. Simon, and R. C. Kessler. 2003. "The Economic Burden of Depression and the Cost-Effectiveness of Treatment." *International Journal of Methods in Psychiatric Research* 12 (1): 22–33.

White, D. L., V. Ratziu, and H. B. El-Serag. 2008. "Hepatitis C Infection and Risk of Diabetes: A Systematic Review and Meta-Analysis." *Journal of Hepatology* 49 (5): 831–44.

Whiteford, H. A., L. Degenhardt, J. Rehm, A. J. Baxter, A. J. Ferrari, and others. 2013. "Global Burden of Disease Attributable to Mental and Substance Use Disorders: Findings from the Global Burden of Disease Study 2010." *The Lancet* 382 (9904): 1575–86.

WHO (World Health Organization). 2011. *Collaborative Framework for Care and Control of Tuberculosis and Diabetes.* Geneva: WHO and International Union Against Tuberculosis and Lung Disease.

———. 2012. *Global Tuberculosis Report 2012.* Geneva: WHO.

———. 2013. *Global Action Plan for the Prevention and Control of Noncommunicable Diseases 2013–2020.* Geneva: WHO.

Wing, R. R., S. Phelan, and D. Tate. 2002. "The Role of Adherence in Mediating the Relationship between Depression and Health Outcomes." *Journal of Psychosomatic Research* 53 (4): 877–81.

Wyatt, C. M., R. R. Arons, P. E. Klotman, and M. E. Klotman. 2006. "Acute Renal Failure in Hospitalized Patients with HIV: Risk Factors and Impact on In-Hospital Mortality." *AIDS* 20 (4): 561–65.

Young, B. A., M. Von Korff, S. R. Heckbert, E. J. Ludman, C. Rutter, and others. 2010. "Association of Major Depression and Mortality in Stage 5 Diabetic Chronic Kidney Disease." *General Hospital Psychiatry* 32 (2): 119–24.

Zhang, Q., H. Xiao, and I. Sugawara. 2009. "Tuberculosis Complicated by Diabetes Mellitus at Shanghai Pulmonary Hospital, China." *Japanese Journal of Infectious Diseases* 62 (5): 390–391.

Chapter 17

Innovations in Community-Based Health Care for Cardiometabolic and Respiratory Diseases

Rohina Joshi, Andre Pascal Kengne, Fred Hersch,
Mary Beth Weber, Helen McGuire, and Anushka Patel

INTRODUCTION

Cardiometabolic conditions (cardiovascular diseases [CVDs], diabetes, and associated chronic kidney disease) and chronic lung diseases are the leading causes of premature mortality and morbidity among adults worldwide, including in many low- and middle-income countries (LMICs). The chronic nature of these conditions imposes a high burden on individuals and societies and creates substantial challenges for traditional health systems.

Prevention and early intervention are crucial. In addition to population-based approaches, key preventive strategies require the extension of health care delivery platforms to the community. This chapter reviews the evidence pertaining to two important strategies for extending health services into communities in LMICs for preventing and managing cardiometabolic and chronic lung conditions and risk factors. The first strategy focuses on task-shifting, defined as assigning health care management and prevention tasks to nonphysicians. A systematic review was performed of the published literature as it relates to cardiometabolic and chronic lung diseases. The second strategy focuses on self-management, with or without support from family or community-based peers. A narrative literature review was performed of literature related to the second strategy, given its broad and diverse focus. While the two strategies seek to extend health care delivery into the community, they are different in that the first strategy involves changing the health workforce structure and delivery of health care, while the second involves educating patients to understand the condition and empowering them to make informed choices in day-to-day management. These detailed reviews are accompanied by two case studies that outline examples of initiatives used in communities in LMICs.

TASK-SHIFTING FOR CARDIOMETABOLIC AND RESPIRATORY DISEASES IN LMICS

In many countries, primary care physicians are the first point of contact and the main providers of health care for individuals with noncommunicable diseases. In LMICs, too few doctors are available, and physician workforce disparities for rural and remote regions are substantial (Kar and others 2008; WHO 2006).

An alternative workforce that is structured around the community and the patient could potentially address this need. *Task-shifting* has been defined as shifting the delivery of services normally performed by physicians to health professionals with a different or lower level of education and training or to persons without formal health education who are trained to perform specific tasks (Lekoubou and others 2010). Task-shifting may be facilitated by medical technology, such as standardized diagnostic equipment linked to electronic decision

Corresponding author: Rohina Joshi, The George Institute for Global Health, University of Sydney, Sydney, Australia; rjoshi@georgeinstitute.org.au.

support, which standardizes the performance and interpretation of certain tasks.

Task-shifting typically occurs in close collaboration with the medical profession (WMA 2009), potentially reducing costs and saving physicians' time (Abegunde and others 2007; Buttorff and others 2012; Mdege, Chindove, and Shehzad 2012). A study in Uganda reporting the potential impact of task-shifting on the costs of antiretroviral therapy and physician supply found that the estimated annual mean costs of follow-up per patient were US$31.68 for physician follow-up, US$24.58 for nurse follow-up, and US$10.50 for pharmacist follow-up (Babigumira and others 2009). In addition, task-shifting is a potentially efficient way to reorganize the workforce by ensuring better specialization and quality of care, allowing physicians to focus on the jobs that cannot be delegated (Callaghan, Ford, and Schneider 2010). A study in Rwanda found that task-shifting from a physician-centered to a nurse-centered model for antiretroviral therapy reduced the demand on physicians' time by 76 percent (Mdege, Chindove, and Shehzad 2012).

Task-shifting in health care began in the 1970s and 1980s, when auxiliary nurses in the Democratic Republic of Congo took on the role of providing health care because of a shortage of physicians. This shift allowed the few available physicians to use their time and expertise to manage people with more complicated diseases. Other LMICs in South Asia and Sub-Saharan Africa have used this approach for childhood conditions (Bang and others 1999; McCollum and others 2010) and for infectious diseases (Fairall and others 2012).

A Cochrane review assessing the performance of nonphysician health workers (NPHWs) in providing maternal and child health services indicated that task-shifting promoted immunization and breastfeeding, improved tuberculosis outcomes, and reduced childhood morbidity and mortality when compared with usual care (Lewin and others 2010). Growing evidence from countries in Sub-Saharan Africa suggests that task-shifting for antiretroviral therapy can help to curb the impact of HIV (human immunodeficiency virus) infection. A systematic review of HIV/AIDS (acquired immune deficiency syndrome) care in Sub-Saharan Africa found that task-shifting offered cost-effective and high-quality care to more patients than physician-centered care (Callaghan, Ford, and Schneider 2010).

Very few studies have examined the role of NPHWs in managing noncommunicable diseases in LMICs. Most of these studies have focused on a single risk factor or disease (Labhardt and others 2010; Lekoubou and others 2010) rather than on integrated disease management.

A Systematic Review

A systematic search was conducted for published studies of interventions that involved shifting tasks to NPHWs for the prevention or management of noncommunicable diseases in LMICs. For the purpose of this review, *NPHWs* were defined as a nurse or health care worker with no formal medical training. *Noncommunicable diseases* were defined as a range of chronic noninfectious conditions, including CVD, diabetes, hypertension, cancer, chronic obstructive pulmonary disease, neurological conditions, and mental health problems. A search was conducted using the following terms: *task-shifting, nonphysician health care workers, community health care worker, hypertension, diabetes, cardiovascular disease, chronic obstructive pulmonary disease, respiratory disease,* and *noncommunicable disease*. The data presented here reflect a subset of identified studies that focus on cardiometabolic and chronic lung diseases.

The databases reviewed were Medline via PubMed and the Cochrane library, and the search was conducted from May 26 to June 13, 2013. The search included all studies available up to and including May 31, 2013. Table 17.1 highlights the inclusion and exclusion criteria used. The review was limited to peer-reviewed, community-based studies in LMICs and studies that involved clinical interventions. Studies focusing on health education or health promotion and hospital-based studies were excluded. Only English-language reports were considered. The quality of studies was assessed on criteria such as study design, method of randomization, and sources of bias; no study was excluded on the basis of study quality. A meta-analysis was not performed because of the high levels of heterogeneity among studies in relation to the task-shifting model under evaluation, types of patients, and outcomes evaluated.

Characteristics of Studies

The search generated 3,009 articles, of which 9 were included in the review. Five studies were conducted in Cameroon, two in India, and two in South Africa (table 17.2). Five studies were based in rural regions, and four studies included both rural and urban regions. Studies involved task-shifting for the management of hypertension, CVD, diabetes, and respiratory diseases. Tasks were shifted predominantly from physicians to nurses (Coleman, Gill, and Wilkinson 1998; Gill and others 2008; Kaufman and others 2012; Kengne and others 2008; Kengne and others 2010; Kengne, Sobngwi, and others 2009; Labhardt and others 2010); there were two examples of shifting to other health workers (Joshi and others 2012; Kar and others 2008).

Table 17.1 Inclusion and Exclusion Criteria for the Systematic Review of Task-Shifting in Cardiometabolic and Respiratory Disease Prevention and Management

Inclusion criteria	Exclusion criteria
• Studies where a task usually performed by physicians is shifted to a different cadre of health care provider	• Studies primarily involving health education or health promotion interventions
• Disease conditions limited to cardiovascular disease, diabetes, hypertension, chronic obstructive pulmonary disease, and respiratory diseases	• Hospital-based studies
• Studies conducted in low- and middle-income countries	
• Intervention studies: randomized control trials, before-and-after studies, and other quasi-experimental studies	
• Community-based studies	
• Peer-reviewed articles	
• Articles in English	

Quality of Studies

Only two of the nine studies were randomized control trials (RCTs). The remaining studies evaluated the effects of the intervention by comparing outcomes before and after implementation in observational studies; these studies provided low-quality evidence of effectiveness. Three of the nine studies did not discuss sources of bias or limitations of the study findings; one did not report the details of the statistical analysis used. Some studies reported more than 40 percent of the patients lost to follow-up, further limiting the reliability of the evaluation findings (Kengne and others 2008; Labhardt and others 2010).

Does Task-Shifting Improve Health Care Effectiveness?

Process of care outcomes. The reviewed studies suggest that trained NPHWs may be able to identify individuals with noncommunicable diseases, including asthma (Coleman, Gill, and Wilkinson 1998), CVD (Joshi and others 2012; Kar and others 2008), hypertension (Coleman, Gill, and Wilkinson 1998; Kengne, Awah, and others 2009; Labhardt and others 2010; Labhardt and others 2011), and diabetes (Coleman, Gill, and Wilkinson 1998; Gill and others 2008; Kengne, Sobngwi, and others 2009; Labhardt and others 2010; Labhardt and others 2011). Findings from studies in which NPHWs were permitted to prescribe medications suggest that trained NPHWs may be able to treat patients according to study protocols for conditions such as asthma (Coleman, Gill, and Wilkinson 1998; Kengne and others 2008), hypertension (Coleman, Gill, and Wilkinson 1998; Kengne, Awah, and others 2009; Labhardt and others 2010; Labhardt and others 2011), and diabetes (Coleman, Gill, and Wilkinson 1998; Gill and others

2008; Kengne, Sobngwi, and others 2009; Labhardt and others 2010; Labhardt and others 2011). Several studies reported improved access to health care at the community level, although the metric used to evaluate access was usually not described (Coleman, Gill, and Wilkinson 1998; Kengne, Sobngwi, and others 2009; Labhardt and others 2010).

Disease control outcomes. Two studies reported disease control outcomes. An observational study from rural South Africa showed that trained NPHWs, with the help of treatment protocols and without the input of physicians, could achieve control in 68 percent of patients with hypertension, 82 percent with diabetes, and 84 percent with asthma, although preintervention rates were not provided for comparison (Coleman, Gill, and Wilkinson 1998). Another observational study from rural South Africa showed that nurses trained in the use of an algorithm could effectively diagnose and manage patients with diabetes, with significant reductions in glycated hemoglobin (HbA1c) described at 18 months, although the observational design limits the ability to ascribe such changes to the intervention (Gill and others 2008).

Treatment concordance. One study examined concordance between physicians and NPHWs for the diagnosis and management of CVD risk, showing a high level of agreement between NPHWs and physicians. The study reported that recommendations for drug therapy made by NPHWs guided by algorithms were the same as those made by physicians in more than 87 percent of patients with prior stroke or myocardial infarction (Joshi and others 2012).

Table 17.2 Summary Data from Published Studies Describing Task-Shifting for Prevention and Management of Cardiometabolic and Respiratory Diseases

Study	Country	Diseases addressed	Study type	Intervention	Outcome	Challenges	Cost-effectiveness analysis
Coleman, Gill, and Wilkinson 1998	South Africa (rural and urban)	Hypertension and diabetes, epilepsy, and asthma	Observational	• Protocol developed based on WHO guidelines • Patients initially screened by a doctor and followed up by NPHWs • Comparator: Usual care before intervention	• BP controlled in 68% of patients; blood glucose controlled in 82% of patients with type 2 diabetes[a] • Better adherence measured by self-report; improved from 79% at the first visit to 87% at the most recent clinic visit	High attrition of patients	No
Kar and others 2008	India (rural, urban, and slum)	Cardiovascular disease	Observational	• NPHWs trained in WHO protocol for CVD risk assessment • Comparator: Usual care before intervention	• Increase in knowledge of NPHWs regarding CVD risk factors and symptoms • Increase in referral of individuals with raised BP • Decrease in systolic BP (154.5–145.6 mmHg), increase in intention to quit tobacco (25.5–60.3%), and reported regular use of antihypertensive medication (34.8–58.3%)	None reported	No
Kengne and others 2008	Cameroon (rural)	Asthma	Observational	• Training of NPHWs for diagnosis and management of asthma • Monthly visit by physician • Patients identified and managed by nurses • Comparator: Usual care before intervention	• Increase in number of days without asthma attack[a]	41% lost to follow-up	No
Gill and others 2008	South Africa (rural)	Diabetes	Observational	• Training of nurses for diagnosis and management of diabetes using an algorithm • Comparator: Usual care	• Reduction in HbA1c from 11.6±4.5% at baseline to 8.7±2.3% at 6 months and 7.7±2.0% at 18 months	26% lost to follow-up	No

table continues next page

Table 17.2 Summary Data from Published Studies Describing Task-Shifting for Prevention and Management of Cardiometabolic and Respiratory Diseases (continued)

Study	Country	Diseases addressed	Study type	Intervention	Outcome	Challenges	Cost-effectiveness analysis
Kengne, Sobngwi, and others 2009	Cameroon (rural and urban)	Hypertension and diabetes	Observational	• Training of NPHWs • Clinical management algorithm • Comparator: Usual care before intervention	• BP decreased by 5.9/3.3 mmHg; fasting glucose decreased by 1.6 mmol/l	High attrition of patients	No
Kengne, Awah, and others 2009	Cameroon (rural and urban)	Hypertension	Observational	• Training of NPHWs • Comparator: Usual care before intervention	• BP decreased by 11.7/7.8 mmHg	High attrition of patients	No
Labhardt and others 2010	Cameroon (rural)	Hypertension and diabetes	Observational	• Training of NPHWs • Provision of equipment (sphygmomanometer, stethoscopes, blood glucose meters) • Drugs • Comparator: Usual care before intervention	• 100% retained equipment; 70% had functional blood glucose meter; 96% used antihypertensives; 72% used oral blood-glucose-lowering drugs[a] • Knowledge of NPHWs significantly improved • BP decreased by 22.8/12.4 mmHg; blood glucose decreased by 3.4 mmol/l	Changes in staff Low case detection High attrition of patients	No
Labhardt and others 2011	Cameroon (rural)	Hypertension and diabetes	RCT	• NPHW-led care. Group 1, treatment contract between patient and nurse plus free medication for a month for every four months of consecutively attended follow-up visits. Group 2, treatment contract plus letters reminding patients of a visit • Comparator: Usual care	• Retention rates in the intervention groups: 60% and 65% in groups 1 and 2, respectively; 29% in control group	50% lost to follow-up across the three arms	No
Joshi and others 2012	India (rural)	CVD (coronary heart disease and stroke)	Cluster RCT	• NPHWs trained to screen individuals at high risk of developing CVD • Algorithm-based care. • Comparator: Usual care	• The proportion of high-risk individuals identified was 12% greater in intervention villages (63.4% vs. 51.4%) • Agreement between the recommendations made by the trained NPHW and physicians was 88.5%	None reported	No

Note: BP = blood pressure; CVD = cardiovascular disease; HbA1c = glycated hemoglobin; mmHg = millimeter of mercury, a unit of pressure; mmol/l = millimoles per liter; NPHW = nonphysician health worker; RCT = randomized control trial; WHO = World Health Organization.

a. Preintervention data unavailable.

Is Task-Shifting Cost-Effective?

None of the studies reported cost-effectiveness outcomes.

What Are the Enablers of and Barriers to the Effectiveness of Task-Shifting Initiatives?

Potential enablers of task-shifting. Health system factors, such as training NPHWs; providing algorithms (Joshi and others 2012); disseminating protocols and guidelines for screening, treatment, and drug titration; and making medications available (Coleman, Gill, and Wilkinson 1998), aided the success of task-shifting interventions. Several studies included a training component specifically designed for NPHWs that involved the development of algorithms and protocols and the provision of training for screening, diagnosis, management, and follow-up for several diseases (Joshi and others 2012; Kengne, Awah, and others 2009; Kengne, Sobngwi, and others 2009; Labhardt and others 2010). Two studies reported significant changes in the knowledge level of NPHWs as a result of training and supervision (Kar and others 2008; Labhardt and others 2010). A study from Cameroon showed that knowledge regarding the choice of correct antihypertensive drugs improved substantially after training (from 17 to 94 percent) and remained high two years after the intervention (95 percent) (Labhardt and others 2010). A study from India indicated that the knowledge levels of NPHWs for CVD increased from 47 to 93 percent after a four-day training program (Kar and others 2008).

The provision of diagnostic and management protocols with treatment algorithms was another key element that appeared to facilitate task-shifting models (Joshi and others 2012; Kengne, Sobngwi, and others 2009). Two studies from South Africa and one from Cameroon developed detailed protocols for hypertension, diabetes, and asthma management based on World Health Organization (WHO) and other international guidelines (Coleman, Gill, and Wilkinson 1998; Gill and others 2008; Kengne, Sobngwi, and others 2009); similar protocols were developed for CVD screening and management in India (Joshi and others 2012; Kar and others 2008). Several studies included a task-sharing model in which physicians were available for consultation in complicated cases (Kengne and others 2010), for confirmation of the diagnosis, and for initiation of CVD treatment (Joshi and others 2012). A cluster RCT in rural Cameroon found that nurse-led facilitators who provided free medications and sent reminder letters retained patients at the end of one year. The retention rates in the two intervention arms were 60 and 65 percent, respectively, compared with 29 percent in the control group (Labhardt and others 2011).

Potential barriers to task-shifting. Potential barriers to successful task-shifting in these studies include poor staff retention, irregular supply of medications, and lack of equipment. A study in Cameroon reported that only 48 percent of the trained NPHWs were retained at the end of the two-year study period; this low rate of retention was primarily due to the transfer of staff to other public health facilities (Labhardt and others 2010). Some primary health centers did not have equipment to measure blood pressure or blood glucose and did not have protocols or guidelines in place to manage noncommunicable diseases (Coleman, Gill, and Wilkinson 1998; Joshi and others 2012; Labhardt and others 2010).

The availability of medications was identified as another challenge. Two studies had to provide the drugs to patients because the first-level health care center did not store sufficient quantities (Coleman, Gill, and Wilkinson 1998; Labhardt and others 2010). A cluster RCT in rural India showed that NPHWs could identify individuals at high risk of CVD with the help of an algorithm, but failed to demonstrate effects on outcomes, such as the number of medications prescribed or blood pressure and cholesterol levels. To obtain treatment, patients had to visit physicians located some distance away because NPHWs did not have authority to prescribe medications (Joshi and others 2012).

Discussion

Subsequent to this systematic review, further relevant information on task-shifting has emerged. An observational study involving Bangladesh, Guatemala, Mexico, and South Africa showed that trained NPHWs could effectively screen and identify patients at high risk of CVD (Gaziano and others 2015), and the concordance of diagnosis between NPHWs and physicians was 97 percent. This study indicated that shifting tasks to NPHWs was both cost-effective and cost saving. In addition, more data have been published in relation to the experiences of task-shifting in Latin America (Abrahams-Gessel and others 2015a, 2015b; Mendoza Montano and others 2015).

The acute shortage and maldistribution of the health workforce in LMICs is a major obstacle to improving outcomes for the prevention and control of cardiometabolic and chronic lung diseases. Historically, reorganizing the workforce for the delivery of maternal and child health significantly improved outcomes (Haines and others 2007). More recently, task-shifting has proved to be a viable and cost-effective option for the management of HIV/AIDS in Sub-Saharan Africa (Callaghan, Ford, and Schneider 2010). High-income countries (HICs) such as Australia, the United Kingdom, and the United States have reengineered their workforces for improved efficiency. For example, tasks such as taking blood samples have been shifted to NPHWs like phlebotomists, who specialize in taking blood samples, freeing up physicians to provide other important services. Nurse practitioners in HICs are increasingly adopting many aspects of health care delivery that were traditionally the domain of physicians.

The adaptation and dissemination of prevention and treatment programs to community settings in the United States has relied heavily on NPHWs, with positive results. A review of translational research projects based on the Diabetes Prevention Program (Ruggiero, Oros, and Choi 2011) concludes that using trained community health workers for patient management and peer education can be as effective as using health professionals. This review suggests that key barriers exist to effective task-shifting for preventing and managing cardiometabolic and respiratory diseases in LMICs (box 17.1).

Although limited, published data suggest that the health workforce needs to be reengineered, in conjunction with changes in the health system.

The WHO, in consultation with experts from a wide range of fields, has formulated a set of 22 recommendations that provide guidance on task-shifting (WHO 2008b). These guidelines, developed in the context of the HIV/AIDS epidemic in Sub-Saharan Africa, have implications for other conditions, including noncommunicable diseases. Not all health care professionals support the concept of task-shifting

(Zachariah and others 2009). Some view task-shifting as creating a competitive environment in which physicians compete with NPHWs for patients (Grumbach and Coffman 1998); others view it as unsafe for patients when care is provided in the absence of close physician supervision (Mullan and Frehywot 2007). The Sixtieth General Assembly of the World Medical Association (WMA) in 2009 adopted a resolution stating that task-shifting is a short-term solution to physician shortages in LMICs that should occur in close consultation with physicians and have patient safety as the central goal. The WMA recommends further research on models of care employing a physician-coordinated task-sharing approach rather than a task-shifting approach (WMA 2009).

More rigorous research clearly is needed to clarify the issues relating to quality of care, patient satisfaction, and health outcomes. Because RCTs are often costly and challenging in these settings, implementation studies using mixed-methods approaches may provide some of this much-needed evidence. Given that NPHWs are a potentially low-cost and sustainable option for managing noncommunicable diseases in resource-constrained settings, future studies should routinely incorporate cost and cost-effectiveness analyses.

Limitations of the Review

None of the studies in this systematic review reported process evaluation data, a critically important component for understanding contextual factors associated with uptake of the intervention that may influence the potential for scale-up. Furthermore, none of the studies discussed the role of incentives and remuneration, and research is needed on optimal workforce conditions for task-shifting. A factor likely to influence the feasibility of these initiatives is their acceptability to patients and communities. In expanding the role of NPHWs in managing chronic illness, a better understanding is needed of, for example, how patients might balance potential concerns about safety and efficacy with lower costs and improved access to care. Qualitative research is needed to address these questions.

This review was restricted to peer-reviewed articles published in English; it may have missed studies published in the gray literature and in languages other than English. No studies reporting negative results were identified, suggesting the possibility of significant publication bias. The low number of studies identified may also reflect the inability to publish because of poor quality. The majority of the study designs reviewed provided relatively poor-quality evidence; future

---

Box 17.1

Barriers to Task-Shifting for the Management of Cardiometabolic and Respiratory Conditions

1. Lack of training of NPHWs in management
2. Inadequate referral pathways
3. Lack of strategies to retain trained staff
4. Inadequate screening and management tools
5. Inability of NPHWs to prescribe or titrate dosages of medications related to management or prevention of conditions.

research on task-shifting should include much more robust evaluations of such strategies.

SELF-MANAGEMENT: ENGAGING PATIENTS AND CAREGIVERS

This section is based on a nonsystematic, narrative review of studies published through September 2013 that involved self-management of cardiometabolic conditions in LMICs. The search was conducted in Medline (Pubmed), Embase (Ovid), and the Cochrane library.

Behavioral changes are needed to prevent and manage cardiometabolic diseases (Newman, Steed, and Mulligan 2004). These changes include implementing healthy lifestyle choices; taking medications on an indefinite basis; and undertaking other preventive actions, including primary prevention of the condition for individuals at risk and secondary prevention of complications for individuals with the condition. To make these changes, individuals and their caregivers must make decisions on a daily basis. The term *self-management* means different things to different people and, occasionally, different things at different times to the same person (McGowan 2005). Self-management has been defined as the ability of the individual to manage the symptoms, treatment, and physical and psychosocial consequences of chronic diseases and to make lifestyle changes related to chronic conditions (Barlow and others 2002). The proponents of this definition stress that effective self-management involves the ability to monitor one's condition and to effect the cognitive, behavioral, and emotional responses required to maintain a satisfactory quality of life (Barlow and others 2002). Self-care is seen as a preventive strategy (Clark and others 1991; Grady and Gough 2014), and self-management includes tasks undertaken by individuals to limit or reduce the impact of disease (Clark and others 1991). We do not make such a differentiation here, given the absence of a clear-cut distinction between risk and disease states for many cardiometabolic conditions and the commonality of strategies for addressing prevention across the continuum of risk exposure.

Self-management strategies for chronic diseases have developed in recognition of the need to shift health care from traditional models of care that place patients in the role of passive recipients to models of care that recognize the pivotal role of patient-provider partnerships in achieving successful prevention and management (Bodenheimer and others 2002). The partnership paradigm embraces two conceptually similar but clinically separable principles: collaborative care and self-management education.

In collaborative care (also known as patient empowerment), providers and patients make health care decisions together. Collaboration entails patients acknowledging their responsibility to manage their conditions and providers encouraging patients to solve their own problems by supplying them with information. Internal motivation, as opposed to external motivation, is the determinant of change. Table 17.3 compares traditional and collaborative care in chronic diseases.

Self-management education occurs in the sphere of patient education and includes a plan to provide patients with problem-solving skills (table 17.4) (Bodenheimer and others 2002; Von Korff and others 1997). A patient with diabetes, for instance, will gain knowledge about diet, physical activity, and drugs that control blood glucose and will acquire technical skills for monitoring blood glucose through traditional patient education.

Self-management interventions seek to address the challenges that individuals face in achieving optimal health goals related to managing their noncommunicable diseases (Newman, Steed, and Mulligan 2004). These interventions vary in population targeted, delivery location, self-management tutors used, mode and format of delivery, and content of the intervention (Barlow and others 2002). Self-management interventions have been implemented as part of multifaceted approaches to chronic care (Arauz and others 2001; Barcelo and others 2010; Faria and others 2013; Galante and others 2012; Thakur and others 2009), and identifying the impact of each component on improving self-management or patient health status is a challenge.

Cardiometabolic Conditions Targeted in Intervention Studies

An overview of selected self-management interventions conducted in LMICs is presented in online annex 17A. Diabetes appears to be the most often targeted condition. This is a global trend, probably because diabetes is one of the conditions for which the evidence base for self-management interventions is more developed (Newman, Steed, and Mulligan 2004). The aims of these interventions tend to be diverse, addressing issues ranging from lifestyle modification to improving glycemic control using medications and coping with symptoms. Interventions in LMICs have also targeted hypertension; obesity; rehabilitation of patients with existing disease, such as coronary heart disease or stroke; and managing overall CVD risk (Fornari and others 2013; Mujica and others 2010).

Table 17.3 Comparison of Traditional and Collaborative Care in Cardiometabolic Diseases

Issue	Traditional care	Collaborative care
What is the relationship between patient and health care provider?	Health care providers tell patients what to do; patients are passive	Expertise is shared with active patients; health care providers are the experts about the disease, and patients are the experts about their lives
Who is the principal caregiver and problem solver? Who is responsible for outcomes?	Health care providers	The patient and health care providers are the principal caregivers; they share responsibility for solving problems and for outcomes
What is the goal?	Compliance with instructions; noncompliance is a personal deficit	Patients set goals, and health care providers help patients to make informed choices; lack of goal achievement is a problem to be solved by modifying strategies
How is behavior changed?	External motivation	Internal motivation; patients gain understanding and confidence to accomplish new behaviors
How are problems identified?	By professionals	By patients (for example, pain or inability to function) and by professionals
How are problems solved?	Health care providers solve problems for patients	Health care providers teach problem-solving skills and help patients to solve problems

Source: Adapted from Bodenheimer and others 2002.

Table 17.4 Comparison of Traditional Education and Self-Management Education

Issue	Traditional patient education	Self-management education
What is taught?	Information and technical skills about the disease	Skills on how to act on problems
How are problems formulated?	Problems reflect inadequate control of the disease	Patients identify problems they experience that may be related to the disease
What is the relationship of education to the disease?	Education is disease specific and teaches relevant information and technical skills	Education provides problem-solving skills that are relevant to the consequences of chronic conditions
What is the theory underlying the education?	Disease-specific knowledge creates behavioral change, which improves clinical outcomes	Greater patient confidence in the capacity to make life-improving changes (self-efficacy) improves clinical outcomes
What is the goal?	Compliance with the behavioral changes taught to improve clinical outcomes	Increased self-efficacy to improve clinical outcomes
Who is the educator?	Health professionals	Health professionals, peer leaders, and other patients, often in group settings

Source: Adapted from Bodenheimer and others 2002.

Theories of Self-Management Interventions

Historically, self-management interventions were based on an educational approach, providing information in a traditional didactic format. The expectation was that the more knowledge people received, the more likely they would be to engage in the behavioral changes required to manage their conditions (Lorig and Holman 2003). This approach is still reported in published models implemented and evaluated in LMICs.

However, with the growing understanding that knowledge alone is not sufficient to promote behavioral change, self-management interventions have increasingly been based on more complex theories (Lorig and Holman 2003; Newman, Steed, and Mulligan 2004). Theoretical models that have commonly been applied to cardiometabolic diseases in LMICs include social cognitive theory, the stress coping model, and the readiness-to-change construct of the transtheoretical model

(Newman, Steed, and Mulligan 2004). The evidence base does not support the use of any one theoretical framework; the appropriateness of each may be highly contextual. Many strategies for self-management interventions for chronic diseases have been based on cognitive behavioral therapy.

Target Populations in Self-Management Interventions

Self-management interventions for cardiometabolic diseases in LMICs have targeted individuals with existing diseases, people with risk factors for disease, family members or companions of persons with or at risk for disease, as well as providers assisting in the delivery of self-management interventions. The intended beneficiaries have often been the direct targets of self-management interventions. However, the complexity of managing multiple risk factors for preventing cardiometabolic diseases suggests that targeting the direct beneficiary alone is insufficient. Alternative approaches have been developed, such as using peer supporters and targeting family members or others. An increasingly adopted innovation is educating children to influence their parents. In Brazil, Fornari and coworkers intervened with schoolchildren to help to lower the cardiovascular risk of their parents (Fornari and others 2013).

Some evidence indicates that family interventions can improve outcomes for individuals with or at risk of chronic diseases (Fisher and Weihs 2000). However, the few available studies in this area have been conducted largely in HICs. In a systematic review of family intervention studies in people with diabetes, Armour and others (2005) found that family interventions were associated with improved diabetes-related knowledge in five studies and a significant improvement in blood glucose control in eight studies. In a trial in Chile that involved 243 patients with type 2 diabetes from three first-level clinics in Santiago, a family-based intervention significantly improved blood glucose control during the first six months of intervention, but not during extended follow-up (Garcia-Huidobro and others 2011). The family-based intervention consisted of two family meetings or visits at home, one individual counseling session, one counseling session with relatives, and one multifamily education session (Garcia-Huidobro and others 2011).

The involvement of health care providers in self-management interventions has often occurred in the context of multidisciplinary teams. Members of these teams include physicians, nurses, dieticians, physical therapists, pharmacists, psychologists, and lay health workers. The use of lay health workers in LMICs is appealing, considering the shortage of trained health workers in these settings. In addition to delivering interventions within health care facilities, NPHWs have been used for community-based interventions, particularly those occurring within households. In the Control of Blood Pressure and Risk Attenuation (COBRA) trial in Pakistan, trained lay health workers delivered a household self-management intervention for controlling blood pressure to several thousand individuals (Jafar and others 2010; Jafar and others 2011).

Pharmacists are another health professional group through which the delivery of self-management interventions is increasingly reported. A review to examine the effects of pharmacist-provided, nondispensing services on patient outcomes, health service use, and costs in LMICs identified 12 relevant studies. The review found that services targeting self-management can improve glucose levels as well as blood pressure and cholesterol levels and may improve the quality of life for patients with diabetes or hypertension. Furthermore, use of pharmacy services appeared to be associated with reduced use of other health care services (Pande and others 2013).

Education in Self-Management

Education is a key element of self-management support and should be targeted to individuals' circumstances (Novak and others 2013). The WHO Working Group on Therapeutic Patient Education has emphasized the importance of patient-centered education for the effective management of chronic diseases (WHO Working Group 1998). Education interventions for cardiometabolic diseases have been delivered using paper-based or electronic support, face-to-face or remote interaction, and individual or group meetings. Multidimensional approaches with both written information and opportunities for in-person education and discussion have been proposed as particularly effective strategies; group settings offer the potential additional benefit of peer support (Novak and others 2013).

A quasi-experimental before-and-after evaluation study in Brazil explored the effect of educational intervention on the outcomes of 51 adults with type 2 diabetes (mean age 57.6 years). The content of the program was informed by the difficulties that providers encountered during patient care. The topics covered were concepts, pathophysiology and treatment of diabetes mellitus, physical activity, nutrition, care and examination of feet, self-monitoring, hypoglycemia, chronic complications, special situations, and family support. The program was delivered via group interactive lectures (20 sessions per group) and complemented by individual consultations for persons with additional needs identified during the group work. Consultations aimed to reinforce the strategies proposed during group meetings. They were conducted with approximately 15 participants who had difficulty maintaining their metabolic control or fitting in the group activities. The program was delivered over a five-month period by a multidisciplinary team including nurses, nutritionists, psychologists, a physical educator, and undergraduate students in nursing and psychology. Participation in the program was associated with improvement in the perceptions of patients regarding their general health status (Faria and others 2013).

In contrast to this high-intensity intervention, a structured public health group-based education program that was administered in two steps to young women (mean age 34 years) in Turkey was associated with significant six-month improvements in dietary habits and reductions in body weight, blood pressure, and prevalence of obesity. However, no economic evaluation was performed to determine cost-effectiveness (Kisioglu and others 2004). The intervention included educating the women about healthy cooking and physical exercise to reduce high blood pressure and weight.

Technology in Self-Management Interventions

Mobile technology applications, such as short message service (SMS) and multimedia message service (MMS), have been suggested as potentially convenient, cost-effective ways of supporting self-management. SMS and MMS programs could overcome barriers to patient education and self-management in LMICs because they are relatively inexpensive and accessible (mobile phone ownership is high and increasing in many LMICs). However, evidence to support their effectiveness remains very limited at the global level. A Cochrane review identified only four relevant studies, all conducted in HICs (de Jongh and others 2012). The review found moderate-quality evidence in support of improvement in individual's self-management capacity for diabetes as well as adherence to medications for diabetes or hypertension. The review further identified significant gaps in evidence regarding the long-term effects, acceptability, costs, and unintended effects of such interventions. A more recent RCT among Indian men with impaired glucose tolerance randomized to receive lifestyle-related SMS demonstrated that the incidence of type 2 diabetes was lower in the intervention group compared with the control (18 percent of participants in the intervention group developed type 2 diabetes compared with 27 percent in the control group; hazard ratio, 0.64; 95% confidence interval, 0.45–0.92; $p = 0.015$) (Ramachandran and others 2013). The use of text messaging to improve self-management is a major focus of

current research, and data relevant to LMIC settings will be increasingly available.

More traditional telecare approaches have also been evaluated. In a short-term randomized trial involving 200 patients with hypertension recruited across clinics in Honduras and Mexico, an intervention comprising automated telephone care management plus home blood pressure monitoring was effective in improving the patients' perception of general health and satisfaction with care. Intervention patients had lower scores for depression and fewer medication-related problems. In the subgroup with high information needs at baseline, the intervention was associated with significant lowering of blood pressure (Piette and others 2012).

The effect of telephone-based self-management support for diabetes control was assessed in two primary care facilities in Chile (Lange and others 2010). The intervention consisted of six telecare self-management support encounters during a 15-month period. Telecare included providing support to participants and motivating them to continue their medications. Information was updated on their electronic health records, which providers could access during the next patient visit. Compared with usual care, participants in the intervention group maintained their blood glucose levels during follow-up, while the control group did not. In the intervention group, perceptions of self-efficacy were higher, compliance with clinic visits was greater, and visits for emergency care were fewer (Lange and others 2010).

Cost-Effectiveness of Self-Management Interventions

Only two studies assessed the cost-effectiveness of self-management interventions in LMICs. The cost-effectiveness of community-based strategies to control blood pressure was evaluated in the COBRA trial in Pakistan (Jafar and others 2011). The COBRA project randomized 1,341 individuals with hypertension in 12 randomly selected centers in Karachi to usual care or one of three intervention programs: (1) combined home health education (HHE) by lay health workers plus trained general practitioners, (2) HHE only, and (3) trained general practitioners only (Jafar and others 2009; Jafar and others 2010). The annual cost per participant was US$3.99 for the combined HHE and trained general practitioners, US$3.34 for HHE alone, and US$0.65 for trained general practitioners alone. The combined HHE and trained general practitioners was the most cost-effective intervention, with an incremental cost-effectiveness ratio of US$25 (95% confidence interval, 6–99) per millimeter of mercury (mmHg, a unit of pressure) reduction in systolic blood pressure (Jafar and others 2011).

The cost-effectiveness of home rehabilitation for ischemic stroke was evaluated in Thailand (Sritipsukho and others 2010). The study randomized 58 patients with ischemic stroke to either home rehabilitation programs or conventional hospital care. The Barthel Index and Modified Rankin Scale were used to evaluate the outcome measures, and success was defined as an improvement by at least one level of the outcome scale. The cost and number of successful cases were greater in the intervention than in the usual care group. For patients with mild or no disability, the incremental cost-effectiveness ratios were 14,212 Thai baht and 24,364 Thai baht, respectively, per one unit of change in the Barthel Index (Sritipsukho and others 2010). The authors found this result to be cost-effective when compared with gross domestic product per capita.

Discussion

Self-management initiatives for cardiometabolic diseases in LMICs and at regional and global levels are in their infancy. Evidence is accumulating from intervention research that supports self-management, but little is known about which components of those interventions work best in LMICs; virtually nothing is known about how to scale up models found to be effective in research settings.

Extensive reviews of self-management intervention studies around the world have identified general components that have been found to work well in diverse settings (de Silva 2011; Novak and others 2013). These components can assist in the development and implementation of strategies for promoting the uptake of self-management for chronic diseases in LMICs (box 17.2). However, for these strategies to be effective, the barriers and facilitators of the implementation, many of which are context specific, must be understood.

Furthermore, different strategies will likely have to be combined for the same condition within any given setting and at different times for the same individual to achieve the desired effect (figure 17.1). In available studies from LMICs, self-management has been implemented as a component of much broader interventions targeting chronic disease prevention and control. Most of these studies did not develop an evaluation framework to tease out the contribution of the self-management component from the overall effect of the intervention.

CONCLUSIONS

Innovative approaches to extending the care of people with cardiometabolic and chronic lung conditions into the community are likely to be crucial components of any suite of strategies to reduce the burden of disease in LMICs. Effective task-shifting to more affordable and community-based health care workers and effective consumer self-management are two important examples. For both, the current evidence base has critical gaps in addressing effectiveness, cost-effectiveness, and key understandings for scale-up, particularly in LMICs. Several large ongoing studies include aspects of self-management and task-shifting; many of these studies involve key stakeholders, including health care providers and patients, in developing the intervention

---

Box 17.2

Elements That Support Self-Management

The following elements support self-management for chronic diseases:

- Involving people in decision making
- Emphasizing problem solving
- Developing care plans as a partnership between service users and professionals
- Setting goals and following up on the extent to which goals are achieved over time
- Promoting healthy lifestyles and educating people about their conditions and how to self-manage

- Motivating people to self-manage using targeted approaches and structured information and support
- Helping people to monitor their symptoms and know when to take appropriate action
- Helping people to manage the social, emotional, and physical impacts of their conditions
- Using proactive follow-up
- Providing opportunities to share and learn from other service users.

Source: Adapted from de Silva 2011.

and in incorporating appropriate frameworks for broad evaluation of effectiveness, cost-effectiveness, acceptability, scalability, and sustainability. Such ongoing and new research is crucial and should provide important insights into practical and affordable community-based models of care in LMICs.

This chapter has provided insights into approaches that have the potential to be effective and scalable as well as factors that might impede or facilitate their utility.

CASE STUDY 17.1: INVESTIGATING AN NPHW-LED CARDIOVASCULAR DISEASE RISK MANAGEMENT MODEL IN RURAL INDIA

Background

Cardiovascular diseases (CVDs) are the major cause of premature death and disability in India, yet few people at risk are able to access best practice health care (WHO 2008a).[1] In India, CVD risk factor levels are high, even in the rural population, which constitutes 70 percent of the total population. CVD is the leading cause of adult deaths in many rural Indian communities (Joshi and others 2006; Kinra and others 2010). Despite the availability of evidence-based guidelines for the prevention of CVD, the use of simple, affordable, preventive treatments (such as smoking cessation strategies and the use of aspirin, low-cost statins, angiotensin-converting enzyme inhibitors, and beta blockers) is very low in these communities (Joshi and others 2009). Numerous barriers exist at different levels of the health system, including lack of facilities, limited access to providers, and high out-of-pocket costs (Rao and others 2011). Mobile Health (mHealth) is a promising strategy for addressing some of these barriers, but very few mHealth interventions have been subject to robust evaluation.

This case study describes an innovative strategy, Systematic Medical Appraisal Referral and Treatment in India (SMARTHealth India), that consists of the following:

- Using a mobile device–based clinical decision support system (CDSS) for CVD risk management
- Shifting tasks from physicians to NPHWs
- Integrating the overall system within the government's primary health care infrastructure in rural India.

The objectives of SMARTHealth were twofold: (1) to develop a valid CVD risk assessment and management algorithm based on best practice national and international recommendations, with a focus on blood pressure management, and (2) to assess utility, preliminary

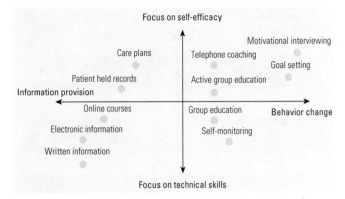

Figure 17.1 Continuum of Strategies to Support Self-Management

Source: Adapted from de Silva 2011.

effectiveness, and acceptability of the system among community members, NPHWs, and physicians.

Methods

A mobile software application (app) was developed to deliver the CDSS, which was based on plain language clinical rules developed from standard guidelines that were subsequently programmed and translated. Formal five-day and one-day training courses were developed for the NPHWs and physicians, respectively, that focused on both the conditions targeted and the delivery of interventions. The algorithm was validated and field tested in 11 villages in Andhra Pradesh; the test involved 11 NPHWs and 3 primary health care physicians. NPHWs are usually female residents of the village with approximately a grade 10 education and are each responsible for an average of 1,000 residents in the village.

The mobile app takes users through a four-step process (patient registration, past medical history and medications, risk factor measurements, and treatment advice). To measure blood pressure, NPHWs and physicians use an automatic monitor to upload readings wirelessly into the app. Blood glucose, cholesterol (if available), height, and weight are entered manually. The treatment advice page provides the 10-year CVD risk for each participant; lifestyle, referral, and follow-up recommendations for NPHWs; and medication recommendations for physicians (figure 17.2).

A mixed-methods evaluation was conducted that consisted of clinical and survey data and in-depth patient and staff interviews to provide an understanding of the barriers to and enablers of use of the system. At the end of the study, all physicians and NPHWs participated in an in-depth interview, and selected community members participated in four village-based focus group discussions in separate groups by gender.

Figure 17.2 Treatment Advice Screen of the Application

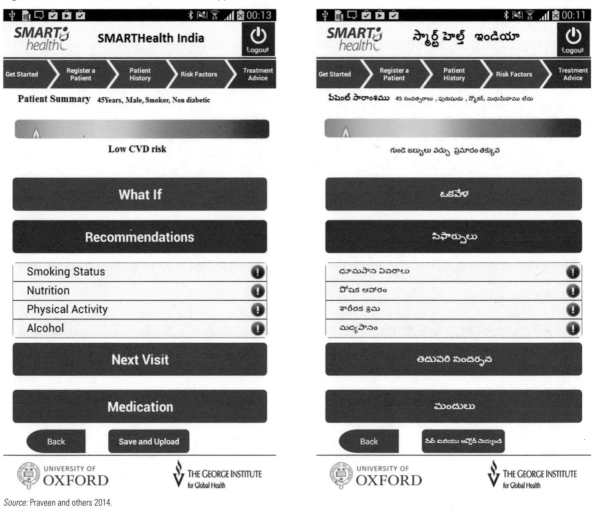

Source: Praveen and others 2014.

Semistructured interviews were conducted by a researcher who was experienced in these field settings and proficient in English and Telugu. Interviews covered the following domains:

- Staff roles and responsibilities
- Patient, NPHW, and doctor satisfaction with using the app
- Staff knowledge and skills
- Impact of CDSS on usual work routines.

Findings

Quantitative Evaluation
During the pilot study, NPHWs and physicians used the CDSS to screen 227 and 65 adults, respectively. The NPHWs identified 39 percent (88) of patients for referral; 78 percent (69) of these referred patients were indicated for blood-pressure-lowering medication (figure 17.3). Only 35 percent (24), however, saw a doctor within one month of referral; of those who did, 42 percent (10) reported continuing medications at a three-month follow-up visit. Physicians identified and recommended 42 percent (10) of patients for blood-pressure-lowering medications. Overall, after three months, only 10 of 69 patients (15 percent) with an indication for blood pressure medications were actually taking them. This pilot demonstrated the need to strengthen the health system if task-shifting strategies are to be successful.

Qualitative Evaluation
All physicians and NPHWs participated in interviews, and four community focus groups were conducted.

Figure 17.3 Assessment and Management Pathway for Patients Screened by NPHWs

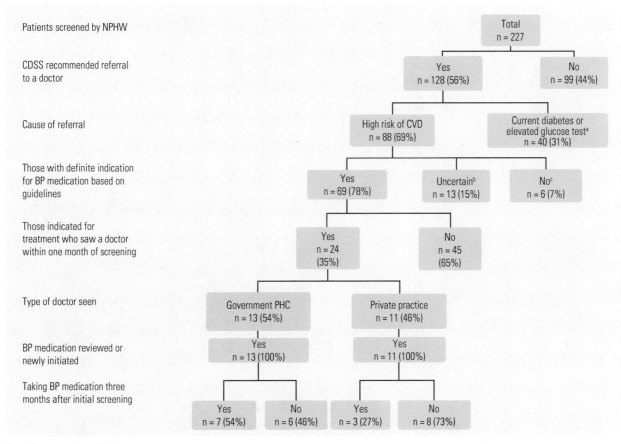

Source: Praveen and others 2014.
Note: NPHW = nonphysician health worker; CDSS = clinical decision support system; BP = blood pressure; CVD = cardiovascular disease; PHC = primary health center.
a. Either patients with a past history of diabetes who were not at elevated CVD risk (n = 9) or patients whose random capillary glucose tests were elevated (n = 31) (excluded from further analysis).
b. Patients diagnosed with peripheral vascular disease but lacking any other data to suggest high CVD risk (excluded from further analysis).
c. Patients with absolute risk of 20–30 percent and BP <140/90 or with absolute risk of 30–40 percent and BP <130/80 are not indicated for medications.

Three interrelated themes emerged from the interviews (figure 17.4):

- The intervention strategy had potential to transform prevailing health care models.
- Task-shifting of CVD screening to NPHWs was the central driver of change.
- Despite high acceptability, actual transformation was limited by system-level barriers, such as access to physicians and medicines.

Conclusions

This feasibility study provided initial insights into the acceptability and preliminary effectiveness of a smartphone CDSS to improve detection, prevention, and management of cardiovascular disease in a first-level

health care facility in India. It incorporated a technological solution with innovative workforce strategies to address the growing CVD epidemic. Broader systems issues, such as the inability of NPHWs to prescribe and dispense essential medications and integration of mHealth strategies within this broader context, are essential factors in maximizing the impact of such approaches.

The intervention strategy has been substantially modified to include a focus on health systems strengthening—providing government support through policy directives, ensuring the availability of essential medications, incorporating recall and reminder systems, modifying provider remuneration incentives, and incorporating a consumer support program for long-term drug adherence. It is being rigorously evaluated for clinical effectiveness and cost-effectiveness in a large cluster

Figure 17.4 Illustration of the Interview Themes in Context of the COM-B Model

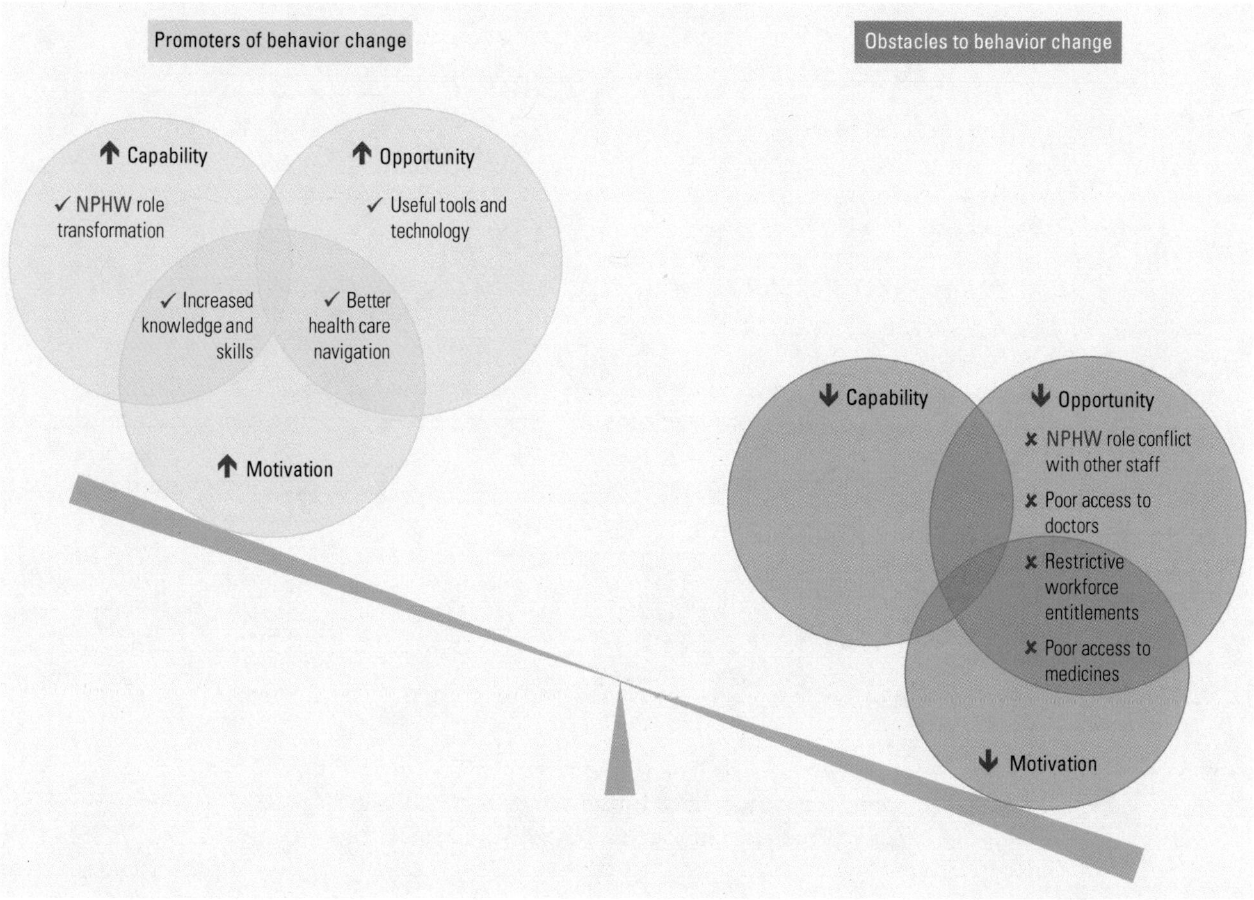

Source: Praveen and others 2014.
Note: NPHW = nonphysician health worker.

randomized trial. If found to be successful, the findings are likely to advance knowledge on scalable strategies to improve access to effective health care for underserved populations in LMICs.

CASE STUDY 17.2: INVESTIGATING A COMMUNITY-BASED DIABETES CARE MODEL: THE MOPOTSYO MODEL IN CAMBODIA

MoPoTsyo Model of Care

More than 325,000 Cambodians have diabetes (IDF 2012) and require access to chronic care.[2] They face four main barriers when seeking services: financial, geographic, informational, and household.

MoPoTsyo is a nonprofit organization that started in 2005 with the goal of empowering people living with diabetes and hypertension to manage their diseases and eliminate the barriers to quality care. Since 2007, MoPoTsyo has screened more than 460,000 adults for diabetes. In 2011, PATH—known as the Program for Appropriate Technology in Health from 1980 until 2014 and now known simply as PATH—selected the MoPoTsyo Patient Information Center in Cambodia as an innovative care model for noncommunicable diseases in low-resource settings. This case study is based on information gathered during PATH's onsite investigation to identify the success factors of MoPoTsyo and its potential for replication.

Currently, 135 peer educators serving 16 districts help to facilitate services for 14,000 people living with diabetes and hypertension. The program includes three components, all managed by core staff at the head office:

a network of peer educators, a revolving drug fund, and contracted physicians.

MoPoTsyo peer educators must be diagnosed with diabetes, complete an intensive six-week course delivered by MoPoTsyo, shadow an experienced peer educator, and pass an examination. Once trained, peer educators lead group screening and information sessions in their homes. These sessions include monitoring blood glucose, blood pressure, heart rate, and weight; providing self-management education; answering member questions; and fostering peer support. Peer educators are organized under a diabetes program manager appointed jointly by MoPoTsyo and the local health authority in each operational district. Robust monitoring of peer educator performance and assurance of consistent quality standards are priorities.

MoPoTsyo procures medicines at international market prices and distributes them to 20 subcontracted community pharmacies, which sell them to MoPoTsyo members at prices fixed below market retail prices. Pharmacies with large sales volumes gain a 5–15 percent profit, and members benefit from a consistent supply of affordable medications.

Outcomes Achieved

An evaluation of 150 randomly selected MoPoTsyo patient records found significant reductions in fasting plasma glucose and out-of pocket expenses (Eggermont 2011; van Pelt and others 2013). The sensitivity and specificity of MoPoTsyo's screening approach, the relative health status of patients screened compared with alternative screening methods, and the operational and logistical implications of diagnosing people earlier in their disease process are being assessed.

Key Success Factors

An Interdisciplinary, Patient-Centered, Team-Based Model of Care

The MoPoTsyo model places the patient at the center, supported by a cross-disciplinary team consisting of a peer educator, a physician, and a pharmacist (Barr and others 2003; WHO 2002). Clearly defined roles, strong relationships, and good communication strategies among team members optimize care. The peer educator coordinates the team and helps patients to navigate the health system.

All team members record symptoms, progress, medical status, and medications in each member's patient care booklet. Peer educators monitor this information, including physicians' orders and patients' adherence to treatment. The booklets serve as identification when members purchase prescribed drugs. This simple information management and coordination system ensures that all team members are informed of the person's health status and care.

Reduced-Cost Community-Level Services

For most Cambodians, diabetes care is difficult; for example, patients often travel long distances for care, and no hospitals offer free diabetes care. MoPoTsyo reduces direct and indirect costs by providing services close to home, using the revolving drug fund, and managing relationships with contracted physicians and pharmacies. Patients pay US$5 for consultation, testing, and transportation, compared with US$30 or more in the private sector. Average monthly medication costs for MoPoTsyo members are US$5.50. Patients report that services and medications are convenient and helpful.

Use of Peer Educators to Enhance Trust and Model Good Disease Management

MoPoTsyo peer educators are viewed as trusted community leaders committed to self-managing their disease. A MoPoTsyo physician reports that many patients have more trust in peer educators than in health care professionals because peer educators set a good example in their lifestyle choices and how they manage their diabetes. Peer educators are not allowed to prescribe or sell medications and do not have a financial stake in medications or services, so patients see them as unbiased. Although peer educators receive a small amount of money as reimbursement for their costs, many report that they are motivated by the desire to manage their disease and the prestige they enjoy educating others to do the same, rather than by the money provided. Many hold jobs in their communities, often in leadership positions. The reputation of the peer educators as respected community members with elevated social status enhances the reputation of MoPoTsyo as a credible organization. Patient trust and respect for MoPoTsyo grows as their health improves.

A Dynamic, Well-Connected Leader

MoPoTsyo's chief executive officer and founder, Maurits van Pelt, has created a strong organization with staff members who are committed to enabling fellow Cambodians to self-manage diabetes and hypertension. MoPoTsyo staff report that van Pelt nurtures a team approach with on-the-job professional development and mentoring. The team has won the support of donors and buy-in from key stakeholders to incorporate the model into the government system.

Conclusion and Implications

The MoPoTsyo model of care offers a promising and affordable approach to the care and management of noncommunicable diseases in low-resource settings and offsets constraints that impede access to care. MoPoTsyo has made services more availabile by centering them in communities, providing medications through contracted pharmacies, and launching a peer education program. It also has provided comprehensive team-based care closer to home at a reduced cost.

ANNEX

The annex to this chapter is as follows. It is available at http://www.dcp-3.org/CVRD.

- Annex 17A. Examples of Self-Management Interventions for Cardiometabolic Conditions in LMICs and the Evaluation of Their Effects

NOTES

World Bank Income Classifications as of July 2014 are as follows, based on estimates of gross national income (GNI) per capita for 2013:

- Low-income countries (LICs) = US$1,045 or less
- Middle-income countries (MICs) are subdivided:
  (a) lower-middle-income = US$1,046 to US$4,125
  (b) upper-middle-income (UMICs) = US$4,126 to US$12,745
- High-income countries (HICs) = US$12,746 or more.

1. This case study was prepared by Devarsetty Praveen, Anushka Patel, Arvind Raghu, Gari D. Clifford, Pallab K. Maulik, Ameer Abdul Mohammad, Kishor Mogulluru, Lionel Tarrasenko, Stephen MacMahon, and David Peiris.
2. This case study was prepared by Claudia Harner-Jay, Ashley Morganstern, Bernhard Weigl, Jennifer Drake, Mary Beth Weber, and Helen C. McGuire.

REFERENCES

Abegunde, D. O., B. Shengelia, A. Luyten, A. Cameron, F. Celletti, and others. 2007. "Can Non-Physician Health-Care Workers Assess and Manage Cardiovascular Risk in Primary Care?" *Bulletin of the World Health Organization* 85 (6): 432–40.

Abrahams-Gessel, S., C. A. Denman, C. M. Montano, T. A. Gaziano, N. Levitt, and others. 2015a. "Lessons from Training and Supervision of Community Health Workers Conducting Population-Based, Noninvasive Screening for CVD in LMIC: Implications for Scaling Up." *Global Heart* 10 (1): 39–44.

———. 2015b. "The Training and Fieldwork Experiences of Community Health Workers Conducting Population-Based, Noninvasive Screening for CVD in LMIC." *Global Heart* 10 (1): 45–54.

Arauz, A. G., G. Sanchez, G. Padilla, M. Fernandez, M. Rosello, and others. 2001. "Community Diabetes Educational Intervention at the Primary Care Level." *Revista Panamericana de Salud Pública* 9 (3): 145–53.

Armour, T. A., S. L. Norris, L. Jack Jr., X. Zhang, L. Fisher, and others. 2005. "The Effectiveness of Family Interventions in People with Diabetes Mellitus: A Systematic Review." *Diabetes Medicine* 22 (10): 1295–305.

Babigumira, J., B. Castelnuovo, M. Lamorde, A. Kambugu, A. Stergachis, and others. 2009. "Potential Impact of Task-Shifting on Costs of Antiretroviral Therapy and Physician Supply in Uganda." *BMC Health Services Research* 9 (1): 192.

Bang, A., R. Bang, S. Baitule, H. Reddy, and M. Deshmukh. 1999. "Effect of Home-Based Neonatal Care and Management of Sepsis on Neonatal Mortality: Field Trial in Rural India." *The Lancet* 354 (9194): 1955–61.

Barcelo, A., E. Cafiero, M. de Boer, A. E. Mesa, M. G. Lopez, and others. 2010. "Using Collaborative Learning to Improve Diabetes Care and Outcomes: The VIDA Project." *Primary Care Diabetes* 4 (3): 145–53.

Barlow, J., C. Wright, J. Sheasby, A. Turner, J. Hainsworth, and others. 2002. "Self-Management Approaches for People with Chronic Conditions: A Review." *Patient Education and Counseling* 48 (2): 177–87.

Barr, V. J., S. Robinson, B. Marin-Link, L. Underhill, A. Dotts, and others. 2003. "The Expanded Chronic Care Model: An Integration of Concepts and Strategies from Population Health Promotion and the Chronic Care Model." *Hospital Quarterly* 7 (1): 73–82. http://www.primaryhealthcarebc.ca/pdf/eccm_article.pdf.

Bodenheimer, T., K. Lorig, H. Holman, and K. Grumbach. 2002. "Patient Self-Management of Chronic Disease in Primary Care." *Journal of the American Medical Association* 288 (19): 2469–75.

Buttorff, C., R. S. Hock, H. A. Weiss, S. Naik, R. Araya, and others. 2012. "Economic Evaluation of a Task-Shifting Intervention for Common Mental Disorders in India." *Bulletin of the World Health Organization* 90 (11): 813–21.

Callaghan, M., N. Ford, and H. Schneider. 2010. "A Systematic Review of Task-Shifting for HIV Treatment and Care in Africa." *Human Resources for Health* 8 (8). doi:10.1186/1478-4491-8-8.

Clark, N. M., M. H. Becker, N. C. Janz, K. Lorig, W. Rakowski, and others. 1991. "Self-Management of Chronic Disease by Older Adults: Review and Questions for Research." *Journal of Aging and Health* 3 (1): 3–27.

Coleman, R., G. Gill, and D. Wilkinson. 1998. "Noncommunicable Disease Management in Resource-Poor Settings: A Primary Care Model from Rural South Africa." *Bulletin of the World Health Organization* 76 (6): 633–40.

de Jongh, T., I. Gurol-Urganci, V. Vodopivec-Jamsek, J. Car, and R. Atun. 2012. "Mobile Phone Messaging for Facilitating Self-Management of Long-Term Illnesses." *Cochrane Database of Systematic Reviews* 12: CD007459.

de Silva, D. 2011. *Evidence: Helping People to Help Themselves; a Review of the Evidence Considering Whether It Is Worthwhile to Support Self-Management.* London: The Health Foundation.

Eggermont, N. 2011. "Evaluation of a Peer-Education Program for Diabetes and Hypertension in Rural Cambodia." Master's Thesis, Universiteit Gent, Institute of Tropical Medicine Antwerp, Antwerp, Belgium. http://www.mopotsyo.org/Thesis%20Natalie_MoPoTsyo%20evaluation.pdf.

Fairall, L., M. O. Bachmann, C. Lombard, V. Timmerman, K. Uebel, and others. 2012. "Task Shifting of Antiretrovhral Treatment from Doctors to Primary-Care Nurses in South Africa (STRETCH): A Pragmatic, Parallel, Cluster-Randomised Trial." *The Lancet* 380 (9845): 889–98.

Faria, H. T., V. S. Veras, A. T. Xavier, C. R. Teixeira, M. L. Zanetti, and others. 2013. "Quality of Life in Patients with Diabetes Mellitus before and after Their Participation in an Educational Program." *Revista da Escola de Enfermagen USP* 47 (2): 348–54.

Fisher, L., and K. L. Weihs. 2000. "Can Addressing Family Relationships Improve Outcomes in Chronic Disease? Report of the National Working Group on Family-Based Interventions in Chronic Disease." *Journal of Family Practice* 49 (6): 561–66.

Fornari, L. S., I. Giuliano, F. Azevedo, A. Pastana, C. Vieira, and others. 2013. "Children First Study: How an Educational Program in Cardiovascular Prevention at School Can Improve Parents' Cardiovascular Risk." *European Journal of Preventive Cardiology* 20 (2): 301–09.

Galante, M., A. Languasco, D. Gotta, S. Bell, T. Lancelotti, and others. 2012. "Venous Thromboprophylaxis in General Surgery Ward Admissions: Strategies for Improvement." *International Journal of Quality in Health Care* 26 (6): 649–56.

Garcia-Huidobro, D., M. Bittner, P. Brahm, and K. Puschel. 2011. "Family Intervention to Control Type 2 Diabetes: A Controlled Clinical Trial." *Family Practice* 28 (1): 4–11.

Gaziano, T. A., S. Abrahams-Gessel, S. Surka, S. Sy, A. Pandya, and others. 2015. "Cardiovascular Disease Screening by Community Health Workers Can Be Cost-Effective in Low-Resource Countries." *Health Affairs* 34 (9): 1538–45.

Gill, G. V., C. Price, D. Shandu, M. Dedicoat, and D. Wilkinson. 2008. "An Effective System of Nurse-Led Diabetes Care in Rural Africa." *Diabetic Medicine* 25 (5): 606–11.

Grady, P. A., and L. L. Gough. 2014. "Self-Management: A Comprehensive Approach to Management of Chronic Conditions." *American Journal of Public Health* 104 (8): e25–31. doi: 10.2105/AJPH.2014.302041. Epub June 12.

Grumbach, K., and J. Coffman. 1998. "Physicians and Nonphysician Clinicians: Complements or Competitors?" *Journal of the American Medical Association* 280 (9): 825–26.

Haines, A., D. Sanders, U. Lehmann, A. K. Rowe, J. E. Lawn, and others. 2007. "Achieving Child Survival Goals: Potential Contribution of Community Health Workers." *The Lancet* 369 (9579): 2121–31.

IDF (International Diabetes Federation). 2012. *IDF Diabetes Atlas,* fifth edition. 2012 update. Brussels: IDF. http://www.idf.org/diabetesatlas/5e/Update2012.

Jafar, T. H., J. Hatcher, N. Poulter, M. Islam, S. Hashmi, and others. 2009. "Community-Based Interventions to Promote Blood Pressure Control in a Developing Country: A Cluster Randomized Trial." *Annals of Internal Medicine* 151 (9): 593–601.

Jafar, T. H., M. Islam, R. Bux, N. Poulter, J. Hatcher, and others. 2011. "Cost-Effectiveness of Community-Based Strategies for Blood Pressure Control in a Low-Income Developing Country: Findings from a Cluster-Randomized, Factorial-Controlled Trial." *Circulation* 124 (15): 1615–25.

Jafar, T. H., M. Islam, J. Hatcher, S. Hashmi, R. Bux, and others. 2010. "Community Based Lifestyle Intervention for Blood Pressure Reduction in Children and Young Adults in Developing Country: Cluster Randomised Controlled Trial." *British Medical Journal* 340 (June 7): C2641.

Joshi, R., M. Cardona, S. Iyengar, A. Sukumar, C. R. Raju, and others. 2006. "Chronic Diseases Now a Leading Cause of Death in Rural India: Mortality Data from the Andhra Pradesh Rural Health Initiative." *International Journal of Epidemiology* 35 (6): 1522–29.

Joshi, R., C. K. Chow, P. K. Raju, K. R. Raju, A. K. Gottumukkala, and others. 2012. "The Rural Andhra Pradesh Cardiovascular Prevention Study." *Journal of the American College of Cardiology* 59 (13): 1188–86.

Joshi, R., C. K. Chow, P. K. Raju, R. Raju, K. S. Reddy, and others. 2009. "Fatal and Nonfatal Cardiovascular Disease and the Use of Therapies for Secondary Prevention in a Rural Region of India." *Circulation* 119 (14): 1950–55. doi:10.1161/CIRCULATIONAHA.108.819201.

Kar, S. S., J. S. Thakur, S. Jain, and R. Kumar. 2008. "Cardiovascular Disease Risk Management in a Primary Health Care Setting of North India." *Indian Heart Journal* 60 (1): 19–25.

Kaufman, J. A., W. Zeng, L. Wang, and Y. Zhang. 2012. "Community-Based Mental Health Counseling for Children Orphaned by AIDS in China." *AIDS Care* 25 (4): 430–37.

Kengne, A. P, P. K. Awah, L. L. Fezeu, E. Sobngwi, and J. C. Mbanya. 2009. "Primary Health Care for Hypertension by Nurses in Rural and Urban Sub-Saharan Africa." *Journal of Clinical Hypertension* 11 (10): 564–72.

Kengne, A. P., L. Fezeu, P. K. Awah, E. Sobngwi, and J. C. Mbanya. 2010. "Task Shifting in the Management of Epilepsy in Resource-Poor Settings." *Epilepsia* 51 (5): 931–32.

Kengne, A. P., E. Sobngwi, L. L. Fezeu, P. K. Awah, S. Dongmo, and J. C. Mbanya. 2008. "Nurse-Led Care for Asthma at Primary Level in Rural Sub-Saharan Africa: The Experience of Bafut in Cameroon." *Journal of Asthma* 45 (6): 437–43.

———. 2009. "Setting-Up Nurse-Led Pilot Clinics for the Management of Non-Communicable Diseases at Primary Health Care Level in Resource-Limited Settings of Africa." *Pan African Medical Journal* 3 (10).

Kinra, S., L. J. Bowen, T. Lyngdoh, D. Prabhakaran, K. S. Reddy, and others. 2010. "Sociodemographic Patterning of Non-Communicable Disease Risk Factors in Rural India: A Cross Sectional Study." *British Medical Journal* 341: C4974. doi:10.1136/Bmj.C4974.

Kisioglu, A. N., B. Aslan, M. Ozturk, M. Aykut, and I. Ilhan. 2004. "Improving Control of High Blood Pressure among

Middle-Aged Turkish Women of Low Socio-Economic Status through Public Health Training." *Croatian Medical Journal* 45 (4): 477–82.

Labhardt, N. D., J. Balo, M. Ndam, J. Grimm, and E. Manga. 2010. "Task Shifting to Non-Physician Clinicians for Integrated Management of Hypertension and Diabetes in Rural Cameroon: A Programme Assessment at Two Years." *BHC Health Service Research* 10 (339). http://www.biomedcentral.com/1472-6963/10/339.

Labhardt, N. D., J. R. Balo, M. Ndam, E. Manga, and B. Stoll. 2011. "Improved Retention Rates with Low-Cost Interventions in Hypertension and Diabetes Management in a Rural African Environment of Nurse-Led Care: A Cluster-Randomised Trial." *Tropical Medicine and International Health* 16 (10): 1276–84.

Lange, I., S. Campos, M. Urrutia, C. Bustamante, C. Alcayaga, and others. 2010. "Effect of a Tele-Care Model on Self-Management and Metabolic Control among Patients with Type 2 Diabetes in Primary Care Centers in Santiago, Chile." *Revista Médica de Chile* 138 (6): 729–37.

Lekoubou, A., P. Awah, L. Fezeu, E. Sobngwi, and A. P. Kengne. 2010. "Hypertension, Diabetes Mellitus, and Task Shifting and Their Management in Sub-Saharan Africa." *International Journal of Environmental Research and Public Health* 7: 353–63.

Lewin, S., S. Munabi-Babigumira, C. Glenton, K. Daniels, X. Bosch-Capblanch, and others. 2010. "The Effect of Lay Health Workers on Mother and Child Health and Infectious Diseases." *Cochrane Database of Systematic Reviews* 3: CD004015. doi:10.1002/14651858.

Lorig, K. R., and H. Holman. 2003. "Self-Management Education: History, Definition, Outcomes, and Mechanisms." *Annals of Behavioral Medicine* 26 (1): 1–7.

McCollum, E. D., G. A. Preidis, M. M. Kabue, E. B. M. Singogo, C. Mwansambo, and others. 2010. "Task Shifting Routine Inpatient Pediatric HIV Testing Improves Program Outcomes in Urban Malawi: A Retrospective Observational Study." *PLoS One* 5 (3): e9626: 10.1371/journal.pone.0009626.

McGowan, P. 2005. "Self-Management." Background Paper for New Perspectives: International Conference on Patient Self-Management. University of Victoria, Centre on Aging, Victoria.

Mdege N. D., S. Chindove, and A. Shehzad. 2012. "The Effectiveness and Cost Implications of Task-Shifting in the Delivery of Antiretroviral Therapy to HIV-Infected Patients: A Systematic Review." *Health Policy and Planning* 28 (3): 223–36. doi:10.1093/heapol/czs058.

Mendoza Montano, C., M. Fort, J. Cruz, and M. Ramírez-Zea. 2015. "Evaluation of a Pilot Hypertension Management Programme for Guatemalan Adults." *Health Promotion International* 31 (2): 363–74. doi: 10.1093/heapro/dau117.

Mujica, V., A. Urzua, E. Leiva, N. Diaz, R. Moore-Carrasco, and others. 2010. "Intervention with Education and Exercise Reverses the Metabolic Syndrome in Adults." *Journal of the American Society of Hypertension* 4 (3): 148–53.

Mullan, F., and S. Frehywot. 2007. "Non-Physician Clinicians in 47 Sub-Saharan African Countries." *The Lancet* 370 (9605): 2158–63.

Newman, S., L. Steed, and K. Mulligan. 2004. "Self-Management Interventions for Chronic Illness." *The Lancet* 364 (9444): 1523–37.

Novak, M., L. Costantini, S. Schneider, and H. Beanlands. 2013. "Approaches to Self-Management in Chronic Illness." *Seminars in Dialysis* 26 (2): 188–94.

Pande, S., J. E. Hiller, N. Nkansah, and L. Bero. 2013. "The Effect of Pharmacist-Provided Non-Dispensing Services on Patient Outcomes, Health Service Utilisation, and Costs in Low- and Middle-Income Countries." *Cochrane Database of Systematic Reviews* 2: CD010398.

Piette, J. D., H. Datwani, S. Gaudioso, S. M. Foster, J. Westphal, and others. 2012. "Hypertension Management Using Mobile Technology and Home Blood Pressure Monitoring: Results of a Randomized Trial in Two Low/Middle-Income Countries." *Telemedicine Journal and e-Health* 18 (8): 613–20.

Praveen, D., A. Patel, A. Raghu, G. D. Clifford, P. K. Maulik, and others. 2014. "SMARTHealth India: Development and Field Evaluation of a Mobile Clinical Decision Support System for Cardiovascular Diseases in Rural India." *JMIR mHealth and uHealth* 2 (4): e54. doi:10.2196/mhealth.3568.

Ramachandran, A., C. Snehalatha, J. Ram, S. Selvam, M. Simon, and others. 2013. "Effectiveness of Mobile Phone Messaging in Prevention of Type 2 Diabetes by Lifestyle Modification in Men in India: A Prospective, Parallel Group, RCT." *The Lancet Diabetes and Endocrinology* 1 (3): 191–98.

Rao, M., K. D. Rao, A. S. Kumar, M. Chatterjee, and T. Sundararaman. 2011. "Human Resources for Health in India." *The Lancet* 377 (9765): 587–98.

Ruggiero, L., S. Oros, and Y. K. Choi. 2011. "Community-Based Translation of the Diabetes Prevention Program's Lifestyle Intervention in an Underserved Latino Population." *The Diabetes Educator* 37 (4): 564–72.

Sritipsukho, P., A. Riewpaiboon, P. Chaiyawat, and K. Kulkantrakorn. 2010. "Cost-Effectiveness Analysis of Home Rehabilitation Programs for Thai Stroke Patients." *Journal of the Medical Association of Thailand* 93 (Suppl 7): S262–70.

Thakur, J. S., S. Pala, Y. Sharma, S. Jain, S. Kumari, and others. 2009. "Integrated Non-Communicable Disease Control Program in a Northern Part of India: Lessons from a Demonstration Project in Low Resource Settings of a Developing Country." *CVD Prevention and Control* 4 (4): 193–99.

van Pelt, M., H. Lucas, C. Men, and O. Vun. 2013. "Yes, They Can: Peer Educators for Diabetes in Cambodia." In *Transforming Health Markets in Asia and Africa: Improving Quality and Access for the Poor*, edited by G. Bloom, B. Kanjilal, H. Lucas, and D. H. Peters, 115–29. New York: Routledge.

Von Korff, M., J. Gruman, J. Schaefer, S. J. Curry, and E. H. Wagner. 1997. "Collaborative Management of Chronic Illness." *Annals of Internal Medicine* 127 (12): 1097–102.

WHO (World Health Organization). 2002. *Innovative Care for Chronic Conditions: Building Blocks for Action Global Report*. Geneva: WHO. http://www.improvingchroniccare.org/downloads/who_innovative_care_for_chronic_conditions.pdf.

———. 2006. *World Health Report 2006: Working Together for Health*. Geneva: WHO.

———. 2008a. *The Global Burden of Diseases, 2004 Update*. Geneva: WHO.

———. 2008b. *Task Shifting: Rational Redistribution of Tasks among Health Workforce Teams; Global Recommendations and Guidelines*. Geneva: WHO.

WHO Working Group on Therapeutic Education. 1998. *Therapeutic Patient Education: Continuing Education Programmes for Health Care Providers in the Field of Prevention of Chronic Diseases*. Copenhagen: WHO.

WMA (World Medical Association). 2009. *WMA Resolution on Task Shifting from the Medical Profession*. New Delhi: WMA.

Zachariah, R., N. Ford, M. Philips, S. Lynch, M. Massaquoi, and others. 2009. "Task Shifting in HIV/AIDS: Opportunities, Challenges, and Proposed Actions for Sub-Saharan Africa." *Transactions of the Royal Society of Tropical Medicine and Hygiene* 103 (6): 549–58.

Chapter 18

Quality Improvement in Cardiovascular Disease Care

Edward S. Lee, Rajesh Vedanthan, Panniyammakal Jeemon,
Jemima H. Kamano, Preeti Kudesia, Vikram Rajan,
Michael Engelgau, and Andrew E. Moran

INTRODUCTION

This chapter reviews the diagnosis and treatment of cardiovascular disease in low- and middle-income countries (LMICs) with a view to improving the quality of care. In keeping with the Institute of Medicine's definition of quality as the "degree to which health services for individuals and population increase the likelihood of desired health outcomes and are consistent with current professional knowledge" (Lohr 1990, 4), the focus is on studies of specific interventions and measurable health outcomes. Because the resources available to support health care delivery in LMICs are scarce, this chapter seeks to improve clinical quality by getting the most out of known effective interventions within the limits of available resources rather than recommending unproven interventions that require early-phase studies or substantial investment to scale up. Clinical quality can be improved anywhere and at any time and doing so need not be expensive.

Quality standards and measures contain principles that can be compared and shared across countries and local settings. However, quality care delivery in low-resource settings does not necessarily mean dissemination and implementation of a universal set of standards—especially those formulated for cardiovascular diseases in

high-income countries (HICs). Standards and interventions should be dictated by context and community capacity. Adaptation to the local setting is necessary for achieving optimal clinical outcomes and patient satisfaction.

A conceptual framework guided this chapter. The authors specified four domains, cutting across two distinct phases of cardiovascular disease (acute versus chronic) and two levels of intervention (health system versus patient-provider) (table 18.1). Health system–level interventions include those directly targeting one or more of the six "building blocks of a health system" as defined by the World Health Organization (2007). Patient-provider-level interventions are focused on influencing patient or provider behavior. Acute phases of cardiovascular disorders, such as acute myocardial infarction, stroke, and limb ischemia, occur unpredictably. Good outcomes demand timely clinical responses, which require adequate and accessible facilities, functional transportation networks, providers prepared to treat cases that present at all hours, and patient awareness of when and how to seek medical attention. In contrast, chronic phases of cardiovascular disorders, such as diabetes mellitus, hypertension, and congestive heart failure, require screening for preclinical risk factors, systematic monitoring for complications, and substantial

Corresponding author: Andrew E. Moran, Division of General Medicine, Columbia University Medical Center, New York, New York, United States; aem35@cumc.columbia.edu.

Table 18.1 Conceptual Framework for Quality of Care for Cardiovascular Diseases

Level	Acute phase	Chronic phase
Health system	• Strategically locate hospitals to reduce treatment delays. • Improve provider skills to deliver high-quality care; provide salary support for health care providers. • Improve access to revascularization services. • Improve transportation to hospital. • Improve population awareness of acute symptoms and means to access acute care. • Formulate and disseminate clinical practice guidelines and standards.	• Formulate and disseminate clinical practice guidelines and standards. • Improve access to health care and medicines. • Train health care providers. • Provide financial support for quality improvement. • Improve infrastructure, including health care facilities and electronic and telephonic communication.
Patient-provider	• Implement clinical practice guidelines using clinical pathway algorithms. • Improve hospital discharge planning and transition to chronic care.	• Educate providers and patients. • Implement clinical practice guidelines. • Improve risk factor monitoring. • Improve treatment adherence.

patient self-care and engagement to initiate and maintain treatment adherence. Good-quality, chronic-phase care may prevent or delay onset of acute-phase manifestations, thereby preventing or delaying disability or death.

Quality interventions are examined at the health care system and patient-provider levels. The authors populated the four domains of this two-by-two framework with potential quality improvement levers based on previous knowledge of the field and examples gleaned from other chapters in this volume. Once the framework was established, a systematic literature review was conducted to identify evidence supporting specific interventions within it. The results are accompanied by detailed narratives of clinical quality improvement efforts for cardiovascular diseases, including the story of a comprehensive community-based cardiovascular disease primary prevention program in Kenya, the experience of an acute coronary syndrome (ACS) clinical pathways intervention in China, and a spotlight on mobile health (m-health) applications around the world.

METHODOLOGY

The methodology for the systematic review, including the electronic search terms used, is detailed in annex 18A. In brief, an electronic search was conducted of the MEDLINE and EMBASE databases to capture published reports of English-language studies on cardiovascular disease care quality improvement studies carried out in LMICs from January 2000 to June 2014. The review identified 49 full text papers that reported on completed, population-based studies with clinically meaningful outcomes. These studies were selected for the review and

assigned to one or more categories in the chapter framework. The chapter highlights 32 of these studies.

SYSTEM-LEVEL INTERVENTIONS

Acute Phase

Timely intervention can dramatically improve the outcomes of acute cardiovascular disease, while delays may result in unnecessary death or disability. System-level factors affect the time to treatment in both the prehospital and hospital phases of an acute event. Before arriving at a hospital, patients educated about the cardinal symptoms of cardiac disease will seek care more quickly and be aware of nearby hospitals or ambulance transport to regional centers. Hours of service availability are critically important. For example, if a patient with an acute cardiovascular event arrives in the middle of the night at a hospital with revascularization services, staff must be available to provide those services. Lack of awareness, lack of acceptability, lack of affordability, and lack of availability are all common barriers that can delay treatment of acute events (see chapter 16 on surgery volume quality in volume 1, Weiser and Gawande 2015).

System-wide planning can overcome barriers to timely and appropriate care for acute cardiovascular disease. The systematic review found limited evidence of interventions to improve system-level, acute-phase care (table 18.2). Poor underlying infrastructure in low-resource settings perhaps presents daunting challenges to reorganizing complex health care delivery systems (Macharia and others 2009). Just as likely, government, nongovernmental, and private sector organizations often introduce system improvements without rigorous systematic study; therefore, the health

Table 18.2 Selected Studies on System-Level, Acute-Phase Quality Improvement Interventions

Quality improvement intervention	Study	Country	Study design	Sample	Observation interval	Quality measures	Results
National health care reform	Nazzal and others 2008	Chile	Retrospective, multicenter	STEMI patients from 10 hospitals that perform thrombolysis as main perfusion therapy	Not reported	Global in-hospital mortality; evidence-based prescribing for patients treated with thrombolysis	10 percentage point absolute increase in use of thrombolysis (50.0% vs. 60.5%); 3.8 percentage point absolute reduction in in-hospital mortality of patients treated with thrombolysis (10.6% vs. 6.8%); 3.4 percentage point absolute reduction in global in-hospital mortality (12.0% vs. 8.6%); adjusted odds ratio for in-hospital mortality, 0.64
Organization of hospitals in hub-and-spoke model	Alexander and others 2013	India	Prospective, multicenter, community-based study	Plan to enroll 1,500 consecutive STEMI patients at participating institutions	Patients to be enrolled over 9 months and followed for 1 year	Before-and-after study of the use of reperfusion therapy, time to reperfusion	Not yet available
Community education program regarding ACS symptoms and treatments	Prabhakaran and others 2008	India	Prospective, nonrandomized study	1,033 ACS patients in 34 hospitals; mean age, 58; males, 71%–78% of total	Follow-up: inpatient hospitalization	No specific outcomes related to community education program	No specific outcomes related to community education program

Note: ACS = acute coronary syndrome; STEMI = ST-elevation myocardial infarction.

effects of system-level changes may go unmeasured or unreported. Randomized comparison studies in low- and middle-income settings may not be conducted because of lack of research capacity, perception of causing unwanted delay in care delivery, "contamination" between intervention and control sites, and ethical concerns.

Alexander and others (2013) reported on a project being launched in the rural region within Tamil Nadu, India, which plans to implement a hub-and-spoke model using existing health care resources to improve the acute ST-elevation myocardial infarction (STEMI) care delivery system. Hub hospitals are capable of delivering timely percutaneous catheter-based reperfusion therapy, while spoke hospitals are primary health care facilities with or without capacity to deliver thrombolytic reperfusion therapy. Hubs and spokes are linked by privately owned professional ambulance services. After an observation phase, the hub-and-spoke program will be implemented, and primary outcomes are expected to change in response to rates of reperfusion therapy and time to coronary reperfusion.

Community-based education initiatives can prime the public by increasing awareness of clinical signs of ACS, stroke, and heart failure and enhance acceptability of acute care solutions in the community. The Kerala Acute Coronary Syndrome Program included community-based health education programs that promoted self-detection of acute coronary disease symptoms, rapid self-referral for treatment, and timely self-administration of aspirin (Prabhakaran and others 2008). The investigators concluded that improved patient awareness contributed to reductions in time-to-thrombolysis achieved by the multicomponent intervention.

No studies were found on the impact of improved geographic and temporal coverage of acute care services, including the impact of building more hospitals within underserved areas or making revascularization more widely available.

Chronic Phase

Most studies in the system-level, chronic-phase category examined the expansion of health insurance coverage (table 18.3). Two studies evaluated the health impact of the Seguro Popular insurance that was rolled out in

Table 18.3 Selected Studies on System-Level, Chronic-Phase Quality Improvement Interventions

Quality improvement intervention	Study	Country	Study design	Sample	Observation interval	Quality measures	Results
Enrollment in Seguro Popular	Bleich and others 2007	Mexico	Cross-sectional, 2005 Mexican national survey	Adults with hypertension; 1,065 uninsured matched with 1,065 insured	Not reported	Self-reported hypertension treatment and control	Adults enrolled in Seguro Popular had higher rates of hypertension treatment (odds ratio 1.5) and controlled blood pressure (odds ratio 1.49)
Enrollment in Seguro Popular	Sosa-Rubi, Galarraga, and Lopez-Ridaura 2009	Mexico	Cross-sectional, 2005–06 Mexican national survey	Adults with diabetes; 425 insured matched with 1,029 uninsured	Not reported	Process outcomes and biological outcomes (hemoglobin A1c)	Adults enrolled in Seguro Popular more likely to have appropriate glucose control (average treatment effect 0.056)
Community-based health insurance	Hendriks and others 2014	Rural Nigeria	Prospective, nonrandom, nonblind; one geographic area with intervention, one control area	Adults with hypertension	Intervention and follow-up for one year	Blood pressure, measured by trained interviewers	Systolic blood pressure decreased by 10.4 mmHg vs. 5.2 mmHg and diastolic blood pressure decreased by 4.3 mmHg vs. 2.2 mmHg in intervention group
Medication subsidy program providing full coverage of antihypertension medications	Yu, Zhang, and Wang 2013	Rural China	Prospective cohort study with propensity-score-matched controls	Low-income, hypertensive adults taking more than one antihypertensive medication (93% taking more than three)	Intervention and follow-up for 18 months	Blood pressure, medication adherence, and health care costs	Intervention arm had a 9 percentage point absolute increase in medication adherence (75% vs. 66%) and lower annual out-of-pocket medical costs overall

Note: mmHg = millimeter of mercury, a measure of pressure.

2002 as part of Mexico's national universal health insurance plan. Seguro Popular covered approximately 50 million low-income people who had no formal health insurance—often because working family members participated in the informal economy. Based on data gathered in Mexican national health and nutrition surveys, Bleich and others (2007) found that, compared with matched hypertensive adults without insurance, Seguro Popular enrollees had 1.5-fold higher odds of receiving hypertension treatment and 1.4-fold higher odds of having controlled blood pressure. A similar study of low-income diabetic patients found those with Seguro Popular insurance were more likely to receive regular blood glucose control monitoring and maintain adequate glucose control compared with their matched, uninsured counterparts (Sosa-Rubi, Galarraga, and Lopez-Ridaura 2009). In rural Nigeria, hypertensive patients living in a district where community-based health insurance was available had significantly lower systolic and diastolic blood pressures, changes not observed in the control group without insurance (Hendriks and others 2014). In rural China, hypertensive patients receiving subsidies to defer medication costs had a 9 percent absolute increase in medication adherence and significantly lower annual out-of-pocket medical costs (Yu, Zhang, and Wang 2013).

System-level quality improvement efforts can lead to measurable improvements in health status in patients with chronic cardiovascular disease. These studies also demonstrate that the health impact of system-level changes can be rigorously evaluated. Researchers can simulate randomization through natural experiments, propensity score matching, or comparison of geographic areas or facilities with and without the intervention. Stepped-wedge trials introduce interventions to couple stepwise active and systematic program implementation with evaluation (Hemming and others 2015). As in the Seguro Popular studies, repeated population-based surveys can be leveraged to measure changes in chronic cardiometabolic disease risk factors and outcomes.

Quality improvement studies will be most feasible where key outcomes are part of, or added to, ongoing surveys.

Many cardiovascular disease patients remain untreated or incompletely treated with standard oral medications for secondary prevention (Yusuf and others 2011). System-level policies to improve the availability and reduce the costs of essential preventive medicines have the potential to extend effective prevention to many more of these patients. No studies were found on the impact of essential medicines designations or pharmaceutical market regulations on the quality of clinical care for

cardiovascular diseases (see chapter 8 in this volume, Dugani and others 2017).

In Sub-Saharan Africa, the substantial infrastructure investment that turned the tide of the human immuno-deficiency virus/acquired immune deficiency syndrome (HIV/AIDS) epidemic is now being leveraged for chronic noncommunicable disease management. Groups like the Kenya-based Academic Model Providing Access to Healthcare (AMPATH) have leveraged the infrastructure established for chronic care to improve hypertension control in the communities they serve (box 18.1).

Box 18.1

Systems and Individuals: The AMPATH Chronic Disease Management Experience in Kenya

In Sub-Saharan Africa, cardiovascular disease (CVD) is the leading cause of death among individuals older than age 30 years (Gaziano and others 2006). In Kenya, atherosclerotic CVD, particularly stroke (Etyang and others 2014), and CVD risk factors, particularly hypertension (Kayima and others 2013), are increasing. To address the rise in noncommunicable diseases, Kenya formed the Division of Noncommunicable Diseases in the Directorate of Preventive and Promotive Health Services within the Ministry of Health. This division has developed a strategic plan for noncommunicable diseases, including hypertension; designated clear targets; and recommended evidence-based interventions.

However, widespread implementation of programs is still lacking. The infrastructure for hypertension management is challenging. Human resources for health are insufficient (WHO 2013), and physicians have traditionally managed hypertension. Stockouts of even the essential medicines on the national formulary are frequent (Manji and others 2012). The availability of hypertension medicines is even less reliable, especially in rural areas. In addition, there is a profound lack of facilities, supplies, and equipment, including sphygmomanometers.

The Academic Model Providing Access to Healthcare (AMPATH)—a collaboration between the Moi University College of Health Sciences, the Moi Teaching and Referral Hospital, and a consortium of North American universities led by Indiana

University—has sought to address both system-level and individual-level factors in an attempt to improve access to high-quality, comprehensive, coordinated, and sustainable care for CVD risk factors such as hypertension and diabetes. AMPATH has established a human immunodeficiency virus/acquired immune deficiency syndrome (HIV/AIDS) care system in western Kenya that has served more than 160,000 patients (AMPATH 2015; Einterz and others 2007). It has also developed a comprehensive chronic disease management program, focusing initially on hypertension and diabetes (Bloomfield and others 2011). The program has several goals:

- Achieve population-wide screening for hypertension and diabetes
- Engage community resources and governance structures
- Achieve geographic decentralization of care services
- Redistribute tasks
- Ensure a consistent supply of essential medicines
- Improve the physical infrastructure of rural health facilities
- Develop an integrated health record to be used at all levels of the health system
- Use mobile health initiatives strategically.

Bringing together all of these components, AMPATH has created an integrated system of chronic disease treatment and prevention services. Nurses in rural dispensaries have received

box continues next page

specialized training and simple clinical algorithms to manage uncomplicated cases of hypertension and diabetes. Community health workers have received structured training to provide health education, link patients to hypertension and diabetes care, and improve retention. Rural clinicians and community health workers are using handheld devices, equipped with clinical decision support and record-keeping functions, to improve the quality of care and the efficiency of follow-up. Novel community-based,

revolving-fund pharmacies (Manji and others 2012) and provider supply networks have been developed to increase the availability of chronic disease medications. The program has also launched a community-based outpatient health insurance program to improve affordability. Finally, implementation research is being conducted to determine which components are or are not working and why to generate lessons for the program and for programs in other low-resource settings worldwide.

PATIENT-PROVIDER-LEVEL INTERVENTIONS

Acute Phase

ACS and acute stroke care have a remarkably strong evidence base, supported by randomized controlled trials of life-saving medications and reperfusion procedures (table 18.4). Professional societies have endorsed clinical practice guidelines that propose to set international quality standards for acute care. However, these quality standards are incompletely implemented even in high-income settings (Aliprandi-Costa and others 2011; Berwanger and others 2012; Cabana and others 1999; Du and others 2014; Fox and others 2002; Hoekstra and others 2002; Pearson, Goulart-Fisher, and Lee 1995). For years, the case for initiatives to improve the quality of ACS care was based on observations of quality gaps in registry studies; only recently has evidence emerged from randomized controlled trials (Flather and others 2011; Tu and others 2009).

Modeling studies have projected that treating ACS patients according to the recommendations of clinical guidelines is cost-effective in LMICs (Megiddo and others 2014; Wang and others 2014; see chapter 8 in this volume [Dugani and others 2017]). However, the gap between current and optimal ACS care appears to be even wider in LMIC hospitals than in HIC hospitals (Berwanger and others 2012; Du and others 2014; Wang and others 2012; Wang and others 2014; Xavier and others 2008). The Kerala Acute Care Syndrome Registry, which studied 25,748 consecutive ACS admissions in hospitals in Kerala, India, over two years, found that 41 percent of STEMI patients reached the health care facility six hours or more after symptom onset (Mohanan and others 2013). Only 41 percent and 13 percent of STEMI patients received reperfusion therapy using thrombolytics or percutaneous

coronary interventions, respectively. The study also demonstrated that optimal in-hospital and discharge medical care were delivered in only 40 percent and 46 percent of admissions, respectively, with rural hospitals performing worse than urban ones (Huffman and others 2013). Patients receiving optimal in-hospital medical therapy reported a 21 percent lower rate of major adverse in-hospital cardiovascular events.

Adopting HIC guidelines for LMICs offers a great opportunity both for implementing quality improvement standards and for benchmarking significant improvements in practice and outcomes. The ACS quality improvement studies identified in the review showed some improvements in measures of clinical process, but, like studies in HICs, only equivocal clinical improvements were found.

Berwanger and others (2012) randomized large urban hospitals in Brazil into those offering a multifaceted quality improvement program with educational material, reminders, algorithms, and training visits and those offering usual care. The intervention group had 2.64 higher odds of receiving evidence-based ACS therapy within the first 24 hours following symptom onset. There were no changes, however, in 30-day mortality or in-hospital cardiovascular events. Du and others (2014) randomized large urban Chinese hospitals to implement a U.S.-guidelines-based ACS pathway, along with periodic clinical performance audits and feedback throughout the intervention period (figure 18.1). Hospitals in the intervention arm showed higher rates of discharge for recommended therapies, but no difference in other indicators, including reperfusion in STEMI cases within 12 hours of symptom onset, door-to-needle time, door-to-balloon time, or high-risk patients undergoing angiography. As in Berwanger and others (2012), there were

Table 18.4 Selected Studies of Patient-Provider-Level, Acute-Phase Quality Improvement Interventions

Quality improvement intervention	Study	Country	Study design	Sample	Observation interval	Quality measures	Results
ACS							
Multifaceted quality improvement intervention with educational materials, reminders, algorithms, and training visits	Berwanger and others 2012	Brazil	Prospective, cluster randomized controlled, multicenter study; 17 hospitals randomized to intervention and 17 to routine practice	1,150 ACS patients in 34 public hospitals; mean age, 62	Follow-up of 30 days	Evidence-based therapy (aspirin, clopidogrel, anticoagulants, and statins) for ACS within first 24 hours	Intervention group more likely to receive all eligible acute and discharge medications and higher adherence; no change in 30-day all-cause mortality or in-hospital cardiovascular events
Clinical pathways approved by the American College of Cardiology and American Heart Association	Du and others 2014	China	Prospective, cluster randomized controlled, multicenter study; regional and tertiary urban hospitals with more than 100 ACS patients annually; 32 hospitals in early intervention and 38 hospitals in late intervention	3,500 ACS patients; mean age, 64; males, 67%–72% of total	Follow-up: inpatient hospitalization	Primary outcomes were correct final diagnosis, thrombolysis or angioplasty within 12 hours, door-to-needle time, door-to-balloon time, high-risk patients undergoing angiography, low-risk patients undergoing functional testing, discharge on correct medications, and length of hospital stay	11.6 percentage point absolute increase in discharge rates on recommended therapies (relative risk 1.23); no difference in other primary outcomes, death, or major cardiovascular events
Education program for physicians and community members in detection and optimal management of ACS	Prabhakaran and others 2008	India	Prospective, nonrandomized study; 34 hospitals treating ACS patients in Kerala region	1,033 ACS patients; mean age 58; males, 71%–78% of total	Follow-up: inpatient hospitalization	Use of aspirin, heparin, beta blockers, lipid-lowering agents, calcium channel blockers; time to thrombolysis	Absolute decreases of 43 minutes in symptom-to-door time, 11 minutes in door-to-thrombolysis, and 55 minutes in time-to-thrombolysis; significant increase in use of aspirin, heparin, beta blockers, lipid-lowering agents; reduction in use of calcium channel blockers
Stroke							
Guideline-based structured case program for secondary stroke prevention	Peng and others 2014	China	Prospective, cluster randomized controlled, multicenter study; large regional or tertiary hospitals; 23 hospitals in intervention and 24 in control	1,287 inpatient stroke patients; mean age, 60–61; males, 67%–69% of total	Follow-up of one year	Medication adherence to secondary prevention	Higher adherence to statins (56% vs. 33%); no difference in antiplatelet, antihypertensive, or diabetes mellitus drugs; no difference in composite endpoint (new stroke, ACS, and all-cause death)

Note: ACS = acute coronary syndrome.

Figure 18.1 Clinical Pathways for Acute Coronary Syndrome in Hospitals with and without Catheterization Facilities in the Phase 2 CPACS-2

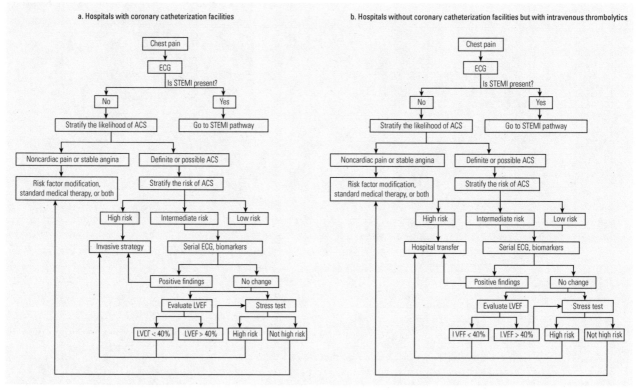

Source: Du and others 2014 (Supplementary Material).
Note: CPACS = Clinical Pathways for Acute Coronary Syndromes; ECG = electrocardiogram; ACS = acute coronary syndrome; STEMI = ST-elevation myocardial infarction; LVEF = left ventricular ejection fraction.

no significant differences in mortality or cardiovascular events. Prabhakaran and others (2008) enrolled 34 hospitals in the Kerala region of India to serve as their own controls in a pre- and postintervention design. After the multifaceted quality improvement intervention, there was a significant median reduction in time-to-thrombolysis of 54 minutes—from 193 to 139 minutes—and a significant increase in the use of evidence-based medications.

In sum, selected studies of quality improvement programs for ACS and stroke care found improvements in some measures of clinical process, but not in clinical outcomes—similar to the pattern commonly found in programs in HICs. Even regarding surrogate measures of process, quality improvement studies yielded variable results. It may be that success depends on the support of health care providers and administrators and tailoring to the specific context of the participating health care system (that is, the availability of treatments and financial protection for patients). Lessons learned from these

programs may be helpful for the design of future patient-provider-level studies on cardiovascular disease (box 18.2). Despite their limitations, these ambitious studies demonstrated that complex quality improvement programs can be implemented in the hospital setting in middle-income countries. No studies were found measuring the impact of physician education on diagnostic accuracy or clinical decision making related to acute cardiovascular disorders.

Chronic Phase

Adherence to life-saving medications and lifestyle changes is suboptimal worldwide, regardless of country income level (Yusuf and others 2011). Since the overwhelming majority of chronic-phase cardiovascular disease patients live in LMICs, where health care resources are limited, optimizing low-cost primary and secondary prevention interventions is critical. Numerous studies have been conducted on a variety of

Acute Care Quality Improvement in Middle-Income Countries: Lessons from the CPACS Study in China

Three acute coronary syndrome (ACS) clinical quality improvement programs were identified, including the second phase of the Clinical Pathways for Acute Coronary Syndromes (CPACS) study conducted in China (Berwanger and other 2012; Du and others 2014; Prabhakaran and others 2008). Following the intervention, CPACS collected data from structured health care provider surveys in all 75 hospitals participating in the initiative and from in-depth semistructured interviews with study coordinators and leaders in 10 of the hospitals. These data were analyzed using quantitative and qualitative methods. The analysis found that provider-level, system-level, and patient-level factors—government and administrative support, hospital resources, and patient health insurance coverage and lack of financial protection—all limited the intervention's impact. Several lessons emerged from the CPACS experience.

Engaging health care providers and hospital administrators. Not all diagnostic and clinical practice guidelines formulated in high-income countries will apply to the local context in low- and middle-income countries. CPACS engaged providers in study hospitals early in the process of planning to involve them as stakeholders and incorporate their recommendations. More than 80 percent of providers attended program training sessions and reported using the ACS pathways in clinical practice, and providers had a generally positive view of the program's objectives. In China, hospital administrators and local governments are powerful arbiters of hospital priorities. Failure to gain support from these high-level officials limited successful implementation of the clinical pathways in some hospitals. For example, hospitals with less administrative buy-in assigned responsibility for collecting and analyzing CPACS data and for following up with patients to students and junior physicians without scaling back their regular academic and administrative obligations.

Overcoming patient-level obstacles. Community education about the signs, symptoms, and treatment of acute cardiovascular disease may be difficult to carry out in large-scale, multisite, hospital-based studies. CPACS found that patient factors limited the effectiveness of the intervention. Patients' insurance circumscribed the treatments reimbursed, and many patients were underinsured or uninsured and found it difficult or impossible to pay out of pocket for treatments considered part of the quality care program. Limited knowledge of coronary heart disease negatively affected patients' participation in discussions regarding informed consent and limited their willingness to pursue long-term secondary prevention after being discharged from the hospital.

interventions to improve the quality of chronic-phase cardiovascular diseases in LMICs (table 18.5). Because patients are ideally prescribed several standard daily oral medications for primary or secondary prevention of cardiovascular disease, achievement of medication adherence, sometimes lifelong, is a key challenge for quality health care worldwide (figure 18.2). Most of the interventions reviewed were related to chronic medication adherence, specifically the use of fixed-dose combination pills, health care delivery supported by mobile communication technology, and task-shifting.

Combination Pills

Many patients with cardiovascular disease are prescribed multiple daily medications. As the number of medications increases, the probability that patients will take all of the prescribed pills declines. For this reason, combining multiple medications into a single pill can improve adherence. Combined low doses of multiple medications in place of higher doses of a single medication also should lower the frequency of side effects.

Thom and others (2013) randomized persons at high risk of cardiovascular disease (CVD) living in India (one of four countries studied) to receive combination pills or the usual multiple-pill therapy. After a mean follow-up of about 15 months, participants taking the combination pills had 25 percent higher absolute adherence and small but significant reductions in both systolic blood pressure and low-density lipoprotein compared with participants randomized to receive

Table 18.5 Selected Studies of Chronic-Phase, Patient-Provider-Level Interventions

Quality improvement intervention	Study	Country or region	Disease	Study design	Sample	Observation interval	Quality measures	Results
Combination pills								
Fixed-dose combination medications	Thom and others 2013	India	CVD, secondary prevention	Prospective, randomized, open-label, multicenter, multinational, blind endpoint trial; 501 patients in intervention, 499 in usual care	Participants with CVD or five-year CVD risk of at least 15%; in all population, mean age, 62 years; males, about 80% of total	Median intervention and follow-up of 15 months	Self-reported adherence to all of aspirin, statin, and two or more medications	25% absolute higher adherence to all four medications (ratio of 1.4); small but statistically significant decreases in systolic blood pressure (−2.6 mmHg) and LDL (6.7 mg/dL)
CVD prevention protocol, including low-dose combination pill with lifestyle modification	Zou and others 2014	Rural China	CVD, secondary prevention	Prospective, nonrandomized, single-center study; pilot before RCT; 153 patients in intervention, no control	Subjects ages 40–74 years with a calculated 10-year CVD risk of 20% or more; mean age 71 years; males, 71% of total	Intervention and follow-up for 3 months	Blood pressure, percent taking CVD medications, self-reported adherence to smoking cessation and salt intake, appointment rates	Significantly higher rates of subjects taking CVD preventive drugs (73% vs. 84%) and reduction in smoking rates (38% vs. 35%); no changes in salt intake or measured blood pressure
Low-dose combination pill, "polycap"	Yusuf and others 2009	India	CVD	Prospective, double-blind, multicenter trial; 2,053 individuals randomized to eight groups; 412 in intervention, about 200 in each of eight groups	Subjects ages 45–80 years without previous CVD but one risk factor	Intervention for 12 weeks; follow-up for 4 weeks post-intervention	Blood pressure, LDL, heart rate, urinary 11-dehydrothromboxane B2	Significant reductions in systolic and diastolic blood pressure (by 7.4 and 5.6 mmHg, respectively) compared with groups not receiving antihypertensives; significant reduction in LDL (by 0.7 millimole per liter) compared with groups not taking simvastatin
Full-dose pills with potassium vs. low-dose combination pills	Yusuf and others 2012	India	CVD	Prospective, randomized, multicenter trial; 257 patients in full-dose group, 261 in low-dose group	Subjects older than age 40 years with blood pressure higher than 130/90 on two consecutive occasions or on antihypertensive medications and with cardiovascular disease or high-risk diabetes	Intervention for 8 weeks; follow-up for 4 weeks postintervention	Blood pressure, heart rate, serum lipids, serum and urinary potassium, and tolerability	Significant reductions in systolic and diastolic blood pressure (by 2.8 mmHg and 1.7 mmHg, respectively); significant reductions in both total cholesterol and LDL; similar rates of discontinuation

table continues next page

Table 18.5 Selected Studies of Chronic-Phase, Patient-Provider-Level Interventions (continued)

Quality improvement intervention	Study	Country or region	Disease	Study design	Sample	Observation interval	Quality measures	Results
Mobile health								
Mobile phone messaging intervention	Ramachandran and others 2013	India	Diabetes	Prospective, multicenter, RCT; 271 subjects in intervention, 266 in control	Men with impaired glucose tolerance; mean age 45–46 years	Mean intervention and follow-up for 20.2 months	Progression to diabetes	9 percentage point absolute reduction in progression to diabetes (18% vs. 27%, hazard ratio 0.64); improved dietary adherence (hazard ratio 0.48)
SMS message about diet, exercise, medication	Goodarzi and others 2012	Iran, Islamic Rep.	Diabetes	Prospective, RCT; 43 subjects in intervention, 38 in control	Subjects with type 2 diabetes; mean age, 51–56 years; males, 21%–24% of total	Intervention and follow-up for 3 months	Laboratory results and questionnaire	0.9 percentage point absolute decrease in hemoglobin A1c; significant decreases in total cholesterol and microalbumin; significant improvement in knowledge, attitude, practice, and self-efficacy
SMS regarding medications and healthy lifestyle changes	Shetty and others 2011	India	Diabetes	Prospective, RCT; 110 subjects in intervention, 105 in control	Subjects with diabetes; mean age, 50 years	Intervention and follow-up for 1 year	Hemoglobin A1c, fasting plasma glucose, lipids	Significant improvement in fasting plasma glucose (185 vs. 166); no significant difference in hemoglobin A1c
Automated phone calls and home blood pressure monitors; e-mail alerts to providers	Piette and others 2012	Honduras; Mexico	Hypertension	Prospective, RCT; primary care clinics; 99 subjects in intervention, 101 in control	Subjects with uncontrolled hypertension; mean age, 58 years; males, 33% of total	Intervention and follow-up for 6 weeks	Blood pressure	No significant effect on systolic blood pressure, but in subgroup analysis, reduction in systolic blood pressure (by 8.8 mmHg) in low-literacy group
Education, counseling, and medical adjustment by nurses via phone calls	Ferrante and others 2010; GESICA Investigators 2005	Argentina	Congestive heart failure	Prospective, multicenter, RCT; 760 patients in intervention, 758 in usual care	Outpatients with stable chronic heart failure; mean age, 65 years; males, 71% of total	Intervention for 1 year; follow-up for 4 years	All-cause mortality and heart failure hospitalization	2 percentage point absolute reduction in composite outcome of mortality or heart failure hospitalization at 3 years (relative risk 0.88); mostly driven by 7 percentage point absolute reduction in heart failure hospitalization at 3 years (relative risk 0.72)

table continues next page

Table 18.5 Selected Studies of Chronic-Phase, Patient-Provider-Level Interventions *(continued)*

Quality improvement intervention	Study	Country or region	Disease	Study design	Sample	Observation interval	Quality measures	Results
Automated SMS message reminders	Khonsari and others 2014	Malaysia	CVD, secondary prevention	Prospective, open-label, single-center, RCT; ACS patients at tertiary teaching hospital; 31 patients in intervention, 31 in control	Participants admitted for ACS; mean age, 58 years; males, 86% of total	Intervention and follow-up for 2 months	Adherence to cardiac medications	Higher medication adherence rate (64.5% vs. 12.9%); intervention group trended toward lower hospital readmission rates (0 vs. 12.9%)
Telephone-based peer support	Rotheram-Borus and others 2012	South Africa	Diabetes	Prospective, single-center, nonrandomized, clinical trial; 22 subjects in intervention	Subjects with diabetes; mean age, 53; all females	Intervention for 3 months; follow-up at end of study and at 3 months postintervention	Blood glucose, body mass index, coping and social support	No significant improvements in clinical measures; blood glucose and diastolic blood pressure increased; social support and coping abilities increased
Task-shifting								
Counseling by pharmacists, telephone reminders	Ramanath and others 2012	India	Hypertension	Prospective, RCT; 26 subjects in intervention, 26 in control	Subjects with hypertension; males, 62%–81% of total	Intervention and follow-up for 1 month	Blood pressure, self-reported medicine adherence	No significant effect on blood pressure; increased self-reported medication adherence
Nurse-led clinic	Kengne and others 2009	Sub-Saharan Africa	Hypertension	Prospective, nonrandomized, no-control study; 5 urban and rural clinics; 454 subjects	Subjects with hypertension; mean age, 53–58 years; males, 41%–55% of total	Median intervention and follow-up for 6 months	Blood pressure	Decrease in systolic and diastolic blood pressure (by 11.7 mmHg and 7.8 mmHg, respectively)
Pharmacist-led hypertension clinic	Erhun, Agbani, and Bolaji 2005	Nigeria	Hypertension	Prospective, randomized cohort trial; state comprehensive health center; 51 subjects	Subjects with uncontrolled hypertension; mean age, 61; males, 29% of total	Intervention and follow-up for 1 year	Blood pressure	Decrease in mean blood pressure from 168/103 at enrollment to 126/80 at fifth visit; no control group
Home visits	Adeyemo and others 2013	Nigeria	Hypertension	Prospective, RCT; rural and urban populations; 280 subjects in intervention, 264 in control	Subjects with hypertension; mean age, 63 years; males, 51%–53% of total	Intervention and follow-up for 6 months	Medication adherence via pill counting or urine test	No difference in adherence

table continues next page

Table 18.5 Selected Studies of Chronic-Phase, Patient-Provider-Level Interventions (continued)

Quality improvement intervention	Study	Country or region	Disease	Study design	Sample	Observation interval	Quality measures	Results
Family-based home health education for patients and training of general practitioners	Jafar and others 2009	Pakistan	Hypertension	Prospective, cluster RCT; geographic census-based clusters; 629 subjects in intervention, 640 in control	Subjects with hypertension; mean age, 54 years; males, 37% of total	Intervention and follow-up for 2 years	Systolic blood pressure	Decrease in systolic blood pressure (by 10.8 mmHg vs. 5.8 mmHg)
Follow-up by nurses	Nesari and others 2010	Iran, Islamic Rep.	Diabetes	Prospective, RCT	Subjects with diabetes; mean age, 51 years; males, 20% in control and 37% in intervention	Intervention and follow-up for 3 months	Hemoglobin A1c	1.87 percentage point absolute decrease in hemoglobin A1c in intervention group; no change in control group; intervention group also saw significantly higher adherence to diet, exercise, and glucose monitoring
Guideline implementation								
Training general practitioners in hypertension management	Qureshi and others 2007	Pakistan	Hypertension	Prospective, cluster RCT; communities in Karachi; 100 subjects in intervention, 100 in control	Subjects with hypertension; mean age, 55 years; males, 38% of total	Intervention and follow-up for 6 weeks	Medication adherence	16 percentage point absolute increase in patient medication adherence (48.1% vs. 32.4%)
Clinical decision support system	Anchala and others 2015	India	Hypertension	Prospective, cluster RCT; eight primary health clusters in each arm; 845 subjects in intervention, 793 in control	Subjects with hypertension; mean age, 54 years; males, 49%–52% of total	Intervention and follow-up for 12 months	Systolic blood pressure, cost-effectiveness	Absolute decrease in systolic blood pressure (by 6.59 mmHg); cost-effectiveness ratio of US$96.01 per systolic blood pressure reduction in intervention and US$36.57 in control

table continues next page

Table 18.5 Selected Studies of Chronic-Phase, Patient-Provider-Level Interventions (continued)

Quality improvement intervention	Study	Country or region	Disease	Study design	Sample	Observation interval	Quality measures	Results
Education of general practitioners regarding management guidelines including meetings, reminders, medical record summary, and patient result cards	Reutens and others 2012	Asia	Diabetes	Prospective, multinational, cluster RCT; 50 subjects in intervention, 49 in control	Asia-Pacific general practitioners; mean age, 44 years; males, 50%–57% of total	Intervention and follow-up for 12 months	Patient hemoglobin A1c, blood pressure, lipids	No significant difference in hemoglobin A1c or other glycemic indexes
Guidelines for diabetes and hypertension incorporated into each chart for providers	Steyn and others 2013	South Africa	Diabetes	Prospective, multicenter, RCT; public sector community health centers; nine centers in intervention, nine in control	Subjects with diabetes or hypertension; 690 in intervention, 686 in control; mean age 58–61 years; males, 72%–83% of total	Intervention and follow-up for 1 year	Blood pressure, A1c	No effect; fewer than 60% of guideline forms used

Note: ACS = acute coronary syndrome; CVD = cardiovascular disease; LDL = low-density lipoprotein; mg/dL = milligram per deciliter; mmHg = millimeters of mercury, a measure of pressure; RCT = randomized controlled trial; SMS = short message service.

Figure 18.2 Number of Drugs Taken for Coronary Heart Disease and Stroke by Individuals in the PURE Study, by Country Income Level, 2003–09

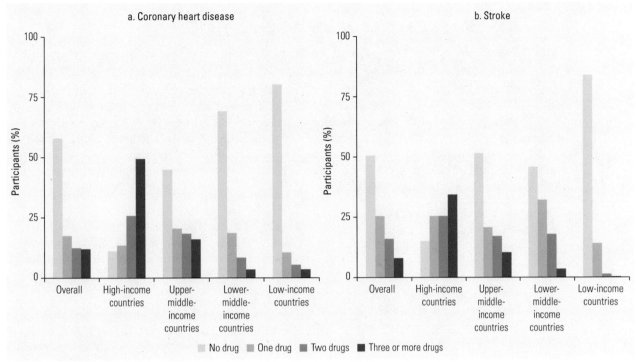

Source: Yusuf and others 2011.
Note: PURE = Prospective Urban Rural Epidemiology.

multiple-pill treatment. Yusuf and others (2009) also found small but significant improvements among Indian subjects at risk for CVD when randomized to receive a combination pill containing multiple blood pressure medications, statins, and aspirin. A follow-up study by Yusuf and others (2012) showed that high-dose combination pills improved blood pressure and lipid control in high-risk Indian subjects compared with low-dose ones with similar rates of tolerability. Zou and others (2014) found that starting high-risk rural Chinese participants on combination pills achieved an 11 percent higher absolute adherence rate.

These trials show that combination pills can improve medication adherence and improve risk factor control in high-risk CVD patients. For this reason, efforts to approve and manufacture combination medications are underway (FDA 2014).

Mobile Communication Technology

Mobile technologies such as cell phones are becoming increasingly available in LMICs and are playing an important role in health promotion (box 18.3). Twelve studies were identified on the role of m-health in the

prevention and treatment of diabetes, hypertension, heart failure, and coronary artery disease. Although not every study demonstrated a significant improvement in clinical care quality, these studies suggest that m-health via text messages and phone calls can be a useful tool for managing chronic cardiovascular conditions in LMICs.

Task-Shifting

Task-shifting refers to the rational redistribution of tasks among health care teams, often from a few highly trained health providers to a larger contingent of providers with less training (see chapter 17 in this volume, Joshi and others 2017; WHO 2008). Six studies were identified evaluating task-shifting for improving patient adherence to prescribed medications. Some studies coupled task-shifting with increased access to affordable or free medications (Erhun, Agbani, and Bolaji 2005; Kengne and others 2009), or family-based home health education and supplemental training of general practitioners (Jafar and others 2009).

Five task-shifting studies targeted hypertensive patients. Kengne and others (2009) carried out a large

Box 18.3

Mobile Health: Harnessing the Communication Revolution in LMICs

Mobile health, also known as *m-health*, uses cell phones and other devices to support public health and clinical care (Kahn, Yang, and Kahn 2010). The number of mobile phone subscriptions reached almost 7 billion by the end of 2014, nearly equaling the number of people in the world, and penetration rates are now 69 percent in Africa, 89 percent in Asia and Pacific, and 90 percent in low- and middle-income countries (LMICs) overall (ITU 2013).

Access to health care providers is a significant challenge in LMICs, especially in rural areas. Kinfu and others (2009) found that it would take 36 years for physicians and 29 years for nurses and midwives to reach the World Health Organization's workforce targets, given current training levels. Voice and short message system (SMS) communication—telemedicine—allows providers to interact with more patients over a wider geographic area, increasing cost efficiency.

Ferrante and others (2010) conducted a multicenter, randomized controlled trial of patients with chronic congestive heart failure in Argentina. Nurses called patients, adjusting their medications depending on their symptoms and providing counseling and education. Patients in the intervention arm had a 20 percent relative risk reduction in all-cause mortality and heart failure hospitalizations at the end of the study (GESICA Investigators 2005). After three years, they continued to have fewer heart failure hospitalizations, higher medication adherence rates, and better quality-of-life scores (Ferrante and others 2010). Similarly, Nesari and others (2010) found that nurse phone calls to Iranian diabetic subjects led to significant improvements in hemoglobin A1c and healthy lifestyle changes.

LMICs often have limited postal and landline capabilities. Landlines require physical wires or fiber optic cable networks, which are prohibitively expensive to build without significant capital investments, and mobile technology allows LMICs to catch up to high-income countries without significant investments.

Affordable and reliable communication channels can be leveraged to better manage chronic conditions. Automated SMS messages led to improved glycemic control in Indians with prediabetes and diabetes (Ramachandran and others 2013; Shetty and others 2011), lower hemoglobin A1c in Iranian diabetics (Goodarzi and others 2012), and higher medication adherence rates in Malaysian ACS patients after hospital discharge (Khonsari and others 2014). All four studies included only participants with access to mobile phones with SMS-receiving capabilities.

Telemonitoring refers to remotely monitoring patients who are at different locations from the health provider. This field has grown dramatically since medical devices, such as blood pressure machines and glucometers, have become more affordable and capable of sending data to health providers over the Internet.

Piette and others (2012) studied the effect of automated phone calls and home blood pressure monitors in Hondurans and Mexicans with uncontrolled hypertension. While persons in the general intervention group did not show any improvement, those with low literacy had significantly lower blood pressure after the intervention. The Minerva Telecardio Project is researching the effect of electrocardiogram machines in remote towns in Brazil. These machines can record and send information to a cardiologist for interpretation. Andrade and others (2011) found that using these machines is more cost-effective than referring patients to another city.

Technological advances are not without inherent risks. Technology has made information vastly more accessible and shareable, but connectivity creates opportunities for abuse. Developed countries, such as the United States, have strict laws regarding health information that are enforced by government institutions and courts. Such legal precedents and infrastructure have not yet been set up in many LMICs.

M-health is not a replacement for patient-provider encounters but a facilitator of existing relationships. LMICs need to continue investing in their networks of medical providers and hospitals for m-health to be effective. Overall, m-health is a promising field of innovation for managing cardiovascular disease and will grow even more rapidly once smartphones with broadband capability become more prevalent in LMICs.

trial of hypertensive participants enrolled in a nurse-led clinic in Cameroon. Erhun, Agbani, and Bolaji (2005) evaluated the role of pharmacist-led clinics for patients with hypertension in Nigeria. Adeyemo and others (2013) randomized Nigerian participants with hypertension to clinic-based care with home visits or to clinic-based care only. Jafar and others (2009) conducted a cluster, randomized controlled trial of two interventions—home health education provided by health aides and training of general practitioners—in a population of Pakistani patients with hypertension. Regardless of the approach, intensified team-based care led to improved hypertension control.

Nesari and others (2010), the single study on diabetes, showed that having nurses call patients regularly to reinforce lifestyle changes and adjust medication doses led to a significant decrease in hemoglobin A1c. The intervention group increased adherence to lifestyle changes and glucose monitoring.

Guideline Implementation or Provider Education

Health care provider education and implementation of guidelines have the potential to standardize, improve, and sustain quality of care for cardiovascular and other conditions in LMICs. Studies of the impact of physician education and guideline dissemination yielded mixed results. Qureshi and others (2007) found that physician education through workshops and guideline dissemination led to significant improvements in patient care. Anchala and others (2015) revealed that providing physicians with a clinical decision support system for undertaking guideline-based hypertension management led to significant reductions in systolic blood pressure. However, Reutens and others (2012) and Steyn and others (2013) showed conflicting results and highlighted that guideline dissemination alone did not lead to actual implementation. Imposing guidelines without first gaining buy-in from providers may be a recipe for failure. Allocating time for education and feedback and strategically inserting guideline information into the flow of clinical practice may increase the chance that guidelines are actually implemented.

CONCLUSIONS

This chapter surveys the evidence on quality improvement in cardiovascular disease care at the system and patient-provider levels. An impressive amount of research on quality improvement has been carried out in LMICs—although not all approaches reviewed were consistently effective (figures 18.3 and 18.4). The innovative approaches taken by these programs demonstrate

that it is not simply a matter of adapting HIC programs to LMICs: innovations to improve the quality of clinical care may originate precisely in low-resource environments. For example, the concept of shifting health care tasks to lay health workers originated in LMICs as a means to address the limited supply of medical doctors. As the AMPATH experience demonstrates (box 18.1), implementing a comprehensive approach to quality improvement, at both the system and patient-provider levels, is feasible in LMICs.

The majority of studies in this review focused on chronic cardiovascular disease and chronic risk factors such as hypertension and diabetes. At the system level, expanded health insurance coverage was found to improve the control of hypertension and diabetes. These powerful findings likely stem from improved access to care and financial protection from out-of-pocket health expenditures. Pharmaceutical supply regulation, drug price regulation, and essential medication designations are all potentially powerful system-level interventions, but their impact on cardiovascular disorders has yet to be studied.

At the patient-provider level, increased intensity of care—however delivered or by whom—was consistently found to improve chronic disease or risk factor outcomes. Intensification involved a team-based approach that included extra health care provider input, such as shifting tasks to pharmacists, dieticians, or nurses; phone counseling; smartphone-based reminders; or home visits. There were no head-to-head comparative effectiveness studies between these approaches, and multiple approaches often were combined (for example, implementing both task-shifting and patient education), so no one approach stands out as better than the others. Care intensification inevitably requires up-front investment, but this investment may be offset by improved downstream health outcomes for cardiovascular disease. A modeling study by Gaziano and others (2014) projected that, despite the added costs of hiring community health workers to manage hypertension in South Africa, increased intensity of care may offset this investment by averting expensive hospital admissions and chronic disease complications.

The studies reviewed for this chapter were often limited in ways that require cautious interpretation of their results. Because of the diversity of interventions and conditions, effect sizes could not be summarized in a meta-analysis. First, it is possible that the studies were published because of their positive results, and, because of the heterogeneity of interventions and targets, it was not possible to evaluate evidence of publication bias. Second, most studies were very short term (less than 12 months), and sustaining intervention effects may be

Figure 18.3 Examples of Acute-Phase Cardiovascular Disease Quality Improvement Interventions Identified in the *DCP3* Systematic Review

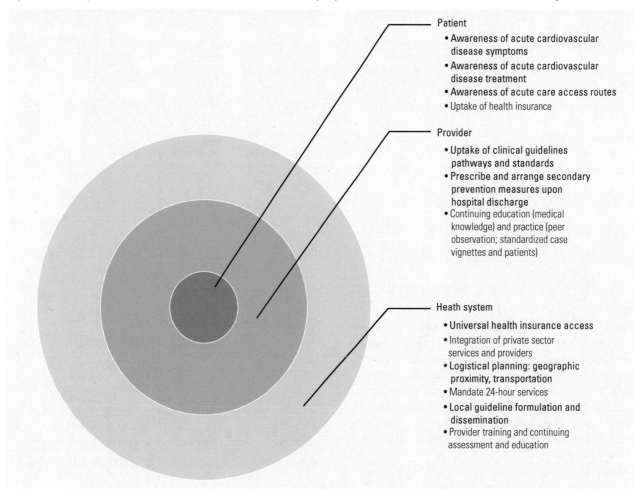

Patient
- Awareness of acute cardiovascular disease symptoms
- Awareness of acute cardiovascular disease treatment
- Awareness of acute care access routes
- Uptake of health insurance

Provider
- Uptake of clinical guidelines pathways and standards
- Prescribe and arrange secondary prevention measures upon hospital discharge
- Continuing education (medical knowledge) and practice (peer observation; standardized case vignettes and patients)

Heath system
- Universal health insurance access
- Integration of private sector services and providers
- Logistical planning: geographic proximity, transportation
- Mandate 24-hour services
- Local guideline formulation and dissemination
- Provider training and continuing assessment and education

Note: DCP3 = Disease Control Priorities (third edition). Types of interventions targeting three levels of acute-phase cardiovascular disease prevention and management. Bulleted items in bold type were supported by evidence from the review. Bulleted items not in bold type indicate that no supporting evidence was found in the review and these interventions are potential areas for further research.

difficult in real clinical settings. As in HICs, most investigators studied clinical process measures and did not report on hard clinical outcomes, which may lead to gaming the system (via an inappropriately strong focus on reaching surrogate targets to the neglect of measures that improve meaningful outcomes) and other unintended consequences when these interventions are introduced into routine practice.

Although all of the studies measured some change in the quality of care, and some reported on the number of provider contacts and specified the technology or medications used, none reported on the costs or cost-effectiveness of these interventions. When resources are limited, the call to improve or restructure existing services may be tempered by the perception that implementation will be costly and not worth the effort—or at least not as attractive as an alternative policy with more immediate returns on investment.

Cost and quality-of-life measurement and cost-effectiveness analyses can be important guides in assessing the net benefits of quality improvement programs in limited-resource contexts. Modeling studies can extend the results of short-term interventions and surrogate clinical measures by simulating a range of likely downstream disease outcomes. At the very least, future studies need to report on intervention inputs as measured by "units"—including the number of providers, contacts between patients and providers, medications, and education classes and teachers—so that clinics and health organizations can "cost out" interventions when seeking the best ones for their settings. Collecting data elements common to implementation research, such as acceptability, sustainability, local context, and affordability, will help ensure that both positive and negative studies will guide implementation and future research.

Figure 18.4 Examples of Chronic-Phase Cardiovascular Disease Quality Improvement Interventions Identified in the *DCP3* Systematic Review

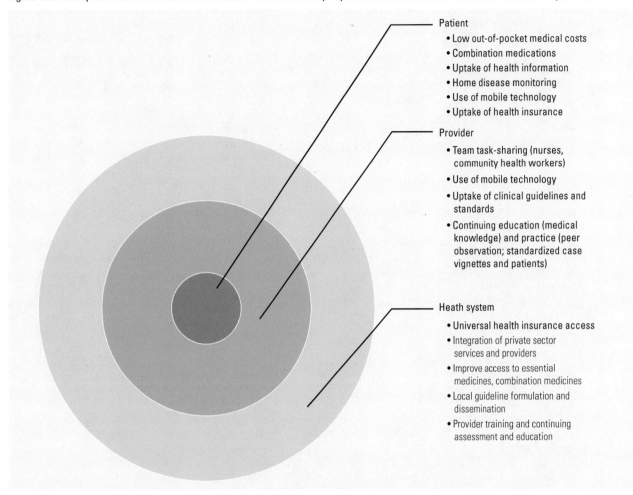

Patient
- Low out-of-pocket medical costs
- Combination medications
- Uptake of health information
- Home disease monitoring
- Use of mobile technology
- Uptake of health insurance

Provider
- Team task-sharing (nurses, community health workers)
- Use of mobile technology
- Uptake of clinical guidelines and standards
- Continuing education (medical knowledge) and practice (peer observation; standardized case vignettes and patients)

Heath system
- Universal health insurance access
- Integration of private sector services and providers
- Improve access to essential medicines, combination medicines
- Local guideline formulation and dissemination
- Provider training and continuing assessment and education

Note: DCP3 = Disease Control Priorities (third edition). Types of interventions targeting three levels of chronic-phase cardiovascular disease prevention and management. Bulleted items in bold are supported by evidence from the review. Bulleted items not in bold type indicate that no supporting evidence was found in the review and these interventions are potential areas for further research.

The majority of cardiovascular disease patients now live in LMICs, and demographic trends virtually guarantee that the number and proportion will grow in coming decades. To ensure that each of these patients receives long-term treatment and control, it is essential to draw on promising research on clinical quality improvement and make the most of the resources directly at hand.

ANNEX

The annex to this chapter is as follows. It is available at http://www.dcp-3.org/CVRD.

- Annex 18A. Systematic Review Methods and Complete Search Results

NOTES

World Bank Income Classifications as of July 2014 are as follows, based on estimates of gross national income (GNI) per capita for 2013:

- Low-income countries (LICs) = US$1,045 or less
- Middle-income countries (MICs) are subdivided:
  (a) lower-middle-income = US$1,046 to US$4,125
  (b) upper-middle-income (UMICs) = US$4,126 to US$12,745
- High-income countries (HICs) = US$12,746 or more.

Funding: AEM was supported by a grant from the U.S. National Heart, Lung, and Blood Institute career development award (K08 HL089675-01). Rajesh Vedanthan was supported by a grant from the Fogarty International Center of the U.S. National Institutes of Health (K01 TW 009218-05).

Panniyammakal Jeemon is supported by a Wellcome Trust, Department of Biotechnology India Alliance clinical and public health intermediate career fellowship.

Disclaimer: None of the authors have conflicts to declare. The views expressed in this article are those of the authors and do not necessarily represent the views of the National Heart, Lung, and Blood Institute; the National Institutes of Health; or the U.S. Department of Health and Human Services. The funders had no role in study design, data collection and analysis, decision to publish, or preparation of the manuscript.

REFERENCES

Adeyemo, A., B. O. Tayo, A. Luke, O. Ogedegbe, R. Durazo-Arvizu, and others. 2013. "The Nigerian Antihypertensive Adherence Trial." *Journal of Hypertension* 31 (1): 201–7.

Alexander, T., S. M. Victor, A. S. Mullasari, G. Veerasekar, K. Subramaniam, and others. 2013. "Protocol for a Prospective, Controlled Study of Assertive and Timely Reperfusion for Patients with ST-Segment Elevation Myocardial Infarction in Tamil Nadu: The TN-STEMI Programme." *BMJ Open* 3 (12): e003850.

Aliprandi-Costa, B., I. Ranasinghe, V. Chow, S. Kapila, C. Juergens, and others. 2011. "Management and Outcomes of Patients with Acute Coronary Syndromes in Australia and New Zealand, 2000–2007." *Medical Journal of Australia* 195 (3): 116–21.

AMPATH (Academic Model Providing Access to Healthcare). 2015. "Our Model." AMPATH. http://www.ampathkenya .org/our-model.

Anchala, R., S. Kaptoge, H. Pant, E. Di Angelantonio, O. H. Franco, and others. 2015. "Evaluation of Effectiveness and Cost-Effectiveness of a Clinical Decision Support System in Managing Hypertension in Resource-Constrained Primary Health Care Settings: Results from a Cluster Randomized Trial." *Journal of the American Heart Association* 4 (1): e001213.

Andrade, M. V., A. C. Maia, C. S. Cardoso, M. B. Alkmim, and A. L. Ribeiro. 2011. "Cost-Benefit of the Telecardiology Service in the State of Minas Gerais: Minas Telecardio Project." *Arquivos Brasileiros de Cardiologia* 97 (4): 307–16.

Berwanger, O., H. P. Guimarães, L. N. Laranjeira, A. B. Cavalcanti, A. A. Kodama, and others. 2012. "Effect of a Multifaceted Intervention on Use of Evidence-Based Therapies in Patients with Acute Coronary Syndromes in Brazil." *Journal of the American Medical Association* 307 (19): 2041–49.

Bleich, S. N., D. M. Cutler, A. S. Adams, R. Lozano, and C. J. Murray. 2007. "Impact of Insurance and Supply of Health Professionals on Coverage of Treatment for Hypertension in Mexico: Population-Based Study." *BMJ* 335 (7625): 875.

Bloomfield, G. S., S. Kimaiyo, E. J. Carter, C. Binanay, G. R. Corey, and others. 2011. "Chronic Noncommunicable Cardiovascular and Pulmonary Disease in Sub-Saharan Africa: An Academic Model for Countering the Epidemic." *American Heart Journal* 161 (5): 842–47.

Cabana, M. D., C. S. Rand, N. R. Powe, A. W. Wu, M. H. Wilson, and others. 1999. "Why Don't Physicians Follow Clinical Practice Guidelines? A Framework for Improvement." *Journal of the American Medical Association* 282 (15): 1458–65.

Du, X., R. Gao, F. Turnbull, Y. Wu, Y. Rong, and others. 2014. "Hospital Quality Improvement Initiative for Patients with Acute Coronary Syndromes in China: A Cluster Randomized, Controlled Trial." *Circulation, Cardiovascular Quality, and Outcomes* 7 (2): 217–26.

Dugani, S. B., A. E. Moran, R. O. Bonow, and T. A. Gaziano. 2017. "Ischemic Heart Disease: Cost-Effective Acute Management and Secondary Prevention." In *Disease Control Priorities* (third edition): Volume 5, *Cardiovascular, Respiratory, and Related Disorders*, edited by D. Prabhakaran, S. Anand, T. A. Gaziano, J.-C. Mbanya, Y. Wu, and R. Nugent. Washington, DC: World Bank.

Einterz, R. M., S. Kimaiyo, H. N. Mengech, B. O. Khwa-Otsyula, F. Esamai, and others. 2007. "Responding to the HIV Pandemic: The Power of an Academic Medical Partnership." *Academic Medicine* 82 (8): 812–18.

Erhun, W. O., E. O. Agbani, and E. E. Bolaji. 2005. "Positive Benefits of a Pharmacist-Managed Hypertension Clinic in Nigeria." *Public Health* 119 (9): 792–98.

Etyang, A. O., K. Munge, E. W. Bunyasi, L. Matata, C. Ndila, and others. 2014. "Burden of Disease in Adults Admitted to Hospital in a Rural Region of Coastal Kenya: An Analysis of Data from Linked Clinical and Demographic Surveillance Systems." *The Lancet Global Health* 2: e216–24.

Ferrante, D., S. Varini, A. Macchia, S. Soifer, R. Badra, and others. 2010. "Long-Term Results after a Telephone Intervention in Chronic Heart Failure: DIAL (Randomized Trial of Phone Intervention in Chronic Heart Failure) Follow-Up." *Journal of the American College of Cardiology* 56 (5): 372–78.

Flather, M. D., D. Babalis, J. Booth, A. Bardaji, J. Machecourt, and others. 2011. "Cluster-Randomized Trial to Evaluate the Effects of a Quality Improvement Program on Management of Non–ST-Elevation Acute Coronary Syndromes: The European Quality Improvement Programme for Acute Coronary Syndromes (EQUIP-ACS)." *American Heart Journal* 162 (4): 700–7.e1.

Fox, K. A., S. G. Goodman, W. Klein, D. Brieger, P. G. Steg, and others. 2002. "Management of Acute Coronary Syndromes: Variations in Practice and Outcome; Findings from the Global Registry of Acute Coronary Events (GRACE)." *European Heart Journal* 23: 1177–89.

Gaziano, T. A., M. Bertram, S. M. Tollman, and K. J. Hofman. 2014. "Hypertension Education and Adherence in South Africa: A Cost-Effectiveness Analysis of Community Health Workers." *BMC Public Health* 14 (240).

Gaziano, T. A., K. S. Reddy, F. Paccaud, S. Horton, and V. Chaturvedi. 2006. "Cardiovascular Disease." In *Disease Control Priorities in Developing Countries*, second edition, edited by D. T. Jamison, J. G. Breman, A. R. Measham, G. Alleyne, M. Claeson, D. B. Evans, P. Jha, A. Mills, and P. Musgrove, 645–62. Washington, DC: World Bank and Oxford University Press.

GESICA Investigators. 2005. "Randomised Trial of Telephone Intervention in Chronic Heart Failure: DIAL Trial." *BMJ* 331 (7514): 425.

Goodarzi, M., I. Ebrahimzadeh, A. Rabi, B. Saedipoor, and M. A. Jafarabadi. 2012. "Impact of Distance Education via Mobile Phone Text Messaging on Knowledge, Attitude, Practice, and Self-Efficacy of Patients with Type 2 Diabetes Mellitus in Iran." *Journal of Diabetes and Metabolic Disorders* 11 (10).

Hemming, K., T. P. Haines, P. J. Chilton, A. J. Girling, and R. J. Lilford. 2015. "The Stepped-Wedge Cluster Randomised Trial: Rationale, Design, Analysis, and Reporting." *BMJ* 350: h391.

Hendriks, M. E., F. W. Wit, T. M. Akande, B. Kramer, G. K. Osagbemi, and others. 2014. "Effect of Health Insurance and Facility Quality Improvement on Blood Pressure in Adults with Hypertension in Nigeria: A Population-Based Study." *JAMA Internal Medicine* 174 (4): 555–63.

Hoekstra, J. W., C. V. Pollack Jr., M. T. Roe, E. D. Peterson, R. Brindis, and others. 2002. "Improving the Care of Patients with Non-ST-Elevation Acute Coronary Syndromes in the Emergency Department: The CRUSADE Initiative." *Academic Emergency Medicine: Official Journal of the Society for Academic Emergency Medicine* 9 (11): 1146–55.

Huffman, M. D., D. Prabhakaran, A. K. Abraham, M. N. Krishnan, A. C. Nambiar, and others. 2013. "Optimal In-Hospital and Discharge Medical Therapy in Acute Coronary Syndromes in Kerala: Results from the Kerala Acute Coronary Syndrome Registry." *Circulation, Cardiovascular Quality, and Outcomes* 6 (4): 436–43.

ITU (International Telecommunication Union). 2013. *The World in 2014: ICT Facts and Figures*. Geneva: ITU.

Jafar, T. H., J. Hatcher, N. Poulter, M. Islam, S. Hashmi, and others. 2009. "Community-Based Interventions to Promote Blood Pressure Control in a Developing Country: A Cluster Randomized Trial." *Annals of Internal Medicine* 151 (9): 593–601.

Joshi, R., A. P. Kengne, F. Hersch, M. B. Weber, H. McGuire, and A. Patel. 2017. "Innovations in Community-Based Health Care for Cardiometabolic and Respiratory Diseases." In *Disease Control Priorities* (third edition): Volume 5, *Cardiovascular, Respiratory, and Related Disorders*, edited by D. Prabhakaran, S. Anand, T. A. Gaziano, J.-C. Mbanya, Y. Wu, and R. Nugent. Washington, DC: World Bank.

Kahn, J. G., J. S. Yang, and J. S. Kahn. 2010. "'Mobile' Health Needs and Opportunities in Developing Countries." *Health Affairs* 29 (2): 252–58.

Kayima, J., R. K. Wanyenze, A. Katamba, E. Leontsini, and F. Nuwaha. 2013. "Hypertension Awareness, Treatment, and Control in Africa: A Systematic Review." *BMC Cardiovascular Disorders* 13 (54).

Kengne, A. P., P. K. Awah, L. L. Fezeu, E. Sobngwi, and J.-C. Mbanya. 2009. "Primary Health Care for Hypertension by Nurses in Rural and Urban Sub-Saharan Africa." *Journal of Clinical Hypertension* 11 (10): 564–72.

Khonsari, S., P. Subramanian, K. Chinna, L. A. Latif, L. W. Ling, and others. 2014. "Effect of a Reminder System Using an Automated Short Message Service on Medication Adherence Following Acute Coronary Syndrome." *European Journal of Cardiovascular Nursing* 14 (2): 170–79. doi:10.1177/1474515114521910.

Kinfu, Y., M. R. Dal Poz, H. Mercer, and D. B. Evans. 2009. "The Health Worker Shortage in Africa: Are Enough Physicians and Nurses Being Trained?" *Bulletin of the World Health Organization* 87 (3): 225–30.

Lohr, K. N., ed. 1990. *Medicare: A Strategy for Quality Assurance.* Vol. 1. Washington, DC: National Academies Press.

Macharia, W. M., E. K. Njeru, F. Muli-Musiime, and V. Nantulya. 2009. "Severe Road Traffic Injuries in Kenya, Quality of Care and Access." *African Health Sciences* 9 (2): 118–24.

Manji, I., S. Lukas, R. Vedanthan, B. Jakait, and S. Pastakia. 2012. "Community-Based Approaches to Reduce Medication Stock Outs in Western Kenya." Paper prepared for the Science of Eliminating Health Disparities Summit, Washington, DC, December 17–19.

Megiddo, I., S. Chatterjee, A. Nandi, and R. Laxminarayan. 2014. "Cost-Effectiveness of Treatment and Secondary Prevention of Acute Myocardial Infarction in India: A Modeling Study." *Global Heart* 9 (4): 391–98.e3.

Mohanan, P. P., R. Mathew, S. Harikrishnan, M. N. Krishnan, G. Zachariah, and others. 2013. "Presentation, Management, and Outcomes of 25,748 Acute Coronary Syndrome Admissions in Kerala, India: Results from the Kerala ACS Registry." *European Heart Journal* 34 (2): 121–92.

Nazzal, N. C., T. P. Campos, H. R. Corbalan, Z. F. Lanas, J. J. Bartolucci, and others. 2008. "The Impact of Chilean Health Reform in the Management and Mortality of ST Elevation Myocardial Infarction (STEMI) in Chilean Hospitals." *Revista Medica de Chile* 136 (10): 1231–39.

Nesari, M., M. Zakerimoghadam, A. Rajab, S. Bassampour, and S. Faghihzadeh. 2010. "Effect of Telephone Follow-Up on Adherence to a Diabetes Therapeutic Regimen." *Japan Journal of Nursing Science* 7 (2): 121–28.

Pearson, S. D., D. Goulart-Fisher, and T. H. Lee. 1995. "Critical Pathways as a Strategy for Improving Care: Problems and Potential." *Annals of Internal Medicine* 123 (12): 941–48.

Peng, B., J. Ni, C. S. Anderson, Y. Zhu, Y. Wang, and others. 2014. "Implementation of a Structured Guideline-Based Program for the Secondary Prevention of Ischemic Stroke in China." *Stroke* 45 (2): 515–19.

Piette, J. D., H. Datwani, S. Gaudioso, S. M. Foster, J. Westphal, and others. 2012. "Hypertension Management Using Mobile Technology and Home Blood Pressure Monitoring: Results of a Randomized Trial in Two Low/Middle-Income Countries." *Telemedicine Journal and e-Health* 18 (8): 613–20.

Prabhakaran, D., P. Jeemon, P. P. Mohanan, U. Govindan, Z. Geevar, and others. 2008. "Management of Acute Coronary Syndromes in Secondary Care Settings in Kerala: Impact of a Quality Improvement Programme." *National Medical Journal of India* 21 (3): 107–11.

Qureshi, N. N., J. Hatcher, N. Chaturvedi, and T. H. Jafar. 2007. "Effect of General Practitioner Education on Adherence to Antihypertensive Drugs: Cluster Randomised Controlled Trial." *BMJ* 335 (7628): 1030.

Ramachandran, A., C. Snehalatha, J. Ram, S. Selvam, M. Simon, and others. 2013. "Effectiveness of Mobile Phone Messaging in Prevention of Type 2 Diabetes by Lifestyle Modification in Men in India: A Prospective, Parallel-Group, Randomised Controlled Trial." *The Lancet Diabetes and Endocrinology* 1 (3): 191–98.

Ramanath, K. V., D. B. S. S. Balaji, C. H. Nagakishore, S. Mahesh Kumar, and M. Bhanuprakash. 2012. "A Study on Impact of Clinical Pharmacist Interventions on Medication Adherence and Quality of Life in Rural Hypertensive Patients." *Journal of Young Pharmacists* 4 (2): 95–100.

Reutens, A. T., R. Hutchinson, T. Van Binh, C. Cockram, C. Deerochanawong, and others. 2012. "The GIANT Study, a Cluster-Randomised Controlled Trial of Efficacy of Education of Doctors about Type 2 Diabetes Mellitus Management Guidelines in Primary Care Practice." *Diabetes Research and Clinical Practice* 98 (1): 38–45.

Rotheram-Borus, M. J., M. Tomlinson, M. Gwegwe, W. S. Comulada, N. Kaufman, and others. 2012. "Diabetes Buddies: Peer Support through a Mobile Phone Buddy System." *Diabetes Educator* 38 (3): 357–65.

Shetty, A. S., S. Chamukuttan, A. Nanditha, R. K. Raj, and A. Ramachandran. 2011. "Reinforcement of Adherence to Prescription Recommendations in Asian Indian Diabetes Patients Using Short Message Service (SMS): A Pilot Study." *Journal of the Association of Physicians of India* 59 (November): 711–14.

Sosa-Rubi, S. G., O. Galarraga, and R. Lopez-Ridaura. 2009. "Diabetes Treatment and Control: The Effect of Public Health Insurance for the Poor in Mexico." *Bulletin of the World Health Organization* 87 (7): 512–19.

Steyn, K., C. Lombard, N. Gwebushe, J. M. Fourie, K. Everett-Murphy, and others. 2013. "Implementation of National Guidelines, Incorporated within Structured Diabetes and Hypertension Records at Primary Level Care in Cape Town, South Africa: A Randomised Controlled Trial." *Global Health Action* 6: 20796.

Thom, S., N. Poulter, J. Field, A. Patel, D. Prabhakaran, and others. 2013. "Effects of a Fixed-Dose Combination Strategy on Adherence and Risk Factors in Patients with or at High Risk of CVD." *Journal of the American Medical Association* 310 (9): 918–29.

Tu, J. V., L. R. Donovan, D. S. Lee, J. T. Wang, P. C. Austin, and others. 2009. "Effectiveness of Public Report Cards for Improving the Quality of Cardiac Care: The EFFECT Study; a Randomized Trial." *Journal of the American Medical Association* 302 (21): 2330–37.

U.S. FDA (United States Food and Drug Administration). 2014. "Briefing Document: Cardiovascular and Renal Drugs Advisory Committee Meeting." U.S. FDA, Washington, DC.

Wang, M., A. E. Moran, J. Liu, P. G. Coxson, P. A. Heidenreich, and others. 2014. "Cost-Effectiveness of Optimal Use of Acute Myocardial Infarction Treatments and Impact on Coronary Heart Disease Mortality in China." *Circulation, Cardiovascular Quality, and Outcomes* 7 (1): 78–85.

Wang, N., D. Zhao, J. Liu, C. Yu, W. Wang, and others. 2012. "Impact of Heart Failure on In-Hospital Outcomes of Acute Coronary Syndrome Patients in China: Results from the Bridging the Gap on CHD Secondary Prevention in China (BRIG) Project." *International Journal of Cardiology* 160 (1): 15–19.

Weiser, T., and A. Gawande. 2015. "Excess Surgical Mortality: Strategies for Improving Quality of Care." In *Disease Control Priorities* (third edition): Volume 1, *Essential Surgery*, edited by H. T. Debas, A. Gawande, D. T. Jamison, M. E. Kruk, and C. N. Mock. Washington, DC: World Bank.

WHO (World Health Organization). 2007. *Everybody's Business: Strengthening Health Systems to Improve Health Outcomes*. WHO's Framework for Action. Geneva: WHO.

———. 2008. *Task Shifting: Global Recommendations and Guidelines*. Geneva: WHO.

———. 2013. *Global Health Workforce Statistics, the 2013 Update*. Geneva: WHO.

Xavier, D., P. Pais, P. J. Devereaux, C. Xie, D. Prabhakaran, and others. 2008. "Treatment and Outcomes of Acute Coronary Syndromes in India (CREATE): A Prospective Analysis of Registry Data." *The Lancet* 371 (9622): 1435–42.

Yu, B., X. Zhang, and G. Wang. 2013. "Full Coverage for Hypertension Drugs in Rural Communities in China." *American Journal of Managed Care* 19 (1): e22–29.

Yusuf, S., S. Islam, C. K. Chow, S. Rangarajan, G. Dagenais, and others. 2011. "Use of Secondary Prevention Drugs for Cardiovascular Disease in the Community in High-Income, Middle-Income, and Low-Income Countries (the PURE Study): A Prospective Epidemiological Survey." *The Lancet* 378 (9798): 1231–43.

Yusuf, S., P. Pais, R. Afzal, D. Xavier, K. Teo, and others. 2009. "Effects of a Polypill (Polycap) on Risk Factors in Middle-Aged Individuals without Cardiovascular Disease (TIPS): A Phase II, Double-Blind, Randomised Trial." *The Lancet* 373 (9672): 1341–51.

Yusuf, S., P. Pais, A. Sigamani, D. Zavier, R. Afzal, and others. 2012. "Comparison of Risk Factor Reduction and Tolerability of a Full-Dose Polypill (with Potassium) Versus Low-Dose Polypill (Polycap) in Individuals at High Risk of Cardiovascular Diseases: The Second Indian Polycap Study (TIPS-2) Investigators." *Circulation, Cardiovascular Quality, and Outcomes* 5 (4): 463–71.

Zou, G., X. Wei, W. Gong, J. Yin, J. Walley, and others. 2014. "Evaluation of a Systematic Cardiovascular Disease Risk Reduction Strategy in Primary Health Care: An Exploratory Study from Zhejiang, China." *Journal of Public Health* 37 (2): 241–50.

Chapter 19

Costs and Cost-Effectiveness of Interventions and Policies to Prevent and Treat Cardiovascular and Respiratory Diseases

Thomas A. Gaziano, Marc Suhrcke, Elizabeth Brouwer, Carol Levin, Irina Nikolic, and Rachel Nugent

INTRODUCTION

The risk factors and disease conditions covered in this volume of *Disease Control Priorities* constitute the majority of the health burden facing middle- and high-income countries (MICs and HICs, respectively) today and are fast approaching a majority of the burden in low-income countries (LICs). Previous editions of *Disease Control Priorities*, published in 1993 and 2006, acknowledged the importance of cardiovascular and related diseases (CVRDs) to the future health and economic well-being of populations in low- and middle-income countries (LMICs) and singled out tobacco taxes and treatment of heart disease with low-cost generics as high-priority, cost-effective interventions. With some exceptions, most of the conclusions about cost-effectiveness were extrapolated from analyses done in HICs (Rodgers and others 2006) and from modeling, because of the paucity of economic analysis of interventions for CVRDs using LMIC data. In 2012, the World Health Organization (WHO) reviewed the cost-effectiveness of noncommunicable disease (NCD) interventions, based on a limited number of modeled studies. The results were used to develop the WHO Best Buys for interventions recommended in the NCD Global Action Plan (WHO 2011).

By 2016, when the WHO updated its review of cost-effectiveness evidence, considerably more LMIC data were available. This chapter also benefits from a larger universe of economic analyses on the conditions and risk factors covered in the chapters in this volume—both from models and from experience. Some recent systematic reviews have examined evidence on the cost-effectiveness of interventions to tackle CVRDs in LMICs (for example, Shroufi and others 2013; Suhrcke, Boluarte, and Niessen 2012; Wiseman and others 2016). These reviews found modest, but growing, evidence of the cost-effectiveness of CVRD interventions in these settings and noted a bias in favor of research on personal medical interventions over population-level interventions.

The chapter catalogues the results of dozens of high-quality, cost-effectiveness analyses for cardiovascular disease (CVD), diabetes, respiratory, and kidney-related conditions and risk factors (hereafter termed CVRDs)—much of it with country-specific data. It begins by summarizing the available literature on population-level health and intersectoral policies to address the major risks in LMICs and discusses some methodological issues in these analyses. It then assesses and discusses the cost-effectiveness of personal services

Corresponding author: Thomas A. Gaziano, Brigham and Women's Hospital, Harvard Medical School, Boston, Massachusetts, United States; tgaziano@partners.org.

delivered through various levels of the health system. It is intended to complement the reviews of effective policies and interventions in other chapters with cost-effectiveness results useful for informing decisions about policies, packages, and delivery platforms. The methodology used for the review is described in online annex 19A, along with the detailed results.

POPULATION-LEVEL INTERVENTIONS AND POLICY

This section reviews the cost-effectiveness of fiscal and regulatory policies used to change behavior and address the external costs associated with tobacco consumption, dietary issues such as obesity (Cawley 2015; Suhrcke and others 2006), and physical activity. Overall, the evidence in favor of fiscal and regulatory policies to curb tobacco consumption is, beyond doubt, more convincing than the evidence for diet. Although mass media campaigns show some promise in HICs, at least when focused on specific dietary targets, evidence of their cost-effectiveness is more nuanced. There is little cost-effectiveness data from LMICs on population-level physical activity interventions.

Figure 19.1 summarizes the evidence on cost-effectiveness for population-level interventions. The figure

only captures cost-effectiveness studies that have expressed outcomes in cost per disability-adjusted life years (DALYs) averted. Table 19A.2 in annex 19A provides more detailed results.

Keeping these reservations in mind, figure 19.1 suggests the following conclusions:

- Overall, population-level interventions to address the risk factors for CVRDs appear to have favorable cost-effectiveness ratios. Several—price and nonprice tobacco interventions and nonprice salt regulation—have the potential to be cost saving.
- Of the population-level interventions examined, tobacco taxation and nonprice salt regulation are, on average, considerably more attractive from a cost-effectiveness standpoint than other, often less intrusive, interventions. However, the seeming superiority of nonprice salt regulation is likely to be driven by the extraordinarily positive results of one study (Rubinstein and others 2009).
- A particularly large range of cost-effectiveness ratios is found across the many types of tobacco regulation, due to diversity in policies and variation in costs.

A summary of the cost-effectiveness literature for CVRD risk factors, specifically tobacco and diet, follows. The cost-effectiveness of interventions to deter excess alcohol use is discussed in volume 4, chapter 7 (Medina-Mora and others 2015).

Figure 19.1 Average Cost-Effectiveness of Population-Level Interventions for CVRD Risk Factors, 2000–14

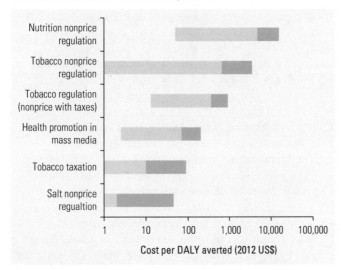

Sources: Based on a systematic literature review of cost-effectiveness ratios for LMICs from 2000 to 2014, including Cecchini and others 2010; Chow, Darley, and Laxminarayan 2007; Higashi and others 2011; Murray and others 2003; Ortegon and others 2012; Ranson and others 2002; Rubinstein and others 2009; Rubenstein and others 2010; Salomon and others 2012.
Note: CVRD = cardiovascular and related disease; DALY = disability-adjusted life year. The bars capture the range of estimated costs per DALY averted from the set of studies reviewed. From each study, the mean estimate is taken as the relevant estimate. The average is the space where the light blue and dark blue bars meet. Light blue represents the range below the average; dark blue represents the range above the average. Negative numbers are not plotted because the x-axis is on a logarithmic scale. Any bars that touch the y-axis have at least one source that found the intervention to be cost saving.

Tobacco Use

Fiscal policies to tackle tobacco-related harm have typically ranked among the most preferred options for addressing CVRDs. In its NCD Best Buys, the WHO ranked the taxation of tobacco as one of the most cost-effective ways to tackle NCDs in LMICs (WHO 2011). This recommendation rests on a considerable body of research regarding effectiveness, but few studies have directly examined the cost-effectiveness of the policy. Ortegon and others (2012) applied the WHO's Choosing Interventions That Are Cost-Effective (CHOICE) model (Tan-Torres Edejer and others 2003) to estimate the cost-effectiveness of 123 single or combined interventions, including tobacco taxation, in two WHO regions with high adult and child mortality—South-East Asia and Sub-Saharan Africa. They found that increasing tobacco taxation to 40 percent to 60 percent of the retail price was among the most favorable of the interventions considered. Previously, Ranson and others (2002) estimated highly favorable cost-effectiveness ratios for increasing tobacco taxation by 10 percent at global and regional levels.

In low- and middle-income regions, they found that such tobacco taxation would cost about US\$4–US\$91 per DALY averted.

Chow, Darley, and Laxminarayan (2007) compared a 10 percent increase in the price of tobacco in India to nicotine replacement therapy and other nonprice interventions, including bans on advertising and promotion of tobacco, dissemination of information on the health consequences of using tobacco, and restrictions on smoking in public and work spaces. The tax increase was estimated to cost US\$13 per DALY averted—a very favorable cost-effectiveness outcome compared with the other interventions analyzed. Similarly, in a modeling exercise for Mexico, Salomon and others (2012) found that increasing the tobacco tax from 60 percent of the retail price of cigarettes to 80 percent had a cost-effectiveness ratio of about US\$22 per DALY averted, which compared very favorably with a ban on advertising, at US\$435 per DALY averted. Higashi and others (2011) obtained similar results for Vietnam.

Modeled evidence suggests that policies regulating tobacco through smoking bans, graphic warning labels, mass media campaigns, advertising bans, and others are generally more cost-effective than personal interventions to reduce tobacco consumption in LMIC settings. However, as with taxation, studies that model regulatory interventions are sensitive to assumptions about the quality of enforcement, the prevalence or intensity of smoking habits, and purchasing patterns.

Two studies modeled tobacco regulation across countries, compared with tobacco taxation. Using a static model, Ranson and others (2002) compared a tobacco tax to nicotine replacement therapy and a combination of other nonprice interventions. A later study (Navarro and others 2014) compared a tobacco tax with a ban on advertising and promotion, dissemination of information on the health consequences of smoking, and restrictions on smoking in public places and workplaces. Results from both of these studies show that nonprice interventions cost between US\$47 and US\$921 per DALY averted in LMICs, which is a less favorable cost-effectiveness result than tobacco taxation (US\$3.9–US\$90.8 per DALY averted), but more attractive than nicotine replacement therapy for individual treatment (US\$363–US\$1,128 per DALY averted).

Ortegon and others (2012) modeled the cost-effectiveness of a set of nonprice population-level interventions for South-East Asia and Sub-Saharan Africa. The population-level tobacco control interventions included restrictions on smoking in public places, advertising bans, warning labels, and consumer information campaigns. The personal interventions included nicotine replacement therapy and physician advice. Of all

of the tobacco and other interventions considered in their analysis, combinations of population-level tobacco interventions were found to be highly cost-effective in both regions. Moreover, the overall set of population-level interventions was more cost-effective than adding individual treatment options (nicotine replacement therapy and physician advice) to the entire package.

Several studies have compared the cost-effectiveness of various tobacco policies in specific countries (or regions of countries), often using similar modeling strategies. Salomon and others (2012) applied the CHOICE model to Mexico to estimate cost-effectiveness of tobacco policies such as excise taxes, advertising bans, indoor air quality laws, and nicotine replacement therapy, as well as combinations of these. A comprehensive advertising ban and enforcement of the air quality law showed favorable cost-effectiveness, whereas nicotine replacement therapy did not. In the incremental analysis, tobacco taxation dominated most other single and combined strategies, with the exception of the "taxation plus ban on advertising" set (which cost US\$435 per DALYs averted).

Higashi and others (2011) modeled the cost-effectiveness of four population-level tobacco interventions in Vietnam: an excise tax increase, graphic warning labels on cigarette packs, mass media campaigns including educational messages for different media, and smoking bans in public or in workplaces. Graphic warning labels on cigarette packs showed the most favorable cost-effectiveness ratios, followed closely by excise tax increases (except for a large tax increase, in which case taxation was the most cost-effective), mass media campaigns, public smoking bans, and workplace smoking bans (table 19.1). The analysis concluded that all

Table 19.1 Costs per Disability-Adjusted Life Year Averted of Population-Level Tobacco Interventions in Vietnam, Exclusive of Potential Cost Offsets (Compared with Status Quo Interventions in Place)

Intervention	Cost per Disability-Adjusted Life Year Averted	
	2007 Vietnamese dong	2012 US\$
Graphic pack warning label	500	0.05
Tax increase maximum (from 55 to 85%)	290	0.03
Tax increase minimum (from 55 to 75%)	4,200	0.41
Tax increase minimum (from 55 to 65%)	8,600	0.83
Smoking ban (public)	67,900	6.56
Smoking ban (work)	336,800	32.53
Mass media campaign	78,300	7.56

Source: Higashi and others 2011.
Note: Cost offset is the savings expected from lower health care costs.

interventions would be cost saving by preventing or reducing spending on future treatment of tobacco-related illness. This study method is unusual, and there is no consensus on whether and how to account for the costs of future unrelated health care (van Baal and others 2011).

Rubinstein and others (2010) modeled the costs and effects of a mass media campaign to promote tobacco cessation among smokers, in addition to population-level salt reduction and four individual, clinical treatment interventions. The mass media campaign produced a cost-effectiveness ratio of US$3,583 per DALY averted, which, while not cost saving (which would require a cost-effectiveness ratio of US$1,582), was still considered good value for money.

Donaldson and others (2011) modeled the cost-effectiveness of an effective prohibition on smoking in public places in Gujarat State in India compared with the current, poorly enforced prohibition of smoking in public places in some districts of the state. The results are expressed in life years (LYs) saved and in heart attacks averted rather than in DALYs averted. A complete ban is highly cost-effective when key variables, including legislation effectiveness, are varied in the sensitivity analyses. Without including medical treatment costs averted, the cost-effectiveness ratio ranges from US$2.4 to US$135.0 per LY saved and US$44.5 to US$464.0 per acute myocardial infarction averted. When including potential future savings in tobacco-related health care costs, the ban becomes cost saving.

In summary, cost-effective policies to reduce tobacco consumption are available. The most favorable policy appears to be a large tax increase on tobacco. Regulatory approaches, including bans on smoking in public places, warning labels, advertising and promotion restrictions, and mass media campaigns, are also attractive from a cost-effectiveness standpoint. All fiscal and regulatory approaches are superior to individual approaches to tobacco reduction.

Diet

Interest has recently increased in the potential use of fiscal policy in many HICs and increasingly in some MICs to improve diets. In addition to changing eating behaviors and reducing obesity, fiscal policies have been justified as a way to eliminate externalities. The argument is made that, whether through health insurance or tax-funded public payment, healthy-weight individuals will subsidize the medical care costs of obese individuals. The higher medical care costs may be passed on to the public in the form of higher payroll or income taxes (Cawley 2015).

For this and other reasons, real-world implementation of fiscal policies to influence dietary behavior is expanding rapidly,[1] yet a considerable amount of research has not yet settled a vigorous debate on the subject. Several recent systematic and nonsystematic reviews of the effectiveness of dietary pricing policies have been published, each with a somewhat different focus (Cabrera Escobar and others 2013; Epstein and others 2012; Eyles and others 2012; Powell and others 2013; Thow, Downs, and Jan 2014). Reflecting wide recognition that diet-related taxation is far more nuanced than tobacco taxation, existing reviews reach varying conclusions regarding the use of fiscal policy to improve diet. For example, according to Thow and others (2010, 1), "Taxes and subsidies on food have the potential to influence consumption considerably and improve health, particularly when they are large," while, according to Cornelsen and others (2015, 18), "There is a very real possibility that [taxes on unhealthy foods and beverages] may not be beneficial after all." The magnitude of the tax or subsidy needed to influence consumption and health, as well as the optimal design of such fiscal policies (that is, what precisely should be taxed or subsidized), is also unclear.[2] In a recent series in *The Lancet* on obesity, Popkin and Hawkes (2015) concluded that taxes on unhealthy food and beverages can reduce obesity by altering preferences.

Some of the variation in the conclusions may be attributed to differences in the scope of each review, given that they tend to differ in regional focus, the precise outcome indicator used, and the type of estimation methodologies used. Part of the problem in developing conclusive evidence is the relatively short real-world experiences with implementing significant fiscal policy measures. Inevitably, most studies rely on analysis of empirical relationships between food prices and food purchases, on analysis of consumption- or diet-related health (for which it is difficult to establish true causal evidence as a proxy for the effect of a policy), or on hypothetical modeling studies (which depend on the assumptions in the model).

Early evidence is mixed. In a short-term evaluation of the first city-level tax on sugar-sweetened beverages (SSBs) in Berkeley, California, Cawley and Frisvold (2015) found relatively little pass-through of the SSB tax to consumers, in that retail prices rose by less than half of the amount of the tax. The direct effect on consumption and obesity is likely to be smaller than expected given that much of the previous literature found or assumed full or even overshifting of taxes.

In contrast, the Mexican SSB tax appears to have had a greater effect on prices and hence on sales and consumption. Grogger (2015) found that the price of SSBs increased by more than the amount of the tax shortly after the policy was implemented. Evaluating the same policy, Colchero and others (2016) concluded that the policy resulted in a 6 percent reduction in purchases (9 percent among low-income groups) and a shift away from SSBs to water and diet drinks.

In light of uncertainty about the effectiveness of diet-related fiscal policies, it is perhaps not surprising that only a few studies have examined their cost-effectiveness, particularly in LMICs. Cecchini and others (2010) modeled obesity prevention policies in LMICs, covering Brazil, China, India, Mexico, and South Africa. Their results indicate that fiscal measures (including increasing the price of food with unhealthy content or reducing the cost of healthy foods rich in fiber) are less expensive per capita than regulatory or individual interventions and are the only measures that were cost saving for all LMICs at both 20- and 50-year time horizons. Additionally, they were cost saving by a magnitude of twice the other interventions considered. Price interventions and regulation appear to produce the largest health gains in the shortest timeframe.

Using a simulation model (relying, in part, on the results of Cabrera Escobar and others 2013), Manyema and others (2014) estimated the effect of a 20 percent tax on SSBs on the prevalence of obesity among adults in South Africa. A 20 percent tax was predicted to reduce energy intake by about 36 kilojoules per day. Obesity was projected to decline 3.8 percent in men and 2.4 percent in women. The number of obese adults was projected to decrease by more than 220,000.

Regulatory and Mass Media Policies

Reducing salt content in manufactured foods through mandatory government regulations or voluntary action from industry is recommended in the WHO Global NCD Action Plan (WHO 2011). In addition to cost-effectiveness of salt regulation, economic analyses have been performed on mass media campaigns and regulation of other undesirable food content, such as trans fatty acids (trans fats) in processed foods. This section reviews those studies.

Salt Consumption

In a wide-ranging application of the CHOICE modeling approach, Murray and others (2003) modeled salt reduction, mass media health education, and individual treatment, as well as various combinations of interventions, in two LMIC regions (South-East Asia, with high rates of adult and child mortality, and Latin America and the Caribbean, with low rates of adult and child mortality) and one high-income region (Europe, with very low rates of adult and child mortality). They found that population-based interventions had more favorable

cost-effectiveness ratios than personalized health service interventions. Voluntary agreements to reduce salt were less cost-effective than legislative measures, with salt reduction legislation estimated to avert one DALY for as little as US$3.74 in South-East Asia and US$2.6 in Latin America and the Caribbean. Combining salt legislation with mass media programs could improve the cost-effectiveness ratio even further. The most cost-effective set of interventions is, however, a mix of population-level preventive interventions and personalized treatments.

Two follow-up studies using the WHO CHOICE model provide multiregional estimates of the cost-effectiveness of salt regulation and other interventions. Asaria and others (2007) modeled the cost and effects of shifting the distribution of risk factors associated with salt intake and tobacco use on chronic disease mortality for 23 countries with 80 percent of the chronic disease burden in LMICs. They showed that, over 10 years (2006–15), implementing these interventions could avert 13.8 million deaths at a cost of less than US$0.40 per person per year in low-income and lower-middle-income countries, and US$0.50–US$1.00 per person per year in upper-middle-income countries (as of 2005). Ortegon and others (2012) provided updated evidence on broadly similar interventions in two WHO regions: South-East Asia and Africa. They modeled the cost-effectiveness of reducing the amount of salt in processed foods via voluntary agreement with industry and via regulation. They concluded that supply-side interventions to reduce salt had less favorable cost-effectiveness ratios than interventions to reduce demand; provide combination drug therapy, either alone or in a multidrug regimen, for high-risk CVD patients (25 percent or more absolute risk of experiencing a cardiovascular event over the next decade); or provide retinopathy screening and glycemic control for patients with diabetes.

The CHOICE model was again used to model salt reduction in Buenos Aires (Rubinstein and others 2009) and in Argentina (Rubinstein and others 2010). The studies modeled similar interventions: reducing the amount of salt in bread via voluntary industry agreements and mass education programs as well as individual treatment options (for example, Murray and others 2003). While broadly similar, the findings for Argentina were more favorable for salt reduction, finding that any approach would be cost saving, while the findings for Buenos Aires showed that voluntary industry salt reduction would cost very little and would have a more favorable cost-effectiveness ratio than a mass media campaign.

Ferrante and others (2012) also assessed the cost-effectiveness of salt reduction in Argentina. They simulated the effects of an intervention that reduced salt content by 5 percent to 25 percent in a wide range of food groups, including bread, bread products, meat products, canned foods, soups, and dressings. This intervention was found to be cost saving while producing substantial improvements in population-wide, diet-related health outcomes. In a study of four countries in the eastern Mediterranean region, Mason and others (2014) evaluated three policies to reduce dietary salt intake—a health promotion campaign, labeling of food packaging, and mandatory reformulation of salt content in processed food—and found that salt reduction may be cost saving, either applied on its own or in combination with other interventions.

Trans Fats Consumption

Several policy guidelines and recommendations, internationally and nationally, have recommended the elimination of trans fatty acids to reduce coronary heart disease worldwide (see chapter 6 in this volume, Afshin and others 2016). The WHO has called for their elimination in its global strategy on diet, physical activity, and health (WHO 2004). Several types of measures to reduce consumption of trans fats have also been implemented, including total bans, mandatory labeling, restaurant bans, and voluntary reformulation (Downs, Thow, and Leeder 2013). So far, very little empirical evaluation of the effectiveness, let alone cost-effectiveness, of these policies has been undertaken. However, some research has used a modeling framework to evaluate some of them.

To the best of our knowledge, the only economic evaluation in an LMIC context is by Chow, Darley, and Laxminarayan (2007), who analyzed the costs and health effects of legislation mandating the replacement of trans fats produced from partial hydrogenation with polyunsaturated fats. This analysis estimated that substituting 2 percent of the energy from trans fats with polyunsaturated fats would cost US$0.50 per adult per year and reduce coronary artery disease by 7 percent over 10 years.

A recent example from an HIC is a modeling study by Allen and others (2015) that simulated costs and effects of three options for restricting the consumption of trans fats in England: a ban on trans fatty acids in processed foods, improved labeling of trans fatty acids, and a ban on trans fats in restaurant foods. The research sought to examine the effects of various approaches across different socioeconomic groups. The expected health effects of a total ban, as well as policies to improve labeling or remove trans fatty acids from restaurant and fast foods, would lead to a considerable reduction in coronary heart disease mortality. The benefits would be larger among lower socioeconomic groups. In addition, the study predicted large cost savings from these policies. Going beyond the usual economic costs, this study included the costs of informal care and lost productivity, among others.

Physical Activity

Increasing physical activity can reduce mortality and improve population health. Governments in many countries have recognized this opportunity, but the evidence on what works best to promote physical activity and what is best value for money is scarce and concentrated largely on HICs. One exception is a study about a comprehensive, school-based intervention program for childhood obesity in China, based on a two-year multiple-center randomized controlled trial. Nutrition-only and physical activity–only interventions were compared with a combined nutritional plus physical activity program (Meng and others 2013). The combined intervention was found to be more cost-effective than either of the single interventions, preventing a case of obesity or overweight for a cost of US$1,519.

Laine and others (2014) reviewed 10 studies from HICs on population-, community-, and individual-level physical activity interventions. Expressing the cost-effectiveness of these studies in dollars per metabolic equivalent of task-hours (MET-h) gained (making comparisons to nonphysical activity interventions impossible), they found that the most efficient interventions to increase physical activity were community rail trails (US$0.006 per MET-h), pedometers (US$0.014 per MET-h), and school health education programs (US$0.056 per MET-h). It is not clear how generalizable these findings are to an LMIC context.

A more encompassing cost-effectiveness review of physical activity by Müller-Riemenschneider, Reinhold, and Willich (2009) identified only eight studies covering 11 intervention strategies, again from HICs only, including, for instance, advice from general practitioners, trail development, promotion of worksite physical activity, and phone delivery of intervention messages. To the extent that any broader patterns could be observed, the more environmental interventions (trail development) and interventions targeted at general practitioners seemed to be the most cost-effective when measured by costs per person becoming physically active.

Lehnert and others (2012) also concluded that environmental approaches have particular promise. They reviewed the long-term cost-effectiveness of obesity prevention interventions, some of which focus on physical activity. Their review focused exclusively on cost-utility analyses, estimating the value for money of interventions as measured by their costs per DALYs averted or quality-adjusted life years (QALYs) gained. Doing so increased the comparability of the results across interventions. The potential downside of relying on such decision-analytic modeling results, however, is that they may be based on a set of assumptions that are not readily appreciated and the point estimate of each cost-utility ratio will be highly uncertain.[3]

Issues in Economic Analysis of Population-Level Health Policies

Research on the cost-effectiveness of population-level preventive interventions is still limited, even in HICs (Schwappach, Boluarte, and Suhrcke 2007), as a result of the methodological challenges of conducting economic evaluations in the public health field (Pitt, Goodman, and Hanson 2016; Weatherly and others 2009). The most binding challenge may be that of attributing potential health effects directly to an intervention, especially when the change is targeted to entire populations or communities, randomized controlled trials are difficult to undertake, and the impact of the intervention takes a long time to emerge. In addition, because many population-level and community-level interventions may be located outside of health care settings, at least part of their costs and consequences are incurred by sectors other than health. These intersectoral costs and consequences may not be taken into account, and how to do so is not obvious (Claxton, Sculpher, and Culyer 2007; Greco, Lorgelly, and Yamabhai 2016). For instance, the cost-effectiveness of tobacco taxation is an unsatisfying concept. First, many of the costs are likely to be incurred by administrative units outside of the health care system, such as the Finance Ministry. Second, while economists agree that the revenues raised by taxes on tobacco are a transfer from consumers to government and thus should not be included in the benefit ledger, it is difficult to measure the efficiency effects of taxation (deadweight loss), and thus tobacco revenues are not usually included in analyses. As such, societal cost-effectiveness or cost-benefit analysis may better capture the full effects of tobacco taxation rather than a purely health system perspective. Results of these different types of economic evaluations are not directly comparable (Claxton and others 2010). Examples of cost-benefit analyses for water, sanitation, and hygiene are reviewed in volume 7, chapter 9 (Hutton and Chase 2017). The chapter by Chang, Jamison, and Horton (2018) in volume 9 discusses cost-benefit methods.

Assessing the impact—effectiveness and cost-effectiveness—of population-level interventions is fraught with challenges that often go beyond those faced in the evaluation of clinical interventions. A major difficulty is that researchers usually need to rely on observational data and modeling studies rather than on randomized studies. Economic modeling is the basis for

cost-effectiveness conclusions in earlier editions of *Disease Control Priorities* and the WHO's CHOICE project.[4]

Moreover, comparability across studies is limited for several reasons. First, the relevant cost-effectiveness threshold for a given intervention in any given country is not clear.[5] Adhering strictly to the widely used rule of thumb of one (or three) times gross domestic product per capita poses the risk that, if the threshold is too high, interventions could displace services and forgo more health than they generate. If the threshold is too low, new interventions could be rejected that would offer a health gain (Revill and Sculpher 2012). Second, because of the limited number of studies for each type of intervention, a single outlier may well tilt the relative ranking one way or another. Third, some types of interventions, such as nonprice regulation of tobacco or salt, may still encompass a wide range of specific interventions and hence widely different cost-effectiveness ratios. Even for more narrowly defined interventions, such as tobacco taxation, the exact magnitude of the tax treatment may differ.

INDIVIDUAL-LEVEL CARE AND MANAGEMENT OF CHRONIC DISEASE

The large reductions in age-adjusted CVD mortality rates in HICs have resulted from three complementary types of interventions. One targets persons with acute or established CVD. A second assesses risk and targets persons with multiple risk factors before their first CVD event. The third uses mass education or policy interventions directed at the entire population to reduce the overall level of risk factors. This section highlights the variety of cost-effective interventions aimed at individuals in different settings, including the community, primary health centers, and hospitals. Much work remains to be done in LMICs to determine the best strategies given limited resources; if implemented, these interventions could help reduce the burden of CVD mortality. Table 19A.3 in online annex 19A lists the cost-effectiveness ratios for many of the most promising interventions used either in the community or at primary health centers that could be or have been adopted in low- and middle-income regions. Table 19A.4 lists the ratios for interventions that occur at primary health centers, first-level hospitals, or advanced-level hospitals and are focused on individuals with established disease.

Community-Based Care

Screening
Primary prevention is paramount for the large number of individuals who are at high risk for CVD. In particular, a significant amount of the reduction in CVD

mortality has come from the control of risk factors (Ford and Capewell 2011). Globally, the major risk factors are poorly controlled. Control rates for hypertension are less than 5 percent. Control rates for lipids are likely even worse, given that many countries do not have the facilities to measure lipids, and statins have become available only recently in low-income regions. For example, several Western European countries have hypertension control rates (blood pressure below 140/90) of less than 10 percent, with Spain having a control rate of less than 5 percent (Wolf-Maier and others 2004). Low control rates reflect low detection rates in addition to lack of drug availability.

Although preventive treatment is available in many LMICs, Mendis and others (2005) found that fewer than 10 percent of members of the community received the recommended care. Awareness, treatment, and control rates of major cardiovascular risk factors such as hypertension must be improved to prevent significant disease. Improved mortality rates require improved awareness of risk, appropriate initiation of treatment when available, and control of risk factors through appropriate follow-up. Major barriers to improving care include crowded primary health centers with long wait times, scarcity of professional health staff, and high costs of traditional screening programs.

Given limited resources, finding low-cost prevention strategies is a top priority. Using prediction rules or risk scores to identify persons at higher risk so as to target specific behavioral or drug interventions is a well-established primary prevention strategy and has proved to be cost-effective in LMICs (Gaziano, Opie, and Weinstein 2006; Gaziano and others 2005). Most methods have included age, sex, hypertension, smoking status, diabetes mellitus, and lipid values; some have included family history (Assmann, Cullen, and Schulte 2002; Conroy and others 2003; Ferrario and others 2005; Wilson and others 1998). See chapter 22 in this volume (Jeemon and others 2017) for a discussion of absolute risk measurement.

More attention is now focused on developing risk scores that would be easy to use without losing predictive discrimination in resource-poor countries. In LICs, a prediction rule that requires a lab test may be too expensive for widespread screening or for any use. In response to this real concern, the WHO released risk prediction charts with and without cholesterol for different regions of the world (Mendis, Lindholm, and others 2007). Pandya, Weinstein, and Gaziano (2011) demonstrated that a risk tool using nonbiometric information (age, systolic blood pressure, body mass index) can screen as effectively as one that uses lab results. Furthermore, the results of the risk tool have been validated in other cohorts in LMICs (Gaziano and

others 2013; Gaziano and others 2016), and the method of assessing absolute risk has proved to be more cost-effective than relying on blood pressure alone (Gaziano and others 2005).

Community Health Workers

Shifting the responsibility for screening to community health workers (CHWs) was shown to be as effective as having nurses or physicians screen for CVD risk in a community study in Bangladesh, Guatemala, Mexico, and South Africa (Gaziano, Abrahams-Gessel, Denman, and others 2015). CHWs using a mobile phone app was found to be life saving in Guatemala (34 lives), Mexico (281 lives), and South Africa (471 lives) per 210,000 adults screened at very cost-effective ratios. Having CHWs conduct screening using a simple tool was much more cost-effective when the primary health system was prepared and equipped to treat persons identified as high risk (Gaziano, Abrahams-Gessel, Surka, and others 2015). In countries like South Africa, where at least half of persons identified as being high risk received medications, the screening intervention was cost saving.

Even in settings such as Guatemala, where fewer than 5 percent of eligible patients received statins, the intervention was still attractive at US$565 per QALY gained. In Mexico, where 36 percent of eligible patients were started on hypertension medications and 18 percent were started on statins, the incremental cost-effectiveness ratio for screening by CHWs was less than US$4 per QALY gained.

CHWs can help improve adherence once individuals are on treatment. Twice yearly visits by a CHW for hypertension and adherence education have a cost-effectiveness ratio of US$320 per QALY gained compared with usual care in South Africa; the cost can be as low as US$17 per QALY gained in an urban setting with shorter distances between homes and as much as US$1,500 per QALY gained in a deep rural setting with greater distances between dwellings (Gaziano and others 2014).

Primary Health Center Care

Much of the screening for cardiometabolic conditions that does not happen in the community can occur in primary health centers, particularly opportunistic hypertension screening. Regardless of the location of the screening, once identified, the bulk of primary prevention for ischemic heart disease and stroke will occur in primary health centers. Furthermore, great overlap occurs in many of the medications used. While many of the interventions for secondary prevention may be initiated in primary care hospitals, once patients are stabilized, they generally receive care at a primary health center.

Much of the management is centered on control of hypertension, blood lipids, and diabetes.

Hypertension and Cholesterol

Control of risk factors is paramount to primary prevention of CVD and a major focus of primary health centers. Blood pressure control has been a cornerstone of the prevention of stroke, ischemic heart disease, and peripheral vascular disease for more than 50 years and is cost-effective in all regions of the world (Rubinstein and others 2010; Wang and others 2011).

Issues regarding the cost-effectiveness of such interventions have recently focused on finding ways to improve the efficiency of identifying who most benefits from treatment, how to improve access to medications, how to improve adherence to medications, and how best to deliver medications. One trend has been to evaluate the overall risk of a patient rather than a single risk factor such as blood pressure. Several studies have shown that it is more cost-effective to identify potential risks based on overall CVD risk than on blood pressure or cholesterol levels alone (Gaziano and others 2005; Lim and others 2007; Rubinstein and others 2010). Similar analyses have been done for cholesterol treatment, and guidelines have been set in both Europe and the United States, while the WHO has moved to global risk-based assessments for initiating statin-based medications. Murray and others (2003) showed that lowering cholesterol for persons at high cardiovascular risk (absolute risk greater than 35 percent) was cost-effective.

Diabetes

The costs associated with mortality and morbidity from diabetes worldwide are staggering. People with diabetes consume two to three times the health care resources of persons without diabetes, and diabetes consumes up to 15 percent of national health care budgets (Zhang and others 2010). Management of persons with diabetes includes control of glucose levels through medications as well as screening for and managing the secondary microvascular complications of diabetes, including retinopathy, nephropathy, and peripheral neuropathy. Although diabetes is associated with increased risk of macrovascular complications, such as strokes and myocardial infarctions, randomized trials have not shown consistent reductions in macrovascular endpoints, and most of the cost-effectiveness literature has focused on microvascular complications.

One study in India found that conducting a telemedicine retinopathy screening program for diabetics in rural areas either once or twice in a lifetime and providing photocoagulation for persons screening positive were cost-effective at US$1,320 and US$1,343 per QALY

gained, respectively (Rachapelle and others 2013). Some interventions, although not studied in LMICs, should receive strong consideration, given the overwhelmingly positive results in HICs.

Intensive treatment of blood pressure in diabetics through the use of generic statins is cost saving, especially for persons older than age 60 years (Li and others 2010). Screening for microalbuminuria five years after the onset of diabetes and treatment with angiotensin-converting enzyme inhibitors (ACEi) is also cost saving for the prevention of end-stage renal disease. Use of angiotensin receptor blockers is cost saving and highly cost-effective in HICs. Other potentially cost-saving interventions include comprehensive foot care to prevent ulcers.

Rheumatic Heart Disease

Acute rheumatic fever remains the most important cause of acquired heart disease in children and young adults in the world (Carapetis, McDonald, and Wilson 2005). Although it is rarely fatal, each case is responsible for the loss of up to 16 years of life and 3 QALYs due to disability (Michaud and Narula 1999). For this reason, the World Heart Federation made the elimination of acute rheumatic fever and control of rheumatic heart disease one of the six main goals in its strategic plan through 2015. In most LMICs, prevention has focused on secondary prevention among persons who have had a previous episode of rheumatic fever. This approach includes life-long treatment with penicillin, either orally or through intramuscular injections.

Secondary prevention in persons without a previous episode of acute rheumatic fever, through screening with echocardiography, was also found to be cost-effective at less than US$100 per QALY gained (Tian and others 2015). In the absence of a vaccine against group A streptococcal infection, primary prevention depends on short-term oral or intramuscular penicillin treatment of patients presenting with acute sore throat (pharyngitis) caused by the infection.

Yet, primary prevention has not been widely adopted in LMICs because of barriers to implementation and cost-effectiveness (Karthikeyan and Mayosi 2009). More recently, investigators have found that using a clinical scoring mechanism not based on lab results followed by intramuscular injection with penicillin for persons judged to be positive would be cost-effective at US$150 per QALY gained for children ages 3–15 years presenting with sore throat in South Africa (Irlam and others 2013).

First-Level Hospital Care

Treatment with aspirin, blood pressure medications, and statins is the cost-effective mainstay for managing the care of persons with a previous stroke or ischemic heart disease event. Unfortunately, use of appropriately recommended medications is extremely low in many countries. Medications such as aspirin, ACEi, beta blockers, and statins have been shown to be cost-effective, with costs less than US$1,000 per DALY averted in all LMIC regions (Gaziano, Opie, and Weinstein 2006; Lim and others 2007). Unfortunately, costs to individuals and access to medications may be limiting the full benefit of life-saving medications. This section discusses methods for improving access and availability as well as adherence. Overcoming these challenges is critical to the primary and secondary prevention that occurs at primary health centers and outpatient care facilities in first-level hospitals.

Drug Availability and Adherence

Several factors are responsible for the low use of medications, including inadequate availability and access to affordable medications, scarcity of health care providers, and complicated medication regimens. In many LMICs, the cost of a month's supply of generic secondary prevention medications ranges from 1.5 to 18.4 times the daily wage of government workers (Mendis, Fukino, and others 2007), and the availability of cardiovascular medications ranges from 25 percent in the public sector to 60 percent in the private sector (Cameron and others 2011; van Mourik and others 2010).

The availability of generic medications was influenced by the Agreement on Trade-Related Aspects of Intellectual Property Rights (TRIPS Agreement) in 1995; the agreement obliged World Trade Organization members to protect pharmaceutical patents for 20 years from their filing (Smith, Lee, and Drager 2009). The subsequent Doha Declaration in 2003 granted nations compulsory licenses to manufacture essential medications domestically without permission of the patent holder, a trend that increased until 2006 (Beall and Kuhn 2012; Correa 2006; Lybecker and Fowler 2009). Canada is the only country to have issued a compulsory license to export generic medications to poorer nations, helping increase the availability of generic medications (Lybecker and Fowler 2009). Other studies have shown that, from 2001 to 2011, generic medications in the private sectors of 19 countries in Latin America, the Middle East, and South Africa accounted for approximately 70 percent to 80 percent of market share, which is larger than in most European countries (Kaplan, Wirtz, and Stephens 2013).

The literature on interventions to improve medication adherence is sparse. Recent reports suggest that lower out-of-pocket expenses, case management, patient education with behavioral support, and mobile phone messaging, supported by broader guidelines and regulatory and communication-based policies, may improve adherence (De Jongh and others 2012; Laba and others 2013; Tajouri, Driver, and Holmes 2014; Viswanathan and others 2012). In this context, the Post-Myocardial Infarction Free Rx Event and Economic Evaluation trial in the United States has shown that eliminating copayments for drugs after a myocardial infarction increases medication adherence to 49.0 percent from 35.9 percent (Choudhry and others 2011). Furthermore, insurance plans that were generous, targeted high-risk patients, offered wellness programs, did not offer disease management programs, and covered medications ordered by mail were associated with a 4 to 5 percentage point higher rate of medication adherence (Choudhry and others 2014). While these studies are promising, future research is needed to determine whether the models could be replicated successfully in LMICs.

One way to address availability and affordability is to give a combination of generic CVD medications (polypill) to all adults with significant risk for CVD (Wald and Law 2003). This single intervention could reduce ischemic heart disease by as much as 50 percent.

The use of a polypill in primary prevention reduces the need for dose titrations, improves adherence, and increases the use of cheap generics in a single formulation (Lonn and others 2010). Several studies have shown reductions in risk factors, such as blood pressure and cholesterol levels (Yusuf and others 2009), and improvements in adherence. The most promising study to date included persons with established heart disease and persons at high risk for CVD. In the UMPIRE (Use of a Multi-drug Pill in Reducing Cardiovascular Events) study, patients who received the fixed-dose combination pill had increased adherence of more than 20 percent and reductions in both cholesterol and blood pressure levels (Thom and others 2013). However, no study has yet been published with reductions in ischemic heart disease or stroke endpoints, although several are underway (Eguzo and Camazine 2013; Lonn and others 2010; Yusuf and others 2009).

The use of a polypill in secondary prevention is less controversial because, even though no trial has proved its efficacy in secondary prevention, multiple trials have shown that the individual component medications (aspirin, statins, beta blockers, and angiotensin II receptor blockers) improve outcomes in patients with known CVD or high levels of risk factors (Lonn and others 2010). A large case-control analysis of 13,029 patients with ischemic heart disease in the United Kingdom indicated that combinations of medications (statin, aspirin, and beta blockers) decrease mortality in patients with known CVD better than single medications (Hippisley-Cox and

Coupland 2005). Finally, the use of combination therapy was shown to be cost-effective in LMICs for both primary and secondary prevention, with the best cost-effectiveness ratio for secondary prevention (Gaziano and others 2005; Lim and others 2007).

Heart Failure

Diuretics are the mainstay treatment for heart failure. They have been shown to be cost-effective for managing hypertension in HICs (Tran and others 2007) and LMICs (Alefan and others 2009), but their cost-effectiveness has not been evaluated for the treatment of heart failure. However, congestive heart failure (CHF) is associated with much higher risks and costs than hypertension, and the relative risk reduction for CHF is similar to that for hypertension, making it safe to infer that diuretics are cost-effective. All other agents for CHF have been compared with a baseline of diuretic therapy. ACEi are an integral part of the treatment of patients with CHF, both reducing costly admissions and prolonging life. Cost-effectiveness studies dating back to the 1990s have shown them to be either highly cost-effective or cost saving in HICs (Butler and Fletcher 1996; Paul and others 1994; Tsevat and others 1995). Their use was found to be cost saving when added to diuretics in all six LMIC regions or to be extremely cost-effective (US$50 per DALY averted) in areas with limited access to hospitals (Gaziano 2005).

Beta blockers are equally integral for managing patients with CHF with reduced ejection fraction. Similar cost-effectiveness results were seen in HICs in the late 1990s for carvedilol and in the early 2000s for metoprolol of less than US$30,000 per QALY gained to as low as US$4,000 per QALY gained (Delea and others 1999; Levy and others 2001). However, these agents cost up to US$500–US$1,000 per year. When analysis was repeated using generic pricing in all six LMIC regions, the incremental cost-effectiveness ratios were extremely favorable, ranging from US$124 to US$219 per DALY averted (Gaziano 2005). Mineralocorticoid agents have a favorable health profile in patients with reduced-systolic-function CHF, reducing both all-cause mortality and hospitalizations. Although eplerenone has proved to be cost-effective in HICs (Weintraub and others 2005), its cost-effectiveness has not been evaluated in LMICs (McKenna and others 2010). One limitation to its use is the need for blood tests to monitor renal function and electrolytes.

Devices such as implantable cardioverter defibrillators for persons with advanced heart failure have been found to be cost-effective in HICs. In LMICs, they have been evaluated in Brazil, with an incremental cost-effectiveness ratio of US$50,000 per QALY gained

(Ribeiro and others 2010). When compared with medical therapy in Brazil, implantable cardiac resynchronization therapy was even more cost-effective, at US$17,700 per QALY gained in 2012 U.S. dollars. When both capabilities were combined in the same device, the incremental cost-effectiveness ratio was nearly US$33,000 per QALY gained (Bertoldi and others 2013). Similar values were found in Argentina (Poggio and others 2012).

Respiratory Conditions

There is relatively little information about the costs of treating and managing respiratory conditions in LMICs. One economic modeling study indicated that chronic obstructive pulmonary disease (COPD) and asthma interventions had poor cost-effectiveness compared with interventions for other chronic conditions because they relied on expensive imported drugs and, in the case of COPD, had relatively few health gains. Only one inhaled corticosteroid was available in the Colombian health insurance plan, and it was the most cost-effective therapy for treating pediatric asthma patients. The next best option cost more than US$55,000 per QALY gained (Rodriguez-Martinez, Sossa-Briceno, and Castro-Rodriguez 2013). Using low-dose inhaled corticosteroids for mild asthma was relatively inexpensive and averted a sizable number of DALYs. Using low-dose inhaled corticosteroids for mild persistent asthma cost about US$2,321 per DALY averted in Sub-Saharan African countries and about US$1,133 per DALY averted in South-East Asian countries. Using low-dose inhaled corticosteroids plus long-acting beta agonists for moderate to persistent asthma cost about US$4,763 per DALY averted in Sub-Saharan Africa and US$1,878 per DALY averted in South-East Asia. Prescription treatment of COPD stage II (inhaled bronchodilator) cost about US$11,000 and US$5,000 in Sub-Saharan Africa and South-East Asia, respectively. While all three interventions had about the same costs per DALY averted in each region, they were much more expensive in Sub-Saharan Africa than in South-East Asia (Stanciole and others 2012).

Acute and Hospital-Based Care

Acute Ischemic Heart Disease

Management of persons with acute myocardial infarction has been shown to be cost-effective in all six LMIC regions. Using aspirin in the acute setting for ST elevation myocardial infarction (STEMI) costs between US$10 and US$20 per QALY gained (Gaziano 2005). Using generic beta blockers costs only US$2 per QALY gained more than using aspirin alone (Gaziano 2005). Using a combination of aspirin, beta blockers, ACEi, and statins in the acute phase was cost-effective in China for acute myocardial infarction, at US$3,100 per QALY gained. Additional treatment of patients with the antiplatelet agent clopidogrel had a higher incremental cost-effectiveness ratio of nearly US$18,000 per QALY gained. Use of unfractionated heparin for patients with acute coronary syndrome was found to be quite cost-effective at US$2,800 per QALY gained.

Generic thrombolytics such as streptokinase can be added for approximately US$700 per QALY gained in an emergency ward capable of administering intravenous medications with physician supervision (Gaziano 2005). Thrombolysis was not evaluated separately in China, but the use of streptokinase in secondary hospitals or percutaneous coronary interventions in hospitals had a combined ratio of approximately US$9,000 per QALY gained (Wang and others 2014). Using primary percutaneous coronary interventions alone for persons with STEMI was US$10,700 per QALY gained in China. In Brazil, delivering thrombolysis with tenecteplase within 60 minutes of an event by paramedics in a prehospital environment was shown to be cost saving (Araujo and others 2008). This intervention requires a highly developed emergency response team with educated paramedics and physicians able to diagnose and rule out contraindications to thrombolysis. Although patients with chest pain should ideally go to an emergency department capable of treating both STEMI and non-STEMI, in areas where advanced emergency transport systems are lacking and where patients seek treatment from their primary doctors, such as in rural India, it is more cost-effective, at US$13 per QALY gained, to use a prehospital electrocardiogram machine than to do nothing (Schulman-Marcus, Prabhakaran, and Gaziano 2010).

Kidney Disease

Like diabetes, patients with chronic kidney disease can gain significant benefits from aggressive blood pressure and lipid control. However, no studies of these interventions have been conducted in LMICs. In particular, patients with chronic kidney disease would benefit particularly from the use of ACEi and statins as well as from screening for proteinuria.

COSTS OF PREVENTION AND TREATMENT OF CVRDs IN LMICs

To complement this review of cost-effectiveness, a systematic literature review was conducted of intervention costs for CVRDs in LMICs from the provider's perspective, given that these costs are poorly understood (Brouwer and Levin 2015). The review focuses on

diabetes, chronic kidney disease, hypertension, stroke, ischemic heart disease, and nonischemic heart disease because of their interrelated risk factors, prevention strategies, and interventions, such as tobacco cessation or hypertension control. Total costs of prevention or treatment per person or per year were inflated to 2012 U.S. dollars for comparability across geographic settings and time periods. The methodology for the review is provided in annex 19A.

The review found that prevention of CVD and related diseases is much less expensive than treatment, although many treatments are cost-effective using standard income thresholds. Most current treatment costs are very high in LMICs, and little is known about the costs of scaling up prevention and early treatment to avoid more catastrophic expenditures. The least expensive interventions were prevention strategies to reduce tobacco use and salt consumption at the population level, while the treatment of chronic kidney disease was the most expensive, followed by surgical interventions for ischemic heart disease. Promotion policies for salt, tobacco, and cholesterol control were inexpensive, at less than US$1.00 per person per year, ranging from about US$0.15 per person per year for mass media campaigns to US$0.80 per person per year for cholesterol control (Ha and Chisholm 2011). The costs of tobacco cessation programs varied, depending on whether individual- or population-based platforms were used. For example, average unit costs ranged from less than US$0.01 per person per year for package warnings in Vietnam (Salomon and others 2012) to US$10,000 per person per year for school-based smoking cessation programs in India (Brown and others 2013). These cost estimates are useful when considering whether to scale up national prevention programs because low per capita costs can quickly translate into high overall program costs depending on the country's population and its geographic distribution.

Treating CVD and its risk factors is complex, in part because of the interrelationship between hypertension, diabetes, and ischemic heart disease and the fact that multiple shared risk factors affect CVD health outcomes. The clinical heterogeneity of CVD can make treatment costs for a single condition much more variable than for infectious or some other chronic diseases. For example, CVD encompasses different types of heart and related diseases, such as hypertension, stroke, and heart failure, with different levels of severity, associated care, and management. Nonetheless, age-adjusted CVD mortality has continued to decline in both HICs and LMICs as a result of an abundance of both policy- and individual-level interventions reviewed in this chapter. As indicated, numerous clinical protocols are available for treating complicated conditions, including different combinations of medications, different diagnostics and imaging technologies, different surgeries, and different requirements for inpatient care and follow-up visits, making cost comparisons between studies all but impossible. Additionally, clinical characteristics, capabilities, and practices vary widely among and within countries; the distribution of costs can vary widely even within a hospital offering different levels of care, such as general, specialty, and intensive care (Khealani and others 2003).

Primary prevention and early management of care can occur at primary care levels with less sophisticated human resource and equipment needs, making local health delivery platforms an attractive option in low-resource settings. There is currently a small but growing body of evidence for CVD treatment and prevention costs in MICs, with fewer in LICs.

CRITICAL RESEARCH GAPS

The lack of data on costs and effectiveness, particularly data from or focused on LMICs, limits the ability of decision makers to plan and allocate resources efficiently and may also result in the underuse of cost-effective interventions (Bloom and others 2014).

Limited evidence of the cost-effectiveness of interventions for cardiometabolic diseases in LMICs largely reflects the limited evidence of intervention effectiveness. The lack of such information makes undertaking cost-effectiveness studies in LMICs very difficult, leading to the use of modeling approaches. It also limits the ability of decision makers to assess whether interventions with demonstrated cost-effectiveness in other countries are likely to be replicable with similar results in a particular country.

Population- and community-level interventions that appear to be the most cost-effective are inherently difficult to evaluate, further complicating assessment. Unlike individual-level interventions, attributing health outcomes to specific interventions is generally difficult, if not impossible. For instance, because interventions can take place outside the health system (for example, through fiscal policy changes or urban planning), assessing their costs can be more difficult than for interventions made through the health system. Nonetheless, the studies discussed in this chapter demonstrate the possibility of producing valuable data.

Additional research is needed on fiscal and regulatory policy changes and other population-level interventions to address the risk factors and burden of cardiometabolic disease. The lack of data on interventions to improve diets and increase physical activity in LMICs is a particular concern.

Comparability is also a concern. Cost data on clinical treatments often reflect experiences in urban areas (more often from middle-income than from low-income countries). Such costs may not be transferable to rural areas and may not be appropriate for making regional or national assessments. Cost comparability would benefit from a more consistent methodology and clear presentation of data on the elements and drivers of cost. Using established, accepted intervention protocols to guide economic evaluations and enable comparability of cost reporting has the potential to improve comparability across studies.

A related issue is the limited availability of longitudinal studies in LMICs, particularly studies concerned with population- and community-level interventions. Without such studies, decision makers will have difficulty both assessing trends, including cost-scale and cost-quality relationships, and prioritizing interventions. This issue is particularly relevant given the significance of generational and age differences for CVD risk factors and intervention strategies in LMICs.

Also needed is research on the costs of scaling up prevention and early treatment in LMICs and the systematic capture of successful experiences and transferable practices in designing and embedding such programs in LMICs, particularly in low-resource settings. In sum, targeted studies focused on LMICs are critical to tailoring responses to CVDs that have actual impacts and are cost-effective. Particularly needed is research on the costs of population-level prevention interventions; low-cost, community-based prevention strategies; strategies for individual-level interventions and platforms to reach low-resource populations; comparable treatment and prevention costs in lower-resource settings; evidence and experience on the design, replicability, scale-up, and implementation costs of interventions in LMICs; and quality data on costs to inform the design, implementation, and scale-up of evidence-based interventions in these countries.

CONCLUSIONS

Many interventions are available for managing cardiovascular, kidney, and respiratory diseases, which account for a large portion of NCDs globally. HICs as well as some LMICs have seen dramatic declines in age-adjusted mortality related to these conditions as a result of many clinical and policy-based interventions. Some interventions have been shown to be cost-effective in both HICs and LMICs, while others need further evaluation.

The burden of CVD is growing in many LMICs, and future research should put greater emphasis on nonclinical interventions. Significant differences in outcome measures and methodologies preclude the ranking of interventions by their degree of cost-effectiveness. Appropriate calibrations should be used when transferring effectiveness estimates from HICs for the purpose of modeling cost-effectiveness in LMICs. In rare instances, studies of CVD risk factors and intervention follow-up are needed. Some pharmaceutical strategies are cost-effective.

Clarification is needed on the diagnostic approach to targeting a single high-risk factor versus absolute risk, the role of patient compliance, and the potential consequences of large-scale medicalization for public health.

ANNEX

The annex to this chapter is as follows. It is available at http://www.dcp-3.org/CVRD.

- Annex 19A. Methods, Framework, and Results

NOTES

World Bank Income Classifications as of July 2014 are as follows, based on estimates of gross national income (GNI) per capita for 2013:

- Low-income countries (LICs) = US$1,045 or less
- Middle-income countries (MICs) are subdivided:
  (a) lower-middle-income = US$1,046 to US$4,125
  (b) upper-middle-income (UMICs) = US$4,126 to US$12,745
- High-income countries (HICs) = US$12,746 or more.

1. As of September 2016, several jurisdictions, including France, Mexico, Berkeley in California, St. Helena, and some islands in the South Pacific, have introduced taxation on SSBs. Hungary has introduced taxes on SSBs, salty condiments, and some snack foods. Finland has introduced taxes on sweets, ice cream, and soft drinks. Norway has introduced taxes on SSBs, chocolate, and sugar. Denmark is the only country that has explicitly introduced (and subsequently withdrawn) a tax on foods high in saturated fat for health purposes (Wareham and Jebb 2015).
2. Two related meta-analyses also provide relevant information on food price elasticities in low, middle-, and high-income countries. While Green and others (2013) focused on own-price elasticities of a range of aggregate food groups, Cornelsen and others (2014) undertook a meta-analysis of cross-price elasticities worldwide. Both studies concluded that changes in food prices have the largest own-price effects in LICs, while cross-price effects are more varied and depend on country income level, reinforcing, undermining, or alleviating own-price effects.
3. For a review of the cost-effectiveness of brief interventions to promote physical activity predominantly in a primary care context, see Vijay and others (2015).

4. For additional examples of economic modeling to inform health priorities, see Vos and others (2010) or various background reports to the United Kingdom's National Institute for Health and Care Excellence public health guidance (Morgovan and others 2010), available for a wide and growing range of topics (https://www.nice.org.uk/guidance/published?type=ph).
5. Countries vary in the opportunity costs they face when using resources for new interventions, with opportunity costs defined as the health gains forgone because resources are not available to deliver interventions elsewhere in the health system. Opportunity costs should—in principle—be reflected in the cost-effectiveness threshold (Revill and others 2015).

REFERENCES

Afshin, A., R. Micha, M. Webb, S. Capewell, L. Whitsel, and others. 2017. "Effectiveness of Dietary Policies to Reduce Noncommunicable Diseases." In *Disease Control Priorities* (third edition): Volume 5, *Cardiovascular, Respiratory, and Related Disorders*, edited by D. Prabhakaran, S. Anand, T. A. Gaziano, J.-C. Mbanya, Y. Wu, and R. Nugent. Washington, DC: World Bank.

Alefan, Q., M. I. M. Ibrahim, T. A. Razak, and A. Ayub. 2009. "Cost-Effectiveness of Antihypertensive Treatment in Malaysia." *Malaysian Journal of Pharmaceutical Sciences* 7 (2): 137–52.

Allen, K., J. Pearson-Stuttard, W. Hooton, P. Diggle, S. Capewell, and others. 2015. "Potential of Trans Fats Policies to Reduce Socioeconomic Inequalities in Mortality from Coronary Heart Disease in England: Cost-Effectiveness Modelling Study." *BMJ* 351 (September 15): h4583.

Araujo, D. V., B. R. Tura, A. L. Brasileiro, H. L. Neto, A. L. Pavao, and others. 2008. "Cost-Effectiveness of Prehospital versus Inhospital Thrombolysis in Acute Myocardial Infarction (Structured Abstract)." *Arquivos Brasileiros de Cardiologia* 90 (2): 91–98.

Asaria, P., D. Chisholm, C. Mathers, M. Ezzati, and R. Beaglehole. 2007. "Chronic Disease Prevention: Health Effects and Financial Costs of Strategies to Reduce Salt Intake and Control Tobacco Use." *The Lancet* 370 (9604): 2044–53.

Assmann, G., P. Cullen, and H. Schulte. 2002. "Simple Scoring Scheme for Calculating the Risk of Acute Coronary Events Based on the 10-Year Follow-Up of the Prospective Cardiovascular Munster (PROCAM) Study." *Circulation* 105 (3): 310–15.

Beall, R., and R. Kuhn. 2012. "Trends in Compulsory Licensing of Pharmaceuticals since the Doha Declaration: A Database Analysis." *PLoS Medicine* 9 (1): e100115.

Bertoldi, E. G., L. E. Rohde, L. I. Zimerman, M. Pimentel, and C. A. Polanczyk. 2013. "Cost-Effectiveness of Cardiac Resynchronization Therapy in Patients with Heart Failure: The Perspective of a Middle-Income Country's Public Health System." *International Journal of Cardiology* 163 (3): 309–15.

Bloom, D. E., E. T. Cafiero-Fonseca, V. Candeias, E. Adashi, L. Bloom, and others. 2014. *Economics of Non-Communicable*

Diseases in India: The Costs and Returns on Investment of Interventions to Promote Healthy Living and Prevent, Treat, and Manage NCDs. Geneva: World Economic Forum; Cambridge, MA: Harvard School of Public Health.

Brouwer, E., and C. Levin. 2015. "Provider Costs for Prevention and Treatment of Cardiovascular and Related Conditions in Low- and Middle-Income Countries: A Systematic Review." *BMC Public Health* 15 (November 26): 1183.

Brown, H. S., III, M. Stigler, C. Perry, P. Dhavan, M. Arora, and others. 2013. "The Cost-Effectiveness of a School-Based Smoking Prevention Program in India." *Health Promotion International* 28 (2): 178–86.

Butler, J. R., and P. J. Fletcher. 1996. "A Cost-Effectiveness Analysis of Enalapril Maleate in the Management of Congestive Heart Failure in Australia." *Australian and New Zealand Journal of Medicine* 26 (1): 89–95.

Cabrera Escobar, M. A., J. L. Veerman, S. M. Tollman, M. Y. Bertram, and K. J. Hofman. 2013. "Evidence That a Tax on Sugar Sweetened Beverages Reduces the Obesity Rate: A Meta-Analysis." *BMC Public Health* 13 (November 13): 1072.

Cameron, A., I. Roubos, M. Ewen, A. K. Mantel-Teeuwisse, H. G. Leufkens, and others. 2011. "Differences in the Availability of Medicines for Chronic and Acute Conditions in the Public and Private Sectors of Developing Countries." *Bulletin of the World Health Organization* 89 (6): 412–21.

Carapetis, J. R., M. McDonald, and N. J. Wilson. 2005. "Acute Rheumatic Fever." *The Lancet* 366 (9480): 155–68.

Cawley, J. 2015. "An Economy of Scales: A Selective Review of Obesity's Economic Causes, Consequences, and Solutions." *Journal of Health Economics* 43 (September): 244–68.

Cawley, J., and D. Frisvold. 2015. "The Incidence of Taxes on Sugar-Sweetened Beverages: The Case of Berkeley, California." Working Paper 21465, National Bureau of Economic Research, Cambridge, MA.

Cecchini, M., F. Sassi, J. A. Lauer, Y. Y. Lee, V. Guajardo-Barron, and others. 2010. "Tackling of Unhealthy Diets, Physical Inactivity, and Obesity: Health Effects and Cost-Effectiveness." *The Lancet* 376 (9754): 1775–84.

Chang, A., D. T. Jamison, and S. Horton. 2018. "Benefit-Cost Analysis." In *Disease Control Priorities* (third edition): Volume 9, *Disease Control Priorities: Improving Health and Reducing Poverty*, edited by D. T. Jamison, R. Nugent, H. Gelband, S. Horton, P. Jha, R. Laxminarayan, and C. N. Mock. Washington, DC: World Bank.

Choudhry, N. K., J. Avorn, R. J. Glynn, E. M. Antman, S. Schneeweiss, and others. 2011. "Full Coverage for Preventive Medications after Myocardial Infarction." *New England Journal of Medicine* 365 (22): 2088–97.

Choudhry, N. K., S. Dugani, W. H. Shrank, J. M. Polinski, C. E. Stark, and others. 2014. "Despite Increased Use and Sales of Statins in India, per Capita Prescription Rates Remain Far below High-Income Countries." *Health Affairs* 33 (2): 273–82.

Chow, J., S. R. Darley, and R. Laxminarayan. 2007. "Cost-Effectiveness of Disease Interventions in India." Discussion Paper dp-07-53, Resources for the Future, Washington, DC.

Claxton, K., M. Sculpher, and A. Culyer. 2007. "Appropriate Methods for the Evaluation of Public Health Interventions." CHE Research Paper 31, Centre for Health Economics, York.

Claxton, K., S. Walker, S. Palmer, and M. Sculpher. 2010. "Appropriate Perspectives for Health Care Decisions." CHE Research Paper 54, Centre for Health Economics, York.

Colchero, M. A., B. M. Popkin, J. A. Rivea, and S. W. Ng. 2016. "Beverage Purchases from Stores in Mexico under the Excise Tax on Sugar-Sweetened Beverages: Observational Study." *BMJ* 352 (January 6): h6704.

Conroy, R. M., K. Pyorala, A. P. Fitzgerald, S. Sans, A. Menotti, and others. 2003. "Estimation of Ten-Year Risk of Fatal Cardiovascular Disease in Europe: The SCORE Project." *European Heart Journal* 24 (11): 987–1003.

Cornelsen, L., R. Green, A. Dangour, and R. Smith. 2015. "Why Fat Taxes Won't Make Us Thin." *Journal of Public Health* 37 (1): 18–23.

Cornelsen, L., R. Green, R. Turner, A. Dangour, B. Shankar, and others. 2014. "What Happens to Patterns of Food Consumption When Food Prices Change? Evidence from a Systematic Review and Meta-Analysis of Food Price Elasticities Globally." *Health Economics* 24 (12): 1548–59.

Correa, C. M. 2006. "Implications of Bilateral Free Trade Agreements on Access to Medicines." *Bulletin of the World Health Organization* 84 (5): 399–404.

De Jongh, T., I. Gurol-Urganci, V. Vodopivec-Jamsek, J. Car, and R. Atun. 2012. "Mobile Phone Messaging for Facilitating Self-Management of Long-Term Illnesses." *Cochrane Database of Systematic Reviews* 12 (December 12): CD007459.

Delea, T. E., M. Vera-Llonch, R. E. Richner, M. B. Fowler, and G. Oster. 1999. "Cost-Effectiveness of Carvedilol for Heart Failure." *American Journal of Cardiology* 83 (6): 890–96.

Donaldson, E. A., H. R. Waters, M. Arora, B. Varghese, P. Dave, and others. 2011. "A Cost-Effectiveness Analysis of India's 2008 Prohibition of Smoking in Public Places in Gujarat." *International Journal of Environmental Research and Public Health* 8 (5): 1271–86.

Downs, S., A. M. Thow, and S. R. Leeder. 2013. "The Effectiveness of Policies for Reducing Dietary Trans Fat: A Systematic Review of the Evidence." *Bulletin of the World Health Organization* 91 (4): 262–69H.

Eguzo, K., and B. Camazine. 2013. "Beyond Limitations: Practical Strategies for Improving Cancer Care in Nigeria." *Asian Pacific Journal of Cancer Prevention* 14 (5): 3363–68.

Epstein, L. H., N. Jankowiak, C. Nederkoorn, H. A. Raynor, S. A. French, and E. Finkelstein. 2012. "Experimental Research on the Relation between Food Price Changes and Food-Purchasing Patterns: A Targeted Review." *American Journal of Clinical Nutrition* 95 (4): 789–809.

Eyles, H., C. Ni Mhurchu, N. Nghiem, and T. Blakely. 2012. "Food Pricing Strategies, Population Diets, and Non-communicable Disease: A Systematic Review of Simulation Studies." *PLoS Medicine* 9 (12): e1001353.

Ferrante, D., J. Konfino, R. Mejia, P. Coxson, A. Moran, and others. 2012. "The Cost-Utility Ratio of Reducing Salt Intake and Its Impact on the Incidence of Cardiovascular Disease in Argentina." *Revista Panamericana de Salud Pública* 32 (4): 274–80.

Ferrario, M., P. Chiodini, L. E. Chambless, G. Cesana, D. Vanuzzo, and others. 2005. "Prediction of Coronary

Events in a Low-Incidence Population: Assessing Accuracy of the CUORE Cohort Study Prediction Equation." *International Journal of Epidemiology* 34 (2): 413–21.

Ford, E. S., and S. Capewell. 2011. "Proportion of the Decline in Cardiovascular Mortality Disease due to Prevention versus Treatment: Public Health versus Clinical Care." *Annual Review of Public Health* 32 (April): 5–22.

Gaziano, T. A. 2005. "Cardiovascular Disease in the Developing World and Its Cost-Effective Management." *Circulation* 112 (23): 3547–53.

Gaziano, T. A., S. Abrahams-Gessel, S. Alam, D. Alam, M. Ali, and others. 2016. "Comparison of Nonblood-Based and Blood-Based Total CV Risk Scores in Global Populations." *Global Heart* 11 (1): 37–46.

Gaziano, T. A., S. Abrahams-Gessel, C. A. Denman, C. M. Montano, M. Khanam, and others. 2015. "An Assessment of Community Health Workers' Ability to Screen for Cardiovascular Disease Risk with a Simple, Non-Invasive Risk Assessment Instrument in Bangladesh, Guatemala, Mexico, and South Africa: An Observational Study." *The Lancet Global Health* 3 (9): e556–63.

Gaziano, T. A., S. Abrahams-Gessel, S. Surka, S. Sy, A. Pandya, and others. 2015. "Cardiovascular Disease Screening by Community Health Workers Can Be Cost-Effective in Low-Resource Countries." *Health Affairs* 34 (9): 1538–45.

Gaziano, T. A., M. Bertram, S. M. Tollman, and K. J. Hofman. 2014. "Hypertension Education and Adherence in South Africa: A Cost-Effectiveness Analysis of Community Health Workers." *BMC Public Health* 14 (March 10): 240.

Gaziano, T. A., L. H. Opie, and M. C. Weinstein. 2006. "Cardiovascular Disease Prevention with a Multidrug Regimen in the Developing World: A Cost-Effectiveness Analysis." *The Lancet* 368 (9536): 679–86.

Gaziano, T. A., A. Pandya, K. Steyn, N. Levitt, W. Mollentze, and others. 2013. "Comparative Assessment of Absolute Cardiovascular Disease Risk Characterization from Non-Laboratory-Based Risk Assessment in South African Populations." *BMC Medicine* 11 (July 24): 170.

Gaziano, T. A., K. Steyn, D. J. Cohen, M. C. Weinstein, and L. H. Opie. 2005. "Cost-Effectiveness Analysis of Hypertension Guidelines in South Africa: Absolute Risk versus Blood Pressure Level." *Circulation* 112 (23): 3569–76.

Greco, G., P. Lorgelly, and I. Yamabhai. 2016. "Outcomes in Economic Evaluations of Public Health Interventions in Low- and Middle-Income Countries: Health, Capabilities, and Subjective Wellbeing." *Health Economics* 25 (1): 83–94.

Green, R., L. Cornelsen, A. D. Dangour, R. Turner, B. Shankar, and others. 2013. "The Effect of Rising Food Prices on Food Consumption: Systematic Review with Meta-Regression." *BMJ* 346 (June 17): f3703.

Grogger, J. 2015. "Soda Taxes and the Prices of Sodas and Other Drinks: Evidence from Mexico." Working Paper 21197, National Bureau of Economic Research, Cambridge, MA.

Ha, D. A., and D. Chisholm. 2011. "Cost-Effectiveness Analysis of Interventions to Prevent Cardiovascular Disease in Vietnam." *Health Policy and Planning* 26 (3): 210–22.

Higashi, H., K. D. Truong, J. J. Barendregt, P. K. Nguyen, M. L. Vuong, and others. 2011. "Cost-Effectiveness of

Tobacco Control Policies in Vietnam: The Case of Population-Level Interventions." *Applied Health Economics and Health Policy* 9 (3): 183–96.

Hippisley-Cox, J., and C. Coupland. 2005. "Effect of Combinations of Drugs on All Cause Mortality in Patients with Ischaemic Heart Disease: Nested Case-Control Analysis." *BMJ* 330 (7499): 1059–63.

Hutton, G., and C. Chase. 2017. "Water Supply, Sanitation, and Hygiene." In *Disease Control Priorities* (third edition): Volume 7, *Injury Prevention and Environmental Health*, edited by C. N. Mock, O. Kobusingye, R. Nugent, and K. Smith. Washington, DC: World Bank.

Irlam, J., B. M. Mayosi, M. Engel, and T. A. Gaziano. 2013. "Primary Prevention of Acute Rheumatic Fever and Rheumatic Heart Disease with Penicillin in South African Children with Pharyngitis: A Cost-Effectiveness Analysis." *Circulation. Cardiovascular Quality and Outcomes* 6 (3): 343–51.

Jeemon, P., R. Gupta, C. Onen, A. Adler, T. A. Gaziano, and others. 2017. "Management of Hypertension and Dyslipidemia for Primary Prevention of Cardiovascular Disease." In *Disease Control Priorities* (third edition): Volume 5, *Cardiovascular, Respiratory, and Related Disorders*, edited by D. Prabhakaran, S. Anand, T. A. Gaziano, J.-C. Mbanya, Y. Wu, and R. Nugent. Washington, DC: World Bank.

Kaplan, W. A., V. J. Wirtz, and P. Stephens. 2013. "The Market Dynamics of Generic Medicines in the Private Sector of 19 Low- and Middle-Income Countries between 2001 and 2011: A Descriptive Time Series Analysis." *PLoS One* 8 (9): e74399.

Karthikeyan, G., and B. M. Mayosi. 2009. "Is Primary Prevention of Rheumatic Fever the Missing Link in the Control of Rheumatic Heart Disease in Africa?" *Circulation* 120 (8): 709–13.

Khealani, B., Z. F. Javed, N. Syed, S. Shafqat, and M. Wasay. 2003. "Cost of Acute Stroke Care at a Tertiary Care Hospital in Karachi, Pakistan." *Journal of Pakistan Medical Association* 53 (11): 552–55.

Laba, T. L., J. Bleasel, J. A. Brien, A. Cass, K. Howard, and others. 2013. "Strategies to Improve Adherence to Medications for Cardiovascular Diseases in Socioeconomically Disadvantaged Populations: A Systematic Review." *International Journal of Cardiology* 167 (6): 2430–40.

Laine, J., V. Kuvaia-Köllner, E. Pietilä, M. Koivuneva, H. Valtonen, and others. 2014. "Cost-Effectiveness of Population-Level Physical Activity Interventions: A Systematic Review." *American Journal of Health Promotion* 29 (2): 71–80.

Lehnert, T., D. Sonntag, A. Konnopka, S. Riedel-Heller, and H. König. 2012. "The Long-Term Cost-Effectiveness of Obesity Prevention Interventions: Systematic Literature Review." *Obesity Reviews* 13 (June): 537–53.

Levy, A. R., A. H. Briggs, C. Demers, and B. J. O'Brien. 2001. "Cost-Effectiveness of Beta-Blocker Therapy with Metoprolol or with Carvedilol for Treatment of Heart Failure in Canada." *American Heart Journal* 142 (3): 537–43.

Li, R., P. Zhang, L. E. Barker, F. M. Chowdhury, and Z. Zhang. 2010. "Cost-Effectiveness of Interventions to Prevent and

Control Diabetes Mellitus: A Systematic Review." *Diabetes Care* 33 (8): 1872–94.

Lim, S. S., T. A. Gaziano, E. Gakidou, K. S. Reddy, F. Farzadfar, and others. 2007. "Prevention of Cardiovascular Disease in High-Risk Individuals in Low-Income and Middle-Income Countries: Health Effects and Costs." *The Lancet* 370 (December 15): 2054–62.

Lonn, E., J. Bosch, K. K. Teo, P. Pais, D. Xavier, and others. 2010. "The Polypill in the Prevention of Cardiovascular Diseases: Key Concepts, Current Status, Challenges, and Future Directions." *Circulation* 122 (2): 2078–88.

Lybecker, K. M., and E. Fowler. 2009. "Compulsory Licensing in Canada and Thailand: Comparing Regimes to Ensure Legitimate Use of the WTO Rules." *Journal of Law and Medical Ethics* 37 (2): 222–39.

Manyema, M., L. Veerman, L. Chola, A. Tugendhaft, B. Sartorius, and others. 2014. "The Potential Impact of a 20% Tax on Sugar-Sweetened Beverages on Obesity in South African Adults: A Mathematical Model." *PLoS One* 9 (8): e105287.

Mason, H., A. Shoaibi, R. Ghandour, M. O'Flaherty, S. Capewell, and others. 2014. "A Cost-Effectiveness Analysis of Salt Reduction Policies to Reduce Coronary Heart Disease in Four Eastern Mediterranean Countries." *PLoS One* 9 (1): e84445.

McKenna, C., J. Burch, S. Suekarran, S. Walker, A. Bakhai, and others. 2010. "A Systematic Review and Economic Evaluation of the Clinical Effectiveness and Cost-Effectiveness of Aldosterone Antagonists for Postmyocardial Infarction Heart Failure." *Health Technology Assessment* 14 (24): 1–162.

Medina-Mora, M. E., M. Monteiro, R. Room, J. Rehm, D. Jernigan, and others. 2015. "Alcohol Use and Alcohol Use Disorders." In *Disease Control Priorities* (third edition): Volume 4, *Mental, Neurological, and Substance Use Disorders,* edited by V. Patel, D. Chisholm, T. Dua, R. Laxminarayan, and M. E. Medina-Mora. Washington, DC: World Bank.

Mendis, S., D. Abegunde, S. Yusuf, S. Ebrahim, G. Shaper, and others. 2005. "WHO Study on Prevention of Recurrences of Myocardial Infarction and Stroke (WHO-PREMISE)." *Bulletin of the World Health Organization* 83 (11): 820–29.

Mendis, S., K. Fukino, A. Cameron, R. Laing, A. Filipe Jr., and others. 2007. "The Availability and Affordability of Selected Essential Medicines for Chronic Diseases in Six Low- and Middle-Income Countries." *Bulletin of the World Health Organization* 85 (4): 279–88.

Mendis, S., L. Lindholm, G. Mancia, J. Whitworth, M. Alderman, and others. 2007. "World Health Organization (WHO) and International Society of Hypertension (ISH) Risk Prediction Charts: Assessment of Cardiovascular Risk for Prevention and Control of Cardiovascular Disease in Low- and Middle-Income Countries." *Journal of Hypertension* 25 (8): 1578–82.

Meng, L., H. Xu, A. Liu, J. van Raaij, W. Bemelmans, and others. 2013. "The Costs and Cost-Effectiveness of a School-Based Comprehensive Intervention Study on Childhood Obesity in China." *PLoS One* 8 (10): e77971.

Michaud, C. R. R., and J. Narula. 1999. "Cost-Effectiveness Analysis of Intervention Strategies for Reduction of the Burden of Rheumatic Heart Disease." In *Rheumatic Fever,* edited by J. Narula, R. Virmani, K. Srinath Reddy, and R. Tandon, 485–97. Washington, DC: American Registry of Pathology.

Morgovan, C., S. Cosma, S. Ghibu, C. Burta, M. Bota, and others. 2010. "Study of Diabetes Mellitus Care Cost in Romania during 2000–2008." *Fundamental and Clinical Pharmacology* 24 (1): 92.

Müller-Riemenschneider, F., T. Reinhold, and S. Willich. 2009. "Cost-Effectiveness of Interventions Promoting Physical Activity." *British Journal of Sports Medicine* 43 (1): 70–76.

Murray, C. J. L., J. A. Lauer, R. C. W. Hutubessy, L. Niessen, N. Tomijima, and others. 2003. "Effectiveness and Costs of Interventions to Lower Systolic Blood Pressure and Cholesterol: A Global and Regional Analysis on Reduction of Cardiovascular-Disease Risk." *The Lancet* 361 (9359): 717–25.

Navarro, J. C., A. C. Baroque II, J. K. Lokin, and N. Venketasubramanian. 2014. "The Real Stroke Burden in the Philippines." *International Journal of Stroke* 9 (5): 640–41.

Ortegon, M., S. Lim, D. Chisholm, and S. Mendis. 2012. "Cost-Effectiveness of Strategies to Combat Cardiovascular Disease, Diabetes, and Tobacco Use in Sub-Saharan Africa and South East Asia: Mathematical Modelling Study." *BMJ* 344 (March 2): e607.

Pandya, A., M. C. Weinstein, and T. A. Gaziano. 2011. "A Comparative Assessment of Non-Laboratory-Based versus Commonly Used Laboratory-Based Cardiovascular Disease Risk Scores in the NHANES III Population." *PLoS One* 6 (5): e20416.

Paul, S. D., K. M. Kuntz, K. A. Eagle, and M. C. Weinstein. 1994. "Costs and Effectiveness of Angiotensin Converting Enzyme Inhibition in Patients with Congestive Heart Failure." *Archives of Internal Medicine* 154 (10): 1143–49.

Pitt, C., C. Goodman, and K. Hanson. 2016. "Economic Evaluation in Global Perspective: A Bibliometric Analysis of the Recent Literature." *Health Economics* 25 (Suppl 1): 9–28.

Poggio, R., F. Augustovsky, J. Caporale, V. Irazola, and S. Miriuka. 2012. "Cost-Effectiveness of Cardiac Resynchronization Therapy: Perspective from Argentina." *International Journal of Technology Assessment in Health Care* 28 (4): 429–35.

Popkin, B. M., and C. Hawkes. 2015. "Sweetening of the Global Diet, Particularly Beverages: Patterns, Trends, and Policy Responses." *The Lancet Diabetes and Endocrinology* 4 (2): 174–86.

Powell, L. M., J. F. Chriqui, T. Khan, R. Wada, and F. J. Chaloupka. 2013. "Assessing the Potential Effectiveness of Food and Beverage Taxes and Subsidies for Improving Public Health: A Systematic Review of Prices, Demand and Body Weight Outcomes." *Obesity Reviews* 14 (2): 110–28.

Rachapelle, S., R. Legood, Y. Alavi, R. Lindfield, T. Sharma, and others. 2013. "The Cost-Utility of Telemedicine to Screen for Diabetic Retinopathy in India." *Ophthalmology* 120 (3): 566–73.

Ranson, M. K., P. Jha, F. J. Chaloupka, and S. N. Nguyen. 2002. "Global and Regional Estimates of the Effectiveness and Cost-Effectiveness of Price Increases and Other Tobacco

Control Policies (Structured Abstract)." *Nicotine and Tobacco Research* 4 (3): 311–19.

Revill, P., J. Ochalek, J. Lomas, R. Nakamura, B. Woods, and others. 2015. "Cost-Effectiveness Thresholds: Guiding Health Care Spending for Population Health Improvement." Centre for Health Economics, University of York. http://www.idsihealth.org/wp-content/uploads/2015/01/CE-Thresholds-iDSI-Working-Group-Final-Report.pdf.

Revill, P., and M. Sculpher. 2012. "Cost-Effectiveness of Interventions to Tackle Non-Communicable Diseases." *BMJ* 344 (March): d7883.

Ribeiro, R. A., S. F. Stella, S. A. Camey, L. I. Zimerman, M. Pimentel, and others. 2010. "Cost-Effectiveness of Implantable Cardioverter-Defibrillators in Brazil: Primary Prevention Analysis in the Public Sector." *Value in Health* 13 (2): 160–68.

Rodgers, A. L., C. Lawes, T. A. Gaziano, and T. Vos. 2006. "The Growing Burden of Risk from High Blood Pressure, Cholesterol, and Bodyweight." In *Disease Control Priorities in Developing Countries*, second edition, edited by D. T. Jamison, J. G. Breman, A. R. Measham, G. Alleyne, M. Claeson, D. B. Evans, P. Jha, A. Mills, and P. Musgrove. Washington, DC: World Bank and Oxford University Press.

Rodriguez-Martinez, C. E., M. P. Sossa-Briceno, and J. A. Castro-Rodriguez. 2013. "Cost-Utility Analysis of the Inhaled Steroids Available in a Developing Country for the Management of Pediatric Patients with Persistent Asthma." *Journal of Asthma* 50 (4): 410–18.

Rubinstein, A., L. Colantonio, A. Bardach, J. Caporale, S. G. Marti, and others. 2010. "Estimation of the Burden of Cardiovascular Disease Attributable to Modifiable Risk Factors and Cost-Effectiveness Analysis of Preventative Interventions to Reduce This Burden in Argentina." *BMC Public Health* 10 (October 20): 627.

Rubinstein, A., S. Garcia Marti, A. Souto, D. Ferrante, and F. Augustovski. 2009. "Generalized Cost-Effectiveness Analysis of a Package of Interventions to Reduce Cardiovascular Disease in Buenos Aires, Argentina." *Cost Effectiveness and Resource Allocation* 7 (May 6): 10.

Salomon, J. A., N. Carvalho, C. Gutierrez-Delgado, R. Orozco, A. Mancuso, and others. 2012. "Intervention Strategies to Reduce the Burden of Non-Communicable Diseases in Mexico: Cost-Effectiveness Analysis." *BMJ* 344 (March 2): e355.

Schulman-Marcus, J., D. Prabhakaran, and T. A. Gaziano. 2010. "Pre-Hospital ECG for Acute Coronary Syndrome in Urban India: A Cost-Effectiveness Analysis." *BMC Cardiovascular Disorders* 10 (March 12): 13.

Schwappach, D., T. Boluarte, and M. Suhrcke. 2007. "The Economics of Primary Prevention of Cardiovascular Disease: A Systematic Review of Economic Evaluations." *Cost Effectiveness and Resource Allocation* 5 (1): 5.

Shroufi, A., R. Chowdhury, R. Anchala, S. Stevens, P. Blanco, and others. 2013. "Cost-Effective Interventions for the Prevention of Cardiovascular Disease in Low- and Middle-Income Countries: A Systematic Review." *BMC Public Health* 13 (March 28): 285.

Smith, R. D., K. Lee, and N. Drager. 2009. "Trade and Health: An Agenda for Action." *The Lancet* 373 (9665): 768–73.

Stanciole, A. E., M. Ortegon, D. Chisholm, and J. A. Lauer. 2012. "Cost-Effectiveness of Strategies to Combat Chronic Obstructive Pulmonary Disease and Asthma in Sub-Saharan Africa and South East Asia: Mathematical Modelling Study." *BMJ* 344 (March 2): e608.

Suhrcke, M., T. A. Boluarte, and L. Niessen. 2012. "A Systematic Review of Economic Evaluations of Interventions to Tackle Cardiovascular Disease in Low- and Middle-Income Countries." *BMC Public Health* 12 (January 3): 2.

Suhrcke, M., R. Nugent, D. Stuckler, and L. Rocco. 2006. "Chronic Disease: An Economic Perspective." Oxford Health Alliance, London.

Tajouri, T. H., S. L. Driver, and D. R. Holmes Jr. 2014. "'Take as Directed': Strategies to Improve Adherence to Cardiac Medication." *Nature Reviews Cardiology* 11 (5): 304–7.

Tan-Torres Edejer, T., R. Balthussen, T. Adam, R. Hutubessy, A. Acharya, and others. 2003. *Making Choices in Health: WHO Guide to Cost-Effectiveness Analysis.* Geneva: WHO.

Thom, S., N. Poulter, J. Field, A. Patel, D. Prabhakaran, and others. 2013. "Effects of a Fixed-Dose Combination Strategy on Adherence and Risk Factors in Patients with or at High Risk of CVD: The UMPIRE Randomized Clinical Trial." *JAMA* 310 (9): 918–29.

Thow, A. M., S. Downs, and S. Jan. 2014. "A Systematic Review of the Effectiveness of Food Taxes and Subsidies to Improve Diets: Understanding the Recent Evidence." *Nutrition Reviews* 72 (9): 551–65.

Thow, A. M., S. Jan, S. Leeder, and B. Swinburn. 2010. "The Effect of Fiscal Policy on Diet, Obesity, and Chronic Disease: A Systematic Review." *Bulletin of the World Health Organization* 88 (8): 609–14.

Tian, M. P., V. S. Ajay, D. B. M. Dunzhu, S. S. Hameed, X. Li, and others. 2015. "A Cluster-Randomized, Controlled Trial of a Simplified Multifaceted Management Program for Individuals at High Cardiovascular Risk (SimCard Trial) in Rural Tibet, China, and Haryana, India." *Circulation* 132 (9): 815–24.

Tran, K., C. Ho, H. Noorani, K. Cimon, A. Hodgson, and others. 2007. *Thiazide Diuretics as First-Line Treatment for Hypertension: Meta-Analysis and Economic Evaluation.* Technology Report 95. Ottawa: Canadian Agency for Drugs and Technologies in Health.

Tsevat, J., D. Duke, L. Goldman, M. A. Pfeffer, G. A. Lamas, and others. 1995. "Cost-Effectiveness of Captopril Therapy after Myocardial Infarction." *Journal of the American College of Cardiology* 26 (4): 914–19.

van Baal, P., T. Feenstra, J. Polder, R. Hoogenveen, and W. Brouwer. 2011. "Economic Evaluation and the Postponement of Health Care Costs." *Health Economics* 20 (4): 432–45.

van Mourik, M. S., A. Cameron, M. Ewen, and R. O. Laing. 2010. "Availability, Price, and Affordability of Cardiovascular Medicines: A Comparison across 36 Countries Using WHO/HAI Data." *BMC Cardiovascular Disorders* 10 (June 9): 25.

Vijay, G. C., E. C. Wilson, M. Suhrcke, W. Hardeman, and S. Sutton. 2015. "Are Brief Interventions to Increase Physical

Activity Cost-Effective? A Systematic Review." *British Journal of Sports Medicine* 50 (7): 408–17.

Viswanathan, M., C. E. Golin, C. D. Jones, M. Ashok, S. J. Blalock, and others. 2012. "Interventions to Improve Adherence to Self-Administered Medications for Chronic Diseases in the United States: A Systematic Review." *Annals of Internal Medicine* 157 (11): 785–95.

Vos, T., R. Carter, J. Barendregt, C. Mihalopoulos, J. Veerman, and others. 2010. *Assessing Cost-Effectiveness in Prevention (ACE–Prevention): Final Report.* Melbourne: University of Queensland; Brisbane: Deakin University.

Wald, N. J., and M. R. Law. 2003. "A Strategy to Reduce Cardiovascular Disease by More Than 80%." *BMJ* 326 (7404): 1419.

Wang, M., A. E. Moran, J. Liu, P. G. Coxson, P. A. Heidenreich, and others. 2014. "Cost-Effectiveness of Optimal Use of Acute Myocardial Infarction Treatments and Impact on Coronary Heart Disease Mortality in China." *Circulation: Cardiovascular Quality and Outcomes* 7 (1): 78–85.

Wang, Y. C., A. M. Cheung, K. Bibbins-Domingo, L. A. Prosser, N. R. Cook, and others. 2011. "Effectiveness and Cost-Effectiveness of Blood Pressure Screening in Adolescents in the United States." *Journal of Pediatrics* 158 (2): 257–64.e7.

Wareham, N., and S. Jebb. 2015. "What Is the Evidence Base for Various Fiscal Measures?" Report on behalf of the MRC Epidemiology Unit and Centre for Diet and Activity Research, University of Cambridge.

Weatherly, H., M. Drummond, K. Claxton, R. Cookson, B. Ferguson, and others. 2009. "Methods for Assessing the Cost-Effectiveness of Public Health Interventions: Key Challenges and Recommendations." *Health Policy* 93 (2–3): 85–92.

Weintraub, W. S., Z. Zhang, E. M. Mahoney, P. Kolm, J. A. Spertus, and others. 2005. "Cost-Effectiveness of Eplerenone Compared with Placebo in Patients with Myocardial Infarction Complicated by Left Ventricular Dysfunction and Heart Failure." *Circulation* 111 (9): 1106–13.

WHO (World Health Organization). 2004. "Global Strategy on Diet, Physical Activity, and Health." WHO, Geneva.

———. 2011. "Scaling up Action against Noncommunicable Diseases: How Much Will It Cost?" WHO, Geneva.

Wilson, P. W., R. B. D'Agostino, D. Levy, A. M. Belanger, H. Silbershatz, and others. 1998. "Prediction of Coronary Heart Disease Using Risk Factor Categories." *Circulation* 97 (18): 1837–47.

Wiseman, V., C. Mitton, M. M. Doyle-Waters, T. Drake, L. Conteh, and others. 2016. "Using Economic Evidence to Set Healthcare Priorities in Low-Income and Lower-Middle-Income Countries: A Systematic Review of Methodological Frameworks." *Health Economics* 25 (Suppl 1): 140–61.

Wolf-Maier, K., R. S. Cooper, H. Kramer, J. R. Banegas, S. Giampaoli, and others. 2004. "Hypertension Treatment and Control in Five European Countries, Canada, and the United States." *Hypertension* 43 (1): 10–17.

Yusuf, S., P. Pais, R. Afzal, D. Xavier, K. Teo, and others. 2009. "Effects of a Polypill (Polycap) on Risk Factors in Middle-Aged Individuals without Cardiovascular Disease (TIPS): A Phase II, Double-Blind, Randomised Trial." *The Lancet* 373 (9672): 1341–51.

Zhang, P., X. Zhang, J. Brown, D. N. R. Vistisen, R. Sicree, and others. 2010. "Global Healthcare Expenditure on Diabetes for 2010 and 2030." *Diabetes Research and Clinical Practice* 87 (3): 293–301.

Chapter 20

Extended Cost-Effectiveness Analyses of Cardiovascular Risk Factor Reduction Policies

David A. Watkins, Rachel Nugent, and Stéphane Verguet

INTRODUCTION

Recent improvements in prevention and treatment have led to marked reductions in age-standardized mortality rates from cardiovascular disease (CVD) in low- and middle-income countries (LMICs). However, because of rapid population growth and aging in these countries, the number of fatal and nonfatal cases of CVD continues to rise (Roth and others 2015). This increase in the absolute burden of CVD is accompanied by an increase in the economic impact of CVD that includes financial risks related to accessing treatment (Bloom and others 2011; Jha and others 2013). The findings from a systematic review indicate incidence of catastrophic health expenditure (CHE) of greater than 70 percent in patients with CVD or stroke in China, India, and Tanzania, and 68 percent in patients with cancer (Huffman and others 2011).

CVD and its risk factors are frequently distributed across populations in different ways. A popular notion is that CVD is a condition of older, urban males; however, evidence suggests that younger individuals in poorer and rural areas are often disproportionately affected (Gaziano 2009). Furthermore, recent studies have shown that the poorest countries and world regions have the highest incidence and case-fatality ratios from CVD, compared with the wealthiest areas. This observation could be due in part to disparities in access to health services in

general and evidence-based interventions in particular (Yusuf and others 2014).

Extended cost-effectiveness analysis (ECEA) is a new economic evaluation method developed as part of the Disease Control Priorities Network grant funded by the Bill & Melinda Gates Foundation and the *Disease Control Priorities, 3rd edition* (*DCP3*, http://www.dcp-3.org). The rationale for ECEA is to extend the scope of cost-effectiveness analysis (CEA) to assess health policies more adequately. CEA centers on the summary metric of incremental cost-effectiveness—cost per amount of health gained—and is a key part of health technology assessment.

ECEA goes beyond simply measuring health outcomes to estimate incremental gains in nonhealth outcomes that are important to health systems, such as financial risk protection (FRP) and distributional consequences like equity and fairness (Verguet, Laxminarayan, and Jamison 2015). ECEA results are usually presented in "dashboard" format, that is, disaggregated into health and nonhealth outcomes per dollar spent on a particular health policy and estimated separately for different socioeconomic groups. ECEA is well designed to respond to the policy questions posed in the *World Health Reports* of 2010 and 2013, specifically, how to move efficiently to universal health coverage (UHC) (WHO 2010, 2013).

Corresponding author: David A. Watkins, Department of Medicine, University of Washington, Seattle, Washington, United States; davidaw@uw.edu.

This chapter summarizes lessons learned from three ECEAs that have been conducted on CVD risk factor reduction policies for *DCP3*. Specifically, it highlights new insights that these ECEAs have provided into the differential impacts of well-established CVD prevention interventions. It also identifies priority issues for future ECEAs to address, and draws some conclusions and implications for public health policy.

SUMMARIES OF THE ECEAs

Each of the three ECEAs on cardiovascular topics addresses a different type of health policy and has a slightly different methodological approach.

- Verguet, Gauvreau, and others (2015) assess an increase in tobacco excise tax in China.
- Watkins and others (2016) assess the regulation of salt content in processed foods in South Africa.
- Verguet, Olson, and others (2015) assess universal public finance of hypertension treatment in Ethiopia as part of a hypothetical bundle of nine health interventions.

The main findings of each of these studies are summarized in table 20.1.

Tobacco Taxation in China

China has the largest number of smokers in the world, and the overwhelming majority of them are male (Yang and others 2008). Cigarette use has become more widespread and affordable over time, which implies that further increases in excise taxes will be necessary to reach target levels recommended by the World Health Organization (WHO) to reduce the prevalence of smoking (IARC 2011). Verguet, Gauvreau, and others (2015) conducted an ECEA with a special focus on the distributional consequences of increased tobacco taxation in

response to the frequently cited concern that taxation disproportionately affects the poor (Remler 2004).

This ECEA used a model to assess the impact on tobacco consumption among male Chinese smokers over a 50-year time horizon following a one-time increase in tobacco prices of 50 percent. The authors estimated health outcomes as reductions in years of life lost (YLL). They also looked at four economic outcomes: increases in excise tax revenues, changes in household expenditure on tobacco, changes in tobacco-related health expenditure, and FRP using the money-metric value of insurance approach (Verguet, Laxminarayan, and Jamison 2015). The model incorporated differential effect sizes of the tax based on empirical studies that have found a gradient in price elasticity of demand for tobacco, wherein the poorest are much more price sensitive (price elasticity range, −0.64 to −1.28) than the wealthiest (price elasticity range, −0.12 to −0.24).

The tobacco tax would result in large health gains and FRP over the 50-year period, with the poorest wealth quintile receiving the plurality of the benefits (table 20.1). The tax would generate US$703 billion in new excise tax revenues (14 percent from the poorest quintile); it would reduce household income by 3.9 percent among the poorest and 0.7 percent among the wealthiest. Tobacco expenditures would increase among all wealth quintiles except the poorest, where they would decrease by US$21 billion. Tobacco-related medical expenditures would also be reduced by US$24 billion (27 percent in the poorest quintile). The money-metric value of insurance was calculated to be US$1.8 billion, with US$1.3 billion realized among the poorest quintile. The insurance value, which measures the reduction in financial risk accruing to segments of the smoking population due to the higher price, is large and significantly pro-poor.

The authors also performed several sensitivity analyses. If price elasticity of demand for tobacco were constant rather than varying across quintiles, the health gains and expenditure changes would even out, and the overall structure of the tax would be more regressive;

Table 20.1 Main Findings of CVD Risk Factors

Study	Health gains	Distribution	FRP
Tobacco in China	231 million YLL averted over 50 years	34% of YLL averted and 74% of insurance gained in poorest quintile	US$1.8 billion value of insurance gained
Salt in South Africa	5,600 deaths and 23,000 cases of CVD averted yearly	Health gains relatively even; FRP mostly benefits middle or upper class, depending on metric used	2,000 cases of poverty or 2,400 cases of CHE averted yearly
Blood pressure in Ethiopia	140 deaths averted over one year	n.a.	1,100 cases of poverty averted over one year

Sources: Verguet, Gavreau, and others 2015; Verguet, Olson, and others 2015; Watkins and others 2016.
Note: CHE = Catastrophic health expenditure; CVD = cardiovascular disease; FRP = financial risk protection; n.a. = not applicable; YLL = years of life lost.

however, FRP would still be concentrated among the lowest two quintiles. If the value of the tax increase were 25 percent instead of 50 percent, the distributional consequences would be the same; however, if the value of the increase were 100 percent, the consequences would be slightly more progressive.

Salt Reduction in South Africa

Comparative risk assessments for burden-of-disease studies have consistently found that high blood pressure is one of the top risk factors in South Africa (Norman and others 2007). The contemporary South African diet is high in salt; although this salt comes largely from processed foods, discretionary use of table salt is also high. In 2013, the South African government began to implement a series of mandatory regulations on the salt content in six key groups of processed foods. In parallel, a public media campaign was initiated to encourage reductions in discretionary salt use (Hofman and Tollman 2013). Watkins and others (2016) conducted an ECEA that examined the impacts of South Africa's comprehensive salt policy.

In the spirit of the comparative risk assessment approach, this ECEA modeled a shift in population blood pressure and a resulting shift in age- and sex-specific rates of CVD. The health outcomes were measured as avertable CVD cases and deaths and comprised stroke, hypertensive heart disease, ischemic heart disease, and end-stage renal disease. The authors looked at four economic outcomes: reductions in government subsidies for the treatment of CVD (mostly for the poor), changes in CVD-related health expenditure, and FRP using two metrics: cases of CHE averted, defined as greater than 10 percent of total household expenditure, and cases of poverty averted using a local poverty line. In this model, the distributional consequences were driven by differences in salt intake and CVD risk due to variations in age, gender, and ethnic composition, as well as blood pressure distribution, by income quintile.

The salt reduction policy, once fully implemented, would reduce CVD deaths by about 11 percent per year compared with current rates. Generally, the health gains would be spread evenly across wealth quintiles, although the poorest quintile would benefit slightly less because of lower baseline CVD risk. Most of the health gains would come from preventing stroke and hypertensive heart disease; ischemic heart disease and hypertensive kidney disease in this population are much smaller contributors. Approximately US$4 million in private out-of-pocket expenditures would be averted, counteracting (but not canceling out) the increase in food prices that could occur if the food industry fully passed along the costs of product reformulation to consumers. Still, the increase

in food prices would constitute less than 1 percent of yearly household food expenditures.

The South African government heavily subsidizes health care for lower-income households. Hence, the salt reduction policy would save about US$51 million yearly in government subsidies for CVD care, creating fiscal space for further investments in health. From the household perspective, the estimated 2,000 cases of poverty or 2,400 cases of CHE averted yearly by the policy would represent a 12 percent to 15 percent increase beyond the FRP that is currently being achieved through government subsidies. It is important to note that these results are context dependent: a country without preexisting CVD care subsidy arrangements would achieve a higher incremental FRP from a similar salt reduction policy. This nuance is likely to be an important consideration in a number of low- and lower-middle-income countries, since CVD care is largely financed out of pocket rather than by governments in many of these countries (Samb and others 2010).

Hypertension Treatment in Ethiopia

The latest health sector development program for Ethiopia clearly emphasizes development of a pathway to UHC (Alebachew, Hatt, and Kukla 2014). In collaboration with the Disease Control Priorities Network, the Ministry of Health is deliberating essential packages of care that will be made universally available through public finance. Verguet, Olson, and others (2015) conducted an ECEA that assessed the tradeoffs between health gains and FRP from public finance of nine illustrative interventions that would be included in this package. Of relevance to this volume, one of their interventions was public finance of antihypertensive medications to individuals at high risk of CVD. In contrast to the other two ECEAs, this analysis did not include considerations of health equity; rather, it focused on the comparative health benefits and FRP per dollar spent on specific publicly financed interventions.

The model used in this study examined the increase in effective treatment rates that would result from a 10 percent increase in coverage in each of nine selected interventions. The nine interventions were rotavirus vaccination, pneumococcal vaccination, measles vaccination, treatment of diarrhea, treatment of pneumonia, treatment of malaria, cesarean section surgery, treatment of tuberculosis, and treatment of hypertension. The small increase in coverage was chosen as a feasible target in the short term—approximately one year—given the short-term constraints in health system capacity.

The policy to reduce hypertension would publicly finance treatment with up to three medications for high-risk individuals, defined as those having greater than

20 percent CVD risk over 10 years. The health outcome was measured as CVD (ischemic heart disease and stroke) deaths averted; the economic outcomes were changes in hypertension expenditure through public finance and in CVD-related health expenditure through better prevention, as well as cases of poverty averted using a local poverty line.

Public finance of hypertension treatment in Ethiopia would cost US$1.3 million yearly, reducing out-of-pocket expenditures on treatment by US$730,000 yearly. The increase in medication use would avert 140 CVD deaths and prevent 1,100 cases of poverty (table 20.1).

When the results of the nine interventions were standardized to health gains and FRP per US$100,000 spent, the financing of hypertension treatment resulted in relatively low health gains compared with highly effective child health interventions such as measles and pneumococcal vaccination. However, the financing of hypertension treatment resulted in relatively high FRP compared with those interventions, since the treatments are much more costly and the out-of-pocket payments averted would be higher. This contrast also held for other adult conditions, such as tuberculosis treatment and cesarean section delivery, which had similarly high costs. Accordingly, this sort of assessment of tradeoffs between health and FRP could be an important step forward for ministries of health deliberating packages of care and seeking to optimize health and nonhealth impacts in the design of health insurance programs.

NEW INSIGHTS FROM THE ECEAs

These ECEAs contribute several novel insights into the CVD cost-effectiveness literature. The tobacco study is one of the first analyses to demonstrate quantitatively that, contrary to popular opinion, tobacco taxation can be progressive, at least when long-term household expenditures—including health expenditures due to the ill effects of smoking—are considered. This new focus on health equity within economic evaluation is especially relevant to countries like China and South Africa that have committed to developing policies that reduce health inequalities and promote economic development.

FRP has traditionally been regarded as a direct objective of health system financing, using public finance to reduce medical impoverishment. Indeed, with the ECEA approach, medical impoverishment and other FRP metrics can be estimated within a cost-effectiveness framework. The incremental FRP per dollar spent can then be compared across interventions to guide decision making around UHC, as was demonstrated in the Ethiopia analysis. At the same time, although tobacco taxation and salt reduction are nonpersonal, population-level interventions, they can—by preventing disease—result in substantial long-term FRP that complements the gain in FRP through public finance of clinical interventions.

An additional implication of the Ethiopia analysis is that adult-onset chronic noncommunicable diseases may be a relatively higher priority for UHC than previously thought. When only cost-effectiveness metrics are included in decision making, child health interventions and others that produce large reductions in mortality often receive highest priority. However, in economic terms, adults contribute more to society than children and receive more income for their work. Furthermore, CVD and other noncommunicable diseases are usually lifelong and expensive to manage. So while the mortality reduction from adult interventions may be much less impressive than for child interventions, the FRP gains may be much more impressive and relatively more attractive as part of a UHC package.

Finally, the distinct advantage of ECEA over CEA in guiding decision making is that ECEA more readily allows health interventions to be compared with interventions in other sectors that also focus on poverty reduction, such as education, transport, and development. This advantage has the potential to elevate the profile of health interventions within ministries of finance.

CROSSCUTTING THEMES OF THE ECEAs

These three ECEAs share additional conclusions. First, ECEAs have usually confirmed the health benefits of CEAs rather than challenged them, mainly because interventions or policies have been selected for ECEAs on the basis of their cost-effectiveness, and many of the inputs into ECEA models are similar to those of CEAs. To date, ECEAs have not been conducted on interventions that are not generally accepted to be cost-effective. In keeping with the findings of the Ethiopia study, future ECEAs may wish to explore costly interventions that do not have large health benefits but may result in substantial FRP, such as the provision of palliative care services (Powell and others 2015).

Second, one important message from these ECEAs is that an aggregated societal approach may miss important transfers and flows of costs and benefits. For example, from a societal perspective, tobacco taxation would conclude that the policy has a very low (or even zero) cost and high effectiveness and is therefore uninteresting as a topic for a CEA. Yet the tax itself has important economic effects on costs and benefits to households and governments separately that may influence policy decisions—as is seen in the discussion about the regressive nature of the tobacco tax in China. Indeed, the whole notion of estimating FRP is predicated on disaggregating costs and analyzing them from multiple perspectives.

LIMITATIONS AND FUTURE RESEARCH TOPICS

The CVD ECEAs also demonstrate two important limitations and unresolved methodological issues that will be important topics for research.

First, a consistent approach is needed to modeling the demand for health care (that is, rates of health service utilization) and changes in demand that might occur as a result of the policy in question. Since ECEAs are often used to assess the impact of public finance, they assume a change in health care–seeking behavior that leads to a change in health outcomes. The salt reduction and hypertension treatment ECEAs both assume constant and homogeneous demand across the population. In a sensitivity analysis, the salt study demonstrates that a lower baseline demand for health care at the population level would not affect estimates of the health gains but would reduce FRP; unfortunately, no empirical literature from South Africa examines what level of health care utilization would be reasonable to assume.

Second, the focus of these ECEAs is on direct medical costs as measured by out-of-pocket expenditures and the economic benefits of reducing such expenditures. However, whether this is an adequate foundation for estimating FRP is not clear. For example, using the poverty and CHE metrics, the salt analysis finds little to no FRP in the poorest quintile of South Africans—all of whom live below the poverty line and receive free or highly subsidized medical care. Yet because the health gains in this quintile were similar to the gains in the wealthier quintiles, it is plausible that productivity would be increased and the risk of impoverishment would be reduced as a direct result of the improvement in health without being mediated through a reduction in out-of-pocket expenses. Apart from these human capital considerations, others have noted that financial risk may take many other forms, including forced borrowing and selling of assets (Ruger 2012). Because of limited microeconomic data in LMICs, no attempts to date have been made to construct FRP metrics around these other economic effects.

In the future, the research agenda for ECEAs on CVD should consider other possible applications that could lend valuable insights. For example, some evidence suggests that lower-income households more frequently borrow money or sell assets (hardship financing) to pay for CVD care (Huffman and others 2011). As this empirical literature grows, it might become feasible to incorporate other FRP metrics, such as hardship financing, that appear to be important for CVD. Also, CVD and its risk factors are known to vary widely by age, gender, and geography. Analyses of CVD policy effects across these strata—instead of, or in addition to, income strata—might provide insights into which sorts of policies facilitate the policy objectives of particular governments, for example, which are significantly pro-female or pro-rural.

CONCLUSIONS

Tobacco taxation, salt reduction, and primary prevention of CVD in high-risk individuals are widely regarded as best buys in global noncommunicable disease policy (WHO 2011). The ECEAs presented in this chapter confirm the findings of previous CEAs, namely, that these interventions are likely to result in large health gains in LMICs.

The ECEAs also present new insights into the broader health system and economic impacts of these interventions. By preventing CVD, nonclinical interventions like population-based tobacco and salt reduction can effectively purchase additional FRP beyond what governments can accomplish through public finance of clinical treatments. ECEAs can examine and address some of the concerns about potential economic distortions caused by health policies, such as the alleged regressivity of tobacco taxes. Incorporating equity and FRP considerations into economic evaluation is a critical methodological advance that speaks directly to the UHC movement and its goals. ECEAs are especially pertinent for CVD and related conditions where financial risk is large according to a growing body of research. Finally, ECEAs have the potential to elevate the priority of CVD interventions through direct comparison with the health and nonhealth impact of interventions for infectious diseases, maternal disorders, injuries, and other conditions. In coming years, this comparative approach may become a standard tool for designing and debating the priority elements of UHC benefits packages.

NOTE

World Bank Income Classifications as of July 2014 are as follows, based on estimates of gross national income (GNI) per capita for 2013:

- Low-income countries (LICs) = US$1,045 or less
- Middle-income countries (MICs) are subdivided:
  (a) lower-middle-income = US$1,046 to US$4,125
  (b) upper-middle-income (UMICs) = US$4,126 to US$12,745
- High-income countries (HICs) = US$12,746 or more.

REFERENCES

Alebachew, A., L. Hatt, and M. Kukla. 2014. "Monitoring and Evaluating Progress towards Universal Health Coverage in Ethiopia." *PLoS Medicine* 11 (9): e1001696.

Bloom, D. E., E. T. Cafiero, E. Jané-Llopis, S. Abrahams-Gessel, L. R. Bloom, and others. 2011. *The Global Economic Burden of Noncommunicable Diseases.* Geneva: World Economic Forum.

Gaziano, T. A. 2009. "Is the Horse Already Out of the Barn in Rural India?" *Circulation* 119 (14): 1850–52.

Hofman, K. J., and S. M. Tollman. 2013. "Population Health in South Africa: A View from the Salt Mines." *The Lancet Global Health* 1 (2): e66–67.

Huffman, M. D., K. D. Rao, A. Pichon-Riviere, D. Zhao, S. Harikrishnan, and others. 2011. "A Cross-Sectional Study of the Microeconomic Impact of Cardiovascular Disease Hospitalization in Four Low- and Middle-Income Countries." *PLoS One* 6 (6): e20821.

IARC (International Agency for Research on Cancer). 2011. *IARC Handbook of Cancer Prevention.* Vol. 14 of *Effectiveness of Tax and Price Policies for Tobacco Control.* Lyon: World Health Organization.

Jha, P., R. Nugent, S. Verguet, D. Bloom, and R. Hum. 2013. "Chronic Disease." In *Global Problems, Smart Solutions: Costs and Benefits,* edited by B. Lomborg, 137–85. Cambridge, U.K.: Cambridge University Press.

Norman, R., D. Bradshaw, M. Schneider, J. Joubert, P. Groenewald, and others. 2007. "A Comparative Risk Assessment for South Africa in 2000: Towards Promoting Health and Preventing Disease." *South African Medical Journal* 97 (8 Pt 2): 637–41.

Powell, R. A., F. N. Mwangi-Powell, L. Radbruch, G. Yamey, E. L. Krakauer, and others. 2015. "Putting Palliative Care on the Global Health Agenda." *The Lancet Oncology* 16 (2): 131–33.

Remler, D. K. 2004. "Poor Smokers, Poor Quitters, and Cigarette Tax Regressivity." *American Journal of Public Health* 94 (2): 225–29.

Roth, G. A., M. H. Forouzanfar, A. E. Moran, R. Barber, G. Nguyen, and others. 2015. "Demographic and Epidemiologic Drivers of Global Cardiovascular Mortality." *New England Journal of Medicine* 372 (14): 1333–41.

Ruger, J. P. 2012. "An Alternative Framework for Analyzing Financial Protection in Health." *PLoS Medicine* 9 (8): e1001294.

Samb, B., N. Desai, S. Nishtar, S. Mendis, H. Bekedam, and others. 2010. "Prevention and Management of Chronic Disease: A Litmus Test for Health-Systems Strengthening in Low-Income and Middle-Income Countries." *The Lancet* 376 (9754): 1785–97.

Verguet, S., C. L. Gauvreau, S. Mishra, M. MacLennan, S. M. Murphy, and others. 2015. "The Consequences of Tobacco Tax on Household Health and Finances in Rich and Poor Smokers in China: An Extended Cost-Effectiveness Analysis." *The Lancet Global Health* 3 (4): 206–16.

Verguet, S., R. Laxminarayan, and D. T. Jamison. 2015. "Universal Public Finance of Tuberculosis Treatment in India: An Extended Cost-Effectiveness Analysis." *Health Economics* 24 (3): 318–32.

Verguet, S., Z. D. Olson, J. B. Babigumira, D. Desalegn, K. A. Johansson, and others. 2015. "Health Gains and Financial Risk Protection Afforded by Public Financing of Selected Interventions in Ethiopia: An Extended Cost-Effectiveness Analysis." *The Lancet Global Health* 3 (5): e288–96.

Watkins, D. A., Z. D. Olson, S. Verguet, R. A. Nugent, and D. T. Jamison. 2016. "Cardiovascular Disease and Impoverishment Averted due to a Salt Reduction Policy in South Africa: An Extended Cost-Effectiveness Analysis." *Health Policy and Planning* 31 (1): 75–82.

WHO (World Health Organization). 2010. *World Health Report 2010: Health Systems Financing: The Path to Universal Coverage.* Geneva: WHO.

———. 2011. *Global Status Report on Noncommunicable Diseases 2010.* Geneva: WHO. http://www.who.int/nmh /publications/ncd_report2010/en/.

———. 2013. *World Health Report 2013: Research for Universal Health Coverage.* Geneva: WHO.

Yang, G., L. Kong, W. Zhao, X. Wan, Y. Zhai, and others. 2008. "Emergence of Chronic Non-Communicable Diseases in China." *The Lancet* 372 (9650): 1697–705.

Yusuf, S., S. Rangarajan, K. Teo, S. Islam, W. Li, and others. 2014. "Cardiovascular Risk and Events in 17 Low-, Middle-, and High-Income Countries." *New England Journal of Medicine* 371 (9): 818–27.

Chapter 21

Priority-Setting Processes for Expensive Treatments for Chronic Diseases

Yuna Sakuma, Amanda Glassman, and Claudia Vaca

INTRODUCTION

Cardiovascular, respiratory, and related chronic disorders are an increasing concern in low- and middle-income countries (LMICs). In 2010, 19 percent (408.7 million) of total disability-adjusted life years (DALYs) and 39 percent (17.0 million) of total deaths in LMICs were attributable to cardiovascular and circulatory diseases, chronic respiratory diseases, diabetes mellitus, and chronic kidney diseases combined. The burden in LMICs accounts for 85 percent and 80 percent of global cardiovascular, respiratory, and related chronic disorder DALYs and deaths, respectively (IHME 2013).

Several treatment options are available for each disease, ranging from generic pharmacologic treatments, such as aspirin for vascular disease, metformin for diabetes, and salbutamol for chronic respiratory disease, to invasive procedures, such as coronary artery bypass graft surgery for vascular disease or kidney transplant for chronic kidney disease. These invasive procedures are often costly and resource intensive, placing a large burden on a country's health care system.

Governments face tough allocation choices for limited public resources across many competing priorities, as each country strives to achieve universal coverage of essential health care services under the Sustainable Development Goals. The large and growing burden of cardiovascular, respiratory, and related chronic disorders forces public

payers to allocate, or at least consider allocating, increasing resources to these diseases and conditions. This chapter explores the difficulty of rationing health resources in LMICs. Governments and public payers may allocate resources using priority-setting policy tools such as essential medicines lists (EMLs), health benefit plans, and health technology assessment (HTA) agencies. Yet, the processes used to arrive at allocation decisions are rarely evidence based, transparent, or participatory.

Furthermore, although the focus of this chapter is on high-cost treatment, the need for a legitimate and evidence-driven priority-setting process applies to all health conditions and diseases, and preventive measures cannot be ignored; the priority-setting process is not complete without considering local evidence on the costs and benefits of both prevention and treatment.

The chapter is divided into three sections. The first section frames the topic of priority setting in health. The second section explores a case study that shows how national essential medicines lists (NEMLs) largely fail to influence prescription shares of types of insulin for which marginal cost-effectiveness has not been fully established in several LMICs. The third section examines a second case study that shows the complexity of the priority-setting process in Thailand's decision to include dialysis in the national health insurance (NHI) plan's benefits package.

Corresponding author: Yuna Sakuma, Center for Global Development, Washington, DC; ysakuma@cgdev.org.

FRAMING THE ISSUES

A fundamental challenge for all health systems is allocating finite resources across the potentially unlimited demand for health services and technologies. This is a rationing problem, regardless of whether it is explicitly addressed as such, because it requires that choices be made regarding how and when services are provided, to whom, and by what mechanism across many dimensions (Ham and Robert 2003). Inevitably some demand goes unmet, which is one source of the intense pressure to provide more services and newer and more sophisticated technologies within any given resource envelope. Efforts to reduce waste, increase quality, and improve efficiency are all responses to this pressure. Expanding health care costs and spending are indications of the same forces.

Conflicts in priority-setting decisions reflect natural features of all societies, including differences in demographics and disease burden as well as cultural preferences and beliefs. In addition, there are no universal answers to the inevitable policy questions, such as the balance of support between preventive and therapeutic measures, or choices between disease control priorities. Insufficient institutional mechanisms for assessing various proffered priorities, evaluating political and economic constraints, and gathering input from citizens and stakeholders make this problem particularly acute for policy makers in LMICs.

The sheer size of the need for treatments for cardiovascular, respiratory, and related chronic disorders in LMICs forces public resources to be allocated to these conditions and ensures that these diseases will be an important concern for policy makers. Although noncommunicable diseases have traditionally been perceived as a high-income health burden, LMICs are increasingly experiencing these problems. Total DALYs and deaths in LMICs attributable to cardiovascular, respiratory, and related chronic disorders increased substantially from 16 percent of total DALYs (377.8 million) and 36 percent of total deaths (15.14 million) in 2000 to 19 percent of total DALYs and 39 percent of total deaths in 2010 (IHME 2013). Additionally, complications that arise from diabetes affect societies more broadly (van Dieren and others 2010). As cardiovascular, respiratory, and related chronic disorder needs grow, the demand for treatment increases. Consequently, the challenge of rationing becomes greater, and prevention efforts become more critical.

Although technical progress can be cost saving and reduce the relative price of health products and services, new technologies can also be costlier—although, ideally, more effective (Martins and Maisonneuve 2006).

Determining the extent of coverage for an intervention requires analysis of the costs and benefits for health. Most LMICs do not incorporate cost-effectiveness evidence, even when available, in spending decisions. Without an explicit rationing mechanism, many LMICs allocate resources to expensive, novel technologies that benefit a small number of people, while not implementing low-cost, highly effective interventions that would benefit a large number of people and provide greater population health gains (Hutubessy and others 2003). In addition, politics can play a role in the process. Industry leaders, health professional associations, and patients themselves are increasingly pressuring health systems to include novel treatments.

For LMICs, affordability is an important perspective. Although many health technologies may be cost-effective when assessed against a gross domestic product (GDP) per capita threshold (Culyer and others 2007; Johannesson and Weinstein 1993; Weinstein and Statson 1977), they may be unaffordable under a given budget constraint, forcing countries to say "no" to putatively cost-effective technologies—or resort to inequitable, implicit rationing methods. Treatments for chronic diseases can be affordable at one stage of a disease but not at another. For example, treatment at an early stage may be cost-effective to the health system, but it may become unaffordable once the disease has progressed. To that end, considering cost-effectiveness of preventive measures, such as screening, is particularly important.

In addition to cost-effectiveness, other values—including fairness, equity, human rights, respect and self-determination, and financial protection—similarly need to be factored into a decision-making framework in an evidence-based way. Although a full discussion is omitted from this chapter, Brock and Wikler (2006) address ethical issues in resource allocation and cost-effectiveness, and the World Health Organization (WHO) Consultative Group on Equity and Universal Health Coverage provides a three-part strategy that countries can use as a guideline for fair, progressive realization of universal health coverage (WHO 2014). Rights-based legal arguments, which have been used in some middle-income countries in Latin America and the Caribbean, have propelled the provision of expensive therapies without directly addressing how much should be spent, how the resources should be used, or what trade-offs might affect equity and health (Kinney and Clark 2004). However, it is important to recognize that many coverage decisions are made with no technical or social goals in mind, no underpinning analysis, and no due process of any kind; this reality is reflected in the case study that follows.

CASE STUDY 1: TYPE 2 DIABETES

This case study examines how NEMLs as a priority-setting mechanism often fail to influence prescription shares of insulin analogs. This case study first discusses the burden of disease, treatment, and guidelines. Second, it discusses NEMLs as a priority-setting mechanism and analyzes prescription data to gauge the effectiveness of NEMLs as a priority-setting tool. It concludes with insights derived from the case study.

Disease Burden and Context

As described in earlier chapters of this volume, diabetes mellitus (type 1 and type 2[1]) accounted for 1.9 percent (46.7 million) of DALYs and 2.4 percent (1.28 million) of deaths in 2010. Type 2 diabetes is a growing global concern, especially in LMICs. In 2009, medications for type 2 diabetes constituted the fourth-largest therapeutic class, generating total global sales of US$30.4 billion (Cohen and Carter 2010). Lower-middle-income countries carry 51.8 percent of the burden of DALYs (24.2 million) and 49.3 percent of deaths (629 million) (IHME 2013). Approximately 90 percent of total diabetes mellitus cases are type 2.

Many pharmacological treatments combat diabetes. Several have been available for many years, such as metformin, which was discovered in the 1950s (Rojas and Gomes 2013). Other agents—such as insulin analogs, which contain small changes to conventional human insulins so that short-acting agents work more rapidly and long-acting agents deliver insulin more slowly—are new and their cost-effectiveness compared with conventional treatments has not yet been established (Cohen and Carter 2010). Newer agents include insulin degludec, an ultra-long-acting insulin analog approved by the European Medicines Agency and the Japanese Pharmaceutical and Medical Devices Agency but rejected by the United States Food and Drug Administration (European Medicines Agency 2014; Japan Pharmaceuticals and Medical Devices Agency 2013; Novo Nordisk 2013). Despite efforts to encourage the use of cost-effective medicines through such instruments as NEMLs and clinical practice guidelines, no insulin is continuously accessible in many LMICs (Beran and Yudkin 2010). As a proportion of all prescriptions, prescriptions for treatments for which cost-effectiveness is not proven, such as insulin analogs, remains high in these countries.

The United Kingdom's National Institute for Health and Care Excellence (NICE) publishes clinical guidelines based on the best available evidence for appropriate care. For the type 2 diabetes patient to achieve target glycemic goals, NICE recommends adjustments in lifestyle as a first step.

If blood glucose levels remain unacceptably high or lifestyle management is inadequate, metformin is recommended as an initial pharmacological therapy. If lifestyle intervention and metformin fail to control blood glucose, the next step is to add a sulfonylurea; with further lack of blood glucose control, insulin can be initiated. Other agents, such as thiazolidinediones, glucagon-like peptide-1 agonists (GLP-1s), dipeptidyl peptidase-4 inhibitors, and sodium-glucose linked transporter-2 inhibitors (SGLT-2s), come later in the treatment paradigm or can be used as substitutes for patients for whom the paradigm may need tailoring (NICE 2009). However, these other agents, known as newer hypoglycemic drugs, are still being evaluated for safety and effectiveness (Karagiannis and others 2012; Pinelli and others 2008; Qaseem and others 2012).

Based on review of the available data, NICE recommends long-acting insulin analogs only to a subset of patients and only if one of the following conditions applies:

- The person needs assistance from a caregiver or health care professional to inject insulin, and use of a long-acting insulin analog (such as insulin detemir or insulin glargine) would reduce the frequency of injections from twice to once daily.
- The person's lifestyle is restricted by recurrent symptomatic hypoglycemic episodes, or the person would otherwise need twice-daily Neutral Protamine Hagedorn (NPH) insulin injections in combination with oral glucose-lowering drugs.
- The person cannot use the device to inject NPH insulin (NICE 2009).

Priority-Setting Mechanism: National Essential Medicines Lists

The EML is among the earliest efforts to provide a basis for explicit priority setting in LMICs. Since 1977, the WHO has published a model list with the intent of informing purchasing decisions by national health officials (van den Ham, Bero, and Laing 2011). The medicines on the list are selected based on public health relevance, evidence on efficacy and safety, and—to some extent—comparative effectiveness so that they satisfy the priority health care needs of the population (van den Ham, Bero, and Laing 2011). The model list—updated every two years based on applications from individuals, governments, pharmaceutical companies, and medical associations—is published online. Countries often create their own versions of EMLs, with infrequent updating. As of 2011, 156 countries had adopted versions of the EML (Glassman and Chalkidou 2012).

In many countries, the adoption of an EML does not lead to the availability of all—or indeed most—of the medicines listed. Surveys undertaken in 36 countries showed that the mean availability of the 15 most frequently surveyed medicines was 38.4 percent in public sector facilities and 64.2 percent in private sector facilities (Cameron and others 2009). The disconnect between the lists, availability, and actual use is likely to be related, at least in part, to the absence of attention and support for an affordability analysis in a specific country's public spending envelope. The WHO's model list includes some hospital and specialist medicines, but many countries seek international advice on how to handle new, higher-cost medications, which—although cost-effective—may be beyond the resources of the health system (PAHO 2010).

The medicines for type 2 diabetes on the 18th WHO EML (updated March 2013) are the following: metformin, NPH insulin, zinc suspension insulin, neutral insulin, glibenclamide, and gliclazide (WHO 2013). Table 21.1 compares the agents on the list with those on the NEMLs of 13 selected countries: Argentina, Brazil, Colombia, the Arab Republic of Egypt, Indonesia, Mexico, Morocco, Pakistan, Peru, the Philippines, South Africa, and República Bolivariana de Venezuela, plus Turkey. The countries were selected based on the availability of IMS MIDAS[2] medical data. Although IMS MIDAS medical data are available for Turkey, the country does not have an NEML.[3]

A comparison of antidiabetic medicines on the WHO model list and on NEMLs shows that in most sampled countries, NEMLs conform closely to WHO recommendations. For human insulins, few countries include other medicines on their NEMLs. Indonesia, the Philippines, South Africa, Thailand, and República Bolivariana de Venezuela include premixed (biphasic) insulin on their NEMLs. Only Argentina and Colombia include any insulin analogs. Argentina's NEML includes insulin aspart (a fast-acting insulin analog); Colombia's NEML includes three fast-acting insulin analogs (insulin aspart, insulin glulisine, and insulin lispro) and two long-acting insulin analogs (insulin glargine and insulin detemir). With the exceptions of Argentina and Colombia, the NEMLs conform closely to the WHO's recommendations.

Priority Setting in Action

This section analyzes prescription data to gauge the effectiveness of NEMLs as a priority-setting tool. It finds a high use of products that are expensive or that are not proven to be cost-effective in many countries. Figure 21.1 shows the proportion of each type of treatment out of total insulin retail prescriptions, which includes human insulins and insulin analogs (Anatomical Therapeutic Chemical Classification System 4 code A10C) for June 2013 from the IMS MIDAS medical database.

Prescription data show high use of insulin analogs in many countries, despite NEML guidance. In several countries, non-analog human insulins make up the vast majority of retail prescriptions, as in Morocco (94.5 percent), Pakistan (90.5 percent), Egypt (79.9 percent), and Peru (75.7 percent).

However, in other countries, insulin analogs make up the majority of the retail prescription market share, even though only Argentina and Colombia include insulin analogs on their NEMLs. Long-acting insulin analogs—insulin glargine and insulin detemir—have the largest share in República Bolivariana de Venezuela (76.2 percent), Brazil (59.3 percent), Mexico (51.7 percent), Colombia (48.5 percent), the Philippines (44.6 percent), and Indonesia (42.8 percent). Fast-acting insulin analogs—insulin glulisine, insulin aspart, and insulin lispro—have the largest share in Turkey (52.3 percent), South Africa (48.7 percent), and Argentina (43.6 percent).

This analysis has several limitations. First, the retail prescription market does not capture the full market and thus does not show the whole picture. However, the results are indicative of extensive use of insulin analogs in a number of countries. Second, not all type 2 diabetes patients undergo insulin therapy, so the analysis captures only part of the patient population. Examining other classes of antidiabetics would be an interesting direction for further research. Third, the data capture only the moving average target of June 2013.[4] Extending the period may provide a different composition of prescriptions and reveal broader trends in adoption and prescription of insulin analogs. Nevertheless, the current analysis provides a snapshot of the insulin market in LMICs that was not previously available in the literature and provides a starting point for follow-on work.

The case study of insulin analogs for the treatment of type 2 diabetes shows that NEMLs do not restrict the prescribing of medicines. In some countries, an NHI formulary—which is the responsibility of health insurers—can supersede an NEML. For example, in Ghana, both an NEML and an NHI formulary exist, but the two do not contain the same drugs. Countries could benefit from synchronizing the two mechanisms to ensure a more coordinated system for priority setting.

NEMLs and NHI formularies should be synchronized for available agents as well as for new products. The insulin analog case study is one example showing that countries would benefit from reviewing both available and novel interventions. A joint report by the International Insulin Foundation and the Health Policy Analysis Centre, with the support of the International Diabetes Federation,

Table 21.1 Antidiabetic Treatments on the WHO and National Essential Medicines Lists

	WHO (2013)	Argentina (2005)	Brazil (2010)	Colombia[a] (2015)	Egypt, Arab Rep.[b] (2006)	Indonesia (2008)	Mexico (2010)	Morocco (2008)	Pakistan (2007)	Peru (20101)	Philippines (2008)	South Africa (2008)	Turkey (No NEML)	Venezuela, RB (2004)
Human insulins and analogs														
Insulin, NPH (isophane)	X	X	X	X	X	X	X	—	X	X	X	X	—	X
Insulin, zinc suspension	X	X	—	X	X	—	X	—	X	—	X	—	—	—
Insulin, soluble (neutral)	X	X	X	X	X	X	X	—	X	X	X	X	—	X
Insulin, premixed (biphasic)	—	—	—	X	—	X	—	—	—	—	X	X	—	X
Insulin aspart	—	—	—	X	—	—	—	—	—	—	—	—	—	—
Insulin detemir	—	—	—	X	—	—	—	—	—	—	—	—	—	—
Insulin glargine	—	—	—	X	—	—	—	—	—	—	—	—	—	—
Insulin glulisine	—	—	—	X	—	—	—	—	—	—	—	—	—	—
Insulin lispro	—	X	—	X	—	—	—	—	—	—	—	—	—	—
Sulfonylureas														
Glibenclamide	X	X	X	X	X	X	X	X	X	X	X	X	—	X
Gliclazide	X	—	X	—	—	—	—	X	—	—	X	X	—	—
Glimepiride	—	—	—	—	—	—	—	X	—	—	—	—	—	—
Glipizide	—	X	—	—	—	X	—	—	—	—	X	—	—	—
Biguanides														
Metformin	X	X	X	X	X	X	X	X	X	X	X	X	—	X
Alpha-glucosidase inhibitors														
Acarbose	—	X	—	X	—	—	—	X	—	—	X	—	—	—

Source: Country-specific national essential medicines lists; available at http://www.who.int/selection_medicines/country_lists/en/.

Note: NPH = Neutral Protamine Hagedorn; WHO = World Health Organization. — = medication is not on the respective WHO or national essential medicines lists.

a. Colombia included insulin analogs in 2011, all others (NPH, zinc, neutral) were included in 2006.

b. For the Arab Republic of Egypt, insulins are listed as Human Insulin Short Acting, Human Insulin Intermediate Acting, and Human Insulin Long Acting.

Figure 21.1 Percentage of Total Human Insulin Retail Prescriptions by Treatment by Country, 2013

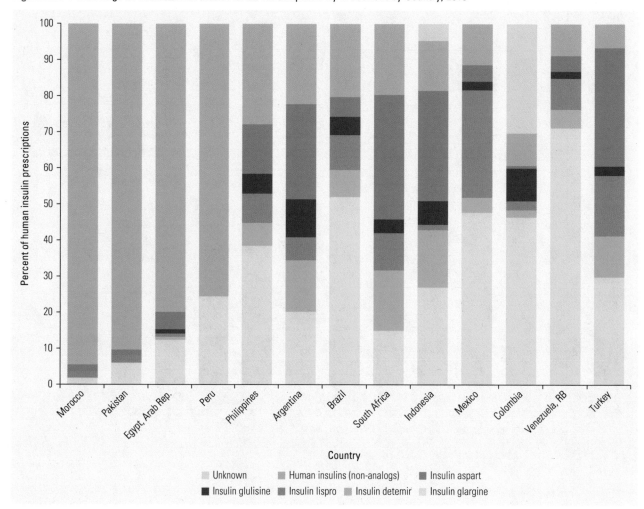

Source: IMS Health 2013.

finds that 57 percent of the Kyrgyz Republic's insulin expenditure goes to insulin analogs. Based on their analysis, switching from an insulin analog to a human insulin could release enough resources to treat twice as many people (Abdraimova and Beran 2009).

Review of available technologies may lead to disinvestment, a process that has traditionally received little attention. Disinvestment involves withdrawing resources, either partially or entirely, from interventions—practices, procedures, pharmaceuticals, or medical devices—that are not cost-effective and do not lead to efficient resource allocation (Elshaug and others 2007). Interest in disinvestment is growing because of budget constraints in countries across all levels of development.

One of NICE's tools for disinvestment is its "do not do" recommendations, a database of clinical practices that NICE's independent advisory board compiles during the process of guidance development, because of

evidence that the practice is not beneficial or lack of evidence to support its continued use (NICE 2012). The database includes several recommendations for type 2 diabetes.

From guidance TA203: Liraglutide (a GLP-1 agonist) 1.8 milligrams daily is not recommended for the treatment of type 2 diabetes.

From guidance CG66: Exenatide (a GLP-1 agonist) is not recommended for routine use in type 2 diabetes.

From guidance TA288: Dapagliflozin (an SGLT-2 inhibitor) in a triple therapy regimen in combination with metformin and a sulfonylurea is not recommended for treating type 2 diabetes, except as part of a clinical trial.

Despite efforts to promote disinvestment, it is difficult to know the extent to which "do not do" lists are implemented given that there is no mandate to adopt the recommendations. A challenge for the United Kingdom's National Health Service is the lack of data on usage beyond the primary care level as well as indication-specific precision (Garner and Littlejohns 2011). Drug utilization studies are critical. In addition, independent information interventions directed at clinicians and patients can reinforce messages of what to do and what not to do. Without these data and interventions, the health system cannot fully determine variations in care and the potential savings from disinvestment.

Case Study Insights

Despite policy makers' attempts to use the NEML as a mechanism to promote cost-effective treatments, insulin analogs make up the majority of retail prescriptions and are purchased in significant quantities by public payers in some countries, with Colombia as a clear example (see also box 21.1). A number of lessons can be drawn from the case study.

Affirming the Role of Cost-Effectiveness Analyses in the Priority-Setting Process

The WHO model list is composed of treatments based on public health relevance, efficacy, safety, and comparative cost-effectiveness, yet the type 2 diabetes treatments on the NEMLs of many countries differ from the model list. In Morocco, the NEML does not include non-analog human insulins, which have been proven cost-effective; the NEMLs of Argentina and Colombia include insulin analogs, which have not been proven to be cost-effective for broad use, at least at the prices currently obtained by different purchasers.

Several reasons could contribute to the discrepancy, such as lack of awareness of the WHO model list or failure to update the NEML to reflect the best available evidence. However, another contributing factor could be that the model list does not reflect country-level cost-effectiveness analyses, and thus cannot be reconciled with the country's public spending envelope. When governments seek to set priorities for the use of limited health resources, including updating an NEML, a global or regional reference is crucial but is only a starting point.

Comparing Priority-Setting Mechanisms and Processes in Similar Countries

Based on the analysis of the 13 NEMLs in this case study, NEMLs differ from each other as well as from the WHO model list. In addition, a comparison of human insulin prescriptions in retail markets shows vastly different compositions across countries, at least of those captured in the IMS MIDAS database. Non-analog insulins make up more than 90 percent of human insulin prescriptions in Morocco and fewer than 10 percent of human insulin prescriptions in Turkey, despite similar epidemiological profiles with respect to population characteristics and diabetes prevalence.

Each country can learn from the priority-setting mechanisms and processes of other countries with similar characteristics, such as region, development status, burden of disease, or health system. In addition to the WHO model list, other countries' NEMLs and processes could serve as good benchmarks when selecting treatments to include on an NEML or in a health benefits package. Data on actual use are helpful to understanding how prescribing levels of various treatments differ between similar countries. NEMLs are easy to obtain online, but obtaining data on actual use is more difficult. It may be costly to obtain use data from a third party; comparing data captured internally by governments requires a large amount of coordination among countries. These data need to be more readily available to enable countries to compare their own priority-setting mechanisms and processes with those in similar countries.

Staying Up to Date on the Market Authorization Process

The case study shows that the composition of human insulin treatment prescriptions is vastly different across countries. Since discrepancies occur between NEMLs and actual prescribing, the prescribing differences between countries are not simply the result of differences in medications listed but can be driven by the entry of new products as part of each country's market authorization process. Once a new product comes to market, the pressure to publicly subsidize it increases.

It is important to be aware of market authorization processes, not only for a single treatment but for the treatment class as a whole. Understanding the market authorization process for classes of drugs in neighboring or similar countries can be useful for managing the pressures on and anticipating the changes to prescribing patterns.

Communicating Priority-Setting Processes and Decisions

In many countries, the actual priority-setting process—for example, exactly how or why a drug is included or excluded from an NEML—is not clear to the public.

Public awareness of the decision-making process and dissemination of the supporting evidence compels a payer or listing entity or the drug regulation entity to remain accountable for its decisions. Accountability mechanisms,

Analog Insulin Pricing and Sales in Colombia

In June 2013, the price per package of Lantus, or insulin glargine, in Colombia was more than twice that in the United Kingdom and several middle-income countries (figure B21.1.1). In 2013, the Colombian government announced that it would regulate several hundred medications based on the international reference price, which benchmarks against the prices of countries such as Argentina, Brazil, Chile, Ecuador, France, Panama, and Spain. Under regulated pricing, the price per package of Lantus is US$45.38; the unregulated price is US$92.23 per 10 milliliter unit. The regulated price is closer to the price in the United Kingdom, although it is still higher than that in other countries.

In 2011, several insulin analogs were included in Colombia's publicly funded health benefits plan, which uses a national essential medicines list as a reference to define the included medicines. Since then, government spending on insulin analogs has accelerated. All insulin analogs except insulin degludec are included in Colombia's national essential medicines list.

Industry- and wholesaler-reported data from a mandatory Ministry of Health system indicate sales to the public sector. These data show rapidly increasing sales of insulin analogs from 2010 to 2013 and a slight decrease in 2014 due to changes in regulation to change the reimbursable price for insulin analogs (figure B21.1.2). Total sales of fast- and long-acting insulin analogs increased by 102 percent and 143 percent, respectively, before 2010 and after the benefits plan was updated in 2012. Long-acting insulin analogs had sales of US$55 million in 2013, more than five times the sales of fast-acting insulin analogs. In the past several years, insulin glargine—a long-acting insulin analog—has had the highest sales among insulin analogs, with US$48 million in 2013, an increase from US$13 million in 2010.

Figure B21.1.1 Price per Package (10 milliliter) of Lantus (Insulin Glargine), 2014

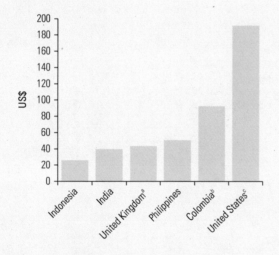

Sources: Colombia: Ministerio de Salud y Protección Social Colombia 2014; Indonesia, India, and the Philippines: MIMS 2014; United Kingdom: British Medical Association and the Royal Pharmaceutical Society of Great Britain 2011; United States: Truven Health Analytics 2014.
a. 2011.
b. Regulated price.
c. Wholesale acquisition cost.

Figure B21.1.2 Insulin Analog Sales to the Institutional Chain, 2010–14

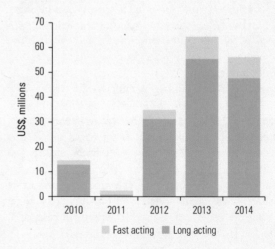

Source: Ministerio de Salud y Protección Social Colombia 2014; SISMED 2014.
Note: Using the average 2013 exchange rate, 1 Col$ = US$0.0005.

such as the appointment of an independent, multidisciplinary committee or the establishment of an appeals process, are discussed in the next section (WHO 2011). These mechanisms reduce the influence of marketing pressures on priority-setting decisions; even if such pressures do have an impact, the mechanisms allow regulators to subsequently manage and minimize the risk of poor prescribing decisions.

The processes for selecting which drugs are on each country's NEML are not clear, especially when they deviate from the WHO model list. For example, Morocco's NEML does not include any non-analog human insulins. Colombia's NEML includes three fast-acting and two long-acting insulin analogs, but Argentina's NEML only includes one insulin analog. Several countries' NEMLs include acarbose, an alpha-glucosidase inhibitor, and glipizide, a sulfonylurea, neither of which are on the WHO model list.

Most countries lack explicit decision-making mechanisms of any kind, but progress has been made. Policy makers in LMICs are increasingly adopting policy instruments that explicitly define, limit, control, or guarantee the particular health technologies, interventions, and benefits that are to be funded and sometimes provided by the government. One approach to explicit priority setting has been to establish HTA entities to assess new and current medical technologies.

CASE STUDY 2: DIALYSIS IN THAILAND

This case study explores Thailand's decision to include dialysis in the benefits package of an NHI plan. First, it discusses the burden of disease, treatment, and health coverage. Second, it discusses HTA agencies as priority-setting mechanisms. Then it examines Thailand's decision to include dialysis using a peritoneal dialysis (PD)–first policy in the Universal Coverage Scheme's (UCS) (box 21.2) benefits package. It concludes with insights from the case study.

Disease Burden and Context

The burden of kidney disease has increased as risk factors such as diabetes and high blood pressure have increased. In LMICs, the DALYs attributable to chronic kidney disease increased by 55 percent between 1990 and 2010 (from 11.0 million to 17.1 million); the number of deaths increased by 87 percent in the same period (from 0.29 million to 0.54 million) (IHME 2013). The increasing trend is notable, although the actual burden-of-disease values, as recognized earlier in this volume, for acute kidney injury, chronic kidney disease, and end-stage renal disease are understudied.

In Thailand, the burden has increased at an accelerated pace—the incidence of end-stage renal disease was 122 per million population (about 8,000 cases) in 2004 and 160 per million population (more than 100,000 cases) in 2007 (Tantivess and others 2013).

Patients with chronic kidney disease require lifetime renal replacement therapy through PD or hemodialysis,[5] if not transplantation—and all interventions come at a high cost. Hemodialysis costs US$12,000 per year, four times higher than the cost per quality-adjusted life year threshold for cost-effectiveness set by the National Health Security Office (NHSO) (Treerutkuarkul 2010). PD costs US$7,300 per year. Instead of receiving treatment as

---

Box 21.2

Health Coverage in Thailand

In Thailand, nearly all citizens have health insurance coverage through three main schemes:

- Social Security Scheme (SSS)
- Civil Servant Medical Benefit Scheme (CSMBS)
- Universal Coverage Scheme (UCS).

SSS and CSMBS cover private and public employees; UCS—launched in 2001 through a reform to Thailand's public health financing system—covers the poor and near-poor. UCS gives each of its 48 million members free care at health centers in their home districts, as well as at contracted hospitals and referrals to second- or third-level hospitals in urban areas.

UCS makes a comprehensive benefits package available to its members. Like SSS, UCS covers outpatient and inpatient care; accident and emergency services; dental and other high-cost care; and diagnostics, special investigations, medicines, and medical supplies. UCS also focuses on prevention by covering clinic-based preventive and health-promotion services in health centers.

prescribed, patients make do through other strategies, such as reducing the frequency of treatment, or they take other measures to fund treatment, such as borrowing money at high interest rates, a common occurrence in poor households (Tantivess and others 2013).

Priority-Setting Mechanism: Health Technology Assessment Agencies

HTA is the systematic appraisal of the properties, effects, or impacts of health technology through a wide range of research methods. In particular, value for money derived from comparative clinical and economic evaluation analysis (cost-effectiveness) is the major component of HTA. Many high-income countries have long used HTA to guide public reimbursement or coverage decisions. Almost all countries have national HTA agencies that prepare evidence dossiers, including cost-effectiveness analyses, as part of the application process for including new medicines for public reimbursement. Since 2005, HTA agencies or units have been established in upper middle-income or new high-income countries, including Brazil, Chile, Colombia, Croatia, Estonia, the Republic of Korea, Malaysia, Poland, Thailand, and Uruguay—and are increasingly influential in providing a basis for the uses of public funding.

The Health Intervention and Technology Assessment Program (HITAP) in Thailand is an autonomous arm of the Ministry of Public Health that provides evidence to support coverage decisions for the UCS benefits package. HITAP is a leader in its use of evidence to manage explicit priority-setting decisions. A highlight of Thailand's health system is that decisions for inclusion or exclusion in the UCS health benefits package are made using an ongoing, explicit priority-setting process by an HTA agency. Thailand's HITAP is sophisticated relative to its counterparts in other middle-income countries for several reasons: a scope beyond the assessment of pharmaceuticals, a deliberative process around HTA, the establishment of a locally relevant cost-effectiveness threshold, and formal stakeholder participation.

Priority Setting in Action

Generally, the UCS benefits package mirrors that of the Social Security Scheme (SSS). However, the SSS and the Civil Servant Medical Benefit Scheme benefits packages have included PD and hemodialysis since 1985 and 1990, respectively, while UCS did not, even though all three schemes rely on public funds. UCS patients—who are typically poor or near-poor—would receive a kidney disease diagnosis and learn that the treatment that

their life depends on would have to be self-financed (Treerutkuarkul 2010).

In the early 2000s, nephrologists and patients made a strong push for inclusion of dialysis in the UCS benefits package on the basis of the equity and financial protection goals of the UCS (Tantivess and others 2013; Treerutkuarkul 2010). At the time, patient groups had not participated in the HTA process; however, for dialysis, an organization called the Thai Kidney Club received support from the HIV/AIDS (human immunodeficiency virus/acquired immune deficiency syndrome) and cancer patient networks, as well as from the Thai Nephrologists Association (Tantivess and others 2013; Treerutkuarkul 2010). Newly in office following a government coup, public health minister Mongkol Na Songkhla sought to identify what forms of therapy should be made available and how dialysis could be financed in a sustainable way.

In response, the NHSO commissioned policy researchers and nephrologists to evaluate the value for money of dialysis. The study found that neither PD nor hemodialysis was cost-effective relative to Thailand's threshold. However, compared with hemodialysis, providing PD would be a relatively cost-effective option. Based on the study's estimates, PD would cost 466,000–497,000 Thai baht (US$15,000) per life year saved or 667,000–700,000 Thai baht (US$21,400) per quality-adjusted life year gained, depending on the patient's age (Teerawattananon, Mugford, and Tangcharoensathien 2007). The infrastructure and human resources needed to treat patients using hemodialysis were concentrated in urban centers, making the treatment inaccessible to rural populations, while PD had a home treatment option (Tantivess and others 2013). Based on the results of the study, the NHSO decided in 2007 to offer PD as a first-line therapy in the UCS benefits package—the PD-first policy.

To make the policy feasible in the long term, the burden of kidney disease had to be controlled. The Ministry of Public Health implemented community screening programs, with financial incentives for community health workers, to boost early detection and treatment of hypertension and diabetes. This effort was accompanied by knowledge strengthening and training to provide information throughout the continuum of care (Tantivess and others 2013).

Despite the measures taken to reduce the burden of kidney disease, the sustainability of this policy is in question. Over the course of 2007–09, the annual incidence of hemodialysis increased by 8 percent (Tantivess and others 2013); the incidence of PD increased by 150 percent (Praditpornsilpa and others 2011). Since 2008, many more patients have received PD—the number of patients grew from less than 1,000 before 2008 to nearly 8,000 per quarter in 2011 (Tantivess and others 2013). By 2012, the number of dialysis units had increased from 23 to 160 and plateaued at this level, with each unit taking on an increasing number of patients (Tantivess and others 2013). Annual budget allocations for dialysis started at US$5 million (160 million Thai baht), or 0.2 percent of the total NHSO budget in 2008, but grew to US$115 million (3.9 billion Thai baht), or 3.4 percent of the total budget in 2012 (Tantivess and others 2013). With continuing increases in the burden of diabetes and hypertension, and most likely kidney disease, the budget for dialysis is likely to increase. Some experts expect that the dialysis budget could be as high as 12 percent of the total budget once access is at full scale (Treerutkuarkul 2010).

Case Study Insights

Thailand is a leader in the universal health coverage movement as evidenced by its early success in reforming the country's health financing system to provide nearly every citizen with health insurance. This health system is supported by a sophisticated HTA agency that sets priorities through an explicit and evidence-driven process. This case study explores the process of including dialysis in the UCS benefits package and some of the considerations involved (a parallel example on South Africa is provided in box 21.3). A few lessons can be drawn from this example.

Acknowledging the Importance of Equity- and Ethics-Related Commitments

Cost-effectiveness and value for money are often key concerns when considering particular interventions to be included or excluded from a benefits package. The decision to include PD in the UCS benefits package was deliberate, based on results from economic evaluations but also considering equity- and ethics-related factors.

The equity-based argument for inclusion of dialysis compared the relative coverage between the UCS and the other two schemes, given that all are supported by public funds. In addition, the UCS aims to reduce catastrophic

---

Box 21.3

Dialysis in South Africa

South Africa's experience with dialysis highlights the challenges with treatment rationing—a difficult decision-making process faced by all countries because the demand for dialysis far exceeds the available resources. Only one of five patients with health insurance or those who are wealthy enough to pay out of pocket for the US$20,000 per year treatment receives dialysis. The remainder rely on public health insurance coverage under a system that has to allocate money to other health priorities.

A dialysis selection committee at each hospital decides which patients will receive coverage for dialysis treatment; there is no explicit decision-making system. Even though apartheid ended in South Africa in 1994, a study finds that white patients were more likely to be accepted for dialysis treatment than nonwhites at Tygerberg between 1988 and 2003. Patients who were to be covered by health insurance for dialysis were selected on the basis of "social worth"—such as income and criminal record—as judged by medical practitioners.

South Africans are working on making the priority-setting process more equitable and transparent. Until 2010, medical staff made decisions based on what they perceived to have been economically beneficial to the hospitals with no involvement by hospital managers. In 2010, provincial officials and medical professionals worked together to create official guidelines for patient selection. A more explicit and accountable system was created. Patients were classified based on medical factors, such as age and body mass index, as well as social factors, such as access to running water and electricity and evidence of financial means to afford transport to a renal unit.

Still, hospitals have to turn away patients. Physicians struggle with the priority-setting process for deciding which patients can receive treatment as well as where they can receive treatment; in addition, they bear the burden of telling the patient.

Sources: Fink 2010; Renal Services Task Team 2010.

expenditures on health for the Thai poor and near-poor. For those who needed dialysis, having to pay large out-of-pocket sums meant that the UCS did not deliver on its promise of financial protection. This case study shows that HTA goes beyond the numbers-based evidence provided by economic analysis by including evidence that involves equity, ethical, social, and legal implications.

Including Input from All Key Stakeholders

The case study shows that the priority-setting process affects many different parties—including policy makers in the Ministry of Public Health, academics, providers in hospitals and health clinics, community health workers, professional associations, and patients. In Thailand, the HTA through HITAP in theory provides an avenue for all stakeholders to play a role in policy change, and this was true for decisions around dialysis.

Through accountability mechanisms such as the appointment of an independent, multidisciplinary committee or establishing an appeals process, the public can take ownership of policy decisions. A transparent priority-setting process via information sharing can limit conflicts between interests (Tantivess and others 2013). For example, physicians recommended coverage of hemodialysis rather than PD based on favorable medical evidence. However, through information sharing—especially of the cost-effectiveness data—and an inclusive process, providers were convinced to accept the decision for PD as first-line therapy.

Incorporating Disease Prevention Measures in the Priority-Setting Process

The burden of noncommunicable disease—specifically cardiovascular, respiratory, and related chronic disorders—will continue to increase in the absence of serious efforts to control risk factors. And because interventions for noncommunicable disease can be expensive and perhaps required for a lifetime, publicly financing these treatments can place a serious burden on a country's economy.

An important component of the UCS is health promotion, and the Thai government continues to invest in such programs. For the early detection and prevention of diabetes and hypertension, the Ministry of Public Health in 2011 launched a US$76 million program of screening measures in 5,500 communities. Still, some in the NHSO consider the health promotion funds to be insufficient and hope to increase efforts to promote healthier lifestyles and prevent noncommunicable diseases overall, not only kidney disease (Treerutkuarkul 2010).

Interventions that target disease prevention cannot be left out of the priority-setting process. When policy makers invest in an expensive curative intervention, it is also important to consider the opportunity cost of investing in preventive interventions. In some cases, treatment alone can be cost-effective but not when coupled with screening.

Using Priority-Setting to Strengthen Overall Health System Capacity

Including an intervention in the benefits package is not just about gathering the evidence and making a decision. For the government to be able to deliver on promises, other parts of the health system must adjust to accommodate new policies. In Thailand, the NHSO encouraged the establishment of clinics that could provide PD in public facilities, particularly first-level hospitals, and partnered with private facilities when it realized that the capacity of public facilities was insufficient (Tantivess and others 2013).

Since 2008, the infrastructure and human resources to accommodate the inclusion of dialysis in the UCS benefits package have been developed. The number of PD clinics increased from 23 to 160 between 2008 and 2012, and the number of nurses trained to care for dialysis patients increased from 56 to 423 during that same period (Tantivess and others 2013). Finding the resources to build the capacity for the provision of dialysis has enabled many to benefit from dialysis coverage under the UCS.

It is not yet clear whether the inclusion of dialysis has had a population health impact, such as improved life expectancy, on the UCS population. As in the previous case study, the Thai dialysis example shows that review of current interventions included in a benefits package, not just new technologies, is crucial in the priority-setting process.

CONCLUSIONS

This chapter brings to light the challenges facing evidence-based resource allocation for health, especially to meet the increasing demand for the treatment of cardiovascular, respiratory, and related chronic disorders. Policy makers in LMICs must weigh prevention, affordability, and ethical considerations in addition to cost-effectiveness when deciding on whom and for what the government will spend. Interventions, both preventive and curative, can be cost-effective, depending on the context, such as disease progression. The priority-setting process can be greatly influenced by political considerations.

The first case study examines prescribing data for human insulin for type 2 diabetes, and reports that, despite being available, an NEML may not have an impact on what treatments physicians actually prescribe and patients actually use. The second case study examines Thailand's decision to include dialysis in the UCS benefits package. Thailand has a sophisticated, explicit priority-setting mechanism—HITAP, its HTA agency—yet, the NHSO still has to make difficult coverage decisions.

Both examples show that countries can benefit from reviewing available interventions in addition to new ones. Crucially, the examples show the importance of institutional capacity in carrying out the process of explicit priority setting to guide technology adoption decisions. Explicit priority setting uses a transparent, deliberative process led by an independent, multidisciplinary committee that considers evidence—as well as other factors, such as inclusiveness—to drive decisions.

A better priority-setting system can provide a fair and transparent mechanism for managing the politics of resource allocation, connect evidence-based decisions to budgets, and create permanent institutional channels for considering resource allocation choices over time.

ACKNOWLEDGMENT

The authors thank Kalipso Chalkidou and Yot Teerawattananon for their contributions and acknowledge the contributions of Sergio Marquez, senior advisor of the Ministry of Health, on medicine pricing policies.

NOTES

World Bank Income Classifications as of July 2014 are as follows, based on estimates of gross national income (GNI) per capita for 2013:

- Low-income countries (LICs) = US$1,045 or less
- Middle-income countries (MICs) are subdivided:
  (a) lower-middle-income = US$1,046–US$4,125
  (b) upper-middle-income (UMICs) = US$4,126–US$12,745
- High-income countries (HICs) = US$12,746 or more.

1. People with type 1 diabetes have a total lack of insulin due to immune system response, while people with type 2 diabetes do not have enough insulin or are insulin resistant.
2. IMS MIDAS medical data show exactly what is being prescribed for a disease or therapy area and is standardized internationally.
3. Many countries, including Turkey, are moving to health insurance formularies that sometimes coexist with and sometimes supersede EMLs, which become defunct and disappear.
4. Average of May, June, and July 2013.
5. Hemodialysis uses an artificial kidney outside the body to filter blood; peritoneal dialysis uses the lining of the abdominal cavity to filter blood.

REFERENCES

Abdraimova, A., and D. Beran. 2009. "Rapid Assessment Protocol for Insulin Access in Kyrgyzstan." Policy Research Document 66, Health Policy Analysis Center, Bishkek, Kyrgyz Republic.

Beran, D., and J. S. Yudkin. 2010. "Looking beyond the Issue of Access to Insulin: What Is Needed for Proper Diabetes Care in Resource Poor Settings." *Diabetes Research and Clinical Practice* 88 (3): 217–21.

British Medical Association and the Royal Pharmaceutical Society of Great Britain. 2011. *British National Formulary* 61. London: BMJ Publishing Group and Pharmaceutical Press.

Brock, D. W., and D. Wikler. 2006. "Ethical Issues in Resource Allocation, Research, and New Product Development." In *Disease Control Priorities in Developing Countries*, second edition, edited by D. T. Jamison, J. G. Breman, A. R. Measham, G. Alleyne, M. Claeson, D. B. Evans, P. Jha, A. Mills, and P. Musgrove, 259–70. Washington, DC: World Bank.

Cameron, A., M. Ewen, D. Ross-Degnan, D. Ball, and R. Laing. 2009. "Medicine Prices, Availability, and Affordability in 36 Developing and Middle-Income Countries: A Secondary Analysis." *The Lancet* 373 (9659): 240–49.

Cohen, D., and P. Carter. 2010. "How Small Changes Led to Big Profits for Insulin Manufacturers." *BMJ* (341): c7139.

Culyer, A. J., C. McCabe, A. Briggs, K. Claxton, M. Buxton, and others. 2007. "Searching for a Threshold, Not Setting One: The Role of the National Institute for Health and Clinical Excellence." *Journal of Health Services Research and Policy* 12 (1): 56–58.

Elshaug, A. G., J. E. Hiller, S. R. Tunis, and J. R. Moss. 2007. "Challenges in Australian Policy Processes for Disinvestment from Existing, Ineffective Health Care Practices." *Australia and New Zealand Health Policy* 4 (23): 1–8.

European Medicines Agency. 2014. "Human Medicines: Tresiba (insulin degludec)." European Medicines Agency, London. http://www.ema.europa.eu/ema/index.jsp?curl =pages/medicines/human/medicines/002498/human _med_001609.jsp&mid=WC0b01ac058001d124.

Fink, S. 2010. "Life and Death Choices as South Africans Ration Dialysis Care." ProPublica, New York.

Garner, S., and P. Littlejohns. 2011. "Do NICE's Recommendations for Disinvestment Add Up?" *BMJ* 343: 349–51.

Glassman, A., and K. Chalkidou. 2012. "Priority-Setting in Health: Building Institutions for Smarter Public Spending." Report of the Priority-Setting Institutions for Global Health Working Group, Center for Global Development, Washington, DC.

Ham, C., and G. Robert. 2003. *Reasonable Rationing: International Experience of Priority Setting in Health Care.* Philadelphia, PA: Open University Press.

Hutubessy, R., R. Baltussen, T. Tan-Torres Edejer, and D. Evans. 2003. "Generalized Cost-Effectiveness Analysis: An Aid to Decision Making in Health." In *Making Choices in Health: WHO Guide to Cost-Effectiveness Analysis*, edited by T. Tan-Torres Edejer, R. Baltussen, T. Adam, R. Hutubessy, A. Acharya, and others, 277–88. Geneva: World Health Organization.

IHME (Institute for Health Metrics and Evaluation). 2013. "Global Burden of Diseases, Injuries, and Risk Factors Study 2010." University of Washington, Institute for Health Metrics and Evaluation, Seattle, WA. http://www.healthdata .org/gbd.

IMS Health. 2013. IMS MIDAS Medical Data.

Japan Pharmaceuticals and Medical Devices Agency. 2013. "New Drugs Approved in FY 2012." Japan Pharmaceuticals and Medical Devices Agency, Tokyo. http://www.pmda.go .jp/english/service/pdf/list/NewdrugsFY2012.pdf.

Johannesson, M., and M. C. Weinstein. 1993. "On the Decision Rules of Cost-Effectiveness Analysis." *Journal of Health Economics* 12 (4): 459–67.

Karagiannis, T., P. Paschos, K. Paletas, D. R. Matthews, and A. Tsapas. 2012. "Dipeptidyl Peptidase-4 Inhibitors for Treatment of Type 2 Diabetes Mellitus in the Clinical Setting: Systematic Review and Meta-Analysis." *BMJ* 344: e1369.

Kinney, E., and B. Clark. 2004. "Provisions for Health and Health Care in the Constitutions of the Countries of the World." *Cornell International Law Journal* 37 (2): 285–355.

Martins, J., and C. Maisonneuve. 2006. "The Drivers of Public Expenditure on Health and Long-Term Care: An Integrated Approach." *Economic Studies* 43, Organisation for Economic Co-operation and Development, Paris.

MIMS (Monthly Index of Medical Specialties). 2014. MIMS Drug Information. https://www.mims.com/.

Ministerio de Salud y Protección Social Colombia. 2014. "Sistema de Informacion de Medicamentos." Bogota.

Moosa, M. R., and M. Kidd. 2006. "The Dangers of Rationing Dialysis Treatment: The Dilemma Facing a Developing Country." *Kidney International* 70 (6): 1107–14.

NICE (National Institute for Health and Care Excellence). 2009. "Type 2 Diabetes: Newer Agents for Blood Glucose Control in Type 2 Diabetes." Short Clinical Guideline 87, NICE, London. http://www.nice.org.uk/nicemedia/pdf /cg87niceguideline.pdf.

———. 2012. "NICE 'Do Not Do' Recommendations." NICE, London. http://www.nice.org.uk/usingguidance /donotdorecommendations/index.jsp.

Novo Nordisk. 2013. "Novo Nordisk Receives Complete Response Letter in the US for Tresiba® and Ryzodeg®." Bagsværd, Denmark. http://www.novonordisk.com/include/asp/exe _news_attachment.asp?sAttachmentGUID=83700060-0ce3 -4577-a35a-f3e57801637d.

PAHO (Pan American Health Organization). 2010. "Access to High-Cost Medicines in the Americas: Situation, Challenges and Perspectives." Technical Series 1—Essential Medicine, Access, and Innovation. PAHO, Washington, DC.

Pinelli, N. R., R. Cha, M. B. Brown, and L. A. Jaber. 2008. "Addition of Thiazolidinedione or Exenatide to Oral Agents in Type 2 Diabetes: A Meta-Analysis." *Annals of Pharmacotherapy* 42 (11): 1541–51.

Praditpornsilpa, K., S. Lekhyananda, N. Premasathian, P. Kingwatanakul, A. Lumpaopong, and others. 2011. "Prevalence Trend of Renal Replacement Therapy in Thailand: Impact of Health Economics Policy." *Journal of the Medical Association of Thailand* 94 (Suppl 4): S1–6.

Qaseem, A., L. L. Humphrey, D. E. Sweet, M. Starkey, and P. Shekelle. 2012. "Oral Pharmacologic Treatment of Type 2 Diabetes Mellitus: A Clinical Practice Guideline from the American College of Physicians." *Annals of Internal Medicine* 156 (3): 218–31.

Renal Services Task Team. 2010. "Guideline: Priority Setting Approach in the Selection of Patients in the Public Sector with End-Stage Kidney Failure for Renal Replacement Treatment in the Western Cape Province." Cape Town, South Africa.

Rojas, L. B. A., and M. B. Gomes. 2013. "Metformin: An Old but Still the Best Treatment for Type 2 Diabetes." *Diabetology and Metabolic Syndrome* 5 (1): 6.

Tantivess, S., P. Werayingyong, P. Chuengsaman, and Y. Teerawattananon. 2013. "Universal Coverage of Renal Dialysis in Thailand: Promise, Progress, and Prospects." *BMJ* 346: f462.

Teerawattananon, Y., M. Mugford, and V. Tangcharoensathien. 2007. "Economic Evaluation of Palliative Management versus Peritoneal Dialysis and Hemodialysis for End-Stage Renal Disease: Evidence for Coverage Decisions in Thailand." *Value Health* 10 (1): 61–72.

Treerutkuarkul, A. 2010. "Thailand: Health Care for All, at a Price." *Bulletin of the World Health Organization* 88 (2): 84–85.

Truven Health Analytics. 2014. Red Book Online. http:// redbook.solutions.aap.org/redbook.aspx.

van den Ham, R., L. Bero, and R. Laing. 2011. "Selection of Essential Medicines." In *World Medicines Situation Report*, third edition. Geneva: World Health Organization.

van Dieren, S., J. Beulens, Y. van der Schouw, D. Grobbee, and B. Neal. 2010. "The Global Burden of Diabetes and Its Complications: An Emerging Pandemic." *European Journal of Preventive Cardiology* 17 (Suppl 1): S3–8.

Weinstein, M. C., and W. B. Statson. 1977. "Foundations of Cost-Effectiveness Analysis for Health and Medical Practices." *New England Journal of Medicine* 296 (13): 716–21.

WHO (World Health Organization). 2011. *Marketing Authorization of Pharmaceutical Products with Special Reference to Multisource (Generic) Products: A Manual for National Medicines Regulatory Authorities (NMRAs).* Geneva: WHO.

———. 2013. "WHO Model List of Essential Medicines, 18th List." WHO, Geneva. http://apps.who.int/iris /bitstream/10665/93142/1/EML_18_eng.pdf.

———. 2014 *Making Fair Choices on the Path to Universal Health Coverage: Final Report of the WHO Consultative Group on Equity and Universal Health Coverage.* Geneva: WHO.

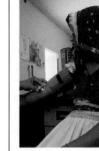

Chapter 22

Management of Hypertension and Dyslipidemia for Primary Prevention of Cardiovascular Disease

Panniyammakal Jeemon, Rajeev Gupta,
Churchill Onen, Alma Adler, Thomas A. Gaziano,
Dorairaj Prabhakaran, and Neil Poulter

INTRODUCTION

Despite declining rates of age-standardized cardiovascular disease (CVD) mortality in high-income countries (HICs) over the past three decades, CVD remains the leading cause of death worldwide (GBD 2013 Mortality and Causes of Death Collaborators 2013). The estimated global cost of CVD in 2010 was US$863 billion, and this cost is expected to rise to US$1,044 billion by 2030 (World Economic Forum 2011). A large proportion of global CVD deaths (about 80 percent) occur in low- and middle-income countries (LMICs). CVD deaths are declining in HICs mainly because of a significant reduction in coronary heart disease (CHD) and in stroke mortality. This decline is largely attributable to changes in population-level risk factors and specific blood pressure (BP) and cholesterol treatments (Björck and others 2015; Davies, Smeeth, and Grundy 2007; Lewsey and others 2015). In this chapter, we discuss antihypertensive and cholesterol-lowering therapies and use of aspirin for primary prevention of CVD. Lifestyle measures such as reductions in smoking and improvements in diet and physical activity are covered in chapter 4 (Roy and others 2017), chapter 5 (Bull and others 2017), and chapter 7 (Malik and Hu 2017) in this volume. Similarly, therapies

to treat ischemic heart disease, therapies to treat chronic heart failure, and therapies to reduce risk in patients with type 1 and type 2 diabetes are described, respectively, in chapter 8 (Dugani and others 2017), chapter 10 (Huffman and others 2017), and chapter 12 (Ali and others 2017) in this volume.

This chapter highlights new findings about the global burden of high BP and lipids. It discusses changing thresholds and targets for BP- and lipid-lowering therapies in the context of newly available evidence from randomized controlled trials (RCTs) and meta-analyses of RCTs. Attention is paid to the adverse effect on blood glucose associated with statin therapy and statin-induced diabetes, the role of ezetimibe in reducing low-density lipoprotein (LDL) cholesterol, and the uncertainty about the risks of aspirin in primary prevention of CVD. We also discuss the available evidence in the context of resource-poor settings and make recommendations.

BURDEN OF HIGH BLOOD PRESSURE

Globally, the population mean BP level has decreased marginally since 1980. From 1980 to 2008, global mean

Corresponding author: Panniyammakal Jeemon, Associate Professor, chronic disease epidemiology, Public Health Foundation of India, New Delhi, India; pjeemon@gmail.com.

age-adjusted systolic blood pressure (SBP) declined from 130.5 millimeters of mercury (mmHg, a measure of pressure) to 128.1 mmHg in men and from 127.2 to 124.4 mmHg in women (Danaei and others 2011). Similarly, the global age-adjusted prevalence of uncontrolled hypertension decreased to 29 percent from 33 percent in men and to 25 percent from 29 percent in women. Despite these changes, high BP has gone from being the fourth-highest risk factor in 1990, as quantified by attributable disability-adjusted life years (DALYs), to the highest risk factor in 2010 (Murray and others 2013). This increase is primarily due to population growth and aging, especially in LMICs, and the consequent rise in the number of people worldwide with uncontrolled hypertension, that is, SBP ≥ 140 mmHg or diastolic blood pressure ≥ 90 mmHg. For example, the number of individuals with uncontrolled hypertension increased from 605 million to 978 million between 1980 and 2008 (Danaei and others 2011). SBP declined largely in HICs, while mean SBP rose in several regions, including East Africa, Oceania, and South and South-East Asia (Danaei and others 2011). Currently, high BP is one of the five leading risk factors of morbidity and mortality in all regions of the world, with the exception of Eastern Sub-Saharan Africa, Oceania, and Western Sub-Saharan Africa (Murray and others 2013).

Furthermore, raised BP (as opposed to hypertension) is among the leading global risk factors for mortality and is responsible for 9.4 million deaths annually (Lim and others 2012). It is independently attributable for at least 45 percent of deaths from ischemic heart disease (IHD) and 51 percent of deaths from stroke. Given this high burden and population aging, hypertension remains an issue of global concern. The estimated total direct and indirect cost of high BP in 2011 was US$46.4 billion and is expected to reach US$274 billion by 2030 (Mozaffarian and others 2015).

BURDEN OF HYPERCHOLESTEROLEMIA

Cholesterol is required to make hormones, vitamin D, and bile acids. Cholesterol also provides cell membrane support. Two kinds of lipoproteins carry cholesterol throughout the body: LDLs (known as bad cholesterol) and high-density lipoproteins (HDLs). A high LDL level often leads to a buildup of cholesterol in the walls of arteries. Globally, hypercholesterolemia, defined as total cholesterol ≥ 190 milligrams per deciliter or ≥ 5.0 millimoles per liter (mmol/L), causes an estimated 2.6 million deaths (4.5 percent of total deaths) and 29.7 million DALYs (2.0 percent of total DALYs) annually (Alwan 2011). More than one-fourth

(29 percent) of DALYs from IHD can be attributed to high total cholesterol, which is the second-leading physiological risk factor for IHD after high BP (Lim and others 2012). Physiologically, LDL is critical to the generation of atherosclerosis.

Mean total serum cholesterol decreased marginally between 1980 and 2008 globally, falling less than 0.1 mmol/L per decade in men and women (Farzadfar and others 2011). The mean age-adjusted total cholesterol level decreased from 4.72 to 4.64 mmol/L (95 percent confidence interval [CI] 4.51–4.76 mmol/L) for men and from 4.83 to 4.76 mmol/L (95 percent CI 4.62–4.91 mmol/L) for women between 1980 and 2008.

In 1990, total cholesterol was ranked fourteenth as a risk factor, as quantified by DALYs, and remained little changed in 2010, when it was ranked fifteenth (Lim and others 2012). The prevalence of elevated total cholesterol was highest in the World Health Organization (WHO) European Region (54 percent for both sexes), followed by the Americas (48 percent for both sexes); the lowest percentages were in the Africa and South-East Asia regions (23 percent and 30 percent, respectively) (Alwan 2011).

INTERVENTIONS FOR THE PRIMARY PREVENTION OF CARDIOVASCULAR DISEASE

CVD encompasses a broad range of vascular conditions comprising IHD (including stable and unstable angina, nonfatal myocardial infarction, and coronary death); heart failure; cardiac arrest; ventricular arrhythmias; sudden cardiac death; rheumatic heart disease; transient ischemic attack; ischemic stroke; subarachnoid and intracerebral hemorrhage; abdominal aortic aneurysm; peripheral artery disease; and congenital heart disease. CHD accounts for the greatest proportion of CVD globally (Mozaffarian and others 2015). However, the incidence and prevalence of CHD vary greatly according to geographic region, gender, and ethnic background. After CHD, cerebrovascular disease or stroke is the second-highest cause of CVD mortality. We focus largely on these two conditions.

Over the past three to four decades, multiple longitudinal follow-up studies have provided valuable insights into the natural history and risk factors associated with the development of and prognosis for CVD (D'Agostino and others 2001; Klag and others 1993; Stamler, Stamler, and Neaton 1993; Vasan and others 2001). More recent data have updated and refined these findings (IOM 2010; Wong 2014). The results of these studies have laid a strong foundation for intervention studies and clinical trials aimed at primary prevention and have resulted in the evolution of hypertension and cholesterol management guidelines. Primary prevention focuses mainly on the modification of risk factors through lifestyle changes, and pharmacological treatment aims to reduce the lifetime risk of developing CHD and stroke. Effective treatments are available to control most cases of hypertension and hypercholesterolemia and thereby to reduce consequent CVD. Although cost-effective interventions are available globally for reducing cardiovascular (CV) risk by addressing hypertension and hypercholesterolemia, there are major gaps in the implementation of current evidence-based interventions, particularly in resource-constrained settings. This section discusses the interventions targeting elevated BP and dyslipidemia (abnormal levels of lipids) for the primary prevention of CVD on the basis of current evidence.

Pharmacotherapy for Treatment of Hypertension

Four important risk factors of CVD—hypertension, dyslipidemia, diabetes, and smoking—are amenable to pharmacological treatment (WHO 2007). Robust RCT-based data show the benefits of lowering BP and LDL cholesterol and of controlling diabetes for preventing CVD (Antonakoudis and others 2007; Marso and others 2016; WHO 2007; Zinman and others 2015).

Meta-analyses have shown (1) that the amount of BP reduction is a more important determinant of the reduction in cardiovascular events than is the choice of drug class and (2) that a combination of at least two drugs is usually needed for long-term control, possibly making the initial choice of drug class less important (Blood Pressure Lowering Treatment Trialists' Collaboration 2000; Staessen and others 2001; Turnbull and Blood Pressure Lowering Treatment Trialists' Collaboration 2003). Currently, the BP of only about 32.5 percent of people treated for hypertension is controlled to targets; this proportion is even lower in low-income (12.7 percent) and lower-middle-income (9.9 percent) countries (Chow and others 2013). Yet lowering CVD risk in half of the people with uncontrolled hypertension, including those untreated and those inadequately treated, would avert an estimated 10 million CV events worldwide over 10 years (Angell, De Cock, and Frieden 2015).

Pharmacological Control of Blood Pressure

Several guidelines on hypertension management have been published since 2013. All current guidelines are consistent and unanimous in recommending nonpharmacological measures to lower BP (for example, weight loss, reduction in alcohol and salt intake) and to reduce CVD

risk (for example, smoking cessation), although there are some differences in the details of these recommendations (for example, reduction in caffeine consumption) (James and others 2014; NICE 2011; WHO 2013).

The thresholds for initiating therapy are largely consistent across sets of guidelines (table 22.1). The most common recommendation is a target of 140/90 mmHg with a few variations based on whether ambulatory BP measurement (ABPM) is used, the absolute estimated CV risk, and age group (James and others 2014; NICE 2011; WHO 2013). Similarly, targets are largely consistent (less than 140/90 mmHg), but again age range affects the recommended target in most guidelines. An exception is the Eighth Joint National Committee (JNC 8) recommendations, which are at odds with all other guidelines and which appear to lack sufficient support to merit compliance with them (James and others 2014).

Recent data from the SPRINT trial have given rise to the question of whether targets should fall further, but the atypical (although probably more robust) method of BP measurement used in that trial (automated unattended office blood pressure) probably exaggerates the benefits attributed to achieving SBP of less than 120 mmHg and more likely relates to SBP of less than 130 mmHg (SPRINT Research Group 2015). Meanwhile, several recent meta-analyses provide conflicting evidence on the merits of lowering BP targets (Thomopoulos, Parati, and Zanchetti 2014a, 2014b, 2014c, 2015; Weber and Lackland 2016; Zanchetti, Thomopoulos, and Parati 2015).

If nonpharmacological interventions have been insufficient to lower BP below the recommended thresholds, the agents recommended for lowering BP are largely restricted to seven drug classes—angiotensin-converting enzyme (ACE) inhibitors, angiotensin receptor blockers, beta blockers, alpha blockers, calcium channel blockers, diuretics, and mineralocorticoid receptor antagonists—with variably strong RCT-based evidence to support their use (table 22.2). Recent statements and guidelines differ in their recommendations for the initial pharmacological treatment of hypertension and for which combinations of two drugs from distinct classes of drugs should be used. Some guidelines suggest initiating therapy with two drugs, particularly for persons with very high initial BP or high CV risk (AAFP 2014; Mancia and others 2013). However, initiating drugs from any of three drug classes—calcium channel blockers, diuretics, or renin-angiotensin system blockers—as first-line monotherapy or low-dose combinations of two drugs is more appropriate in low-resource settings for treating hypertension in general (Bronsert and others 2013).

Table 22.1 Thresholds for Initiating Therapy

Blood pressure (mmHg), except where noted

Indicator	NICE 2011	ESH, ESC 2013	ASH, ISH 2014	AHA, ACC, CDC 2013	2014 hypertension guidelines, JNC 8
Definition of hypertension	≥ 140/90; daytime ABPM (or home BP monitoring) of ≥ 135/85	≥ 140/90	≥ 140/90	≥ 140/90	Not addressed
Drug therapy in low-risk patients after nonpharmacological treatments	≥ 160/100 or daytime ABPM ≥ 150/95	≥ 140/90	≥ 140/90	≥ 140/90	In persons < age 60 years, ≥ 140/90; in persons > age 60 years, ≥ 150/90
Beta blockers as first-line drug	No (step 4)	Yes	No (step 4)	No (step 3)	No (step 4)
Diuretics	Chlorthalidone, indapamide	Thiazides, chlorthalidone, indapamide	Thiazides, chlorthalidone, indapamide	Thiazides	Thiazides, chlorthalidone, indapamide
Initiation of drug therapy with two drugs	Not mentioned	In patients with markedly elevated BP	≥ 160/100	≥ 160/100	≥ 160/100
BP targets	< 140/90; for persons > age 80 years, < 150/90	< 140/90; in patients < age 80 years, SBP of < 140; in fit patients, SBP of < 140; in patients > age 80 years, SBP of 140–150	< 140/90; in patients > age 80 years, < 150/90	< 140/90; lower targets may be appropriate in some patients, including the elderly	In persons < age 60 years, < 140/90; in persons > age 60 years, < 150/90
BP target in patients with diabetes mellitus	Not addressed	< 140/85	< 140/90	< 140/90; lower targets may be considered	< 140/90

Note: ABPM = ambulatory blood pressure measurement; ACC = American College of Cardiology; AHA = American Heart Association; ASH = American Society of Hypertension; BP = blood pressure; CDC = Centers for Disease Control and Prevention; ESC = European Society of Cardiology; ESH = European Society of Hypertension; ISH = International Society of Hypertension; JNC 8 = Eighth Joint National Committee; mmHg = millimeters of mercury, a measure of pressure; NICE = National Institute for Health and Care Excellence; SBP = systolic blood pressure.

Table 22.2 Pharmacological Agents Available as Generics for Controlling Hypertension and Reducing Cardiovascular Risk in Many Countries

Class	Common examples (alphabetic)
Angiotensin-converting enzyme inhibitors	Captopril, enalapril, lisinopril, perindopril, ramipril
Angiotensin receptor blockers	Candesartan, losartan, olmesartan, telmisartan, valsartan
Calcium channel blockers	Amlodipine, cilnidipine, lercanidipine, nifedipine
Diuretics (thiazides and thiazide-like)	Bendroflumethiazide, chlorthalidone, chlorothiazide, hydrochlorothiazide, indapamide
Beta blockers	Atenolol, bisoprolol, carvedilol, metoprolol, nebivolol, propranolol
Mineralocorticoid receptor antagonists	Eplerenone, spironolactone
Alpha blockers	Doxazosin, prazosin
Others	Clonidine, hydralazine, methyldopa, minoxidil, reserpine

Note: Preferred antihypertensive drugs in women of reproductive age with intention for conception and for pregnant and breastfeeding women are methyldopa, nifedipine, and hydralazine.

Combination Therapy for Management of Hypertension

Population and trial-based evidence shows that the majority of patients with hypertension require at least two antihypertensive agents to control BP to currently recommended targets (figure 22.1).

Limited RCT-based evidence is available with which to evaluate the best combination of two antihypertensive agents, as reflected in the inconsistent recommendations of recent hypertension guidelines (table 22.3). However, most guidelines recommend at least one of the possible combinations of three classes: renin-angiotensin system blockers, calcium channel blockers, and diuretics (Weber and others 2014).

For several logical reasons, albeit not based on definitive RCT data, several sets of guidelines (James and others 2014; Mancia and others 2013) recommend initiating therapy with two drugs. The WHO list of essential medicines for antihypertensive drugs includes calcium channel blockers (amlodipine); beta blockers (atenolol, bisoprolol, carvedilol, metoprolol); ACE inhibitors (enalapril); hydrochlorothiazide; hydralazine; and methyldopa. The Sustainable Developmental Goals of the United Nations envisage making these essential medicines available in at least 80 percent of health care facilities by 2030. Similarly, when a combination of drugs is indicated, the use of single-pill combinations of drugs (frequently and often inaccurately described as fixed-dose combinations) is usually recommended in guidelines (AAFP 2014; WHO 2007) based on largely observational data and logic.

Antiplatelet Therapy

In the context of primary prevention, the RCT-based evidence regarding the level of CV risk at which aspirin (or other antiplatelet therapy) provides more good than harm remains uncertain. Trials with huge sample sizes and long-term follow-up are required to establish the evidence for aspirin in primary prevention. Halvorsen and others (2014) proposed a pragmatic step-wise approach for the use of aspirin in primary prevention. It includes assessing both short-term CV risk and bleeding risk simultaneously and then starting low-dose aspirin with caution if the CV risk is 10 percent to 20 percent. However, if there is no bleeding risk and the CV risk is more than 20 percent, aspirin should be started immediately. There is no need to start aspirin if the CV risk is less than 10 percent.

Pharmacotherapy for Lowering of Lipids

Extensive observational and experimental data have confirmed that elevated LDL cholesterol is not only an

Figure 22.1 Average Number of Antihypertensive Agents Used to Try to Reach Blood Pressure Goal in Several Hypertension Trials

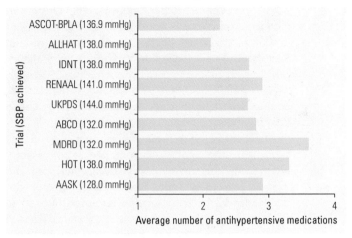

Sources: Bakris 2004; Dahlöf and others 2005.
Note: AASK = African American Study of Kidney Disease and Hypertension; ABCD = Appropriate Blood Pressure Control in Diabetes trial; ALLHAT = Antihypertensive and Lipid-Lowering Treatment to Prevent Heart Attack Trial; ASCOT-BPLA = Anglo-Scandinavian Cardiac Outcomes Trial–Blood Pressure Lowering Arm; HOT = Hypertension Optimal Treatment Study; IDNT = Irbesartan Diabetic Nephropathy Trial; MDRD = Modification of Diet in Renal Disease study; mmHg = millimeters of mercury, a unit of pressure; RENAAL = Reduction of Endpoints in NIDDM with the Angiotensin II Antagonist Losartan study; SBP = systolic blood pressure; UKPDS = U.K. Prospective Diabetes Study.

Table 22.3 Recommended Two-Drug Combinations of Antihypertensive Drugs

NICE	ESH, ESC 2013	ASH, ISH	JNC 8
A + C	A + C	African American	African American
	A + D	A + C	C + D
	C + D	A + D	
		C + D	
		Non-African American	Non-African American
		A + C	A + C
		A + D	A + D
			C + D

Note: A = ACE (angiotensin-converting enzyme) inhibitor or angiotensin receptor blocker; C = calcium channel blocker; D = diuretic (including thiazides or thiazide-like or type); ASH = American Society of Hypertension; ESC = European Society of Cardiology; ESH = European Society of Hypertension; ISH = International Society of Hypertension; JNC 8 = Eighth Joint National Committee; NICE = National Institute for Health and Care Excellence.

independent risk factor for the generation of atherosclerosis and major adverse CV events, but also the pivotal component of the atherosclerotic process (Libby 2000). Data are also compelling, but less consistent, in showing that low HDL cholesterol and high triglycerides are independent risk factors for the generation of major adverse CV events (Miller and others 2011; Toth 2005). Nevertheless, before the introduction of statin therapy in the 1990s, the benefits of lipid-lowering therapy were controversial and the use of lipid-lowering agents was not part of routine practice, except possibly for persons with familial hypercholesterolemia. However, since publication of the results of the Scandinavian Simvastatin Survival Study trial in 1994, which confirmed the significant benefits of lowering lipids with simvastatin for all-cause mortality (Olsson and others 1994), credible doubts about the benefits of statin use have largely disappeared.

The benefits of various statins have been clearly shown in the context of secondary and primary prevention—for strokes and CHD among men and women, persons of young and old age, persons with diabetes and hypertension, and irrespective of baseline CV risk or starting lipid levels (Baigent and others 2010). High-dose statin use has been shown to reduce intravascular atherosclerotic load. Meta-analyses suggest that for every 1.0 mmol/L reduction in LDL cholesterol, there is a 22 percent reduction in CHD mortality and a 29 percent reduction in nonfatal myocardial infarction, and no level below which benefits are not apparent (Baigent and others 2010).

The following lipid-lowering agents for clinical management are currently available:

- Statins
- Ezetimibe
- Fibrates
- Cholesteryl ester transfer protein (CETP) inhibitors
- Fish oils
- Nicotinic acid
- Proprotein convertase subtilisin/kexin type 9 (PCSK9) inhibitors.

Statins constitute the overwhelming majority of lipid-lowering agents in use and hence are the focus of this review.

Statins

The enzyme 3-hydroxy-3-methylglutaryl-coenzyme A (HMG-CoA) reductase is the rate-limiting enzyme for synthesizing cholesterol. HMG-CoA reductase inhibitors (statins) lower LDL cholesterol by, as their name suggests, intrahepatic inhibition of HMG-CoA reductase, which reduces cholesterol biosynthesis and leads to reduced blood levels of LDL cholesterol. Statins also induce small (about 5 percent) increases in serum HDL cholesterol levels and modest (about 20 percent) reductions in serum triglyceride levels.

Side effects (established in RCTs with more than 160,000 patients) include myopathy, rhabdomyolysis (breakdown of skeletal muscle), and increased rates of new-onset diabetes. On the basis of observational data, statin use has also been linked with several other side effects, including myalgia, cognitive impairment, erectile dysfunction, and cataract—none of which has been confirmed in the extensive RCT database. Nevertheless, the link between statin use and side effects has had an unfavorable and inappropriate impact on the use of statins (Schaffer and others 2015). In a review of 39 statin trials, stopping the use of statins as a result of perceived side effects was associated with a significant increase in CV and cerebrovascular events and death rates (Gomez Sandoval, Braganza, and Daskalopoulou 2011).

Statins are currently recommended for all patients with primary lipid disorders, established CVD, or diabetes and, in the context of primary prevention, persons at high levels of estimated absolute risk. The definition of *high* varies across guidelines but has been altered recently in both U.S. and U.K. guidelines to 10-year risk of 7.5 percent and 10 percent, respectively (Rabar and others 2014; Stone and others 2014). All guidelines recommend healthy diets and lifestyles to improve lipid profiles and reduce CV risk. However, guidelines differ in their recommendations regarding the pivotal lipid measurement—LDL cholesterol (Stone and others 2014) or non-HDL cholesterol (Rabar and others 2014)—and whether a target lipid level is appropriate for the use of statins (Stone and others 2014).

Other Lipid-Lowering Agents

Results of individual trials or meta-analyses have undermined the use of fish oils (Kwak and others 2012), fibrates (Katsiki and others 2013; Shipman, Strange, and Ramachandran 2016), CETP inhibitors (Nicholls and others 2011), and nicotinic acid (Kones and Rumana 2015; Tuteja and Rader 2014) for the treatment of dyslipidemia to prevent major adverse CV events. Fibrates, nicotinic acid, and fish oils remain in use by lipid specialists, but on a relatively tenuous basis, for subgroups of patients in whom low HDL cholesterol and high triglycerides predominate (Dierkes, Luley, and Westphal 2007; Shearer, Savinova, and Harris 2012; Zhao and others 2004).

The significant beneficial effect of ezetimibe versus placebo when added to a statin has established this agent as the only evidence-based add-on therapy to statins that helps prevent major adverse CV events in the context of secondary prevention.

In the near future, the first PCSK9 inhibitor to be used in addition to routine high-dose statin therapy may become readily available for secondary prevention purposes (Stoekenbroek, Kastelein, and Huijgen 2015; Yang 2015). The role of these agents in primary prevention where statins are insufficient or not tolerated remains to be established.

Polypills

The most cost-effective way to prevent major adverse CV events is to acknowledge the frequent coexistence of major risk factors—which has a critical impact on absolute risk of a CV event—and therefore to target persons at highest estimated CV risk. Hence, risk assessment is a routine component of the management of risk factors such as raised BP and, particularly, lipid levels (NICE 2011; Räber and others 2015; Stone and others 2014).

Some of the major determinants of CV risk, such as age and sex, are not "treatable," and lipid levels may not be abnormal in a person with mild hypertension. However, if the person is older (for example, 69 years) and a male with mild hypertension, the estimated risk levels may be sufficient (for example, 20 percent risk in the next 10 years) to merit intervention with a statin. Indeed, British guidance recommends using a statin for almost all persons with treated hypertension or diabetes. This routine use of two or more agents has given rise to increased interest in the use of multicomponent pills (polypills). These formulations of two or more agents have been shown to increase compliance and to thereby generate better control of individual risk factors (Castellano and others 2014).

The polypill concept first received attention in an article by Wald and Law (2003). This article proposed the idea of a population-based approach to preventing CVD by giving a single polypill that included six components to all middle-aged persons, with the expectation of preventing 80 percent of heart attacks. The proposed components were a statin, aspirin, folate, and three low doses of BP-lowering agents: a diuretic, an ACE inhibitor, and a beta blocker. Since then, several trials have yielded strong evidence that the use of polypills improves adherence (Webster and others 2013). Additionally, improved adherence was found to be directly associated with a reduction in targeted risk factors. None of these initial trials was designed to detect a difference in outcomes, and no differences in fatal or nonfatal events were demonstrated. In a nested case control analysis of 13,029 patients with IHD in the United Kingdom, however, combinations of drugs such as a statin, aspirin, and a beta blocker rather than single agents decreased mortality in patients with known CVD (Hippisley-Cox and Coupland 2005).

Screening

CVDs are characterized by the commonality and presence of a wide overlap of modifiable and nonmodifiable risk factors. This section focuses on screening for potentially modifiable CVD risk factors, subclinical disease in asymptomatic persons, and clinical disease. Novel or emerging risk factors are not discussed. Screening approaches are guided by simplicity, wide availability, relatively low cost, applicability in resource-limited settings, noninvasiveness, and cost-effectiveness of selected tools; are supported by evidence when available; and are guided by detailed history and thorough clinical examinations whenever applicable.

Screening programs rely on several prerequisites. First, the condition being identified must be serious or lead to serious clinical outcomes; second, preclinical conditions should be common and asymptomatic; and third, early treatment of the condition detected through screening should have proven benefit (Wilson and Jungner 1968). Unfortunately, the inherent imperfection of clinical diagnostic tests introduces uncertainty into their interpretation. The magnitude of diagnostic uncertainty after any test may be quantified by information theory. However, understanding the theory of conditional probability (Bayes's theorem) may not be necessary for applying a screening program effectively in asymptomatic individuals and in medical decision making.

Blood Pressure Screening

BP is a powerful, consistent, independent, and continuous risk factor for CVD and for cerebrovascular and renal diseases (Lewington and others 2002). Observational studies involving more than 1 million individuals have indicated that the number of deaths from CHD and stroke increases progressively and linearly from BP levels as low as 115 mmHg systolic and 75 mmHg diastolic upward in persons of all ages from 40 years to 89 years (Lewington and others 2002). Overall, mortality from CHD and stroke doubles for every 20 mmHg increase in systolic pressure and 10 mmHg increase in diastolic pressure (Franco, Oparil, and Carretero 2004). Correct measurement and interpretation of BP is therefore essential in the accurate diagnosis of hypertension. The use of properly calibrated and validated BP measurement devices with appropriate cuff sizes is essential.

Despite several limitations, office-based BP measurement (OBPM) is the most practical and frequently used method, but home (out-of-office) BP measurement (HBPM) and ABPM are increasingly used and are more valid measurement strategies (Breaux-Shropshire and others 2005). The British National Institute for Health and Care Excellence (NICE) guidelines recommend the use of ABPM to confirm the diagnosis of hypertension if OBPM is elevated, and HBPM when ABPM is unavailable or unaffordable (Krause and others 2011). However, in low-resource settings, the feasible approach currently remains OBPM.

The difference between systolic and diastolic BP (pulse pressure) is a measure of arterial stiffness. Pulse pressure is a significant predictive factor for CVD and chronic kidney disease (Franklin and others 1999; Malone and Reddan 2010). Estimation of pulse pressure is a simple and practical determinant of CV risk, provided that BP measurements have followed standardized approaches.

Lipid Screening

Lipids are perfect targets for CV screening programs, given their central role in atherosclerotic disorders leading to CHD and ischemic stroke. Furthermore, the relationship between atherogenic lipid fractions and subfractions and CHD is continuous, graded, and powerful, with lower thresholds in persons with diabetes mellitus. However, the decision to treat lipids should be guided not by lipid levels alone, but also by the overall CV risk, which is primarily influenced by age, sex, hypertension, smoking, and family history of premature CHD (that is, first-degree male relative with CHD before age 55 years or first-degree female relative with CHD before age 65 years) (Grundy and others 2004).

The most cost-effective method for predicting CHD is measuring the ratio of total cholesterol to HDL cholesterol (Lemieux and others 2001). This test is widely available, well standardized, and comparatively inexpensive and requires no prior fasting. The ratio of total cholesterol to HDL cholesterol is also widely validated in most CHD risk scores. Non-HDL cholesterol, derived by subtracting HDL cholesterol from total cholesterol, is a better predictor than LDL cholesterol. LDL cholesterol is calculated using the Friedewald equation (LDL cholesterol = total cholesterol minus HDL minus triglycerides times 0.2), which applies only to the fasting state and is affected by

hypertriglyceridemia (Fukuyama and others 2008). Direct measurement of LDL cholesterol is technically more challenging and not sufficiently standardized. Besides, different subfractions of LDL cholesterol have different atherogenic potential but have not been shown to have sufficient incremental value to traditional risk factor assessments to merit routine adoption. It is doubtful whether the marginal improvements in CVD prediction gained by including combinations of apolipoprotien B and A1 justify the application of these tools for screening purposes (Di Angelantonio and others 2012). Triglycerides also appear to have relatively smaller predictive power once total cholesterol and HDL cholesterol have been measured and hence do not form a major component of most risk prediction models.

Various guidelines have given wide-ranging target age groups for lipid screening in men and women (NICE 2014; U.S. Preventive Services Task Force 2014). Overall, in low-resource settings, it appears rational to screen all persons for total cholesterol and HDL cholesterol in nonfasting state after age 40 years, but there is evidence to support screening of men and women who are at high risk of CHD starting at age 20 years. Repeat lipid measurements are recommended every three years in persons with atherogenic lipid profiles on prior measurement, but repeat measurement may be every five years in persons with initial lipid levels below the threshold for treatment.

Diabetes Mellitus, Prediabetes, and Gestational Diabetes Screening

Diabetes mellitus fulfills all of the requisites for screening. The methods of measuring glucose both for screening and diagnosing and for managing diabetes are identical. Blood glucose values span a continuum in any population, but there is a threshold above which the risk of potential adverse events is substantial. This threshold is discussed in chapter 12 in this volume (Ali and others 2017). Other methods of screening are listed in table 22.4.

To manage CVD in low-resource settings, the WHO has developed a cost-effective package based on expert opinion (WHO 2002). The proposed strategy starts with CV risk screening by nonphysician health care workers using hypertension as an entry point, with the additional option for using diabetes or smoking as an entry point. This pragmatic approach to managing CVD in low-resource settings reduces absolute CV risk by targeting multiple risk factors at the same time. The potential improvement in health outcomes is manifold compared with the identification and treatment of individual risk factors.

Table 22.4 Screening for Subclinical Cardiovascular Disease and Other Conditions

Method	Purpose
Echocardiography	To detect presence of left ventricular hypertrophy or valvular, myocardial, or pericardial diseases
Coronary artery calcium scanning	To quantify coronary artery calcium and thereby detect significant coronary artery disease
Intraarterial cerebral angiography, carotid duplex ultrasound, magnetic resonance angiography, computed tomography angiography	To measure carotid and coronary artery stenosis
Renal ultrasonography, duplex ultrasound	To test for renal artery stenosis

COST AND COST-EFFECTIVENESS OF INTERVENTIONS

Control of risk factors is paramount to the primary prevention of CVD and a major focus of primary health care. BP control has been a cornerstone of the reduction of stroke, IHD, and peripheral vascular disease for more than 50 years. Its cost-effectiveness is well accepted in all regions (Murray and others 2003; Rosendaal and others 2016; Rubinstein and others 2010; Wang and others 2001). Issues regarding the cost-effectiveness of such interventions have focused more recently on ways to improve the efficiency of identifying who most benefits from treatment, how to improve access to medications, how to improve adherence to medications, and how best to deliver medications. One trend has been to evaluate the overall risk of a patient compared with a single risk factor such as BP. Several studies have shown that it is more cost-effective to choose whom to treat for BP on the basis of the overall CVD risk rather than on the basis of BP or cholesterol level alone (Gaziano and others 2005; Lim and others 2007; Rosendaal and others 2016; Rubinstein and others 2010). Similar analyses have been done for cholesterol treatment, with guidelines in Europe, the United States, and the WHO moving to global risk-based assessments for recommendations regarding when to initiate statin-based medications. Work by Murray and others (2003) showed that efforts to lower cholesterol were cost-effective for persons at high cardiovascular risk (absolute risk more than 35 percent). Efforts to improve adherence to statins by writing longer prescriptions have also been shown to be cost saving and highly cost-effective in South Africa (Gaziano, Cho, and others 2015).

Another way to address the availability and affordability of medications for hypertension and dyslipidemia is to use a combination of generic CVD medications or a polypill for all adults with significant risk for CVD (Wald and Law 2003). This single intervention could reduce IHD events by as much as 50 percent. The potential advantages of a polypill for primary prevention include reduced need for dose titrations (Lonn and others 2010), improved adherence (Thom and others 2014), and availability of cheap generics in a single formulation.

Although several studies have shown reductions in risk factors such as BP and cholesterol (Yusuf and others 2009) and improvement in adherence in association with use of a polypill, no published study has shown reductions in IHD or stroke endpoints, although several studies are under way (Eguzo and Camazine 2013; Lonn and others 2010; Yusuf and others 2009). The use of combination therapy was shown to be cost-effective in LMICs for both primary and secondary prevention, with

the best cost-effectiveness ratio for secondary prevention (Gaziano and others 2005; Lim and others 2007).

Although preventive treatment is available in many LMICs, less than 10 percent of the population receives the recommended care for primary prevention (Mendis and others 2005). Major barriers to improving care include crowded primary health centers with long wait times, scarcity of professional health staff, and high costs of traditional screening programs. In a community study in Bangladesh, Guatemala, Mexico, and South Africa, shifting the responsibility for screening to community health workers (CHWs) using a simple nonlaboratory screening tool was shown to be equally effective when screening for CVD risk as using nurses or physicians (Gaziano, Abrahams-Gessel, Denman, and others 2015). CHWs using the same tool in a mobile phone application could save an estimated 15,000–110,000 lives in Guatemala, Mexico, or South Africa at very cost-effective ratios. Using CHWs to screen for CVD using a simple tool is much more cost-effective when the primary health system is prepared and equipped to treat persons identified as high risk (Gaziano, Abrahams-Gessel, Surka, and others 2015). In countries such as South Africa, where at least half of persons identified as high risk get medications, the screening intervention was cost saving. Even in settings such as Guatemala, where fewer than 5 percent of eligible patients receive statins, the intervention was still attractive at US$565 per quality-adjusted life year (QALY). In Mexico, with initiation rates of 36 percent for hypertension medications and half that for statins, the incremental cost-effectiveness ratio for screening by CHWs was less than US$4 per QALY.

In general, population-based interventions (such as policies to increase excise taxes on tobacco, salt, and trans-fatty acids) are highly cost-effective even in resource-constrained settings because the price elasticity is higher in such settings than in high-income regions (Gaziano and Pagidipati 2013). Multidrug regimens for secondary prevention of CVD are cost-effective even in LMICs, according to WHO standards (Gaziano and Pagidipati 2013). Application of mHealth (mobile health) strategies and involvement of CHWs in CVD screening are considered to be scalable and cost-effective in LMIC settings (Gaziano, Abrahams-Gessel, Surka, and others 2015).

RESEARCH AND DEVELOPMENT

Box 22.1 summarizes important research gaps in the area of BP management, as proposed in two recent sets of guidelines.

Unresolved Issues in the Management of Hypertension Requiring Further Evidence from Randomized Controlled Trials

1. Do the use of home, ambulatory, and office blood pressure (BP) monitoring and BP variability add incremental value to routine clinic BP monitoring for optimizing hypertension management? If so, what levels of each of these measures should be used as thresholds and targets?

2. At what BP levels (BP thresholds) should antihypertensive agents be initiated (if at all) for various subgroups of patients, including young persons (younger than age 40 years), elderly persons (older than age 65 years), persons with white-coat hypertension (high only in medical settings), and persons at relatively low CV risk? The latter subgroup has recently been investigated in the HOPE-3 trial (Lonn and others 2016).

3. How far should BP be lowered (targets) in the general management of hypertension and in specific subgroups? The SPRINT trial (Wright and others 2015) has addressed this question in high-risk hypertensive patients, but the measurement techniques used in the trial make direct translation of results into clinical practice difficult. Meanwhile, meta-analyses of this question have generated conflicting results (Brunström and Carlberg 2016; Ettehad and others 2016; Xie and others 2016).

4. What are the best two-, three-, and four-drug combinations for optimizing BP management for particular ethnic groups? The PATHWAY-2 study (Williams and others 2015) has provided robust evidence that spironolactone is the best fourth-line agent for resistant hypertension (after a renin-angiotensin-system blocker, a calcium channel blocker, and a diuretic have been shown to be inadequate). No data are available to support the best combinations of antihypertensives in each of the major ethnic groups.

5. Beyond the use of spironolactone as a fourth-line agent—for which an alpha blocker and a beta blocker are recommended add-on drugs (NICE 2011)—various devices and interventions, including renal denervation, are undergoing investigation, but no such interventions are currently established.

6. How is BP best measured for patients with atrial fibrillation?

7. How is CV risk best assessed for patients with elevated BP?

8. Can target organ damage be used reliably as a surrogate outcome in trials of hypertension management?

9. Is it possible or reasonable to evaluate lifestyle interventions to lower BP and thereby reduce major adverse CV events in randomized controlled trials?

Source: Based on a summary of recent U.K. and European guidelines (Mancia and others 2013; NICE 2011).

In the area of lipids, given the outstanding benefits associated with the use of statins, future research and development should focus on what can be done for persons who are intolerant of statins and who require additional therapy when statins are inadequate to provide optimal control of dyslipidemia. While modest, albeit significant, benefits have been associated with the addition of ezetimibe to statin therapy (Cannon and others 2015), the results of trials of PCSK9 inhibitors are keenly awaited in this regard because of their large beneficial impact on LDL reduction.

RECOMMENDATIONS FOR RESOURCE-POOR SETTINGS

The World Heart Federation has outlined key strategies for controlling hypertension (Adler and others 2015). A key challenge in the management of hypertension and dyslipidemia is that both conditions are largely asymptomatic for a prolonged period leading up to a cardiovascular event. Therefore, to prevent primary CVD events, an effective screening program is crucial, although screening should be undertaken only when treatment is possible.

Screening for hypertension is simple and costs relatively little. At a minimum, patients attending clinics for any reason should be screened at least once a year (opportunistic screening); screening can also be undertaken opportunistically as part of antenatal care, in the workplace, or in mobile units specifically set up for the purpose. To avoid false positives, screening should ideally involve 24-hour or home-based methods, but in many low-resource settings these methods are not feasible. In low-resource settings, the minimum screening should be serial paired BP readings. In these cases, if the first measurement is normal, a second reading is unnecessary. If the difference between the two readings is greater than 10 mmHg, a third reading should be made and the mean of the last two used. In cases in which the average is greater than 160 mmHg, the patient should be treated immediately (Adler and others 2015). If the patient presents with other extreme conditions (for example, pain), caution should be used in interpreting high BP.

Cholesterol screening is more difficult because it requires the drawing of a blood sample for biochemical evaluation. Given the escalation of CV risk factors, especially after age 35 in men and age 45 in women, screening for lipid disorders is recommended in these groups. However, young men and women should be screened if they are at increased risk of CHD. In low-resource settings, screening should follow a cost-effective, benefit-based, tailored treatment strategy of lowering total cardiovascular risk.

Another long-term barrier to optimizing CVD prevention, given the asymptomatic nature of hypertension and dyslipidemia, is medication adherence. Health care professionals and patients need to understand that BP and cholesterol medications are nearly always required for life and generally should be continued even after achieving target BP and cholesterol levels. Health care professionals and patients need to be educated on nonpharmacological (including heart-healthy diet, weight control, moderate alcohol use, and physical activity) and locally appropriate pharmacological BP control methods. Health care professionals need to be educated on guidelines and, where appropriate, be trained in decision support systems (Anchala and others 2012).

CONCLUSIONS

Elevated BP and total cholesterol levels are leading physiological risk factors for IHD and stroke. Although proven, cost-effective, and acceptable medical and lifestyle interventions exist to prevent and treat hypertension and dyslipidemia, uptake is still unacceptably low in all countries, particularly in resource-poor settings. Guidelines for BP control recommend nonpharmacological measures to lower BP (including salt reduction and weight loss) and to reduce overall CVD risk (including smoking cessation and cholesterol lowering).

The pharmacological interventions recommended for lowering BP include seven drug classes—ACE inhibitors, angiotensin-receptor blockers, alpha blockers, beta blockers, calcium channel blockers, diuretics, and mineralocorticoid receptor antagonists. Although different guidelines make varying recommendations, lowering BP is most important; the means by which this is accomplished are secondary. Many guidelines suggest initiating therapy with two drugs, particularly for persons with high initial BP or high overall risk; this guideline is of particular importance in low-resource settings where it may be difficult to get patients to return for follow-up appointments.

Initiating pharmacological interventions in lipid management should be based not only on the absolute level of lipids but also on the level of total CV risk. It is important to adopt a more cost-effective, benefit-based treatment strategy of lowering total CV risk that is tailored to the individual. Pharmacological interventions recommended for high cholesterol include statins that are off patent, available in generic forms, effective, and safe (Macedo and others 2014).

NOTES

The authors would like to acknowledge the contributions of Shuchi Anand and Debarati Mukherjee in drafting and editing this chapter.

World Bank Income Classifications as of July 2014 are as follows, based on estimates of gross national income (GNI) per capita for 2013:

- Low-income countries (LICs) = US$1,045 or less
- Middle-income countries (MICs) are subdivided:
  (a) lower-middle-income = US$1,046 to US$4,125
  (b) upper-middle-income (UMICs) = US$4,126 to US$12,745
- High-income countries (HICs) = US$12,746 or more.

REFERENCES

AAFP (American Academy of Family Physicians). 2014. "Practice Guidelines: JNC 8 Guidelines for the Management of Hypertension in Adults." *American Family Physician* 90 (7): 503–4.

Adler, A. J., D. Prabhakaran, P. Bovet, D. S. Kazi, G. Mancia, and others. 2015. "Reducing Cardiovascular Mortality through Prevention and Management of Raised Blood Pressure: A World Heart Federation Roadmap." *Global Heart* 10 (2): 111–22.

Ali, M. K., K. R. Siegel, F. Chandrasekar, N. Tandon, P. Aschner, and others. 2017. "Diabetes: An Update on the Pandemic and Potential Solutions." In *Disease Control Priorities* (third edition): Volume 5, *Cardiovascular, Respiratory, and Related Disorders*, edited by D. Prabhakaran, S. Anand, T. A. Gaziano, J.-C. Mbanya, Y. Wu, and R. Nugent. Washington, DC: World Bank.

Alwan, A. 2011. *Global Status Report on Noncommunicable Diseases 2010*. Geneva: World Health Organization.

Anchala, R., M. P. Pinto, A. Shroufi, R. Chowdhury, J. Sanderson, and others. 2012. "The Role of Decision Support System (DSS) in Prevention of Cardiovascular Disease: A Systematic Review and Meta-Analysis." *PLoS One* 7 (10): e47064.

Angell, S. Y., K. M. De Cock, and T. R. Frieden. 2015. "A Public Health Approach to Global Management of Hypertension." *The Lancet* 385 (9970): 825–27.

Antonakoudis, G., L. Poulimenos, K. Kifnidis, C. Zouras, and H. Antonakoudis. 2007. "Blood Pressure Control and Cardiovascular Risk Reduction." *Hippokratia* 11 (3): 114–19.

Baigent, C., L. Blackwell, J. Emberson, L. E. Holland, C. Reith, and others. 2010. "Efficacy and Safety of More Intensive Lowering of LDL Cholesterol: A Meta-Analysis of Data from 170,000 Participants in 26 Randomised Trials." *The Lancet* 376 (9753): 1670–81.

Bakris, G. L. 2004. "The Importance of Blood Pressure Control in the Patient with Diabetes." *American Journal of Medicine* 116 (Suppl 5A): 30S–38S.

Björck, L., S. Capewell, M. O'Flaherty, G. Lappas, K. Bennett, and others. 2015. "Decline in Coronary Mortality in Sweden between 1986 and 2002: Comparing Contributions from Primary and Secondary Prevention." *PLoS One* 10 (5): e0124769.

Blood Pressure Lowering Treatment Trialists' Collaboration. 2000. "Effects of ACE Inhibitors, Calcium Antagonists, and Other Blood-Pressure-Lowering Drugs: Results of Prospectively Designed Overviews of Randomised Trials." *The Lancet* 356 (9246): 1955–64.

Breaux-Shropshire, T. L., E. Judd, L. A. Vucovich, T. S. Shropshire, and S. Singh. 2005. "Does Home Blood Pressure Monitoring Improve Patient Outcomes? A Systematic Review Comparing Home and Ambulatory Blood Pressure Monitoring on Blood Pressure Control and Patient Outcomes." *Integrated Blood Pressure Control* 8 (July 3): 43–49.

Bronsert, M. R., W. G. Henderson, R. Valuck, P. Hosokawa, and K. Hammermeister. 2013. "Comparative Effectiveness of Antihypertensive Therapeutic Classes and Treatment Strategies in the Initiation of Therapy in Primary Care Patients: A Distributed Ambulatory Research in Therapeutics Network (DARTNet) Study." *Journal of the American Board of Family Medicine* 26 (5): 529–38.

Brunström, M., and B. Carlberg. 2016. "Effect of Antihypertensive Treatment at Different Blood Pressure Levels in Patients with Diabetes Mellitus: Systematic Review and Meta-Analyses." *BMJ* 352 (February): i717.

Bull, F., S. Goenka, V. Lambert, and M. Pratt. 2017. "Physical Activity for the Prevention of Cardiometabolic Disease."

In *Disease Control Priorities* (third edition): Volume 5, *Cardiovascular, Respiratory, and Related Disorders*, edited by D. Prabhakaran, S. Anand, T. A. Gaziano, J.-C. Mbanya, Y. Wu, and R. Nugent. Washington, DC: World Bank.

Cannon, C. P., M. A. Blazing, R. P. Giugliano, A. McCagg, J. A. White, and others. 2015. "Ezetimibe Added to Statin Therapy after Acute Coronary Syndromes." *New England Journal of Medicine* 372 (25): 2387–97.

Castellano, J. M., G. Sanz, J. L. Peñalvo, S. Bansilal, A. Fernández-Ortiz, and others. 2014. "A Polypill Strategy to Improve Adherence." *Journal of the American College of Cardiology* 64 (20): 2071–82.

Chow, C. K., K. K. Teo, S. Rangarajan, S. Islam, R. Gupta, and others. 2013. "Prevalence, Awareness, Treatment, and Control of Hypertension in Rural and Urban Communities in High-, Middle-, and Low-Income Countries." *Journal of the American Medical Association* 310 (9): 959–68.

D'Agostino, R. B. Sr., S. Grundy, L. M. Sullivan, P. Wilson, and CHD Risk Prediction Group. 2001. "Validation of the Framingham Coronary Heart Disease Prediction Scores: Results of a Multiple Ethnic Groups Investigation." *Journal of the American Medical Association* 286 (2): 180–87.

Dahlöf, B., P. S. Sever, N. R. Poulter, H. Wedel, D. G. Beevers, and others. 2005. "Prevention of Cardiovascular Events with an Antihypertensive Regimen of Amlodipine Adding Perindopril as Required versus Atenolol Adding Bendroflumethiazide as Required, in the Anglo-Scandinavian Cardiac Outcomes Trial–Blood Pressure Lowering Arm (ASCOT-BPLA): A Multicentre Randomised Controlled Trial." *The Lancet* 366 (9489): 895–906.

Danaei, G., M. M. Finucane, J. K. Lin, G. M. Singh, C. J. Paciorek, and others. 2011. "National, Regional, and Global Trends in Systolic Blood Pressure since 1980: Systematic Analysis of Health Examination Surveys and Epidemiological Studies with 786 Country-Years and 5.4 Million Participants." *The Lancet* 377 (9765): 568–77.

Davies, A. R., L. Smeeth, and E. M. D. Grundy. 2007. "Contribution of Changes in Incidence and Mortality to Trends in the Prevalence of Coronary Heart Disease in the U.K.: 1996–2005." *European Heart Journal* 28 (17): 2142–47.

Di Angelantonio, E., P. Gao, L. Pennells, S. Kaptoge, M. Caslake, and others. 2012. "Lipid-Related Markers and Cardiovascular Disease Prediction." *Journal of the American Medical Association* 307 (23): 2499–506.

Dierkes, J., C. Luley, and S. Westphal. 2007. "Effect of Lipid-Lowering and Anti-Hypertensive Drugs on Plasma Homocysteine Levels." *Vascular Health Risk Management* 3 (1): 99–108.

Dugani, S. B., A. E. Moran, R. O. Bonow, and T. A. Gaziano. 2017. "Ischemic Heart Disease: Cost-Effective Management and Secondary Prevention." In *Disease Control Priorities* (third edition): Volume 5, *Cardiovascular, Respiratory, and Related Disorders*, edited by D. Prabhakaran, S. Anand, T. A. Gaziano, J.-C. Mbanya, Y. Wu, and R. Nugent. Washington, DC: World Bank.

Eguzo, K., and B. Camazine. 2013. "Beyond Limitations: Practical Strategies for Improving Cancer Care in Nigeria." *Asian Pacific Journal of Cancer Prevention* 14 (5): 3363–68.

Ettehad, D., C. A. Emdin, A. Kiran, S. G. Anderson, T. Callender, and others. 2016. "Blood Pressure Lowering for Prevention of Cardiovascular Disease and Death: A Systematic Review and Meta-Analysis." *The Lancet* 387 (10022): 957–67.

Farzadfar, F., M. M. Finucane, G. Danaei, P. M. Pelizzari, M. J. Cowan, and others. 2011. "National, Regional, and Global Trends in Serum Total Cholesterol since 1980: Systematic Analysis of Health Examination Surveys and Epidemiological Studies with 321 Country-Years and 3.0 Million Participants." *The Lancet* 377 (9765): 578–86.

Franco, V., S. Oparil, and O. A. Carretero. 2004. "Hypertensive Therapy: Part I." *American Heart Association Journal* 109 (24): 2953–58.

Franklin, S. S., S. A. Khan, N. D. Wong, M. G. Larson, and D. Levy. 1999. "Is Pulse Pressure Useful in Predicting Risk for Coronary Heart Disease? The Framingham Heart Study." *Circulation* 100 (4): 354–60.

Fukuyama, N., K. Homma, N. Wakana, K. Kudo, A. Suyama, and others. 2008. "Validation of the Friedewald Equation for Evaluation of Plasma LDL-Cholesterol." *Journal of Clinical Biochemistry and Nutrition* 43 (1): 1–5.

Gaziano, T. A., S. Abrahams-Gessel, C. A. Denman, C. M. Montano, M. Khanam, and others. 2015. "An Assessment of Community Health Workers' Ability to Screen for Cardiovascular Disease Risk with a Simple, Non-Invasive Risk Assessment Instrument in Bangladesh, Guatemala, Mexico, and South Africa: An Observational Study." *The Lancet Global Health* 3 (9): e556–63.

Gaziano, T. A., S. Abrahams-Gessel, S. Surka, S. Sy, A. Pandya, and others. 2015. "Cardiovascular Disease Screening by Community Health Workers Can Be Cost-Effective in Low-Resource Countries." *Health Affairs* 34 (9): 1538–45.

Gaziano, T. A., S. Cho, S. Sy, A. Pandya, N. S. Levitt, and others. 2015. "Increasing Prescription Length Could Cut Cardiovascular Disease Burden and Produce Savings in South Africa." *Health Affairs* 34 (9): 1578–85.

Gaziano, T. A., and N. Pagidipati. 2013. "Scaling Up Chronic Disease Prevention Interventions in Lower- and Middle-Income Countries." *Annual Review of Public Health* 34 (January 7): 317–35.

Gaziano, T. A., K. Steyn, D. J. Cohen, M. C. Weinstein, and L. H. Opie. 2005. "Cost-Effectiveness Analysis of Hypertension Guidelines in South Africa: Absolute Risk versus Blood Pressure Level." *Circulation* 112 (23): 3569–76.

GBD 2013 Mortality and Causes of Death Collaborators. 2013. "Global, Regional, and National Age–Sex Specific All-Cause and Cause-Specific Mortality for 240 Causes of Death, 1990–2013: A Systematic Analysis for the Global Burden of Disease Study 2013." *The Lancet* 385 (9963): 117–71.

Gomez Sandoval, Y.-H., M. V. Braganza, and S. S. Daskalopoulou. 2011. "Statin Discontinuation in High-Risk Patients: A Systematic Review of the Evidence." *Current Pharmaceutical Design* 17 (33): 3669–89.

Grundy, S. M., J. I. Cleeman, C. N. B. Merz, H. B. Brewer, L. T. Clark, and others. 2004. "Implications of Recent Clinical Trials for the National Cholesterol Education Program Adult Treatment Panel III Guidelines." *Circulation* 110 (2): 104–6.

Halvorsen, S., F. Andreotti, J. M. ten Berg, M. Cattaneo, S. Coccheri, and others. 2014. "Aspirin Therapy in Primary Cardiovascular Disease Prevention: A Position Paper of the European Society of Cardiology Working Group on Thrombosis." *Journal of the American College of Cardiology* 64 (3): 319–27.

Hippisley-Cox, J., and C. Coupland. 2005. "Effect of Combinations of Drugs on All Cause Mortality in Patients with Ischaemic Heart Disease: Nested Case-Control Analysis." *BMJ* 330 (7499): 1059–63.

Huffman, M. D., G. A. Roth, K. Sliwa, C. W. Yancy, and D. Prabhakaran. 2017. "Heart Failure." In *Disease Control Priorities* (third edition): Volume 5, *Cardiovascular, Respiratory, and Related Disorders,* edited by D. Prabhakaran, S. Anand, T. A. Gaziano, J.-C. Mbanya, Y. Wu, and R. Nugent. Washington, DC: World Bank.

IOM (Institute of Medicine). 2010. *Promoting Cardiovascular Health in the Developing World: A Critical Challenge to Achieve Global Health.* Washington, DC: National Academies Press.

James, P. A., S. Oparil, B. L. Carter, W. C. Cushman, C. Dennison-Himmelfarb, and others. 2014. "Evidence-Based Guideline for the Management of High Blood Pressure in Adults: Report from the Panel Members Appointed to the Eighth Joint National Committee (JNC 8)." *Journal of the American Medical Association* 311 (5): 507–20.

Katsiki, N., D. Nikolic, G. Montalto, M. Banach, D. P. Mikhailidis, and others. 2013. "The Role of Fibrate Treatment in Dyslipidemia: An Overview." *Current Pharmaceutical Design* 19 (17): 3124–31.

Klag, M. J., D. E. Ford, L. A. Mead, J. He, P. K. Whelton, and others. 1993. "Serum Cholesterol in Young Men and Subsequent Cardiovascular Disease." *New England Journal of Medicine* 328 (5): 313–18.

Kones, R., and U. Rumana. 2015. "Current Treatment of Dyslipidemia: Evolving Roles of Non-Statin and Newer Drugs." *Drugs* 75 (11): 1201–28.

Krause, T., K. Lovibond, M. Caulfield, T. McCormack, and B. Williams. 2011. "Management of Hypertension: Summary of NICE Guidance." *BMJ* 343 (August 25): d4891.

Kwak, S. M., S.-K. Myung, Y. J. Lee, and H. G. Seo. 2012. "Efficacy of Omega-3 Fatty Acid Supplements (Eicosapentaenoic Acid and Docosahexaenoic Acid) in the Secondary Prevention of Cardiovascular Disease: A Meta-Analysis of Randomized, Double-Blind, Placebo-Controlled Trials." *Archives of Internal Medicine* 172 (9): 686–94.

Lemieux, I., B. Lamarche, C. Couillard, A. Pascot, B. Cantin, and others. 2001. "Total Cholesterol/HDL Cholesterol Ratio vs. LDL Cholesterol/HDL Cholesterol Ratio as Indices of Ischemic Heart Disease Risk in Men." *Archives of Internal Medicine* 161 (22): 2685.

Lewington, S., R. Clarke, N. Qizilbash, R. Peto, and R. Collins. 2002. "Age-Specific Relevance of Usual Blood Pressure to Vascular Mortality: A Meta-Analysis of Individual Data for One Million Adults in 61 Prospective Studies." *The Lancet* 360 (9349): 1903–13.

Lewsey, J. D., K. D. Lawson, I. Ford, K. A. A. Fox, L. D. Ritchie, and others. 2015. "A Cardiovascular Disease Policy Model That Predicts Life Expectancy Taking into Account Socioeconomic Deprivation." *Heart* 101 (3): 201–8.

Libby, P. 2000. "Changing Concepts of Atherogenesis." *Journal of Internal Medicine* 247 (3): 349–58.

Lim, S. S., T. A. Gaziano, E. Gakidou, K. S. Reddy, F. Farzadfar, and others. 2007. "Prevention of Cardiovascular Disease in High-Risk Individuals in Low-Income and Middle-Income Countries: Health Effects and Costs." *The Lancet* 370 (9604): 2054–62.

Lim, S. S., T. Vos, A. D. D. Flaxman, G. Danaei, K. Shibuya, and others. 2012. "A Comparative Risk Assessment of Burden of Disease and Injury Attributable to 67 Risk Factors and Risk Factor Clusters in 21 Regions, 1990–2010: A Systematic Analysis for the Global Burden of Disease Study 2010." *The Lancet* 380 (9859): 2224–60.

Lonn, E. M., J. Bosch, P. López-Jaramillo, J. Zhu, L. Liu, and others. 2016. "Blood-Pressure Lowering in Intermediate-Risk Persons without Cardiovascular Disease." *New England Journal of Medicine* 374 (21): 2009–20.

Lonn, E., J. Bosch, K. K. Teo, P. Pais, D. Xavier, and others. 2010. "The Polypill in the Prevention of Cardiovascular Diseases: Key Concepts, Current Status, Challenges, and Future Directions." *Circulation* 122 (20): 2078–88.

Macedo, A. F., F. C. Taylor, J. P. Casas, A. Adler, D. Prieto-Merino, and others. 2014. "Unintended Effects of Statins from Observational Studies in the General Population: Systematic Review and Meta-Analysis." *BMC Medicine* 12 (March): 51.

Malik, V., and F. Hu. 2017. "Weight Management." In *Disease Control Priorities* (third edition): Volume 5, *Cardiovascular, Respiratory, and Related Disorders,* edited by D. Prabhakaran, S. Anand, T. A. Gaziano, J.-C. Mbanya, Y. Wu, and R. Nugent. Washington, DC: World Bank.

Malone, A. F., and D. N. Reddan. 2010. "Pulse Pressure: Why Is It Important?" *Peritoneal Dialysis International* 30 (3): 265–68.

Mancia, G., R. Fagard, K. Narkiewicz, J. Redon, A. Zanchetti, and others. 2013. "ESH/ESC Guidelines for the Management of Arterial Hypertension: The Task Force for the Management of Arterial Hypertension of the European Society of Hypertension (ESH) and of the European Society of Cardiology (ESC)." *European Heart Journal* 34 (28): 2159–219.

Marso, S. P., G. H. Daniels, K. Brown-Frandsen, P. Kristensen, J. F. E. Mann, and others. 2016. "Liraglutide and Cardiovascular Outcomes in Type 2 Diabetes." *New England Journal of Medicine* 375 (4): 311–22.

Mendis, S., D. Abegunde, S. Yusuf, S. Ebrahim, G. Shaper, and others. 2005. "WHO Study on Prevention of REcurrences of Myocardial Infarction and StrokE (WHO-PREMISE)." *Bulletin of the World Health Organization* 83 (11): 820–28.

Miller, M., N. J. Stone, C. Ballantyne, V. Bittner, M. H. Criqui, and others. 2011. "Triglycerides and Cardiovascular Disease: A Scientific Statement from the American Heart Association." *Circulation* 123 (20): 2292–333.

Mozaffarian, D., E. J. Benjamin, A. S. Go, D. K. Arnett, M. J. Blaha, and others. 2015. "Heart Disease and Stroke Statistics—2015 Update: A Report from the American Heart Association." *Circulation* 131 (4): e29–322.

Murray, C. J. L., J. A. Lauer, R. C. W. Hutubessy, L. Niessen, N. Tomijima, and others. 2003. "Effectiveness and Costs of Interventions to Lower Systolic Blood Pressure and Cholesterol: A Global and Regional Analysis on Reduction of Cardiovascular-Disease Risk." *The Lancet* 361 (9359): 717–25.

Murray, C. J. L., T. Vos, R. Lozano, M. Naghavi, A. D. Flaxman, and others. 2013. "Disability-Adjusted Life Years (DALYs) for 291 Diseases and Injuries in 21 Regions, 1990–2010: A Systematic Analysis for the Global Burden of Disease Study 2010." *The Lancet* 380 (9859): 2197–23.

NICE (National Institute for Health and Care Excellence). 2011. "Hypertension in Adults: Diagnosis and Management." NICE, London.

———. 2014. "Cardiovascular Disease: Risk Assessment and Reduction, Including Lipid Modification." NICE, London.

Nicholls, S. J., H. B. Brewer, J. J. P. Kastelein, K. A. Krueger, M.-D. Wang, and others. 2011. "Effects of the CETP Inhibitor Evacetrapib Administered as Monotherapy or in Combination with Statins on HDL and LDL Cholesterol: A Randomized Controlled Trial." *Journal of the American Medical Association* 306 (19): 2099–109.

Olsson, A. G., J. McMurray, G. Thorgeirsson, C. Spaulding, J. Slattery, and others. 1994. "Randomised Trial of Cholesterol Lowering in 4444 Patients with Coronary Heart Disease: The Scandinavian Simvastatin Survival Study (4S)." *The Lancet* 344 (8934): 1383–89.

Rabar, S., M. Harker, N. O'Flynn, and A. S. Wierzbicki. 2014. "Lipid Modification and Cardiovascular Risk Assessment for the Primary and Secondary Prevention of Cardiovascular Disease: Summary of Updated NICE Guidance." *BMJ* 349 (July): g4356.

Räber, L., M. Taniwaki, S. Zaugg, H. Kelbæk, M. Roffi, and others. 2015. "Effect of High-Intensity Statin Therapy on Atherosclerosis in Non-Infarct-Related Coronary Arteries (IBIS-4): A Serial Intravascular Ultrasonography Study." *European Heart Journal* 36 (8): 490–500.

Rosendaal, N. T. A., M. E. Hendriks, M. D. Verhagen, O. A. Bolarinwa, E. O. Sanya, and others. 2016. "Costs and Cost-Effectiveness of Hypertension Screening and Treatment in Adults with Hypertension in Rural Nigeria in the Context of a Health Insurance Program." *PLoS One* 11 (6): e0157925.

Roy, A., I. Rawal, S. Jabbour, and D. Prabhakaran. 2017. "Tobacco and Cardiovascular Disease: A Summary of Evidence." In *Disease Control Priorities* (third edition): Volume 5, *Cardiovascular, Respiratory, and Related Disorders,* edited by D. Prabhakaran, S. Anand, T. A. Gaziano, J.-C. Mbanya, Y. Wu, and R. Nugent. Washington, DC: World Bank.

Rubinstein, A., L. Colantonio, A. Bardach, J. Caporale, S. G. Martí, and others. 2010. "Estimation of the Burden of Cardiovascular Disease Attributable to Modifiable Risk Factors and Cost-Effectiveness Analysis of Preventative Interventions to Reduce This Burden in Argentina." *BMC Public Health* 10 (1): 627.

Schaffer, A. L., N. A. Buckley, T. A. Dobbins, E. Banks, and S.-A. Pearson. 2015. "The Crux of the Matter: Did the ABC's Catalyst Program Change Statin Use in Australia?" *Medical Journal of Australia* 202 (11): 591–94.

Shearer, G. C., O. V. Savinova, and W. S. Harris. 2012. "Fish Oil: How Does It Reduce Plasma Triglycerides?" *Biochimica et Biophysica Acta* 1821 (5): 843–51.

Shipman, K. E., R. C. Strange, and S. Ramachandran. 2016. "Use of Fibrates in the Metabolic Syndrome: A Review." *World Journal of Diabetes* 7 (5): 74–88.

SPRINT Research Group. 2015. "A Randomized Trial of Intensive versus Standard Blood-Pressure Control." *New England Journal of Medicine* 373 (22): 2103–16.

Staessen, J. A., J.-G. Wang, L. Thijs, E. Casiglia, P. Spolaore, and others. 2001. "Cardiovascular Protection and Blood Pressure Reduction: A Meta-Analysis." *The Lancet* 358 (9290): 1305–15.

Stamler, J., R. Stamler, and J. D. Neaton. 1993. "Blood Pressure, Systolic and Diastolic, and Cardiovascular Risks: U.S. Population Data." *Archives of Internal Medicine* 153 (5): 598–615.

Stoekenbroek, R. M., J. J. Kastelein, and R. Huijgen. 2015. "PCSK9 Inhibition: The Way Forward in the Treatment of Dyslipidemia." *BMC Medicine* 13 (1): 258.

Stone, N. J., J. Robinson, A. H. Lichtenstein, C. N. Bairey Merz, D. M. Lloyd-Jones, and others. 2014. "2013 ACC/AHA Guideline on the Treatment of Blood Cholesterol to Reduce Atherosclerotic Cardiovascular Risk in Adults: A Report of the American College of Cardiology/American Heart Association Task Force on Practice Guidelines." *Journal of the American College of Cardiology* 129 (25, Suppl 2): S1–S45.

Thom, S., J. Field, N. Poulter, A. Patel, D. Prabhakaran, and others. 2014. "Use of a Multidrug Pill in Reducing Cardiovascular Events (UMPIRE): Rationale and Design of a Randomised Controlled Trial of a Cardiovascular Preventive Polypill-Based Strategy in India and Europe." *European Journal of Preventive Cardiology* 21 (2): 252–61.

Thomopoulos, C., G. Parati, and A. Zanchetti. 2014a. "Effects of Blood Pressure Lowering on Outcome Incidence in Hypertension: 1; Overview, Meta-Analyses, and Meta-Regression Analyses of Randomized Trials." *Journal of Hypertension* 32 (12): 2285–95.

———. 2014b. "Effects of Blood Pressure Lowering on Outcome Incidence in Hypertension: 2; Effects at Different Baseline and Achieved Blood Pressure Levels—Overview and Meta-Analyses of Randomized Trials." *Journal of Hypertension* 32 (12): 2296–304.

———. 2014c. "Effects of Blood Pressure Lowering on Outcome Incidence in Hypertension: 3; Effects in Patients at Different Levels of Cardiovascular Risk—Overview and Meta-Analyses of Randomized Trials." *Journal of Hypertension* 32 (12): 2305–14.

———. 2015. "Effects of Blood Pressure Lowering on Outcome Incidence in Hypertension: 4; Effects of Various Classes of Antihypertensive Drugs—Overview and Meta-Analyses." *Journal of Hypertension* 33 (2): 195–211.

Toth, P. P. 2005. "Cardiology Patient Page: The Good Cholesterol, High-Density Lipoprotein." *Circulation* 111 (5): e89–e91.

Turnbull, F., and the Blood Pressure Lowering Treatment Trialists' Collaboration. 2003. "Effects of Different Blood-Pressure-Lowering Regimens on Major Cardiovascular Events: Results of Prospectively-Designed Overviews of Randomised Trials." *The Lancet* 362 (9395): 1527–35.

Tuteja, S., and D. J. Rader. 2014. "Dyslipidaemia: Cardiovascular Prevention—End of the Road for Niacin?" *Nature Reviews Endocrinology* 10 (11): 646–47.

U.S. Preventive Services Task Force. 2014. "Lipid Disorders in Adults (Cholesterol, Dyslipidemia): Screening." U.S. Preventive Services Task Force, Rockville, MD.

Vasan, R. S., M. G. Larson, E. P. Leip, J. C. Evans, C. J. O'Donnell, and others. 2001. "Impact of High-Normal Blood Pressure on the Risk of Cardiovascular Disease." *New England Journal of Medicine* 345 (18): 1291–97.

Wald, N. J., and M. R. Law. 2003. "A Strategy to Reduce Cardiovascular Disease by More Than 80%." *BMJ* 326 (7404): 1419.

Wang, Y. C., A. M. Cheung, K. Bibbins-Domingo, L. A. Prosser, N. R. Cook, and others. 2001. "Effectiveness and Cost-Effectiveness of Blood Pressure Screening in Adolescents in the United States." *Journal of Pediatrics* 158 (2): 257–64.e1–7.

Weber, M. A., and D. T. Lackland. 2016. "Hypertension: Cardiovascular Benefits of Lowering Blood Pressure." *National Reviews Nephrology* 12 (4): 202–4.

Weber, M. A., E. L. Schiffrin, W. B. White, S. Mann, L. H. Lindholm, and others. 2014. "Clinical Practice Guidelines for the Management of Hypertension in the Community: A Statement by the American Society of Hypertension and the International Society of Hypertension." *Journal of Hypertension* 32 (1): 3–15.

Webster, R., A. Patel, L. Billot, A. Cass, C. Burch, and others. 2013. "Prospective Meta-Analysis of Trials Comparing Fixed-Dose Combination-Based Care with Usual Care in Individuals at High Cardiovascular Risk: The SPACE Collaboration." *International Journal of Cardiology* 170 (1): 30–35.

WHO (World Health Organization). 2002. "WHO CVD-Risk Management Package for Low- and Medium-Resource Settings." WHO, Geneva.

———. 2007. *Prevention of Cardiovascular Disease: Guidelines for Assessment and Management of Cardiovascular Risk.* Geneva: WHO.

———. 2013. "A Global Brief on Hypertension: Silent Killer, Global Public Health Crisis." WHO, Geneva.

Williams, B., T. M. MacDonald, S. Morant, D. J. Webb, P. Sever, and others. 2015. "Spironolactone versus Placebo, Bisoprolol, and Doxazosin to Determine the Optimal Treatment for Drug-Resistant Hypertension (PATHWAY-2): A Randomised, Double-Blind, Crossover Trial." *The Lancet* 386 (10008): 2059–68.

Wilson, J., and Y. Jungner. 1968. "Principles and Practice of Screening for Disease." Public Health Paper, WHO, Geneva.

Wong, N. D. 2014. "Epidemiological Studies of CHD and the Evolution of Preventive Cardiology." *Nature Reviews Cardiology* 11 (5): 276–89.

World Economic Forum. 2011. *The Global Economic Burden of Non-Communicable Diseases.* Geneva: World Economic Forum.

Wright, J. T., J. D. Williamson, P. K. Whelton, J. K. Snyder, K. M. Sink, and others. 2015. "A Randomized Trial of Intensive versus Standard Blood-Pressure Control." *New England Journal of Medicine* 373 (22): 2103–16.

Xie, X., E. Atkins, J. Lv, A. Bennett, B. Neal, and others. 2016. "Effects of Intensive Blood Pressure Lowering on Cardiovascular and Renal Outcomes: Updated Systematic Review and Meta-Analysis." *The Lancet* 387 (10017): 435–43.

Yang, E. 2015. "PCSK9 Inhibitors: Are We on the Verge of a Breakthrough?" *Clinical Pharmacology and Therapeutics* 98 (6): 590–601.

Yusuf, S., P. Pais, R. Afzal, D. Xavier, K. Teo, and others. 2009. "Effects of a Polypill (Polycap) on Risk Factors in Middle-Aged Individuals without Cardiovascular Disease (TIPS): A Phase II, Double-Blind, Randomised Trial." *The Lancet* 373 (9672): 1341–51.

Zanchetti, A., C. Thomopoulos, and G. Parati. 2015. "Randomized Controlled Trials of Blood Pressure Lowering in Hypertension: A Critical Reappraisal." *Circulation Research* 116 (6): 1058–73.

Zhao, X. Q., J. S. Morse, A. A. Dowdy, N. Heise, D. Deangelis, and others. 2004. "Safety and Tolerability of Simvastatin Plus Niacin in Patients with Coronary Artery Disease and Low High-Density Lipoprotein Cholesterol (the HDL Atherosclerosis Treatment Study)." *American Journal of Cardiology* 93 (3): 307–12.

Zinman, B., C. Wanner, J. M. Lachin, D. Fitchett, E. Bluhmki, and others. 2015. "Empagliflozin, Cardiovascular Outcomes, and Mortality in Type 2 Diabetes." *New England Journal of Medicine* 373 (22): 1–12.

DCP3 Series Acknowledgments

Disease Control Priorities, third edition *(DCP3)* compiles the global health knowledge of institutions and experts from around the world, a task that required the efforts of over 500 individuals, including volume editors, chapter authors, peer reviewers, advisory committee members, and research and staff assistants. For each of these contributions we convey our acknowledgment and appreciation. First and foremost, we would like to thank our 32 volume editors who provided the intellectual vision for their volumes based on years of professional work in their respective fields, and then dedicated long hours to reviewing each chapter, providing leadership and guidance to authors, and framing and writing the summary chapters. We also thank our chapter authors who collectively volunteered their time and expertise to writing over 170 comprehensive, evidence-based chapters.

We owe immense gratitude to the institutional sponsor of this effort: The Bill & Melinda Gates Foundation. The Foundation provided sole financial support of the Disease Control Priorities Network (DCPN). Many thanks to Program Officers Kathy Cahill, Philip Setel, Carol Medlin, Damian Walker and (currently) David Wilson for their thoughtful interactions, guidance, and encouragement over the life of the project. We also wish to thank Jaime Sepúlveda for his longstanding support, including chairing the Advisory Committee for the second edition and, more recently, demonstrating his vision for *DCP3* while he was a special advisor to the Gates Foundation. We are also grateful to the University of Washington's Department of Global Health and successive chairs King Holmes and Judy Wasserheit for providing a home base for the *DCP3* Secretariat, which included intellectual collaboration, logistical coordination, and administrative support.

We thank the many contractors and consultants who provided support to specific volumes in the form of economic analytical work, volume coordination, chapter drafting, and meeting organization: the Center for Disease Dynamics, Economics & Policy; Center for Chronic Disease Control; Centre for Global Health Research; Emory University; Evidence to Policy Initiative; Public Health Foundation of India; QURE Healthcare; University of California, San Francisco; University of Waterloo; University of Queensland; and the World Health Organization.

We are tremendously grateful for the wisdom and guidance provided by our advisory committee to the editors. Steered by Chair Anne Mills, the advisory committee ensures quality and intellectual rigor of the highest order for *DCP3*.

The National Academies of Sciences, Engineering, and Medicine, in collaboration with the Interacademy Medical Panel, coordinated the peer-review process for all *DCP3* chapters. Patrick Kelley, Gillian Buckley, Megan Ginivan, Rachel Pittluck, and Tara Mainero managed this effort and provided critical and substantive input.

World Bank Publishing provided exceptional guidance and support throughout the demanding production and design process. We would particularly like to thank Carlos Rossel, Mary Fisk, Nancy Lammers, Rumit Pancholi, Deborah Naylor, and Sherrie Brown for their diligence and expertise. Additionally, we thank Jose de Buerba, Mario Trubiano, Yulia Ivanova, and Chiamaka Osuagwu of the World Bank for providing professional counsel on communications and marketing strategies.

Several U.S. and international institutions contributed to the organization and execution of meetings that supported the preparation and dissemination of *DCP3*.

We would like to express our appreciation to the following institutions:

- University of Bergen, consultation on equity (June 2011)
- University of California, San Francisco, surgery volume consultations (April 2012, October 2013, February 2014)
- Institute of Medicine, first meeting of the Advisory Committee to the Editors (March 2013)
- Harvard Global Health Institute, consultation on policy measures to reduce incidence of noncommunicable diseases (July 2013)
- National Academy of Medicine, systems strengthening meeting (September 2013)
- Center for Disease Dynamics, Economics & Policy (Quality and Uptake meeting, September 2013; reproductive and maternal health volume consultation, November 2013)
- National Cancer Institute, cancer consultation (November 2013)
- Union for International Cancer Control, cancer consultation (November 2013, December 2014)
- Harvard T. H. Chan School of Public Health, economic evaluation consultation (September 2015)
- University of California, Berkeley School of Public Health, and Stanford Medical School, occupational and environmental health consultations (December 2015).

Carol Levin provided outstanding governance for cost and cost-effectiveness analysis. Stéphane Verguet added valuable guidance in applying and improving the extended cost-effectiveness analysis method. Elizabeth Brouwer, Kristen Danforth, Nazila Dabestani, Shane Murphy, Zachary Olson, Jinyuan Qi, and David Watkins provided exceptional research assistance and analytic assistance. Brianne Adderley ably managed the budget and project processes, while Jennifer Nguyen, Shamelle Richards, and Jennifer Grasso contributed exceptional project coordination support. The efforts of these individuals were absolutely critical to producing this series, and we are thankful for their commitment.

Volume and Series Editors

VOLUME EDITORS

Dorairaj Prabhakaran

Dorairaj Prabhakaran, MD, DM (Cardiology), MSc, FRCP, FNASc, is a cardiologist and epidemiologist, with special interest in genetic epidemiology. Until recently, he was Professor at All India Institute of Medical Sciences; he currently heads the Center for Chronic Disease Control and is Professor of Chronic Disease Epidemiology at the Public Health Foundation of India. He is the Head of the Center of Excellence–Center for Cardio-metabolic Risk Reduction in South Asia (CoE-CARRS) located in the Public Health Foundation of India and funded by the National Heart, Lung, and Blood Institute. He is also a consultant to the World Bank, the World Health Organization (WHO), and other international organizations and is a reviewer for several international and national journals. He is associate editor of *Journal of Epidemiology and Community Health* and member of the Editorial Advisory Board of Clinical Science. He has more than 100 publications in several high-impact journals, such as the *New England Journal of Medicine, The Lancet,* the *Journal of the American Medical Association,* and the *Journal of American College of Cardiology.*

Shuchi Anand

Shuchi Anand, MD, is an Instructor of Medicine at Stanford University School of Medicine, with a research focus on chronic kidney disease epidemiology and management in low-resource settings. She is a former Fogarty Scholar, and a current recipient of National Institute for Diabetes and Digestive and Kidney Diseases Career Development award. She is studying epidemiology and management of chronic kidney disease in urban India, dialysis practices in China, and the epidemic of chronic kidney disease in Sri Lanka.

Thomas A. Gaziano

Thomas A. Gaziano, MD, MSc, is jointly appointed to the Divisions of Cardiovascular Medicine and Social Medicine and Health Inequalities at Brigham & Women's Hospital, Harvard Medical School, and the Department of Health Policy and Management, Harvard T. H. Chan School of Public Health, Cambridge, Massachusetts. He is certified as a Diplomat in Internal Medicine and Cardiovascular Diseases and has expertise in the treatment of cardiovascular diseases (CVD) in low- and middle-income countries, including the epidemiology and management of its risk factors. His research includes the development of decision analytic models to assess the cost-effectiveness of various screening, prevention, and management decisions. His international experience includes two years at Oxford University South Africa as the first *Lancet* International Fellow and four months in India evaluating CVD epidemiology and cost-effective strategies for its management. He has served as a consultant and author for the Disease Control Priorities Project organized by the World Bank; the WHO; and the Fogarty International Center, National Institutes of Health, and has been funded by the Bill & Melinda Gates Foundation.

Jean-Claude Mbanya

Jean-Claude Mbanya is Professor of Medicine and Endocrinology at the Faculty of Medicine and Biomedical Sciences, University of Yaoundé, Cameroon; Consultant Physician, Director of the Health in

Transition Research Group, and Director of the National Obesity Centre, University of Yaoundé, Cameroon; and Chief of the Endocrinology and Metabolic Diseases Unit at the Hospital Central in Yaoundé. Professor Mbanya served as President of the International Diabetes Federation (IDF) from 2009 to 2012. He was instrumental in the IDF-led Unite for Diabetes campaign, which led to the passage of the United Nations Day Resolution on Diabetes in December 2006. He now steers IDF strategic direction to encourage governments to implement policies for the treatment, care, and prevention of diabetes. His research mainly focuses on cultural diabetes-related factors, which are often unique to the Sub-Saharan African countries and communities he studies. His practice and research have largely contributed to increase the world's awareness on diabetes in this region.

Rachel Nugent

Rachel Nugent is Vice President for Global Noncommunicable Diseases at RTI International. She was formerly a Research Associate Professor and Principal Investigator of the DCPN in the Department of Global Health at the University of Washington. Previously, she served as Deputy Director of Global Health at the Center for Global Development, Director of Health and Economics at the Population Reference Bureau, Program Director of Health and Economics Programs at the Fogarty International Center of the National Institutes of Health, and senior economist at the Food and Agriculture Organization of the United Nations. From 1991 to 1997, she was associate professor and department chair in economics at Pacific Lutheran University.

Yangfeng Wu

Yangfeng Wu is the Director of The George Institute, China. He is also the Executive Associate Director, Peking University Clinical Research Institute. A cardiovascular specialist, Professor Wu is responsible for the scientific program in China, which includes all areas of noncommunicable disease and injuries. Professor Wu has made valuable contributions to reduce the impact of cardiovascular disease in the region with his work at Fu Wai Hospital; the WHO Collaborating Center in Cardiovascular Disease Prevention, Control, and Research, China; and Peking University. While the director of the WHO Collaborating Center in Cardiovascular Disease Prevention, Control, and Research in China, he has reported on hypertension control in low- and middle-income countries, including reducing salt intake in populations.

SERIES EDITORS

Dean T. Jamison

Dean T. Jamison is an Emeritus Professor of Global Health at the University of Washington and an Emeritus Professor of Global Health Sciences at the University of California, San Francisco. He previously held academic appointments at Harvard University and the University of California, Los Angeles, and he was an economist on the staff of the World Bank, where he was lead author of the World Bank's *World Development Report 1993: Investing in Health*. He was the lead editor of *DCP2*. He holds a PhD in economics from Harvard University and is an elected member of the Institute of Medicine of the U.S. National Academies. He recently served as Co-Chair and Study Director of *The Lancet's* Commission on Investing in Health.

Rachel Nugent

See the list of Volume Editors.

Hellen Gelband

Hellen Gelband is an independent global health policy expert. Her work spans infectious disease, particularly malaria and antibiotic resistance, and noncommunicable disease policy, mainly in low- and middle-income countries. She has conducted policy studies at Resources for the Future, the Center for Disease Dynamics, Economics & Policy, the (former) Congressional Office of Technology Assessment, the Institute of Medicine of the U.S. National Academies, and a number of international organizations.

Susan Horton

Susan Horton is Professor at the University of Waterloo and holds the Centre for International Governance Innovation (CIGI) Chair in Global Health Economics in the Balsillie School of International Affairs there. She has consulted for the World Bank, the Asian Development Bank, several United Nations agencies, and the International Development Research Centre, among others, in work conducted in over 20 low- and middle-income countries. She led the work on nutrition for the Copenhagen Consensus in 2008, when micronutrients were ranked as the top development priority. She has served as associate provost of graduate studies at the University of Waterloo, vice-president academic at Wilfrid Laurier University in Waterloo, and interim dean at the University of Toronto at Scarborough.

Prabhat Jha

Prabhat Jha is the founding director of the Centre for Global Health Research at St. Michael's Hospital and holds Endowed and Canada Research Chairs in Global Health in the Dalla Lana School of Public Health at the University of Toronto. He is lead investigator of the Million Death Study in India, which quantifies the causes of death and key risk factors in over two million homes over a 14-year period. He is also Scientific Director of the Statistical Alliance for Vital Events, which aims to expand reliable measurement of causes of death worldwide. His research includes the epidemiology and economics of tobacco control worldwide.

Ramanan Laxminarayan

Ramanan Laxminarayan is Vice President for Research and Policy at the Public Health Foundation of India, and he directs the Center for Disease Dynamics, Economics & Policy in Washington, DC, and New Delhi. His research deals with the integration of epidemiological models of infectious diseases and drug resistance into the economic analysis of public health problems. He was one of the key architects of the Affordable Medicines Facility–malaria, a novel financing mechanism to improve access and delay resistance to antimalarial drugs. In 2012, he created the Immunization Technical Support Unit in India, which has been credited with improving immunization coverage in the country. He teaches at Princeton University.

Charles N. Mock

Charles N. Mock, MD, PhD, FACS, has training as both a trauma surgeon and an epidemiologist. He worked as a surgeon in Ghana for four years, including at a rural hospital (Berekum) and at the Kwame Nkrumah University of Science and Technology (Kumasi). In 2005–07, he served as Director of the University of Washington's Harborview Injury Prevention and Research Center. In 2007–10, he worked at the WHO headquarters in Geneva, where he was responsible for developing the WHO's trauma care activities. In 2010, he returned to his position as Professor of Surgery (with joint appointments as Professor of Epidemiology and Professor of Global Health) at the University of Washington. His main interests include the spectrum of injury control, especially as it pertains to low- and middle-income countries: surveillance, injury prevention, prehospital care, and hospital-based trauma care. He was President (2013–15) of the International Association for Trauma Surgery and Intensive Care.

Contributors

Alma Adler
Department of Non-communicable Disease Epidemiology, London School of Hygiene & Tropical Medicine, London, United Kingdom

Ashkan Afshin
Institute for Health Metrics and Evaluation, University of Washington, Seattle, Washington, United States

Vamadevan S. Ajay
Centre for the Control of Chronic Conditions; Public Health Foundation of India, New Delhi, India

Mohammed K. Ali
Rollins School of Public Health, Emory University, Atlanta, Georgia, United States

Shuchi Anand
Stanford University School of Medicine, Stanford, California, United States

Eric Bateman
Division of Pulmonology, Department of Medicine, University of Cape Town, South Africa

Janet Bettger
Department of Orthopaedic Surgery, Duke University; Duke Clinical Research Institute; Duke Global Health Institute, Durham, North Carolina, United States

Robert O. Bonow
Center for Cardiovascular Innovation, Feinberg School of Medicine, Northwestern University, Chicago, Illinois, United States

Elizabeth Brouwer
University of Washington, Seattle, Washington, United States

Gene Buhkman
Department of Global Health & Social Medicine, Harvard University; Division of Cardiovascular Medicine, Harvard Medical School; Partners in Health, Boston, Massachusetts, United States

Fiona Bull
Centre for the Built Environment and Health, The University of Western Australia, Crawley, Western Australia, Australia

Peter Burney
National Heart & Lung Institute, Imperial College London, London, United Kingdom

Simon Capewell
Institute of Psychology, Health and Society, University of Liverpool, Liverpool, United Kingdom

Juliana Chan
MRC Epidemiology Unit, University of Cambridge, Cambridge, United Kingdom; Hong Kong Institute of Diabetes and Obesity; International Diabetes Federation Centre of Education; The Chinese University of Hong Kong–Prince of Wales Hospital, Hong Kong SAR, China

Eeshwar K. Chandrasekar
Emory University School of Medicine, Atlanta, Georgia, United States

Jie Chen
Shanghai Advanced Institute of Finance, Shanghai Jiao Tong University, Shanghai, China

Michael H. Criqui
Division of Preventive Medicine, Department of Family Medicine and Public Health, University of California–San Diego School of Medicine, La Jolla, California, United States

John Dirks
Gairdner Foundation (Emeritus President);
Massey College, University of Toronto, Toronto,
Ontario, Canada

Chandrasagar B. Dugani
Department of Medicine, and Division of Cardiology,
Brigham and Women's Hospital; Harvard Medical
School, Boston, Massachusetts, United States;
St. Michael's Hospital; University of Toronto,
Toronto, Ontario, Canada

Michael Engelgau
Center for Translation Research and Implementation
Science, National Heart Lung and Blood Institute,
National Institutes of Health, Bethesda, Maryland,
United States

Meguid El Nahas
Sheffield Kidney Institute; Global Kidney Academy,
Sheffield, United Kingdom

Caroline H. D. Fall
MRC Lifecourse Epidemiology Unit, University of
Southampton, Southampton, United Kingdom

Valery Feigin
National Institute of for Stroke and Applied
Neurosciences, Auckland University of Technology,
Auckland, New Zealand

F. Gerald R. Fowkes
Usher Institute of Population Health Sciences and
Informatics, University of Edinburgh, Edinburgh,
United Kingdom

Thomas A. Gaziano
Harvard Medical School, Harvard T. H. Chan School of
Public Health; Brigham and Women's Hospital, Boston,
Massachusetts, United States

Amanda Glassman
Center for Global Development, Washington, DC,
United States

Shifalika Goenka
Public Health Foundation of India, New Delhi, India

Rajeev Gupta
Fortis Escorts Hospital, New Delhi, India

Babar Hasan
Department of Paediatric and Child Health, The Aga
Khan University, Karachi, Pakistan

Fred Hersch
School of Public Health, Sydney Medical School,
University of Sydney, Sydney, Australia

Frank Hu
Harvard T. H. Chan School of Public Health, Boston,
Massachusetts, United States

Mark D. Huffman
Feinberg School of Medicine, Northwestern University,
Chicago, Illinois, United States

Samer Jabbour
Faculty of Health Sciences, American University of
Beirut, Beirut, Lebanon

Deborah Jarvis
National Heart & Lung Institute, Imperial College
London, London, United Kingdom

Panniyammakal Jeemon
Center for Control of Chronic Conditions, Public
Health Foundation of India, New Delhi, India

Rohina Joshi
The George Institute for Global Health; Faculty of
Medicine, University of Sydney, Sydney, Australia

Jemima H. Kamano
Department of Medicine, Moi University School of
Medicine; The Academic Model Providing Access to
Healthcare, Eldoret, Kenya

Andre Pascal Kengne
South African Medical Research Council, Tygerberg,
South Africa

Preeti Kudesia
Health, Nutrition, and Population Global Practice,
World Bank, Washington, DC, United States

R. Krishna Kumar
Department of Pediatric Cardiology, Amrita Institute
of Medical Sciences and Research Centre, Cochin, India

Kalyanaraman Kumaran
MRC Lifecourse Epidemiology Unit, University of
Southampton, Southampton, United Kingdom;
Epidemiology Research Unit, CSI Holdsworth
Memorial Hospital, Mysore, India

Estelle V. Lambert
Division of Exercise Science and Sports Medicine,
Department of Human Biology, Faculty of Health Sciences,
University of Cape Town, Cape Town, South Africa

Edward S. Lee
Keck School of Medicine, University of Southern
California, Los Angeles, California, United States

Carol Levin
Department of Global Health, University of
Washington, Seattle, Washington, United States

Chaoyun Li
Global Health Research Center, Duke Kunshan
University, Kunshan, China

Rong Luo
The George Institute for Global Health, Peking
University Health Science Center, Beijing, China

Matthew Magee
Georgia State University School of Public Health,
Atlanta, Georgia, United States

Vasanti S. Malik
Department of Nutrition, Harvard T. H. Chan School
of Public Health, Boston, Massachusetts, United States

J. Antonio Marin-Neto
Medical School of Ribeirão Preto, University of São
Paulo, São Paulo, Brazil

Guy Marks
South Western Sydney Clinical School, University of
New South Wales, Liverpool, New South Wales,
Australia

Bongani Mayosi
Faculty of Health Sciences, University of Cape Town,
Cape Town, South Africa

Jean-Claude Mbanya
Faculty of Medicine and Biomedical Sciences,
University of Yaoundé, Yaoundé, Cameroon

Helen McGuire
PATH, Seattle, Washington, United States

Renata Micha
Friedman School of Nutrition Science and Policy, Tufts
University, Boston, Massachusetts, United States

J. Jaime Miranda
CRONICAS Center of Excellence for Chronic Diseases,
Universidad Peruana Cayetano Heredia,
Lima, Peru

Pablo Aschner Montoya
MRC Epidemiology Unit, University of Cambridge,
Cambridge, United Kingdom; Javeriana University
School of Medicine; San Ignacio University Hospital;
Colombian Diabetes Association, Bogotá, Colombia

Andrew E. Moran
Division of General Medicine, Department of
Medicine, Columbia University Medical Center, New
York, New York, United States

Dariush Mozaffarian
Friedman School of Nutrition Science & Policy, Tufts
University, Boston, Massachusetts, United States

Saraladevi Naicker
School of Clinical Medicine, University of the
Witwatersrand, Johannesburg, South Africa

Nadraj G. Naidoo
University of Cape Town, Cape Town, South Africa

K. M. Venkat Narayan
Rollins School of Public Health, Emory University,
Atlanta, Georgia, United States

Irina Nikolic
Division of Health, Nutrition, and Population Global
Practice, World Bank, Washington, DC, United States

Rachel Nugent
Research Triangle Institute International, Research
Triangle Park, North Carolina; Research Triangle
Institute, Seattle, Washington, United States

Martin O'Donnell
National University of Ireland Galway, Galway, Ireland

Churchill Onen
Diabetes Association of Botswana, Gaborone,
Botswana

Clive Osmond
MRC Lifecourse Epidemiology Unit, University of
Southampton, Southampton General Hospital,
Southampton, United Kingdom

Anushka Patel
University of Sydney, Sydney, Australia

Rogelio Perez-Padilla
National Institute of Respiratory Diseases of Mexico,
Mexico City, Mexico

Neil Poulter
National Heart & Lung Institute, Imperial College
London, London, United Kingdom

Dorairaj Prabhakaran
Centre for Chronic Disease Control; Public Health
Foundation of India, New Delhi, India

Michael Pratt
National Center for Chronic Disease Prevention
and Health Promotion, Centers for Disease Control
and Prevention; Emory University, Atlanta, Georgia,
United States

Miriam Rabkin
ICAP at Columbia, Mailman School of Public Health,
Columbia University, New York, New York,
United States

Vikram Rajan
World Bank, New Delhi, India

Anis Rassi
Anis Rassi Hospital, Goiânia, Brazil

Anis Rassi Jr.
Anis Rassi Hospital, Goiânia, Brazil

Ishita Rawal
Centre for Chronic Disease Control, New Delhi, India

Giuseppe Remuzzi
Istituto di Ricerche Farmacologiche Mario Negri,
Centro Maria Astori; Bergamo, Italy

Miguel Riella
Evangelic School of Medicine; Evangelic University
Hospital; Pro-Renal Brazil Foundation Curitiba, Parana,
Brazil

Greg A. Roth
Division of Cardiology, Department of Medicine,
School of Medicine, University of Washington, Seattle,
Washington, United States

Ambuj Roy
All India Institute of Medical Sciences, New Delhi,
India

Adolfo Rubinstein
South American Center of Excellence in Cardiovascular
Health; Institute for Clinical Effectiveness and Health
Policy; School of Medicine, University of Buenos Aires,
Buenos Aires, Argentina

Yuna Sakuma
Center for Global Development, Washington, DC,
United States

Uchechukwu K. A. Sampson
National Heart, Lung, and Blood Institute, National
Institutes of Health, Bethesda, Maryland, United States

Karen R. Siegel
Emory University, Atlanta, Georgia, United States

Karen Sliwa
Hatter Institute for Cardiovascular Research in Africa,
University of Cape Town, Cape Town, South Africa

Marc Suhrcke
Centre for Health Economics, University of York, York,
United Kingdom

Nikhil Tandon
All India Institute of Medical Sciences; Centre for
Chronic Disease Control, New Delhi, India

Bernadette Thomas
Institute for Health Metrics and Evaluation, University
of Washington, Seattle, Washington, United States

Claudia Vaca
Ministry of Health, Bogotá, Colombia

Rajesh Vedanthan
Icahn School of Medicine at Mount Sinai, New York,
New York, United States

Stéphane Verguet
Department of Global Health and Population, Harvard
T. H. Chan School of Public Health, Boston,
Massachusetts, United States

David A. Watkins
Departments of Medicine and Global Health, University
of Washington, Seattle, Washington, United States

Michael Webb
Stanford University, Palo Alto, California, United States

Mary Beth Weber
Emory Global Diabetes Research Center, Hubert
Department of Global Health, Emory University,
Atlanta, Georgia, United States

Laurie Whitsel
American Heart Association, Washington, DC,
United States

Gary Wong
Prince of Wales Hospital, The Chinese University of
Hong Kong, Shatin, Hong Kong SAR, China

Yangfeng Wu
The George Institute for Global Health, Peking
University Health Science Center; Department of
Epidemiology and Biostatistics, Peking University
School of Public Health, Beijing, China

Lijing L. Yan
Global Health Research Center, Duke Kunshan
University; The George Institute for Global Health,
Peking University Health Science Center, Beijing, China

Clyde W. Yancy
Feinberg School of Medicine, Northwestern University,
Chicago, Illinois, United States

Ping Zhang
Centers for Disease Control and Prevention, Atlanta,
Georgia, United States

Dong Zhao
Department of Epidemiology, Beijing Anzhen Hospital,
Capital Medical University, Beijing, China

Yishan Zhu
National School of Development, Peking University,
Beijing, China

Advisory Committee to the Editors

Reviewers

Olusoji Adeyi
Director, Health, Nutrition, and Population Global Practice, World Bank, Washington, DC, United States

Kamel Ajlouni
The National Center for Diabetes, Endocrinology and Genetics; The University of Jordan, Amman, Jordan

Wael K. Al-Delaimy
University of California–San Diego, La Jolla, California, United States

Valter Cordeiro Barbosa Filho
Research Centre in Physical Activity and Health, Federal University of Santa Catarina, Florianópolis, Brazil

Robert Beaglehole
International Public Health Consultants, Auckland, New Zealand

Digambar Behera
Department of Pulmonary Medicine, Postgraduate Institute of Medical Education & Research; WHO Collaborating Centre for Research and Capacity Building in Chronic Respiratory Diseases, Chandigarh, India

Liwei Chen
Clemson University, Clemson, South Carolina, United States

Valentin Fuster
The Mount Sinai Medical Hospital; Mount Sinai Heart; Icahn School of Medicine at Mount Sinai, New York, New York, United States

Guillermo Garcia-Garcia
Hospital Civil de Guadalajara "Fray Antonio Alcalde," University of Guadalajara Health Sciences Center, Guadalajara, Mexico

Scott Kahan
National Center for Weight and Wellness, Washington, DC, United States; Johns Hopkins Bloomberg School of Public Health, Baltimore, Maryland, United States

Jonathan Kaltman
National Heart, Lung, and Blood Institute, National Institutes of Health, Bethesda, Maryland, United States

Eduardo M. Krieger
Heart Institute, Medical School of the University of São Paulo (InCor-FMUSP), São Paulo, Brazil

Harriet V. Kuhnlein
Centre for Indigenous Peoples' Nutrition and Environment and School of Dietetics and Human Nutrition, McGill University, Montreal, Canada

Anuradha Lala
Icahn School of Medicine at Mount Sinai; The Zena and Michael A. Wiener Cardiovascular Institute, Mount Sinai Hospital, New York, New York, United States

Naomi Levitt
University of Cape Town; Chronic Disease Initiative for Africa, Cape Town, South Africa

Carlos Mendoza Montano
Institute of Nutrition of Central America and Panama (INCAP); INCAP Research Center for the Prevention of Chronic Diseases, Guatemala City, Guatemala

George A. Mensah
National Heart, Lung, and Blood Institute, National Institutes of Health, Bethesda, Maryland, United States

Andrew J. Mirelman
Centre for Health Economics, University of York, York, United Kingdom

Monica L. Mispireta
School of Nursing, Idaho State University, Pocatello, Idaho, United States

Jorge A. Motta
National Secretary Science, Technology and Innovation, Panama City, Panama

Jagat Narula
Journal of the American College of Cardiology, Washington, DC, United States; Arnhold Institute for Global Health at Mount Sinai; Icahn School of Medicine at Mount Sinai; Mount Sinai West and Mount Sinai St. Luke's Hospitals, New York, New York, United States

Frida Ngalesoni
University of Bergen, Bergen, Norway

Ole Frithjof Norheim
University of Bergen, Bergen, Norway

Pekka Puska
National Institute for Health and Welfare (THL), Helsinki, Finland

Cristina Rabadan-Diehl
Office of the Americas, Office of Global Affairs, United States Department of Health and Human Services, Washington, DC, United States

K. Srinath Reddy
Public Health Foundation of India, New Delhi, India

Rebecca Reynolds
University of Edinburgh, Edinburgh, United Kingdom

Jonathan M. Samet
Keck School of Medicine, University of Southern California (USC); USC Institute for Global Health, Los Angeles, California, United States

John W. Stanifer
Duke University; Duke Clinical Research Institute; Duke Global Health Institute, Durham, North Carolina, United States

Nigel Unwin
Chronic Disease Research Centre, University of the West Indies, Barbados; MRC Epidemiology Unit, Cambridge University, Cambridge, United Kingdom

Martin Veller
University of the Witwatersrand, Johannesburg, South Africa

S. Goya Wannamethee
University College London Medical School, London, United Kingdom

Kremlin Wickramasinghe
Nuffield Department of Population Health, University of Oxford, Oxford, United Kingdom

Edwina H. Yeung
Eunice Kennedy Shriver National Institute of Child Health and Human Development, National Institutes of Health, Bethesda, Maryland, United States

Policy Forum Participants

The following individuals provided valuable insights to improve this volume's key findings through participation in the Disease Control Priorities-World Health Organization, Eastern Mediterranean Regional Office policy forum on Cardiovascular Disease and Diabetes, in Geneva, Switzerland, on November 14, 2015. The forum was organized by Dr. Ala Alwan, Regional Director, World Health Organization, and member of the DCP3 Advisory Committee to the Editors.

Ala Alwan
Regional Director Emeritus, World Health Organization Regional Office for the Eastern Mediterranean, Cairo, Arab Republic of Egypt

Fawzi Amin
Secretary General, Bahrain Red Crescent Society; Former Director General of Primary Health Care and Assistant Undersecretary, Ministry of Health, Manama, Bahrain

Walid Ammar
Director General, Ministry of Public Health, Beirut, Lebanon

Karim Aoun
Director General, Ministry of Health, Tunisia; Professor in Parasitology, Medical School of Tunis, Tunis, Tunisia

Nooshin Mohd Bazargani
Deputy Head of Dubai Heart Centre, Dubai, United Arab Emirates; Board Member of World Heart Federation, Geneva, Switzerland; Chair, CVD Prevention Group of Emirates Cardiac Society, Abu Dhabi, United Arab Emirates

Suraya Dalil
Permanent Representative of the Government of the Islamic Republic of Afghanistan to the United Nations, Geneva, Switzerland; Former Minister of Health, Kabul, Afghanistan

Reida M. A. Elaokley
Minister of Health, Ministry of Health, El-Beida, Libya

Hassen Ghannem
Director, Tunisia Center of Excellence to Combat Chronic Diseases, Department of Epidemiology, University Hospital Farhat Hached, Sousse, Tunisia

Assad Hafeez
Director General of Health, Ministry of National Health Services, Regulation, and Coordination, Islamabad, Pakistan

Ali bin Talib Al Hinai
Undersecretary for Planning, Ministry of Health, Muscat, Oman

Didier Houssin
President, High Council for the Evaluation of Research and Higher Education, Paris, France; Former Director General for Health, Ministry of Health, Paris, France

Azhar Mahmood Kayani
Consultant Cardiologist, Army Medical College, Rawalpindi, Pakistan

Sa'ad Kharabsheh
Former Minister of Health, Amman, Jordan

Bagher Ardeshir Larijani
Deputy Minister for Education; Head of High Level
NCD Council, Ministry of Health and Medical
Education, Tehran, Islamic Republic of Iran

Pekka Puska
Former Director General, The National Institute for
Health and Welfare, Helsinki, Finland

Ali Faraj Al-Qaraghuli
Senior Consultant Cardiologist, Al Oyoun Hospital,
Amman, Jordan

Junaid Razzak
Director, Telemedicine Programme and Senior Advisor
Global Health, Department of Emergency Medicine,
Johns Hopkins University School of Medicine; Department

of International Health, Bloomberg School of Public
Health, Johns Hopkins University, Baltimore, Maryland,
United States; Visiting Faculty, Department of Emergency
Medicine, Aga Khan University, Karachi, Pakistan

Qasim Bin Ahmad Al Salimi
Director General, The Royal Hospital,
Muscat, Oman

Amirhossein Takian
Deputy Acting Minister for International Affairs,
Ministry of Health and Medical Education, Tehran,
Islamic Republic of Iran

Mohammed Hamad J. Al-Thani
Director of Public Health, Department of Public
Health, Ministry of Public Health, Doha, Qatar

Index

Boxes, figures, maps, notes, and tables are indicated by b, f, m, n, and t following page numbers.

A

abdominal obesity, 28–29. *See also* obesity/
    overweight
Academia de Cidade (Brazil), 90*b*
Academic Model Providing Access to Healthcare
    (AMPATH), 331
ACE inhibitors. *See* angiotensin-converting enzyme
    inhibitors
ACE Obesity Study, 127–29, 128*t*
acute coronary syndrome (ACS), 136, 140–43,
    328–29, 333–35, 338, 340, 360
acute kidney injury (AKI), 15, 178, 235–39,
    237*b*, 242, 383
acute rheumatic fever (ARF), 197–200, 357
ADA. *See* American Diabetes Association
adherence to treatment
    chronic respiratory diseases, 270, 272–73
    community-based care and, 315, 321
    cost-effectiveness of interventions and, 358
    costs and, 356–58
    diabetes, 218, 223
    heart failure, 182, 186
    hypertension, 163, 395, 397
    integrated care and, 296–97
    ischemic heart disease, 142, 144, 146
    obesity interventions, 126
    quality of care and, 330, 333, 334–36, 338–39, 341
    rheumatic heart disease, 198, 202
    stroke, 160
Adler, Alma, 389
adolescence, BMI in, 42–43
Africa. *See also specific countries*
    congenital heart disease in, 194
    cost-effectiveness of interventions in, 353
    diabetes in, 211, 216

    diet and nutrition in, 106
    heart failure in, 175, 185
    ischemic heart disease in, 138–40, 142–43
    kidney disease in, 236
    obesity/overweight in, 120
    priority-setting for treatments in, 379
    quality of care in, 338, 340, 342
    rheumatic heart disease in, 200
    tobacco use in, 68
Afshin, Ashkan, 101
Agita São Paulo (Brazil), 90*b*
AIDS. *See* HIV/AIDS
Ajay, Vamadevan S., 23, 287
AKI. *See* acute kidney injury
Ali, Mohammed K., 209, 287
Allen, K., 110
Alzheimer's disease, 64–65
American College of Cardiology, 174*b*
American College of Sports Medicine, 89
American Diabetes Association (ADA), 85, 214–15, 217
American Heart Association, 162, 174*b*
American Stroke Association, 162
AMPATH (Academic Model Providing Access to
    Healthcare), 331
Amrita Institute of Medical Sciences (India), 196
Anand, Shuchi, 1, 235
angina, 136
angiotensin-converting enzyme (ACE) inhibitors, 12,
    141, 178–79, 181–84, 186, 215, 242, 247, 393, 395
angiotensin receptor blockers (ARBs), 7, 15, 142, 145,
    178, 215, 219, 222, 242–43, 247, 357, 391–92
antibiotics, 237, 274–76
anticoagulation therapies, 164–65, 179, 186
antihypertensive treatments, 163, 165, 186, 393
antiplatelet therapy, 166, 393

aortic artery disease, 66
ARBs. *See* angiotensin receptor blockers
ARF. *See* acute rheumatic fever
Argentina
    Chagas disease in, 204
    cost-effectiveness of interventions in, 353, 359
    diet and nutrition in, 108, 110
    heart failure in, 184
    ischemic heart disease in, 141, 147
    priority-setting for treatments in, 378–83
    quality of care in, 342
    stroke in, 165
Armour, T. A., 314
arrhythmia, 64, 66, 178
Asaria, P., 110
aspirin, 141–46, 164, 166, 179, 185, 254, 329, 333, 336,
    341, 357–59, 375, 389, 393, 395
asthma
    assessment, 271–72
    barriers to care, 272–73
    burden of disease, 263–65
    community-based care, 307–8
    diagnosis, 271
    management of, 272, 277, 308, 310
    mortality and morbidity trends, 27
    pharmacological management, 272
    prevention, 269
    risk factors, 263–65
    symptoms, 27, 271–72
atenolol, 8, 142, 178, 392–93
atherosclerosis, 58*b*
atherothrombosis, 58*b*
atrial fibrillation, 64, 66, 160–64, 179, 197, 398
Australia
    Chagas disease in, 203
    chronic respiratory diseases in, 264
    community-based care in, 305, 311
    diabetes in, 216
    diet and nutrition in, 106
    ischemic heart disease in, 144, 146
    obesity/overweight in, 126–27, 129
    physical activity in, 87–88

B
Bakshi, K. D., 196
Bangladesh
    cardiometabolic disease in, 46–47
    community-based care in, 310
    cost-effectiveness of interventions in, 356
    hypertension in, 397
bariatric surgery, 127
Barker, D. J. P., 37, 39
Barthel Index, 168, 316

Bateman, Eric, 263
Belarus
    breastfeeding promotion in, 47
    ischemic heart disease in, 138
beta blockers, 6, 9–10, 141–46, 163, 177–79, 181,
    183–86, 254, 317, 333, 358–59, 391–93, 395
Bettger, Janet, 157
bidi smoking, 68. *See also* tobacco use
birth weight
    cardiometabolic disease and, 37–40, 43–46, 48
    low birth weight, 30–31, 37, 39, 43–45, 241, 267–68
bisphenol, 44
blood pressure (BP)
    cardiometabolic disease and, 39–40, 42, 44–47
    community-based care and, 308–10, 314–15,
      319, 321
    cost-effectiveness of interventions, 356–58
    diabetes and, 214, 216–17
    integrated care and, 295, 297
    kidney disease and, 243–44
    management of, 389, 391–92, 395, 397–98
    physical activity and, 84–85, 91
    quality of care and, 330, 336–38, 340
    as risk factor, 28–30
    stroke and, 161, 163–65, 166
    tobacco use and, 60, 62–63, 66, 70
BMI. *See* body mass index
body fat. *See also* obesity/overweight
    cardiometabolic disease and, 40–41
    obesity/overweight and, 117–18
    physical activity and, 91
body mass index (BMI)
    cardiometabolic disease and, 37, 39, 41–43, 47–48
    chronic respiratory diseases and, 264
    diet and, 104
    integrated care and, 292
    obesity/overweight and, 117–19, 123, 128
    physical activity and, 83–86
    priority-setting for treatments, 385
Bonow, Robert O., 135
Boston University, 241*b*
BP. *See* blood pressure
Brazil
    Chagas disease in, 204
    chronic respiratory diseases in, 278
    community-based care in, 314
    community-based physical activity programs in, 90*b*
    cost-effectiveness of interventions in, 16, 353,
      359–60
    diabetes in, 10, 213
    diet and nutrition in, 110
    heart failure in, 184
    ischemic heart disease in, 139, 141–42

kidney disease in, 236, 240, 244
    obesity/overweight in, 118, 120–21, 124–25,
        127, 130
    physical activity in, 14, 82, 87, 89, 92–93
    priority-setting for treatments in, 378–80,
        382, 384
    quality of care in, 332, 342
    rheumatic heart disease in, 201
    stroke in, 163
    tobacco use in, 68
breastfeeding, 44, 47
bronchiectasis, 268–69, 276
bronchodilators, 274
Brouwer, Elizabeth, 349
Bukhman, Gene, 191
Bulgaria, ischemic heart disease in, 138
Bull, Fiona, 79
burden of disease
    asthma, 263–65
    Chagas disease, 203
    chronic obstructive pulmonary disease (COPD),
        263–67
    chronic respiratory diseases, 263–69, 266–67f
    congenital heart disease (CHD), 191–92
    diabetes, 209–12, 377
    dyslipidemia, 390
    heart failure, 173–77, 175–76t, 176f
    hypertension, 389–90
    ischemic heart disease (IHD), 136–40, 137m,
        138–39f
    obesity/overweight, 117–18
    peripheral artery disease (PAD), 256
    physical activity and inactivity, 80–81f, 80–82
    rheumatic heart disease (RHD), 197
    stroke, 157–59
Burney, Peter, 263

C
CABG (coronary artery bypass graft), 143, 185
calcium channel blockers, 163, 179, 333, 391–93
Callender, T., 181b
Cambodia
    community-based care in, 320–21
    diabetes in, 217
    integrated care in, 294
    kidney disease in, 239–40
Cameroon
    community-based care in, 306, 308–10
    quality of care in, 343
    tobacco use in, 68
Canada
    cost-effectiveness of interventions in, 358
    ischemic heart disease in, 143–45

    kidney disease in, 235, 237
    obesity/overweight in, 126
    physical activity in, 87, 92–93
cancer, 210
Capewell, Simon, 70, 101
carbohydrates, 121–22
cardiac resynchronization therapy (CRT), 141, 147,
    180, 183–84, 186, 359
cardiometabolic disease, 37–55. See also specific
    conditions
    bisphenol A and, 44
    breastfeeding and, 44, 47
    childhood weight gain and growth, 47–48
        BMI in adulthood, 43
        BMI in childhood and adolescence, 42–43
        height in childhood, 43
        weight and BMI in infancy, 42
    community-based care, 312–14, 316
    cost-effectiveness of interventions, 361
    developmental origins of health and disease,
        39–40, 40f
        adjustments, 45
        confounding issues, 45
        genetic effects, 45
        measurement errors, 45
    fuel-mediated teratogenesis and, 40–41
    genetic effects, 45
    gestational diabetes and, 40–41, 41f, 47
    integrated care and, 296
    interventions, 46–48
        cost-effectiveness, 361
    maternal obesity and, 40–41, 41f, 47
    maternal smoking and, 44
    micronutrient supplementation, 46–47
    nutritional interventions in pregnancy, 46–47
    physical activity and, 79, 81, 82–86, 87, 89, 91
    phytoestrogens and, 44
    polychlorinated biphenyls and, 44
    public health implications, 48–49
    risk factors, 37–39, 38f
cardiomyopathy, 8, 27, 173–75, 183–84, 193
cardiovascular, respiratory, and related disorders
        (CVRDs). See also specific conditions
    framework for addressing, 9, 32–33, 33f
    mortality and morbidity trends, 24–25, 24t,
        25–26f, 26t
    risk factors
        adolescence determinants, 31–32
        alcohol use, 30
        dyslipidemia, 28
        early childhood determinants, 9, 30–31
        high blood pressure, 29
        middle childhood determinants, 31–32

modifiable, 28–30
nonmodifiable, 27–28
obesity/overweight, 29
physical inactivity, 29–30
reducing, 32
social and ecological determinants, 30–32, 33
tobacco use, 28
cardiovascular disease (CVD). *See also* cardiovascular,
  respiratory, and related disorders (CVRDs);
  ischemic heart disease (IHD)
  mortality rates, 4
  tobacco use and, 57–78. *See also* tobacco use
    CVD mortality rates and, 64
    CVD outcomes and, 63–67, 64*b*, 64*f*
    CVD pathophysiology and mechanisms, 58–62,
      59–60*f*
    CVD risk factors, 62–63
carotid and cerebrovascular diseases, 65
carotid endarterectomy, 165
carotid stenosis surgery, 166
catecholamines, 58–59, 61–62, 66
Cawley, J., 109
CCC (chronic Chagas cardiomyopathy), 202–4
CD. *See* Chagas disease
CDSS (clinical decision support system), 317–19, 343
Cecchini, M., 110
Centers for Disease Control and Prevention, 392
Chagas disease (CD), 191, 202–4
  burden of disease, 203
  heart failure and, 173, 176
  interventions, 203
    cost-effectiveness, 203–4
  natural history, 202–3
  pathogenesis, 202–3
  risk factors, 27
Chan, Juliana, 209
Chandrasekar, Eeshwar, 209
CHD. *See* coronary heart disease
Chen, Jie, 157
children
  asthma and, 263–64
  BMI
    in childhood and adolescence, 42–43
    in infancy, 42
  cardiometabolic disease and, 47–48
  height in childhood, 43
  mortality rates, 49, 110, 350, 353
  obesity/overweight, 31–32, 44, 47, 125,
    127–28, 354
  weight gain and growth, 42–43, 47–48
Chile
  community-based care in, 314–15
  ischemic heart disease in, 142

obesity/overweight in, 124–25
  priority-setting for treatments in, 382, 384
China
  congenital heart disease in, 191, 194
  cost-effectiveness of interventions in, 353–54,
    360, 369–70, 372–73
  diabetes in, 210, 213, 217
  diet and nutrition in, 106, 110
  health care costs in, 8
  integrated care in, 289–91, 293, 295
  ischemic heart disease in, 137, 140–42
  kidney disease in, 236, 240, 243, 245
  obesity/overweight in, 118, 120–22, 124–27, 129–30
  peripheral artery disease in, 8–9
  physical activity in, 12, 82
  quality of care in, 335
  stroke in, 157, 159, 162–64, 166–67
cholesterol. *See also* dyslipidemia
  cardiometabolic disease and, 46
  community-based care and, 317
  cost-effectiveness of interventions, 356–58
  high-density lipoprotein (HDL), 29, 46, 61–62,
    390, 396
  integrated care and, 297
  low-density lipoprotein (LDL), 28, 61–62, 85, 146,
    163, 335–36, 340, 389–91, 394, 396
  management of, 389–90, 397
  physical activity and, 85
  as risk factor, 28–30
  tobacco use and, 61–62
chronic bronchitis, 264, 268–69
chronic Chagas cardiomyopathy (CCC), 202–4
chronic kidney disease (CKD), 235, 239–45
  diabetes and, 210–12, 214, 220
  epidemiology of, 239
  hypertension and, 9, 396
  integrated care and, 288, 294
  interventions, 241, 243–44*t*
    cost-effectiveness, 13, 245–46, 360
    renal replacement therapy, 245–46, 245*f*
    screening, 245, 246*b*
  pharmacological interventions, 242
  policy implications, 246–47, 247*t*
  prevalence, 240
  priority-setting for treatments, 375, 383
  tobacco use and, 64, 66–67
chronic obstructive pulmonary disease (COPD)
  burden of disease, 263–67
  clinical course and management, 273–74, 277
  community-based care and, 306–7
  cost-effectiveness of interventions, 13, 359
  diagnosis, 273
  heart failure and, 175

mortality and morbidity trends, 27–28
pharmacological management, 274–75
prevention, 269
primary care centers and, 15
risk factors, 263–67
tobacco use and, 65
chronic respiratory diseases, 263–86, 264*t*.
    See also specific conditions
    asthma, 263–65
        assessment, 271–72
        barriers to care, 272–73
        diagnosis, 271
        pharmacological management, 272
    bronchiectasis, 268–69, 276
    burden of disease, 263–69, 266–67*f*
    chronic airway obstruction and COPD, 265–66
        clinical course and management, 273–74
        diagnosis, 273
        pharmacological management, 274–75
    chronic bronchitis, 268–69
    community-based care and, 305–6, 310
    idiopathic low FVC, 266–68, 275
    interventions
        cost-effectiveness, 359
        management, 271–76
        primary prevention, 269, 269*b*
        principles of care, 270, 270*b*
    mortality and morbidity rates, 23–25, 27–29
    restrictive lung disease and fibrosis, 268
        diagnosis, 275
        treatment, 275–76
    risk factors, 31, 33
    systems and organization of care, 276–78,
        277*t*, 278*b*
    tobacco use and, 66
cigar and cigarette smoking. *See* tobacco use
Civil Servant Medical Benefit Scheme (CSMBS,
    Thailand), 383
CKD. *See* chronic kidney disease
claudication, 64, 253–54, 256–58
clinical decision support system (CDSS),
    317–19, 343
clinical interventions
    community-based care and, 306
    cost-effectiveness, 10, 355, 372
    diabetes, 218
    obesity, 129
cognitive rehabilitation, 168
collaborative care, 294, 297, 312–13
Colombia
    community-based physical activity
        programs in, 90*b*
    physical activity in, 14, 87, 89, 92–93

priority-setting for treatments in, 378–82, 384
community-based health care, 305–26
    case studies, 317–22, 318–20*f*
    rheumatic heart disease (RHD), 199
    self-management, 312–16, 313*t*, 316*b*, 317*f*
        cost-effectiveness, 315–16
        education in, 314–15
        target populations, 314
        technology for, 315
        theories of, 313–14
    stroke, 164
    task-shifting, 305–12, 307–9*t*, 311*b*
congenital heart disease (CHD), 191–96
    burden of disease, 191–92
    categories of, 191, 192*t*
    curative care and treatment, 15, 194–95
    hypertension and, 390
    interventions, 192–94
        cost-effectiveness, 195–96
        neonatal screening, 194
        prenatal screening, 193–94, 193*t*
        prevention, 192–93
        screening, 193–94, 195–96
    palliative care and treatment, 194–95
    prevalence rate, 191
    risk factors, 26, 192
    treatment, 194–95
        access to, 10, 15
        cost-effectiveness, 195–96
Congleton, T. M., 162
Consortium for the Epidemic of Nephropathy in
    Central America and Mexico, 241*b*
Consortium of Health-Orientated Research in
    Transitioning Societies, 42, 49
Control of Blood Pressure and Risk Attenuation
    (COBRA), 314
COPD. *See* chronic obstructive pulmonary disease
Cornelson, L., 362n2
coronary artery bypass graft (CABG), 143, 185
Coronary Artery Risk Development in Young Adults
    Study, 85
coronary heart disease (CHD). *See also* heart failure;
        ischemic heart disease
    cardiometabolic disease and, 37, 40, 42–45, 48
    community-based care, 312
    cost-effectiveness of interventions, 354
    diabetes and, 210–11, 214
    diet and, 102–4
    hypertension and, 389–90, 394–96
    integrated care and, 288, 294
    ischemic heart disease and, 137
    physical activity and, 82–83, 83*f*, 86–87
    quality of care and, 335, 341

risk factors, 29
stroke and, 160, 163
tobacco use and, 64–70
coronary vasoconstriction, 58*b*
corticosteroids, 272, 274–75
cost
    cardiometabolic disease interventions, 49
    Chagas disease (CD) interventions, 203–4
    chronic respiratory disease interventions, 270,
        272, 277
    community-based care, 306, 308–9, 314–16
    congenital heart disease interventions, 194–95
    diabetes interventions, 211–12, 214–15,
        218–19, 224
    health care, generally, 57, 65–66, 86–87, 109,
        124, 140
    heart failure interventions, 178, 180–81, 183–84
    hypertension interventions, 397
    indirect, 87, 140, 159, 195, 212, 321, 390
    ischemic heart disease, 140, 143
    kidney disease interventions, 235, 238, 244–47
    obesity/overweight interventions, 124, 125, 127–31
    peripheral artery disease interventions, 258
    physical activity interventions, 86–87, 89, 91–92
    prevention, 360–61
    priority-setting for treatments and, 383–84
    quality of care and, 343–44
    rheumatic heart disease interventions, 201–2
    stroke interventions, 166, 168
    treatment, 9–17, 360–61
cost-effectiveness of interventions, 10–13, 11*b*
    acute and hospital-based care, 359–60
    Chagas disease, 203–4
    cholesterol, 357
    chronic kidney disease (CKD), 245–46
    community-based care, 355–56
    congenital heart disease (CHD), 195–96
    diabetes, 217–19, 220*t*, 357
    diet and nutrition, 109–11, 352–53
    dyslipidemia, 397
    extended cost-effectiveness analyses (ECEAs),
        11, 16, 369–73
    first-level hospital care, 357–59
    heart failure, 183–84, 185*t*, 359
    hypertension, 357, 370*t*, 371–72, 397
    individual-level interventions, 355–60
        acute and hospital-based care, 359–60
        cholesterol, 357
        community-based care, 355–56
        diabetes, 357
        first-level hospital care, 357–59
        heart failure, 359
        hypertension, 357, 370*t*, 371–72

ischemic heart disease, 359–60
    kidney disease, 360
    medication availability and adherence, 358–59
    primary health center care, 356–57
    respiratory conditions, 359
    rheumatic heart disease, 357
    screening, 355–56
    ischemic heart disease, 145, 359–60
    kidney disease, 238, 360
    mass media policies, 353–55
    medication availability and adherence, 358–59
    obesity/overweight, 127–30, 128*t*, 130*t*
    peripheral artery disease (PAD), 258–60
    physical activity, 91–92, 354–55
    population-level interventions, 350–55, 350*f*
        diet and nutrition, 352–53
        mass media policies, 353–55
        physical activity, 354–55
        regulatory policy, 353–55
        salt consumption, 353–54, 370*t*, 371
        tobacco use, 350–52, 351*t*, 370–71, 370*t*
        trans fats consumption, 353–54
    primary health center care, 356–57
    ratios, 12, 92, 110, 130, 350, 352–53, 355
    regulatory policy, 353–55
    respiratory conditions, 359
    rheumatic heart disease, 201–2, 357
    salt consumption, 353–54, 370*t*, 371
    screening, 355–56
    self-management, 315–16
    stroke, 165, 168
    threshold for, 130, 355, 384
    tobacco use, 350–52, 351*t*, 370–71, 370*t*
    trans fats consumption, 353–54
counseling, dietary, 47, 86
Criqui, Michael H., 253
Critchley, J. A., 70
critical limb ischemia, 257–58
cyclophosphamide, 242

D
D'Alessandro, A., 66
DALYs (disability-adjusted life-years)
    Chagas disease and, 203–4
    congenital heart disease and, 191–92
    cost-effectiveness of interventions and, 11–12,
        350–54, 358–59
    diabetes and, 211–12
    diet and, 104, 110
    heart failure and, 184–85
    hypertension and, 390
    ischemic heart disease and, 135, 137, 139–40, 145
    obesity/overweight and, 127–30

physical activity and, 87
priority-setting for treatments and, 375, 377, 383
rheumatic heart disease and, 197
risk factors and, 4, 25, 27–29
stroke and, 157–58, 169
death rates. *See* mortality rates
dementia, 64–65, 82, 86
Denmark
cardiometabolic disease in, 47
diabetes in, 215
diet and nutrition in, 108
integrated care in, 292–93
taxation of unhealthy foods and beverages in, 362n1
depression
community-based care and, 315
diabetes and, 210, 212, 214, 217, 288, 295, 297
integrated care and, 287–88
physical activity and, 83, 86–87
risk factors, 30
stroke and, 158–59, 161, 167
developmental origins of health and disease (DOHaD) for cardiometabolic disease, 39–40, 40*f*
adjustments, 45
confounding issues, 45
genetic effects, 45
interventions, 37, 39–40, 49
measurement errors, 45
diabetes, 209–34
burden of disease, 209–12, 377
cancer and, 210
cardiometabolic disease and, 39, 42
chronic kidney disease (CKD) and, 210
community-based care, 314
complications of, 6, 12, 210–11, 215, 219
coronary heart disease (CHD) and, 210
depression and, 217, 288, 295, 297
diagnosis, 215–16
diet and, 104
disability and, 211–12
end-stage renal disease (ESRD) and, 210, 241–42
heart failure and, 210
HIV/AIDS and, 292–94, 293*t*
hypertension and, 9, 240, 308–9, 320–21, 331–32, 340, 343, 384, 392, 394, 396
integrated care and, 289–93
interventions, 9, 213–15, 217, 220
cost-effectiveness, 217–19, 220*t*, 356, 357
management, 144, 214–15, 216, 220, 308
prevention, 213–14, 216, 219
priorities, 221, 221–23*t*
screening, 213, 215, 219, 396

ischemic heart disease and, 136
knowledge gaps, 221, 223
management of, 144, 214–15, 216, 220, 308
maternal, 39, 48, 192
mental health and, 287–88
mortality and morbidity trends, 27, 211–12, 211*t*
obesity/overweight and, 122
physical activity and, 84–85, 84–85*f*
prevalence rate, 48, 63, 109, 209–10, 214, 216, 288–90, 292, 381
prevention, 12, 213, 216–18, 221, 223
priority-setting for treatments, 375, 377
quality of care and, 327
risk factors, 24–26
stroke and, 159–60, 210
tobacco use and, 63
treatment, 216–17
tuberculosis and, 288–92, 289*f*, 290–91*t*
Diabetes Prevention Program (DPP), 84, 216, 222, 311
diabetic retinopathy, 215, 220–21
diagnosis
chronic obstructive pulmonary disease (COPD), 273
diabetes, 215–16
heart failure, 173
peripheral artery disease (PAD), 253–54
stroke, 162
dialysis, 15, 64, 210, 235–40, 242–43, 375
Diep, L., 83
diet and nutrition, 101–15
carbohydrates, 121–22
cardiometabolic disease and, 39, 43, 46
chronic respiratory diseases and, 264, 267, 271
community-based care, 314
counseling, 47, 86
fatty acids, 14, 102, 104, 143, 353–54
folate deficiency, 192
grains, 102–4, 122, 124–25, 131
interventions, 105–9, 105*t*
cost-effectiveness, 109–11, 352–53
fiscal policies, 107, 107*t*
local food environment, 108
mass media campaigns, 105–7
multicomponent interventions, 109
organizational settings, 107–8
pregnancy and, 46–47
taxation of unhealthy beverages and foods, 108–9
trans fats restrictions, 108
micronutrients, 46–47, 121–22
obesity/overweight and, 117–18, 121–24, 127–28, 131
risk factors, 102–5, 103–4*t*
salt consumption, 16, 110, 163, 165, 353–54, 370*t*, 371–73

stroke and, 160–61

sugar and sugar-sweetened beverages (SSBs), 11–13, 17, 102–9, 119, 123–28, 131, 222, 266, 352–53

trans fats consumption, 14, 102, 104, 106, 108, 353–54

vegetables, 13, 28, 32–33, 103–8, 124–26, 129, 131, 160–62, 169, 266

digital health strategies, 164–65

digoxin, 178–79, 186

Dirks, John, 235

disability

chronic respiratory diseases and, 276

community-based care and, 316–17

cost-effectiveness of interventions, 11, 16–17, 357

diabetes and, 211–12

heart failure and, 174, 184

integrated care and, 288

ischemic heart disease and, 135

primary care centers and, 3–4b

quality of care and, 328

risk factors, 25–28

stroke and, 157–58, 160–61, 166–67

diuretics, 6, 15, 163, 177, 181, 183–84, 186, 359, 391–93, 395

DOHaD. *See* developmental origins of health and disease

Doll, R., 64

DPP. *See* Diabetes Prevention Program

drugs. *See* pharmacological interventions

Dugani, Sagar B., 135

dyslipidemia

burden of disease, 390

cost-effectiveness of interventions, 397

interventions, 393–95

polypills, 395

screening, 396

statins, 394. *See also* statins

tobacco use and, 62

E

East Asia and Pacific. *See also specific countries*

congenital heart disease in, 192

diabetes in, 220

heart failure in, 176, 185

ischemic heart disease in, 137–38, 141

kidney disease in, 245

peripheral artery disease in, 256

stroke in, 157

ECEAs (extended cost-effectiveness analyses), 11, 16, 369–73

echocardiography, 173, 178, 182, 184, 186, 194, 199, 201, 357, 396

Egypt, Arab Republic of

diabetes in, 210

priority-setting for treatments in, 378–79

tobacco use in, 68

e-Health, 164

ejection fraction, 177–78, 181–82

electronic nicotine delivery systems (electronic cigarettes), 69

El Nahas, Meguid, 235

El Salvador, kidney disease in, 241b

EMLs. *See* essential medicines lists

endothelial dysfunction, 58–62, 58b

endovascular therapy, 257–58

end-stage renal disease (ESRD), 235, 239–42

diabetes and, 210, 215, 219–20, 241–42

dialysis, 242

epidemiology of, 240

hypertension and, 241–42

interventions, 241–42

cost-effectiveness, 357, 371

prevalence, 240

priority-setting for treatments, 383

transplantation, 243–44

treatment, 242–45

Engelgau, Michael, 327

ESRD. *See* end-stage renal disease

essential medicines lists (EMLs), 375, 377–78

estimated glomerular filtration rate (eGFR), 239

Ethiopia

cost-effectiveness of interventions in, 370–71

hypertensive treatment in, 16, 371–72

rheumatic heart disease in, 197

Europe and Central Asia. *See also specific countries*

diabetes in, 211, 220

heart failure in, 174, 176, 185

ischemic heart disease in, 138–39

kidney disease in, 245

peripheral artery disease in, 256–57, 259

European Medicines Agency, 377

exercise. *See* physical activity

extended cost-effectiveness analyses (ECEAs), 11, 16, 369–73

F

Fall, Caroline H. D., 37

fatty acids, 14, 102, 104, 143, 353–54

FCTC. *See* Framework Convention on Tobacco Control

Feigin, Valery, 157

Ferrante, D., 110

fibrinogen, 61–62, 67

fibrosis and restrictive lung disease, 268, 275–76

Figueira, F. R., 84

financial risk protection (FRP), 2, 9, 11, 16–17, 369–73

Finland
    cardiometabolic disease in, 42–43, 45, 48
    diabetes in, 213, 216
    diet and nutrition in, 105, 109
    kidney disease in, 238
    physical activity in, 92–93
    taxation of unhealthy foods and
        beverages in, 362n1
Finnish Diabetes Prevention Trial, 84
fiscal policies, 13–14, 107, 350, 352
folic acid, 46–47, 166, 192
food advertising and labeling, 105, 123, 124–25,
        129–31
Food and Drug Administration (U.S.), 274
Football Fans in Training program, 91
forced vital capacity (FVC), 265–68, 275
Forouhi, N. G., 290
Forsdahl, A., 37
Fowkes, F. Gerald R., 253
Framework Convention on Tobacco
        Control (FCTC), 9, 32, 70, 144
Framingham Heart study, 23, 165
France
    diet and nutrition in, 107–8
    ischemic heart disease in, 137
    obesity/overweight in, 125
    priority-setting for treatments in, 382
    taxation of unhealthy foods and
        beverages in, 362n1
Freeman, S. D., 162
free trade agreements, 119
Freinkel, N., 40
Friends of Aldo Castenada Foundation, 196
Frisvold, D., 109
FRP. See financial risk protection
fuel-mediated teratogenesis, 40–41
FVC (forced vital capacity), 265–68, 275

G
The Gambia, nutrition during pregnancy in, 46
Garrett, S., 92
Gaziano, Thomas A., 1, 135, 349, 389
GDM. See gestational diabetes mellitus
gender issues
    physical activity, 80, 91b
    tobacco use, 65
generic medications, 8, 17, 145–46, 358
genetics
    developmental origins of health and disease
        (DOHaD), 45
    obesity/overweight, 123
    tobacco use and, 62
George, J., 238

gestational diabetes
    cardiometabolic disease and, 40–41, 41f, 47
    congenital heart disease and, 196
    defined, 209
    screening for, 217, 396
GFR (glomerular filtration rate), 239, 243–44
Glassman, Amanda, 375
Global Advocacy for Physical Activity Initiative, 88
Global Burden of Disease (GBD) Study, 102, 135, 174.
        See also burden of disease
Global Initiative for Asthma (GINA), 270–73
Global Initiative for Chronic Obstructive Lung Disease
        (GOLD), 265
Global Physical Activity Questionnaire (GPAQ), 81
Global Registry of Acute Coronary Events, 142
Global Strategy on Diet, Physical Activity and Health
        (WHO), 92, 107
glomerular filtration rate (GFR), 239, 243–44
Goenka, Shifalika, 79
GOLD (Global Initiative for Chronic Obstructive Lung
        Disease), 265
GPAQ (Global Physical Activity Questionnaire), 81
grains, 102–4, 122, 124–25, 131
Green, R., 362n2
Guatemala
    cardiometabolic disease in, 46
    community-based care in, 310
    cost-effectiveness of interventions in, 356
    hypertension in, 397
Gulf Registry of Acute Coronary Events, 142, 143
Gupta, Rajeev, 389

H
Harikrishnan, S., 181b
Hasan, Babar, 191
Hawkesworth, S., 46
HCV (hepatitis C virus), 293
HDL. See high-density lipoprotein
health care costs. See also cost
    diet and nutrition, 109
    ischemic heart disease in, 140
    obesity/overweight, 124
    physical activity and, 86–87
    tobacco use and, 57, 65–66
health care providers
    community-based care and, 305, 307, 313–14, 316
    integrated care and, 297
    ischemic heart disease and, 136, 145
    obesity/overweight and, 130–31
    physical activity and, 88
    quality of care and, 328, 334–35, 342
    rheumatic heart disease and, 200
    stroke and, 162, 164, 166–67

health technology assessment (HTA), 369, 375, 384, 386
heart disease. *See* congenital heart disease; coronary
　　heart disease; ischemic heart disease
heart failure, 173–90
　　burden of disease, 173–77, 175–76*t*, 176*f*
　　causes, 173
　　diabetes and, 210
　　diagnosis, 173
　　health service arrangements, 180–82
　　interventions, 177–80, 183*t*
　　　　angiotensin-converting enzyme (ACE)
　　　　　　inhibitors, 178, 184
　　　　angiotensin receptor blockers, 178
　　　　anticoagulants, 179
　　　　beta blockers, 177–78, 184
　　　　case management, 180
　　　　cost-effectiveness, 183–84, 185*t*, 359
　　　　devices, 180, 184
　　　　digoxin, 178–79
　　　　diuretics, 177, 183–84
　　　　exercise-based rehabilitation, 179–80
　　　　inotropes, 179
　　　　mineralocorticoid receptor antagonists,
　　　　　　178, 184
　　　　noninvasive positive pressure
　　　　　　ventilation, 179
　　　　pharmacological, 177–79
　　mortality rates, 174, 175*t*
　　prevalence rates, 174, 176*t*
　　stages and classes of, 174*b*
　　tobacco use and, 58, 62, 64–65, 68, 70
hemodialysis, 15, 239, 245–46, 383–84
hemorrhagic stroke, 15, 30, 65, 83, 159–61, 165, 169
Henry Ford Exercise Testing Project, 85
hepatitis C virus (HCV), 293
Hersch, Fred, 305
HHE (home health education), 315, 343
high blood pressure. *See* hypertension
high-density lipoprotein (HDL), 29, 46, 61–62,
　　390, 396
high-income countries (HICs)
　　cardiometabolic disease in, 39, 41–42, 44
　　cardiovascular, respiratory, and related disorders
　　　　(CVRDs) in, 24–26, 30
　　Chagas disease in, 203–4
　　chronic respiratory diseases in, 269–71
　　community-based care in, 311
　　congenital heart disease in, 191–95
　　cost-effectiveness of interventions in, 12,
　　　　14–15, 349–50, 354–55
　　diabetes in, 213–15, 217–20
　　heart failure in, 173–74, 183–84
　　hypertension in, 389–90

integrated care in, 292
ischemic heart disease in, 135–37, 143–45
obesity/overweight in, 117, 119–21
peripheral artery disease in, 253–58
physical activity in, 80, 86–89
quality of care in, 341–42, 344–45
stroke in, 157, 162–63, 168–69
HITAP (Health Intervention and Technology
　　Assessment Program), 384
HIV/AIDS
　　chronic respiratory diseases and, 269, 278
　　community-based care, 306
　　diabetes and, 217, 223, 292–94, 293*t*
　　integrated care and, 287, 290, 292–94
　　ischemic heart disease (IHD) and, 135–36
　　kidney disease and, 236, 240
　　priority-setting for treatments, 384
　　quality of care and, 331
home health education (HHE), 315, 343
homocysteine-lowering therapy, 166
Howard, K., 245
HTA (health technology assessment), 369, 375,
　　384, 386
Hu, Frank B., 117
Huffman, Mark D., 173, 203
Hungary
　　diet and nutrition in, 108
　　taxation of unhealthy foods and beverages in, 362n1
hypercholesterolemia, 390. *See also* dyslipidemia
hypersensitivity pneumonitis, 264, 268, 275–76
hypertension, 389–404
　　burden of disease, 389–90
　　diabetes and, 9, 240, 308–9, 320–21, 331–32, 340,
　　　　343, 384, 394
　　end-stage renal disease (ESRD) and, 241–42
　　interventions, 9, 390–93, 392–93*t*, 393*f*, 398*b*
　　　　antiplatelet therapy, 393
　　　　combination therapy, 393
　　　　cost-effectiveness, 357, 370*t*, 371–72, 397
　　　　pharmacological, 391
　　　　screening, 395–96
　　tobacco use and, 62–63
　　treatment, 330, 370, 372

I

ICDs. *See* implantable cardioverter defibrillators
ICERs. *See* incremental cost-effectiveness ratios
IDF. *See* International Diabetes Federation
idiopathic low FVC, 266–68, 275
idiopathic pulmonary fibrosis (IPF), 268, 275–76
IHD. *See* ischemic heart disease
IMAI (Integrated Management of Adolescent and
　　Adult Health), 277

impaired glucose tolerance (IGT), 37, 41, 84–85, 109, 210, 214, 315
implantable cardioverter defibrillators (ICDs), 15, 141, 147, 180, 183–84, 359
incremental cost-effectiveness ratios (ICERs)
    Chagas disease, 204
    community-based care, 315–16, 356
    congenital heart disease, 195
    diabetes, 217, 219–20
    heart failure, 179, 184–85, 359
    ischemic heart disease (IHD), 141, 143, 145, 147, 360
    kidney disease, 245
    rheumatic heart disease, 201–2
India
    cardiometabolic disease in, 39, 41–42
    community-based care in, 308–10, 317
    congenital heart disease in, 194, 196
    cost-effectiveness of interventions in, 11–12, 351–53
    diabetes in, 213, 216–18
    health care costs in, 8
    heart failure in, 181, 181b
    hypertension in, 389
    integrated care in, 289–90
    kidney disease in, 244
    obesity/overweight in, 121, 124, 126–27, 129–30
    physical activity in, 80, 82
    priority-setting for treatments in, 382
    quality of care in, 329, 334–35
    rheumatic heart disease in, 200–202
    stroke in, 167–68
    tobacco use in, 57
Indonesia
    integrated care in, 291
    priority-setting for treatments in, 378–80, 382
infectious diseases. See also specific diseases
    chronic respiratory diseases and, 269
    community-based care, 306
    congenital heart disease and, 196
    cost-effectiveness of interventions, 373
    diabetes and, 210, 212, 223
    integrated care and, 288–89
    kidney disease and, 237, 240
inflammation of vascular tissue, 58b, 61–62
Inglis, S. C., 180
inhaled corticosteroids, 7, 9, 12, 15, 271–72, 274, 359
in-hospital mortality
    heart failure, 179–81
    ischemic heart disease, 143
    kidney disease, 235–36
    quality of care and, 329

inotropes, 179
insulin
    cardiometabolic disease and, 39, 43, 46–47
    cost-effectiveness of, 12
    diabetes treatment, 212, 214, 218, 222
    integrated care and, 292
    obesity/overweight and, 122
    priority-setting processes and, 375, 377–79
    tobacco use and, 61, 63
insulin resistance
    cardiometabolic disease and, 39, 41, 43, 45–46
    obesity/overweight and, 118
    physical activity and, 86
    tobacco use and, 59–61, 63
integrated care, 287–97, 294–95t, 295f, 298t
    adherence to treatment and, 296–97
    blood pressure (BP) and, 295, 297
    body mass index (BMI) and, 292
    cardiometabolic disease and, 296
    cholesterol and, 297
    chronic kidney disease (CKD) and, 288, 294
    chronic respiratory diseases, 277–78
    coronary heart disease (CHD) and, 288, 294
    depression and, 287–88
    diabetes and, 289–93
    disability and, 288
    health care providers and, 297
    HIV/AIDS and, 287, 290, 292–94
    infectious diseases and, 288–89
    insulin and, 292
    kidney disease and, 294
    obesity/overweight and, 292
    physical activity and, 288
    primary care centers and, 295, 297
    relative risk (RR) and, 292–93
    risk factors and, 287–88, 292
    self-management interventions, 295
    tuberculosis and, 287–92, 294
Integrated Management of Adolescent and Adult Health (IMAI), 277
INTERHEART study, 28, 65, 67, 68
intermittent claudication, 256–57
International Agency for Research on Cancer, 144
International Charter on Cardiovascular Prevention and Rehabilitation, 147
International Diabetes Federation (IDF), 27, 209–12, 214–15, 288, 290, 320, 378
International Physical Activity Questionnaire, 81
International Society of Nephrology, 237b
International Society of Peritoneal Dialysis, 239
International Study of Asthma and Allergies in Childhood, 264

International Union Against Tuberculosis and Lung Disease, 289
INTERSTROKE study, 28, 65, 159
interventions
cardiometabolic disease, 46–48
Chagas disease, 203
chronic kidney disease (CKD), 241, 243–44*t*
cost-effectiveness, 245–46
renal replacement therapy, 245–46, 245*f*
screening, 245, 246*b*
chronic respiratory diseases
management, 271–76
primary prevention, 269, 269*b*
principles of care, 270, 270*b*
congenital heart disease (CHD), 192–94
cost-effectiveness, 195–96
neonatal screening, 194
prenatal screening, 193–94, 193*t*
prevention, 192–93
screening, 193–94, 195–96
diabetes, 9, 213–15, 217, 220
cost-effectiveness, 217–19, 220*t*, 357
management, 214–15
prevention, 213–14, 216, 219
priorities, 221, 221–23*t*
screening, 213, 215, 219, 396
diet and nutrition, 105–9, 105*t*
cost-effectiveness, 109–11, 352–53
fiscal policies, 107, 107*t*
local food environment, 108
mass media campaigns, 105–7
multicomponent interventions, 109
organizational settings, 107–8
taxation of unhealthy beverages and foods, 108–9
trans fats restrictions, 108
dyslipidemia, 393–95
cost-effectiveness, 397
polypills, 395
screening, 396
statins, 394
end-stage renal disease (ESRD), 241–42
essential package, 6–7*t*, 15–16
heart failure, 177–80, 183*t*
angiotensin-converting enzyme (ACE) inhibitors, 178, 184
angiotensin receptor blockers, 178
anticoagulants, 179
beta blockers, 177–78, 184
case management, 180
cost-effectiveness, 183–84, 185*t*, 359
devices, 180, 184
digoxin, 178–79

diuretics, 177, 183–84
exercise-based rehabilitation, 179–80
inotropes, 179
mineralocorticoid receptor antagonists, 178, 184
noninvasive positive pressure ventilation, 179
pharmacological, 177–79
hypertension, 9, 390–93, 392–93*t*, 393*f*, 398*b*
antiplatelet therapy, 393
combination therapy, 393
cost-effectiveness, 357, 370*t*, 371–72, 397
pharmacological, 391
screening, 395–96
ischemic heart disease (IHD), 140–47, 141–42*t*
access to medications, 145–46
acute management, 140, 142–43, 147
cardiac rehabilitation, 147
cardiac resynchronization therapy, 147
cost-effectiveness, 145, 359–60
implantable cardioverter defibrillators, 147
individual-level, 144–45
population-level, 144
secondary prevention, 143–46
kidney disease, 237
cost-effectiveness, 238, 360
mental health, 296–97
obesity/overweight, 123–27, 131*t*
agricultural policies, 124
bariatric surgery, 127
cost-effectiveness, 127–30, 128*t*, 130*t*
food advertising, 125
food labeling, 124–25
mass media campaigns, 125
nutritional policies, 124
pharmacological strategies, 126–27
prevention, 117, 122–24, 130–31
school-based interventions, 125–26
urban planning and design, 126
weight-loss diets, 126
workplace interventions, 125–26
patient-provider-level interventions, 332–43, 333*t*, 334*f*, 335*b*, 336–40*t*, 341*f*, 342*b*
acute phase, 332–34
chronic phase, 334–43
mobile communication technology and, 341, 342*b*
task-shifting, 341, 343
peripheral artery disease (PAD), 256–58
cost-effectiveness, 258–60
critical limb ischemia, 257–58
intermittent claudication, 256–57
physical activity, 87–91
community-based programs, 90*b*, 91
cost-effectiveness, 91–92, 354–55

primary health care, 88–89
public education campaigns, 89
sports systems and programs, 89, 91
transport and urban design, 89
whole-of-school programs, 88
prevention, 13–14
restrictive lung disease and fibrosis, 275–76
rheumatic heart disease (RHD), 197–201, 198t
cardiac surgery, 198–99
community-based programs, 199
cost-effectiveness, 201–2, 357
echocardiography, 199
primary prevention, 197
primordial prevention, 199
public policy, 200, 200t
secondary prevention, 198, 201
surgical care platforms, 199–200
system-level interventions, 328–31, 329–30t,
331–32b
acute phase, 328–29
chronic phase, 329–31
IPF. See idiopathic pulmonary fibrosis
Iran
kidney disease in, 244
obesity/overweight in, 125
quality of care in, 337, 339
stroke in, 161, 168
tobacco use in, 68
Irlam, J., 201
ischemic heart disease (IHD), 135–56
burden of disease, 136–40, 137m, 138–39f
cardiometabolic disease and, 38
heart failure and, 173–77, 179, 181, 184–85
HIV/AIDS and, 136
hypertension and, 389–90, 395, 397
interventions, 140–47, 141–42t
access to medications, 145–46
acute management, 140, 142–43, 147
cardiac rehabilitation, 147
cardiac resynchronization therapy, 147
cost-effectiveness, 12, 145, 356–58, 359–60,
371–72
implantable cardioverter defibrillators, 147
individual-level, 144–45
population-level, 144
secondary prevention, 143–46
manifestations of, 136
medications
access to, 145–46
adherence, 146–47
mortality and morbidity trends, 26, 27f
risk factors, 136
tobacco use and, 67–68, 144

ischemic stroke, 159–62
community-based care, 316
hypertension and, 390, 396
mortality and morbidity rates, 27
primary care centers and, 15
risk factors, 30
tobacco use and, 65
treatment, 165–66

J
Jabbour, Samer, 57
Janssen, I., 87
Japan
Chagas disease in, 203
diabetes in, 213
diet and nutrition in, 106
ischemic heart disease in, 137
obesity/overweight in, 126
stroke in, 165
tobacco use in, 67
Jarvis, Deborah, 263
Jeemon, Panniyammakal, 327, 389
Joint National Committee on Prevention, Detection,
Evaluation, and Treatment of High Blood
Pressure, 163
Joseph, K. S., 48
Joshi, Rohina, 305

K
Kamano, Jemima H., 327
Katzmarzyk, P. T., 87
Kengne, Andre Pascal, 305
Khatibzadeh, S., 177
kidney disease, 235–52. See also chronic kidney disease
(CKD); end-stage renal disease (ESRD)
etiology, 236–37
hypertension and, 393
integrated care and, 294
interventions, 237
cost-effectiveness, 238, 360
mortality and morbidity rates, 24–26, 236, 236t
policy implications, 238–39, 238–39t
prevalence, 235–36
priority-setting for treatments, 383–86, 383b, 385b
tobacco use and, 63–64
Kidney Help Trust of Chennai, 246b
Korea, Republic of
diet and nutrition in, 106
ischemic heart disease in, 137
obesity/overweight in, 125
priority-setting for treatments in, 384
Kramer, M., 48
Kudesia, Preeti, 327

Kumar, R. Krishna, 191
Kumaran, Kalyanaraman, 37
Kwan, G. F., 183
Kyrgyz Republic
    diabetes in, 212
    priority-setting for treatments in, 380

L
LABAs (long-acting beta2-agonists), 272, 274
Laine, J., 92
La Isla Foundation, 241*b*
Lambert, Vicki, 79
Latin America and Caribbean.
        See also specific countries
    Chagas disease in, 203–4
    community-based care in, 310
    cost-effectiveness of interventions in, 353, 358
    diabetes in, 211–12, 216, 220
    diet and nutrition in, 110
    heart failure in, 176, 185
    ischemic heart disease in, 138–40, 142–43
    kidney disease in, 236, 244–45
    peripheral artery disease in, 257, 259–60
    physical activity in, 88
    priority-setting for treatments in, 376
    rheumatic heart disease in, 200
    stroke in, 157
LDL. *See* low-density lipoprotein
Lee, Edward S., 327
leukotriene receptor antagonists, 272
Levin, Carol, 349
Levy, D., 67
Li, Chaoyun, 157
LICs. *See* low-income countries
Lifestyle in Pregnancy and Offspring study, 47
life years (LYs)
    cost-effectiveness of interventions and, 11, 350,
        352, 354
    diabetes and, 211
    diet and, 103–4
    hypertension and, 390
    ischemic heart disease and, 135, 137
    obesity/overweight and, 127
    physical activity and, 87
    priority-setting for treatments and, 375
    stroke and, 157
lipids. *See also* cholesterol; dyslipidemia
    diabetes and, 214
    hypertension and, 394–96
    interventions, 166
    oxidation and tobacco use, 61
    stroke and, 164
LMICs. *See* low- and middle-income countries

London Stroke Carers Training Course (LSCTC), 167
long-acting beta2-agonists (LABAs), 272, 274
Look AHEAD study, 218
low- and middle-income countries (LMICs)
    cardiometabolic disease in, 39, 41–44
    cardiovascular, respiratory, and related disorders
        (CVRDs) in, 23–30, 32–33
    Chagas disease in, 202–4
    chronic respiratory diseases in, 263–64, 271–72,
        276–77
    community-based care in, 305–6, 310–17
    congenital heart disease in, 191–96
    cost-effectiveness of interventions in, 12–14,
        349–51, 353
    diabetes in, 209–10, 212–13, 215–16, 218–21,
        223–24
    diet and nutrition in, 108, 110
    heart failure in, 179–81, 181*b*, 183–84
    integrated care in, 288–90, 294–97
    ischemic heart disease in, 135–37
    obesity/overweight in, 118–22, 124–27
    peripheral artery disease in, 253–54, 256, 258, 260
    physical activity in, 87–89
    primary care centers in, 16–17
    priority-setting for treatments in, 375–78
    quality of care in, 341–43
    rheumatic heart disease in, 197–202
    stroke in, 157–59, 161–69
low birth weight
    cardiometabolic disease in, 37, 39, 43–45
    chronic respiratory diseases and, 267–68
    kidney disease and, 241
    as risk factor, 30–31
low-density lipoprotein (LDL)
    ischemic heart disease and, 146
    management of, 389–91, 394, 396
    physical activity and, 85
    quality of care and, 335–36, 340
    as risk factor, 28
    stroke and, 163
    tobacco use and, 61–62
low-income countries (LICs)
    cardiovascular, respiratory, and related disorders
        (CVRDs) in, 24–26, 28–30
    cost-effectiveness of interventions in, 9–10, 13,
        356, 373
    diet and nutrition in, 107
    ischemic heart disease in, 139, 141–42, 146
    kidney disease in, 236
    primary care centers in, 16
    quality of care in, 341, 345
    rheumatic heart disease in, 201
    stroke in, 169

Lubinga, S. J., 202
Luo, Rong, 157
LYs. *See* life years

M

Magee, Matthew, 287
Malawi
  chronic respiratory diseases in, 278
  integrated care in, 294
Malaysia
  ischemic heart disease in, 143
  priority-setting for treatments in, 384
  quality of care in, 342
Malik, Vasanti S., 117
Marin-Neto, J. Antonio, 191
Marks, Guy, 263
mass media campaigns
  cost-effectiveness of interventions and,
    350–53, 360
  diet and nutrition, 105–7
  ischemic heart disease, 144
  obesity/overweight, 124–25, 129–31
  physical activity, 89
  stroke, 162
Maternal and Infant Nutrition Interventions in
    Matlab (MINIMat), 46, 47
maternal obesity, 40–41, 41*f*, 47
maternal tobacco use, 44
Mauritius
  diabetes in, 210
  diet and nutrition in, 106, 109
  ischemic heart disease in, 144
Mayosi, Bongani, 191
Mbanya, Jean-Claude, 1, 209
McGuire, Helen, 305
medication. *See* adherence to treatment;
    pharmacological interventions
mental health
  depression, 30, 83, 86–87, 158–59, 161, 167,
    210, 212, 214, 217, 287–88, 315
  diabetes and, 287–88
  interventions, 296–97
metformin, 218
Mexico
  chronic respiratory diseases in, 278
  community-based care in, 310, 315
  cost-effectiveness of interventions in, 10–12, 351,
    353, 356
  diabetes in, 218
  diet and nutrition in, 108, 110
  hypertension in, 397
  integrated care in, 291
  kidney disease in, 241–43, 245–46

obesity/overweight in, 119–20, 124–25, 127, 130
  priority-setting for treatments in, 378–80
  quality of care in, 330, 337, 342
  stroke in, 163
  taxation of unhealthy foods and beverages in,
    12, 362n1
  tobacco use in, 68
Micha, Renata, 101
micronutrients, 46–47, 121–22
MICs. *See* low- and middle-income countries;
    middle-income countries
Middle East and North Africa. *See also*
    specific countries
  congenital heart disease in, 192
  cost-effectiveness of interventions in, 358
  diabetes in, 210–11, 220
  heart failure in, 185
  ischemic heart disease in, 138–39, 142–43, 146
  kidney disease in, 244–45
  peripheral artery disease in, 257, 259–60
  physical activity in, 81, 92
middle-income countries (MICs). *See also* low- and
    middle-income countries
  cardiovascular, respiratory, and related disorders
    (CVRDs) in, 23–29
  chronic respiratory diseases in, 263–64
  congenital heart disease in, 196, 198
  cost-effectiveness of interventions in, 9–13,
    352–53, 371
  diet and nutrition in, 108, 110
  heart failure in, 181
  ischemic heart disease in, 139, 141–43
  kidney disease in, 236
  peripheral artery disease in, 255–56
  physical activity in, 80
  primary care centers in, 15, 16
  priority-setting for treatments in, 377
  quality of care in, 334–35, 345
  stroke in, 168–69
mineralocorticoid receptor antagonists, 178, 184
Miranda, J. Jaime, 157
mitral regurgitation, 147
mobile communication technology, 341, 342*b*
Model List of Essential Medicines (WHO), 9, 14, 145,
    147, 177
Montoya, Pablo Aschner, 209
MoPoTsyo Model of Care (Cambodia), 320–22
Moran, Andrew E., 67, 135, 327
morbidity rates
  asthma, 27
  cardiovascular, respiratory, and related disorders
    (CVRDs), 24–25, 24*t*, 25–26*f*, 26*t*
  chronic obstructive pulmonary disease (COPD), 27

chronic respiratory diseases, 23–25, 27–29
diabetes, 27, 211–12, 211*t*
ischemic heart disease (IHD), 26, 27*f*
ischemic stroke, 27
kidney disease, 24–26
peripheral artery disease (PAD), 26–27, 256, 257–58*f*, 259–60*f*
stroke, 26, 27*f*, 157, 158*m*, 160, 162, 211, 389
Morocco, priority-setting for treatments in, 378–81
mortality rates, 4–8, 8*f*
asthma, 27
cardiovascular, respiratory, and related disorders (CVRDs), 24–25, 24*t*, 25–26*f*, 26*t*, 30
cardiovascular disease, 4, 64
children, 49, 110, 350, 353
chronic obstructive pulmonary disease (COPD), 27–28
chronic respiratory diseases, 23–25, 27–29
diabetes, 27, 211–12, 211*t*
heart failure, 174, 175*t*
ischemic heart disease, 26, 27*f*, 138, 140, 144
ischemic stroke, 27
kidney disease, 24–26, 236, 236*t*, 244
peripheral artery disease, 26–27, 256–58, 257–60*f*
premature mortality, 25, 57, 82, 87, 211, 305
rheumatic heart disease, 197
stroke, 26, 27*f*, 157, 158*m*, 160, 162, 168, 211, 389
movement therapy, 168
Mozaffarian, Dariush, 101
Multicenter Automated Defibrillator Implantation Trial, 66
multicomponent interventions
diabetes, 217
diet and nutrition, 105, 109
obesity, 125
quality of care, 329
Murray, C. J., 110
mycophenolate mofetil, 242
myocardial infarction, 136
myocardial ischemia, 58*b*
myocarditis, 8, 27, 173–75

N
NAFTA (North American Free Trade Agreement), 119
Naicker, Saraladevi, 235
Naidoo, Nadraj G., 253
Narayan, K. M. Venkat, 209, 287
National Autonomous University of Nicaragua at Léon, 241*b*
national essential medicines lists (NEMLs), 375, 377–79, 381–83, 386
National Health and Nutrition Examination Survey, 67

National Health Security Office (NHSO, Thailand), 383–84
National Institutes of Health (NIH), 162
National Kidney Foundation, 241
NEMLs. *See* national essential medicines lists
Nepal, cardiometabolic disease in, 46
nephropathy, 27
neuropathy, 27, 219
Neutral Protamine Hagedorn (NPH) insulin, 377, 379
New York Heart Association, 174*b*
New Zealand
diet and nutrition in, 106–7
obesity/overweight in, 126
physical activity in, 87–88
stroke in, 164
Ng, S. W., 82
Nicaragua, kidney disease in, 241*b*
nicotine, 28, 58, 60–63, 66, 68–69, 254. *See also* tobacco use
nicotine replacement therapy (NRT), 144–45, 271, 351
Nigeria
diabetes in, 218
kidney disease in, 240, 242
quality of care in, 343
stroke in, 161
Nikolic, Irina, 349
noninvasive positive pressure ventilation, 179
North American Free Trade Agreement (NAFTA), 119
Norway
diet and nutrition in, 108
taxation of unhealthy foods and beverages in, 362n1
NRT (nicotine replacement therapy), 144–45, 271, 351
Nugent, Rachel, 1, 349, 369
nutrition. *See* diet and nutrition

O
obesity/overweight, 117–34
behavioral change and, 121
burden of, 117–18
cardiometabolic disease and, 40–41, 41*f*, 43–44, 47, 48
cardiovascular, respiratory, and related disorders (CVRDs) and, 29–31
children, 127–28
chronic respiratory diseases and, 264
community-based care, 312
congenital heart disease and, 193–94
diabetes and, 209, 213–14
diet and, 102, 109, 121–23
genetic factors, 123
income status and, 119–20
integrated care and, 292

interventions, 123–27, 131*t*
    agricultural policies, 124
    bariatric surgery, 127
    cost-effectiveness, 12–13, 127–30, 128*t*, 130*t*,
        350, 352–54
    food advertising, 125
    food labeling, 124–25
    mass media campaigns, 125
    nutritional policies, 124
    pharmacological strategies, 126–27
    prevention, 117, 122–24, 130–31
    school-based interventions, 125–26
    urban planning and design, 126
    weight-loss diets, 126
    workplace interventions, 125–26
  ischemic heart disease and, 136, 144
  maternal, 40–41
  physical activity and, 79, 83, 85–86, 120–21
  prevalence, 41, 118–19, 122–23, 315, 353
  risk factors, 118–23, 119*f*
  sociocultural norms and, 121
  socioeconomic status and, 119–20
  stroke and, 160–61, 169
  trade liberalization and, 119
  urbanization and, 120
occupational therapy, 168
Oceania
  hypertension in, 390
  ischemic heart disease in, 137
  peripheral artery disease in, 256, 260
O'Donnell, Martin, 157
Olasky, S. J., 67
Onen, Churchill, 389
Organisation for Economic Co-operation and
    Development (OECD), 13, 127, 129–30, 130*t*
organ transplantation, 243–44
Ortegon, M., 110
Osmond, Clive, 37
oxidative stress, 58*b*

P

PAD. *See* peripheral artery disease
Pakistan
  community-based care in, 314–15
  cost-effectiveness of interventions in, 12
  diet and nutrition in, 106
  integrated care in, 290
  ischemic heart disease in, 140
  kidney disease in, 244
  priority-setting for treatments in, 378–80
palliative care and treatment, 194–95
passive smoking, 28
Patel, Anushka, 86, 305

PATH (Program for Appropriate Technology in
    Health), 320
patient-provider-level interventions
  acute phase, 332–34
  chronic phase, 334–43
  mobile communication technology and, 341, 342*b*
  quality of care, 332–43, 333*t*, 334*f*, 335*b*, 336–40*t*,
    341*f*, 342*b*
  task-shifting, 341, 343
PD. *See* peritoneal dialysis
Pedersen, J., 40
percutaneous coronary interventions (PCI), 12, 141,
    143, 147, 360
Perez-Padilla, Rogelio, 263
peripheral artery disease (PAD), 253–62
  burden of disease, 256
  causes, 253–54
  diagnosis, 253–54
  epidemiology, 254
  hypertension and, 390
  interventions, 256–58
    cost-effectiveness, 258–60
    critical limb ischemia, 257–58
    intermittent claudication, 256–57
  ischemic heart disease and, 136
  mortality and morbidity trends, 24, 26–27, 256,
    257–58*f*, 259–60*f*
  prevalence, 254, 255–56*f*
  risk factors, 253, 254, 256, 260
  tobacco use and, 64, 66
peritoneal dialysis (PD), 15, 236–39, 237*b*, 242,
    383–86
Peru
  obesity/overweight in, 125
  priority-setting for treatments in, 378–80
pharmacological interventions
  chronic kidney disease (CKD), 242
  chronic obstructive pulmonary disease (COPD),
    274–75
  generic medications, 8, 17, 145–46, 358
  heart failure, 177–79
  hypertension, 391
  ischemic heart disease, 145–47
  obesity/overweight, 126–27
  stroke, 163
Philippines
  cost-effectiveness of interventions in, 12
  priority-setting for treatments in, 378–80, 382
physical activity, 79–100
  cardiometabolic disease and, 40, 47, 82–86
  cardiovascular, respiratory, and related disorders
    (CVRDs) and, 28, 30–31
  community-based care and, 312, 314

coronary heart disease and, 82–83, 83*f*
defined, 80*b*
diabetes and, 84–85, 84–85*f*, 222–23
diet and, 104–5
economic costs of inactivity, 86–87
exercise-based rehabilitation, 179–80
gender issues, 91*b*
hypertension and, 389
integrated care and, 288
interventions, 14, 87–91
    community-based programs, 90*b*, 91
    cost-effectiveness, 12, 91–92, 350, 354–55
    primary health care, 88–89
    public education campaigns, 89
    sports systems and programs, 89, 91
    transport and urban design, 89
    whole-of-school programs, 88
ischemic heart disease and, 136
obesity/overweight and, 119–23, 125–28
policy implications, 92–93
prevalence and burden of inactivity, 80–81*f*,
    80–82
sedentary activity and sitting, 86
stroke and, 83–84, 160–62, 165, 169
physical therapy, 168
phytoestrogens, 44
pipe smoking, 68
polychlorinated biphenyls, 44
polypills, 146, 163–64, 395
Popkin, B. M., 82
population-level interventions
    cost-effectiveness, 13, 349–51, 355, 361, 372
    diabetes, 223
    diet and nutrition, 101, 109–10
    ischemic heart disease, 140, 144
    obesity/overweight, 123, 131
Poulter, Neil, 389
Prabhakaran, Dorairaj, 1, 23, 57, 101, 173, 287, 389
Practical Approach to Lung Health in South Africa
    (PALSA), 278*b*
Pratt, Michael, 79, 87
prediabetes, 12, 210, 213–14, 216–17, 342, 396
pregnancy. *See also* gestational diabetes
    cardiometabolic disease and, 37, 39, 41, 44, 46–49
    cardiovascular, respiratory, and related disorders
        (CVRDs) and, 30, 31
    Chagas disease and, 203
    chronic respiratory diseases and, 267, 269
    congenital heart disease and, 192–93
    obesity/overweight and, 40–41, 41*f*, 47, 118
    prenatal screening, 193–94, 193*t*
    rheumatic heart disease and, 197
    tobacco use and, 44

prevalence
    chronic kidney disease (CKD), 240
    congenital heart disease (CHD), 191
    diabetes, 48, 63, 109, 209–10, 214, 216, 288–90,
        292, 381
    end-stage renal disease (ESRD), 240
    heart failure, 174, 176*t*
    kidney disease, 235–36
    obesity/overweight, 41, 118–19, 122–23, 315, 353
    peripheral artery disease (PAD), 254, 255–56*f*
    physical activity and inactivity, 80–81*f*, 80–82
prevention
    asthma, 269
    chronic obstructive pulmonary disease
        (COPD), 269
    congenital heart disease (CHD), 192–93
    cost-effectiveness, 13–14
    diabetes, 12, 213–14, 216–19, 221, 223
    heart failure, 179
    ischemic heart disease (IHD), 143–46
    obesity/overweight, 117, 122–24, 130–31
    rheumatic heart disease (RHD), 197, 198, 199, 201
    statins as, 394–95
    stroke, 161–65, 179, 357
        antiplatelet therapy, 166
        atrial fibrillation control, 164
        blood pressure control, 166
        carotid stenosis surgery, 166
        community-based education, 164
        cost-effectiveness, 165
        digital health strategies, 164–65
        family support, 166–67
        high blood pressure, 163
        homocysteine-lowering therapy, 166
        lipid-lowering therapy, 166
        pharmaceutical treatments, 163
        polypill use, 163–64
        primary, 162–65
        secondary, 166–67
        self-management, 166–67
        sodium reduction, 163
        tobacco use reduction, 162
primary care centers, 12, 14–16. *See also* quality
    of care
    chronic obstructive pulmonary disease (COPD)
        and, 15, 273–74
    chronic respiratory diseases and, 270, 276–78,
        277*t*, 278*b*
    community-based care and, 305, 310
    cost-effectiveness, 356–57
    heart failure, 180–82
    hypertension and, 397
    improvement of, 3*b*

integrated care and, 295, 297
kidney disease and, 242, 244
obesity/overweight and, 129
physical activity and, 88–89
role of, 14–16
priority-setting for treatments, 375–88
diabetes, 377–83, 379t, 380f, 382b
dialysis, 383–86, 383b, 385b
Program for Appropriate Technology in
Health (PATH), 320
Promotion of Breastfeeding Intervention Trial
(Belarus), 47
prothrombotic state, 58b, 61
pulmonary thromboembolism, 276

Q

QALYs (quality-adjusted life years)
cost-effectiveness of interventions and, 12, 354,
356–57, 359–60
diabetes and, 218–19
heart failure and, 184
hypertension and, 397
ischemic heart disease and, 141–43, 145–47
kidney disease and, 238, 245
peripheral artery disease and, 258
physical activity and, 91–92
priority-setting for treatments and, 383–84
rheumatic heart disease and, 201
quality of care, 327–48
conceptual framework, 327, 328t
patient-provider-level interventions, 332–43, 333t,
334f, 335b, 336–40t, 341f, 342b
acute phase, 332–34
chronic phase, 334–43
mobile communication technology and,
341, 342b
task-shifting, 341, 343
system-level interventions, 328–31, 329–30t,
331–32b
acute phase, 328–29
chronic phase, 329–31

R

Rajan, Vikram, 327
Rassi, Anis, 191
Rassi, Anis, Jr., 191
Rawal, Ishita, 57
Reduction of Atherothrombosis for Continued
Health (REACH), 146
rehabilitation from stroke, 167–68, 167–68t
relative risk (RR)
cardiometabolic disease, 38
diet and nutrition, 104

heart failure and, 178–80, 183
integrated care and, 292–93
obesity/overweight and, 129
peripheral artery disease, 258
physical activity and, 83–84, 86
quality of care and, 337
stroke, 159–60, 163, 165
tobacco use and, 63, 65–68, 70
Remuzzi, Giuseppe, 235
renal replacement therapy (RRT), 237–38, 240,
245–47, 245f, 383
respiratory diseases, chronic, 140, 263, 269–70,
274, 276, 375
restrictive lung disease and fibrosis, 268, 275–76
retinopathy, 27, 215
RF. See rheumatic fever
RHD. See rheumatic heart disease
rheumatic fever (RF), 6, 197–98, 200, 357
rheumatic heart disease (RHD), 197–202
burden of disease, 197
cardiovascular, respiratory, and related disorders
(CVRDs) and, 27
heart failure nad, 176–77
hypertension and, 390
interventions, 197–201, 198t
cardiac surgery, 198–99
community-based programs, 199
cost-effectiveness, 13, 201–2, 357
echocardiography, 199
primary prevention, 197
primordial prevention, 199
public policy, 200, 200t
secondary prevention, 198, 201
surgical care platforms, 199–200
mortality rates, 197
natural history, 197
pathogenesis, 197
risk factors, 197
Riella, Miguel, 235
risk factors, 9–10
alcohol use, 30
asthma, 263–65
cardiometabolic disease, 37–39, 38f, 41
cardiovascular, respiratory, and related disorders
(CVRDs), 28–32
cardiovascular disease, 62–63
Chagas disease, 27
chronic obstructive pulmonary disease (COPD),
263–67
chronic respiratory diseases, 31, 33,
263–68
congenital heart disease, 26, 192–93, 196
coronary heart disease, 29

cost-effectiveness of interventions and, 355–58,
     360–61
depression, 30
diabetes, 24–26, 160, 209–10, 215–17
diet and nutrition, 14, 102–5, 103–4t, 122, 161
disability, 25–28
dyslipidemia, 28
early childhood determinants, 30–31
heart failure, 174
high blood pressure, 29, 159
hypertension, 390–91, 397
integrated care and, 287–88, 292
ischemic heart disease, 136, 140
ischemic stroke, 30
kidney disease, 240–41
middle childhood determinants, 31–32
modifiable, 23, 28–30, 159–61, 192, 196
nonmodifiable, 27–28, 395
obesity/overweight, 29, 118–23, 119f, 129, 161
peripheral artery disease (PAD), 253, 254, 256, 260
physical inactivity, 29–30, 86, 161
rheumatic heart disease (RHD), 197
social and ecological determinants, 30–32, 33
stroke, 28–29, 65, 70, 83, 157, 159–61, 159–60t,
     163–64, 166, 169
tobacco use, 28, 63, 65–66, 70, 160
rituximab, 242
Rivero-Ayerza, M., 180
Roth, Greg A., 173
Rotterdam Study, 66
Roux, L., 91
Roy, Ambuj, 57
RR. See relative risk
RRT. See renal replacement therapy
Rubinstein, Adolfo, 101
Russian Federation
     ischemic heart disease in, 138
     obesity/overweight in, 127, 130
     stroke in, 161
     tobacco use in, 68
Rwanda
     heart failure in, 183, 184t
     integrated care in, 294

S
Sakuma, Yuna, 375
salt consumption, 16, 110, 163, 165, 353–54, 370t,
     371–73
Sampson, Uchechukwu K. A., 253
screening
     chronic kidney disease (CKD), 245, 246b
     congenital heart disease (CHD), 193–94, 195–96
          neonatal screening, 194

prenatal screening, 193–94, 193t
     cost-effectiveness, 355–56
     diabetes, 213, 215, 219, 396
     dyslipidemia, 396
     hypertension, 395–96
     stroke, 161–62
secondary prevention
     cardiovascular, respiratory, and related disorders
          (CVRDs), 28, 32
     community-based care and, 312
     cost-effectiveness, 14–15, 356–59
     diabetes, 221
     hypertension, 394, 397
     ischemic heart disease, 135, 137, 139–41, 143,
          145–47
     peripheral artery disease, 258
     physical activity, 79, 83
     quality of care and, 331, 333
     rheumatic heart disease, 197–203
     stroke, 157, 161, 166, 169
     tobacco use, 70
secondhand smoke, 28, 58–59, 61–62, 67, 70, 144
sedentary activity, 86
Seguro Popular (Mexico), 329–30
self-management interventions
     chronic respiratory diseases, 275
     community-based care and, 305, 312–16, 313t,
          316b, 317f
     cost-effectiveness, 315–16
     diabetes, 212, 214, 217–18, 220
     education in, 214, 312–13, 314–15
     heart failure, 182
     integrated care, 295
     stroke, 166–67
     target populations, 314
     technology for, 315
     theories of, 313–14
self-monitoring of blood glucose (SMBG), 12, 214,
     217–18, 220
short message service (SMS), 315, 337,
     340, 342
Siegel, Karen R., 209
Singapore, diet and nutrition in, 105–6
Sliwa, Karen, 173
Small, C. W., 162
SMBG. See Self-Monitoring of Blood Glucose
smokeless tobacco, 68–69
smoking. See tobacco use
sodium. See salt consumption
Soudarssanane, M. B., 201
South Africa
     chronic respiratory diseases in, 278b
     community-based care in, 306–8, 310

cost-effectiveness of interventions in, 12, 353,
356–58
diabetes in, 213
diet and nutrition in, 107, 110
hypertension in, 397
integrated care in, 290, 292–93
ischemic heart disease in, 136, 140, 142, 144–46
kidney disease in, 242, 244
obesity/overweight in, 120, 124, 127, 130
primary care centers in, 16
priority-setting for treatments in, 378, 380, 385
quality of care in, 343
rheumatic heart disease in, 199, 201
South Asia. *See also specific countries*
cardiometabolic disease in, 39
cardiovascular, respiratory, and related disorders
(CVRDs) in, 26, 28, 30
chronic respiratory diseases in, 264
community-based care in, 306
diabetes in, 211, 216, 220
heart failure in, 185
hypertension in, 390
ischemic heart disease in, 140–41
kidney disease in, 244–45
obesity/overweight in, 117
rheumatic heart disease in, 197
stroke in, 157
tobacco use in, 68–70
South-East Asia. *See also specific countries*
cardiovascular, respiratory, and related disorders
(CVRDs) in, 26
chronic respiratory diseases in, 264
cost-effectiveness of interventions in, 350–51,
353, 359
diabetes in, 211
diet and nutrition in, 110
hypertension in, 390
ischemic heart disease in, 137–38
kidney disease in, 240
peripheral artery disease in, 256
physical activity in, 80–81
tobacco use in, 68
Spain
cost-effectiveness of interventions in, 356
ischemic heart disease in, 146
priority-setting for treatments in, 382
speech therapy, 168
sports systems and programs, 79–80, 85, 87–91
Sri Lanka, kidney disease in, 240, 241*b*
SSBs. *See* sugar and sugar-sweetened beverages
statins. *See also* dyslipidemia
cost-effectiveness, 12, 356–58, 360
diabetes and, 219, 224

ischemic heart disease and, 141–43, 145–46
peripheral artery disease and, 254
primary care centers and, 15
for primary prevention, 394–95
quality of care and, 333, 336, 341
stroke and, 163, 165–66
ST-elevation myocardial infarction (STEMI), 136,
143, 329, 334, 359–60
Stevenson, C. R., 290
streptococcal pharyngitis, 197, 200–201
stroke, 157–72. *See also* ischemic stroke
burden of disease, 157–59
cardiometabolic disease and, 37
cardiovascular, respiratory, and related disorders
(CVRDs) and, 23–24, 26–30
community-based care and, 309, 312
cost-effectiveness of interventions, 12, 356–58,
360, 369, 371–72
diabetes and, 160, 210–11, 214
diagnosis, 162
diet and, 103–4, 161
disability and, 158
hypertension and, 159, 390–91, 394–95, 397
ischemic heart disease and, 136–37
modifiable risk factors, 159–61
mortality and morbidity, 26, 27*f*, 157, 158*m*, 160,
162, 211, 389
obesity/overweight and, 161
peripheral artery disease and, 253–54
physical activity and, 82, 83–84, 86–87, 161
prevention, 161–65, 179, 357
antiplatelet therapy, 166
atrial fibrillation control, 164
blood pressure control, 166
carotid stenosis surgery, 166
community-based education, 164
cost-effectiveness, 165
digital health strategies, 164–65
family support, 166–67
high blood pressure, 163
homocysteine-lowering therapy, 166
lipid-lowering therapy, 166
pharmaceutical treatments, 163
polypill use, 163–64
primary, 162–65
secondary, 166–67
self-management, 166–67
sodium reduction, 163
tobacco use reduction, 162
primary care centers and, 15
quality of care and, 327, 329, 331, 333, 341
risk factors, 28–29, 65, 70, 83, 159–60*t*, 159–61,
163–64

screening, 161–62
surveillance, 161
tobacco use and, 63–65, 67–68, 160, 162
treatment, 165–66
cognitive rehabilitation, 168
cost-effectiveness, 168
physical, occupational, or movement therapy, 168
rehabilitation, 167–68, 167–68t
speech therapy, 168
Stroke Riskometer (mobile app), 165
structural heart diseases, 191–208
Chagas disease, 202–4. *See also* Chagas disease
congenital heart disease, 191–96. *See also* congenital heart disease
rheumatic heart disease, 197–202. *See also* rheumatic heart disease
Sub-Saharan Africa. *See also specific countries*
community-based care in, 306, 311
cost-effectiveness of interventions in, 350–51, 359
diabetes in, 211–12
heart failure in, 174, 176–77, 181
hypertension in, 390
ischemic heart disease in, 138–41
kidney disease in, 245
peripheral artery disease in, 254, 256–57, 259–60
quality of care in, 331
rheumatic heart disease in, 197, 199, 202
tobacco use in, 68
sugar and sugar-sweetened beverages (SSBs), 11–13, 17, 102–9, 119, 123–28, 131, 222, 266, 352–53
Suhrcke, Marc, 101, 349
suicide, 288
Sustainable Development Goals, 2, 23, 375
Sustainable Kidney Foundation, 237b
Sweden
diet and nutrition in, 108
physical activity in, 88
Switzerland
diabetes in, 212
diet and nutrition in, 108
integrated care in, 293
obesity/overweight in, 125
physical activity in, 79
sympathetic stimulation, 58b
system-level interventions
acute phase, 328–29
chronic phase, 329–31
quality of care in, 328–31, 329–30t, 331–32b

T
Taiwan
integrated care in, 291, 293
obesity/overweight in, 121, 125

Tandon, Nikhil, 209
Tanzania
cost-effectiveness of interventions in, 369
health care costs in, 8
kidney disease in, 237b, 238–39
task-shifting
community-based health care, 305–12, 307–9t, 311b
patient-provider-level interventions, 341, 343
taxation
of tobacco use, 9, 13, 16, 144–45, 162, 350–52, 355, 372–73
of unhealthy beverages and foods, 11–12, 108–9, 124
telemedicine, 315
television watching, 79, 106, 120–21, 125, 127–28
Thailand
community-based care in, 316
ischemic heart disease in, 141, 144–45
kidney disease in, 245, 247
obesity/overweight in, 125
primary care centers in, 15
priority-setting for treatments in, 375, 378
stroke in, 163, 167–68
Thai Registry in Acute Coronary Syndrome (TRACS), 143
thirdhand smoke, 67–68
Thomas, Bernadette, 235
thrombolysis, 143, 254, 329, 333, 360
thrombosis, 60–61, 164
tiotropium, 272
tissue plasminogen activator (tPA), 165
tobacco use, 57–78
aortic artery disease and, 66
arrhythmia and, 66
cardiovascular, respiratory, and related disorders (CVRDs) and, 26, 28–30, 31–32
cardiovascular disease and
health outcomes, 63–67, 64b, 64f
mortality rates, 64
pathophysiology and mechanisms, 58–62, 59–60f
risk factors, 62–63
carotid and cerebrovascular diseases and, 65
cessation benefits, 69–70, 70b
chronic kidney disease and, 66–67
chronic respiratory diseases and, 265, 271
community-based care and, 308
coronary heart disease and, 65
cost-effectiveness of interventions, 350–52, 351t, 353, 355, 360, 370–71, 370t
diabetes and, 63, 210, 215
diet and, 110
dyslipidemia and, 62
forms of, 67t, 68–69

global mandate for reducing, 57–58

health consequences of, 351

heart failure and, 65

hypertension and, 62–63, 397

ischemic heart disease and, 142, 143–45

maternal smoking and cardiometabolic disease, 39, 44

obesity/overweight and, 130

peripheral artery disease and, 66, 255–56

secondhand smoke, 67

smoking cessation, 62, 144, 221, 224, 258, 263, 265, 336, 391

socioeconomic variables, 69

stroke and, 65, 159–60, 162, 169

taxation of, 9, 13, 16, 144–45, 162, 350–52, 355, 372–73

thirdhand smoke, 67–68

TRACS (Thai Registry in Acute Coronary Syndrome), 143

Trade-Related Aspects of Intellectual Property Rights (TRIPS) Agreement (1995), 145

Training Programme for Caregivers of Inpatients after Stroke, 167

trans fats consumption, 14, 102, 104, 106, 108, 353–54

transportation systems design, 89

treatment

congenital heart disease (CHD), 194–95

cost-effectiveness, 195–96

end-stage renal disease (ESRD), 242–45

hypertension, 330, 370, 372

kidney disease, 383–86, 383b, 385b

priority-setting for, 383–86, 383b, 385b

stroke, 165–66

cognitive rehabilitation, 168

cost-effectiveness, 168

physical, occupational, or movement therapy, 168

rehabilitation, 167–68, 167–68t

speech therapy, 168

TRIPS (Trade-Related Aspects of Intellectual Property Rights) Agreement (1995), 145

Trivandrum heart failure registry, 181b

tuberculosis

chronic respiratory diseases and, 264, 267–69, 275

cost-effectiveness of interventions, 371

diabetes and, 288–92, 289f, 290–91t

integrated care and, 287–92, 294

kidney disease and, 244

Turkey

community-based care in, 315

obesity/overweight in, 120

priority-setting for treatments in, 378–81

U

Uganda

community-based care in, 306

surgical treatment in, 10

UHC. *See* universal health coverage

Ukraine, ischemic heart disease in, 138

United Kingdom

cardiometabolic disease in, 37–38, 41, 48

chronic respiratory diseases in, 263, 268

community-based care in, 311

congenital heart disease in, 195

cost-effectiveness of interventions in, 358

hypertension in, 395

obesity/overweight in, 118, 124–26, 130

peripheral artery disease in, 258

physical activity in, 82, 87–89

primary care centers in, 14

priority-setting for treatments in, 382

stroke in, 164

tobacco use in, 62, 66

United Kingdom National Institute for Health and Care Excellence, 377

United Nations, 91–92, 393

United Nations High-level Meeting on Non-Communicable Diseases, 295

United States

Chagas disease in, 203

community-based care in, 311

congenital heart disease in, 191, 195

cost-effectiveness of interventions in, 357–58, 369

diabetes in, 209–10, 213, 216–18

diet and nutrition in, 101, 105, 107–9

heart failure in, 179

integrated care in, 287, 291–95

ischemic heart disease in, 141, 143–44, 146–47

kidney disease in, 238, 240, 242, 244–46

obesity/overweight in, 117–22, 124–26

physical activity in, 82, 88

priority-setting for treatments in, 382

rheumatic heart disease in, 199

stroke in, 159, 164

universal health coverage (UHC), 4, 16–17, 23, 344–45, 369, 371–72, 376, 385

University of Colorado at Denver, 241b

urban planning and design, 89, 120, 126

Uruguay

ischemic heart disease in, 144

kidney disease in, 244

priority-setting for treatments in, 384

V

Vaca, Claudia, 375

Vaidyanathan, B., 191

van Pelt, Maurits, 321
Vedanthan, Rajesh, 327
vegetables, 13, 28, 32–33, 103–8, 124–26, 129, 131, 160–62, 169, 266
Venezuela, República Bolivariana de
    insulin costs in, 10
    priority-setting for treatments in, 378
Verguet, Stéphane, 369
Vietnam
    chronic respiratory diseases in, 264
    congenital heart disease in, 194
    cost-effectiveness of interventions in, 11, 351, 360
    tobacco use in, 68

W

waterpipe smoking, 68
Watkins, David A., 1, 23, 191, 201, 202, 369
Webb, Michael, 101
Weber, Mary Beth, 305
weight. *See* birth weight; body mass index; obesity/ overweight
weight-loss diets, 126
Whitsel, Laurie, 101
WHO. *See* World Health Organization
WHO Choosing Interventions that are Cost-Effective (WHO-CHOICE), 110
WHO Study on Prevention of Recurrences of Myocardial Infarction and Stroke (WHO-PREMISE), 145
Will, J. C., 63
women. *See* gender issues; pregnancy
Wong, Gary, 263
worksite interventions, 105, 129–30

World Health Assembly, 57
World Health Organization (WHO)
    on cardiovascular, respiratory, and related disorders (CVRDs), 23–31
    on chronic respiratory diseases, 277–78
    on community-based care, 308–11
    on congenital heart disease, 191–92
    on cost-effectiveness of interventions, 13–15, 353–57, 369–70
    on diabetes, 211
    on diet and nutrition, 107–9
    on heart failure, 174–75, 182*b*
    on hypertension, 390–91, 396–97
    on integrated care, 288–90
    on ischemic heart disease, 145
    on obesity interventions, 117–18, 129–30, 130*t*
    on physical activity, 79–81, 92
    on priority-setting for treatments, 376–79
    on rheumatic heart disease, 197–201
    on tobacco use, 57
World Medical Association, 311
Wu, Yangfeng, 1, 157

Y

Yan, Lijing L., 157
Yancy, Clyde W., 173
Yeates, Karen, 237*b*

Z

Zhang, Ping, 209
Zhao, Dong, 157
Zhu, Yishan, 157

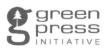

Percent Reduction in Premature Mortality 2003–2013

Legend:
- Less than or equal to 10.00%
- 10.01%–15.00%
- 15.01%–19.00%
- 19.01%–22.49%
- Greater than or equal to 22.50%
- No data

Premature mortality is defined as death before age 70. The map groups countries by percentage reduction in premature mortality rates in the decade from 2003. Ole F. Norheim and others propose a goal for 2030 of a 40 percent reduction in premature mortality from what would have resulted at 2010 death rates ("Avoiding 40% of the Premature Deaths in Each Country, 2010–30: Review of National Mortality Trends to Help Quantify the UN Sustainable Development Goal for Health," *The Lancet*, September 19, 2014, doi:10.1016/S0140-6736(14)61591-9). Countries in green had rates of reduction in 2003–2013 high enough to meet that 40 percent goal.